HEALTHCARE FINANCE

Fourth Edition

HEALTHCARE
FINANCE

An Introduction to
Accounting and
Financial Management

Fourth Edition

Louis C. Gapenski

AUPHA
HAP

Your board, staff, or clients may also benefit from this book's insight. For more information on quantity discounts, contact the Health Administration Press Marketing Manager at (312) 424-9470.

This publication is intended to provide accurate and authoritative information in regard to the subject matter covered. It is sold, or otherwise provided, with the understanding that the publisher is not engaged in rendering professional services. If professional advice or other expert assistance is required, the services of a competent professional should be sought.

The statements and opinions contained in this book are strictly those of the author and do not represent the official positions of the American College of Healthcare Executives, of the Foundation of the American College of Healthcare Executives, or of the Association of University Programs in Health Administration.

12   11   10   09   08   5   4   3   2

Library of Congress Cataloging-in-Publication Data

Gapenski, Louis C.
    Healthcare finance : an introduction to accounting and financial
management / Louis C. Gapenski.—4th ed.
        p. cm.
    Includes bibliographical references and index.
    ISBN 978-1-56793-280-5 (alk. paper)
    1. Health facilities—Finance—Textbooks. 2. Health
facilities—Accounting—Textbooks. I. Title.
[DNLM: 1. Financial Management, Hospital. 2. Accounting. 3. Capital
    Financing. 4. Health Facilities—economics. WX 157 G211h 2007]
    RA971.3.G3695 2007
    362.1068'1—dc22   2007015110

The paper used in this publication meets the minimum requirements of American National Standards for Information Sciences—Permanence of Paper for Printed Library Materials, ANSI Z39.48-1984. ∞™

Acquisitions manager: Janet Davis; Project manager: Jane Calayag

Health Administration Press
A division of the Foundation
    of the American College of
    Healthcare Executives
One North Franklin Street
Suite 1700
Chicago, IL 60606
(312) 424-2800

Association of University Programs
    in Health Administration
2000 N. 14th Street
Suite 780
Arlington, VA 22201
(703) 894-0940

BRIEF CONTENTS

DETAILED CONTENTS

PART III Managerial Accounting

PREFACE

S ome 20 years ago, after years of teaching corporate finance and writing related textbooks and casebooks, I began teaching healthcare financial management in the University of Florida's Master of Health Administration (MHA) program. The move prompted me to write my first healthcare finance textbook, *Understanding Health Care Financial Management*. The book was designed for use in health services administration financial management courses in which students had prerequisite courses in both accounting and corporate finance. In general, such courses are case courses, so this book served primarily as a reference tool when working healthcare finance cases.

In recent years, I expanded my healthcare finance teaching to include other courses in traditional, nontraditional, and clinician-oriented programs in which students do not have a formal educational background in healthcare finance. Finance courses in these programs require a book that provides basic information on foundation topics. Furthermore, these courses often are part of programs that contain just one healthcare finance course, so the course must cover both accounting and financial management. In reviewing the books available for use in such courses, I found some that were strong in accounting and others that were strong in financial management; however, I could not find one that gave equal emphasis to both components of healthcare finance. This situation prompted me to write *Healthcare Finance: An Introduction to Accounting and Financial Management*.

Concept of the Book

My goal in writing this book was to create a text that introduces students to the most important principles and applications of healthcare finance, with roughly equal coverage of accounting and financial management. Furthermore, because the book is intended for use primarily in clinical and health services administration programs, in which students are trained primarily for professional positions within healthcare providers, its focus is on healthcare finance as practiced within such organizations. The examples within the book are based on such organizations as hospitals, medical practices, clinics, home health agencies, nursing homes, and managed care organizations.

Another consideration in writing the book is that most readers would be seeing the material for the first time. Thus, it is very important that the material be explained as clearly and succinctly as possible. I have tried very hard to create a book that readers will find user-friendly—one that they will enjoy reading and can learn from on their own. If students don't find a book interesting, understandable, and useful, they won't read it.

The book begins with an introduction to healthcare finance and a description of the current financial environment in which providers operate. From there, it takes students through the basics of financial and managerial accounting. Here, my goal is not to turn clinicians or generalist managers into accountants, but to present those accounting concepts that are most critical to managerial decision making. The book then discusses the basic foundations of financial management before progressing to demonstrate how healthcare managers can apply financial management theory and principles to help make better decisions, where *better* is defined as decisions that promote the financial well-being of the organization.

Intended Market and Use

The book is not targeted for specific types of educational programs. Rather, it is designed to teach students, in one course, the fundamental concepts of healthcare finance, including both accounting and financial management, with emphasis on provider organizations. Thus, the book can be used in a wide variety of settings: undergraduate and graduate programs, traditional and executive programs, on-campus and distance learning programs, and even independently for professional development.

The key to the book's usefulness is not the educational program but the focus of the course. If the course is a stand-alone course designed to cover both healthcare accounting and financial management, the book will fit. In fact, the book can be easily used across a two-course healthcare finance sequence, especially in modular programs where each course is two credit hours. Typically, such a sequence begins with an accounting course and ends with a financial management course. This book, supplemented by cases (and possibly readings), would work well in such a sequence. The ideal casebook for use here is *Cases in Healthcare Finance* by Louis C. Gapenski, which is part of Health Administration Press's healthcare finance series. The casebook contains 30 cases that focus on the topics contained in this textbook, along with eight ethics mini-cases that can be used to highlight ethical issues in a healthcare finance setting.

The book should also be useful to practicing healthcare professionals who, for one reason or another, must increase their understanding of healthcare finance. Such professionals include clinicians who have some management responsibilities as well as line managers who now require additional finance skills. Finally, many members of financial staffs, especially those who work exclusively in a single area, such as patient accounts, would benefit from having a broader understanding of finance principles and hence would find this book useful.

Changes in the Fourth Edition

Since the publication of the third edition of this book, I have used it numerous times in various settings. In addition, I have received many comments from users at other universities. The overall reaction of students, other professors, and the marketplace in general has been overwhelmingly positive—every comment received indicates that the basic concept of the book is sound. Even so, nothing is perfect, and the healthcare environment is evolving at a dizzying pace. Thus, many changes have been made to the book; the most important of which are listed here:

- The book was updated and clarified throughout. Particular care was taken to include the most recent information on reimbursement and to update the real-world examples. In addition, there is no doubt that text material improves as it is repeatedly edited. Like all books, the third edition had some rough spots, and considerable effort was expended to improve these discussions.
- Kristin L. Reiter of the University of North Carolina at Chapel Hill reviewed and suggested improvements to the six financial and managerial accounting chapters. Her educational and professional background in healthcare accounting compliments my background in healthcare financial management.
- Three new online resources for students have been added: (1) Chapter 19: Distributions to Owners: Bonuses, Dividends, and Repurchases; (2) Chapter 20: Capitation, Rate Setting, and Risk Sharing; and (3) Online Appendixes: Financial Ratios and Operating Indicator Ratios.
- Many students, as well as instructors, have asked that a glossary be added to the book. This edition has one.
- New sections have been added or existing sections have been expanded for the following topics: municipal bond pools, cost of capital for not-for-profit and small businesses, modified internal rate of return, supply chain management, current challenges for healthcare managers, and health savings accounts.
- The lecture presentation software was updated and improved based on continuous usage and suggestions from adopters and students alike.

All in all, these changes improve the quality and value of the book without affecting its basic concept and approach to learning.

Ancillary Materials for Instructors

Two important teaching aids are available online for instructors who use this book. To request access to online instructor resources, please email hap1@ ache.org.

- **Instructor's Manual.** A comprehensive online manual is available to instructors who adopt the book. The manual includes a sample course outline and solutions to the end-of-chapter questions and problems.
- **Lecture Presentation Software.** A set of PowerPoint© slides that cover all the essential issues contained in each chapter is also available. Concepts, graphs, tables, lists, and calculations are presented in about 40 slides per chapter, much as an instructor might present them on a blackboard. However, the slides are more crisp, clear, and colorful than a blackboard, and can be displayed on a screen almost instantaneously. Furthermore, hard copies of the slides can be provided to students for use as lecture notes. Many instructors will find these slides useful, either as is or customized to best meet the situation at hand.

Ancillary Materials for Students

Three new instructional tools are now available to students at the Health Administration Press Book Companion website at ache.org/books /HCFinance4.

- **Chapter 19.** This chapter discusses distributions to owners of for-profit businesses, including dividends, bonuses, and stock repurchases. It is not included in the book because many of the students who use the text will work at not-for-profit organizations.
- **Chapter 20.** Chapter 20 provides additional information on capitation, rate setting, and risk sharing. It is not included in the book because these topics, for the most part, are beyond the scope of an introductory text.
- **Online Appendixes.** These appendixes provide a much more compete list of financial and operating indicator ratios and their definitions. These could not be included in the text because they would greatly increase the length and cost of the book.

Acknowledgments

This book reflects the efforts of many people. First and foremost, I would like to thank Mark Covaleski of the University of Wisconsin, who made significant contributions to the accounting content of the book. In fact, without his materials, advice, and counsel, the book could not have been written. In addition, Anna McAleer of Arcadia University (formerly Beaver College) provided many useful comments for improving both the text and the Instructor's Manual.

Colleagues, students, and staff at the University of Florida provided inspirational support, as well as more tangible support, during the development and class testing of the text. Also, the Health Administration Press staff was instrumental in ensuring the quality and usefulness of the book.

Finally, Kristin Reiter's review of the financial and managerial accounting chapters both improved the readability of these chapters and ensured the validity of the material.

Errors in the Book

In spite of the significant effort that has been expended by many individuals on this book, it is safe to say that some errors exist. In an attempt to create the most error-free and useful book possible, I strongly encourage both instructors and students to write me at the address below with comments and suggestions for improving the book. I certainly welcome your input.

Conclusion

In the environment faced by healthcare providers today, good finance is more important than ever to the economic well-being of the enterprise. Because of its importance, managers of all types and at all levels should be thoroughly grounded in finance principles and applications; but this is easier said than done. I hope that *Healthcare Finance: An Introduction to Accounting and Financial Management* will help you understand the finance problems currently faced by healthcare providers and, more importantly, that it will provide guidance on how best to solve them.

Louis C. Gapenski, Ph.D.
Box 100195
Health Science Center
University of Florida
Gainesville, Florida 32610–0195

September 2007

The Healthcare Environment

Two factors make the provision of health services different from other services. First, many providers are organized as not-for-profit corporations as opposed to being investor owned. Second, payment for services typically is made by third parties rather than by the patients who receive the services. By focusing on these differences, Part I provides students with unique background information that creates the framework for the practice of healthcare finance.

The first chapter discusses the institutional setting for the delivery of healthcare services, including the organization and role of the finance staff, health services settings, and information on the book itself and its use.

The second chapter focuses on alternative forms of business organization and ownership, the third-party payer system, and alternative reimbursement methodologies. It is essential that healthcare managers understand who the payers are and what payment methods are used, because these external factors have a profound influence on the practice of healthcare finance.

INTRODUCTION TO HEALTHCARE FINANCE

Learning Objectives

After studying this chapter, readers will be able to:

- Define the term *healthcare finance* as it is used in this book.
- Discuss the structure of the finance department, the role of finance in health services organizations, and how this role has changed over time.
- Describe the major players in the health services industry.
- List the key issues currently facing healthcare managers.
- Describe the organization of this book and the learning aids contained in each chapter.

Introduction

In today's healthcare environment, where financial realities play an important role in business decision making, it is vital that managers at all levels understand the basic concepts of healthcare finance and how these concepts are used to enhance the financial well-being of the organization. In this chapter, we introduce readers to the book, including its goals and organization. Furthermore, we present some basic background information about healthcare finance and the health services system. We sincerely hope that this book will be a significant help to you in your quest to increase your professional competency in the very important area of healthcare finance.

Defining Healthcare Finance

What is healthcare finance? Surprisingly, there is no single answer to that question because the definition of the term depends, for the most part, on the context in which it is used. Thus, in writing this book, our first step was to decide how to define "healthcare finance."

We began by examining the *healthcare sector* of the economy, which is second in size only to the real estate sector and consists of a diverse collection of industries that involve, either directly or indirectly, the healthcare of the population. The major industries in the healthcare sector include:

- **Health services.** The health services industry consists of *providers* of health services, including medical practices, hospitals, clinics, nursing homes, and home health care agencies.
- **Health insurance.** The health insurance industry, which makes most of the payments to health services providers, includes government programs and commercial insurers as well as self-insurers. Also included here are managed care companies, such as health maintenance organizations (HMOs), which incorporate both insurance and health services (provider) functions.
- **Medical equipment and supplies.** These industries include the makers of durable medical equipment, such as diagnostic equipment and wheelchairs, and expendable medical supplies, such as disposable surgical instruments and bandages.
- **Pharmaceuticals and biotechnology.** These industries develop and market drugs and other therapeutic products.
- **Other.** This category includes a diverse collection of businesses ranging from consulting firms to educational institutions to government and private research agencies.

Most users of this book will become (or already are) managers at health services organizations, or at companies such as insurance and consulting firms that deal directly with health services organizations. Thus, to create a book that has the most value to its primary users, we focus on finance as it applies within the health services industry. Of course, the principles and practices of finance cannot be applied in a vacuum but must be based on the realities of the current healthcare environment, including how health services are financed. Furthermore, insurance involves payment to healthcare providers; much of managed care involves utilization management of healthcare providers, either directly or through contracts; and most consulting work is done for providers; so the material in this book is also relevant for managers in other industries related to health services.

Now that we have defined the healthcare focus of this book, the term *finance* must be defined. Finance, as the term is used within the health services industry, and as it is used in this book, consists of both the accounting and the financial management functions. (In many settings, accounting and financial management are separate disciplines.) *Accounting,* as its name implies, concerns the recording, in financial terms, of economic events that reflect the operations, resources, and financing of an organization. In general, the purpose of accounting is to create and provide to interested parties, both internal and external, useful information about an organization's financial status and operations.

Whereas accounting provides a rational means by which to measure a business's financial performance and assess operations, *financial management,* or *corporate finance,* provides the theory, concepts, and tools necessary to help managers make better financial decisions. Of course, the boundary between accounting and financial management is blurred; certain aspects of accounting involve decision making, and much of the application of financial management theory and concepts requires accounting data.

1. What is meant by the term *healthcare finance*?
2. What is the difference between accounting and financial management?

Self-Test Questions

Purpose of the Book

Many books cover the general topics of accounting and financial management, so why is a book needed that focuses on health services finance? The reason is that while all industries have certain individual characteristics, the health services industry is truly unique. For example, the provision of healthcare services is dominated by *not-for-profit* organizations, both private and governmental, and such entities are inherently different from *investor-owned* businesses. Also, the majority of payments made to healthcare providers are not made by the individuals who use the services but by *third-party payers* (e.g., an employer, commercial insurance company, or government program). Throughout the book, the ways in which the unique features of the health services industry influence the application of finance principles and practices are emphasized.

This book is designed to introduce students to healthcare finance, which has two important implications. First, the book assumes no prior knowledge of the subject matter; thus, the book is totally self-contained, with each topic explained from the beginning in basic terms. Furthermore, because clarity is so important when concepts are first introduced, the chapters have been written in an easy-to-read fashion. None of the topics are inherently difficult, but new concepts often take some effort to understand. This process is made easier by the writing style used.

Second, because this book is introductory, it contains a broad overview of healthcare finance. The good news here is that the book presents virtually all the important healthcare finance principles that are used by managers in health services organizations. The bad news is that the large number of topics covered prevents us from covering principles in great depth or including a wide variety of illustrations. Thus, students who use this book are not expected to fully understand every nuance of every finance principle and practice that pertains to every type of health services organization. Nevertheless, this book provides a sufficient knowledge of healthcare finance so that readers will be better able to function as managers, judge the quality of financial analyses performed by others, and incorporate sound principles and practices into their own personal finance decisions.

Naturally, an introductory finance book does not contain everything that a healthcare financial manager must know to competently perform his or her job. Nevertheless, the book is useful even for those working in finance positions within health services organizations because it presents an overview of the finance function. Often, when one is working in a specific area of finance, it is too easy to lose sight of the context of one's work. This book will help provide that context.

Self-Test Questions
1. Why is it necessary to have a book dedicated to healthcare finance?
2. What is the purpose of the book?

The Role of Finance in Health Services Organizations

The primary role of finance in health services organizations, as in all businesses, is to plan for, acquire, and utilize resources to maximize the efficiency and value of the enterprise. As we discuss in the next section, the two broad areas of finance—accounting and financial management—are separate functions in larger organizations, although the accounting function usually is carried out under the direction of the organization's chief financial officer and hence falls under the overall category of finance.

In general, finance activities include:

- **Planning and budgeting.** First and foremost, business finance involves evaluating the financial effectiveness of current operations and planning for the future. *Budgets* play an important role in this process.
- **Financial reporting.** For a variety of reasons, it is important for businesses to record and report to outsiders the results of operations and current financial status. This is typically accomplished by a set of *financial statements*.
- **Capital investment decisions.** Although capital investment is more important to senior management, managers at all levels must be concerned with the capital investment decision process. Such decisions, which are called *capital budgeting* decisions, focus on the acquisition of land, buildings, and equipment. They are the primary means by which businesses implement strategic plans, and hence they play a key role in a business's financial future.
- **Financing decisions.** All organizations must raise *capital* to buy the assets necessary to support operations. Such decisions involve the choice between internal and external funds, the use of debt versus equity capital, the use of long-term versus short-term debt, and the use of lease versus conventional financing. Although senior managers typically make financing decisions, these decisions have ramifications for managers at all levels.

- **Working capital management.** An organization's current, or short-term, assets, such as cash, marketable securities, receivables, and inventories, must be properly managed both to ensure operational effectiveness and to reduce costs. Generally, managers at all levels are involved to some extent in short-term asset management, which is often called *working capital management.*
- **Contract management.** In today's healthcare environment, health services organizations must negotiate, sign, and monitor contracts with managed care organizations and third-party payers. The financial staff typically has primary responsibility for these tasks, but managers at all levels are involved in these activities and must be aware of their effects on operating decisions.
- **Financial risk management.** Many financial transactions that take place to support the operations of a business can themselves increase the business's risk. Thus, an important finance activity is to control financial risk.

These specific finance activities often are summarized by the "four Cs": costs, cash, capital, and control. The measurement and minimization of *costs* is vital to the financial success of any business. Rampant costs, as compared to revenues, usually spell doom for any business. A business can be profitable but still face a crisis due to a shortage of *cash*. Cash is the "lubricant" that makes the wheels of a business run smoothly—without it, the business grinds to a halt. *Capital* are the funds used to acquire land, buildings, and equipment. Without capital, businesses would not have the physical resources needed to provide goods and services. Finally, a business must be under *control* to ensure that its resources are being wisely employed and protected for future use.

In times of high profitability and abundant financial resources, the finance function tends to decline in importance. Thus, when most healthcare providers were reimbursed on the basis of costs incurred, the role of finance was minimal. At that time, the most critical finance function was cost accounting because it was more important to account for costs than it was to control them. In response to payer (primarily Medicare) requirements, providers (primarily hospitals) churned out a multitude of reports both to comply with regulations and to maximize revenues. The complexities of cost reimbursement meant that a large amount of time had to be spent on cumbersome accounting, billing, and collection procedures. Thus, instead of focusing on value-adding activities, most finance work focused on bureaucratic functions.

In recent years, however, providers have been redesigning their finance functions to recognize the changes that have occurred in the health services industry. Although billing and collections remain important, to be of maximum value to the enterprise today the finance function must support cost-containment efforts, managed care and other payer contract negotiations, joint venture decisions, and integrated delivery system participation.

In essence, finance must help lead organizations into the future rather than merely record what has happened in the past.

In this book, the emphasis is on the finance function, but there are no unimportant functions in health services organizations. Senior executives must understand a multitude of other functions, such as marketing, facilities management, and human resource management, in addition to finance. Still, all business decisions have financial implications, so all managers—whether in operations, marketing, personnel, or facilities—must know enough about finance to properly incorporate any financial implications into decisions made within their own specialized areas.

Self-Test Questions	1. What is the role of finance in today's health services organizations?
	2. What are the "four Cs"?
	3. How has this role changed over time?

The Structure of the Finance Department

The size and structure of the finance department within health services organizations depend on the type of provider and its size. Still, the finance department within larger provider organizations generally follows the model described here.

The head of the finance department holds the title *chief financial officer (CFO)*, or sometimes *vice president–finance*. This individual typically reports directly to the organization's *chief executive officer (CEO)* and is responsible for all finance activities within the organization. The CFO directs two senior managers who help manage finance activities. First is the *comptroller* (pronounced, and sometimes spelled, "controller"), who is responsible for accounting and reporting activities such as routine budgeting, preparation of financial statements, payables management, and patient accounts management. For the most part, the comptroller is involved in those activities covered in Chapters 3 through 8 of this text. Second is the *treasurer*, who is responsible for the acquisition and management of capital (funds). Treasurer activities include the acquisition and employment of capital, cash and debt management, lease financing, financial risk management, and endowment fund management (within not-for-profits). In general, the treasurer is involved in those activities discussed in Chapters 11 through 18 of this text.

Of course, in larger organizations, the comptroller and treasurer have managers with responsibility for specific functions, such as the *patient accounts manager*, who reports to the comptroller, and the *cash manager*, who reports to the treasurer. In very small businesses, many of the finance responsibilities are combined and assigned to just a few individuals. In the smallest health services organizations, the entire finance function is managed by one person, often called the *business (practice) manager*.

1. Briefly describe the typical structure of the finance department within a health services organization.

Self-Test Question

Health Services Settings

Health services are provided in numerous settings, including hospitals, ambulatory care facilities, long-term care facilities, and even at home. Before the 1980s, most health services organizations were freestanding and not formally linked with other organizations. Those that were linked tended to be part of horizontally integrated systems that controlled a single type of healthcare facility such as hospitals or nursing homes. Recently, however, many health services organizations have diversified and become vertically integrated either through direct ownership or contractual arrangements.

Hospitals

Hospitals provide diagnostic and therapeutic services to individuals who require more than several hours of care, although most hospitals are actively engaged in ambulatory (walk-in) services as well. To ensure a minimum standard of safety and quality, hospitals must be licensed by the state and undergo inspections for compliance with state regulations. In addition, most hospitals are accredited by the *Joint Commission* (formerly called the *Joint Commission on Accreditation of Healthcare Organizations [JCAHO]*). Joint Commission accreditation is a voluntary process that is intended to promote high standards of care. Although the cost to achieve and maintain compliance with standards can be substantial, accreditation provides eligibility for participation in the Medicare program, and hence most hospitals seek accreditation.

Recent environmental and operational changes have created significant challenges for hospital managers. For example, many hospitals are experiencing decreasing admission rates and shorter lengths of stay, which results in excess capacity. At the same time, hospitals have been pressured to give discounts to managed care plans, to limit the growth in patient charges, and to assume greater risk in their contracts with third-party payers. Because of the changing environmental and increasing cost-containment pressures, the number of hospitals (and beds) has declined in recent years.

Hospitals differ in function, length of patient stay, size, and ownership. These factors affect the type and quantity of assets, services offered, and management requirements and often determine the type and level of reimbursement. Hospitals are classified as either general acute care facilities or specialty facilities. *General acute care hospitals* provide general medical and surgical services and selected acute specialty services. General acute care hospitals are short-stay facilities and account for the majority of hospitals. *Specialty hospitals*, such as psychiatric, children's, women's, rehabilitation, and cancer, limit admission of patients to specific ages, sexes, illnesses, or conditions. The number of specialty hospitals has grown significantly in the past few decades because of the increased need for such services.

Hospitals vary in size, from fewer than 25 beds to more than 1,000 beds; general acute care hospitals tend to be larger than specialty hospitals. Small hospitals, those with fewer than 100 beds, tend to be located in rural areas. Many rural hospitals have experienced financial difficulties in recent years because they have less ability than larger hospitals to lower costs in response to ever-tighter reimbursement rates. Most of the largest hospitals are academic health centers or teaching hospitals, which offer a wide range of services, including tertiary services. (*Tertiary care* is highly specialized and technical in nature, with services for patients with unusually severe, complex, or uncommon problems.)

Hospitals are classified by ownership as private not-for-profit, investor owned, and governmental. *Governmental hospitals*, which make up 25 percent of all hospitals, are broken down into federal and public (nonfederal) entities. *Federal hospitals*, such as those operated by the military services or the Department of Veterans Affairs, serve special purposes. *Public hospitals* are funded wholly or in part by a city, county, tax district, or state. In general, federal and public hospitals provide substantial services to indigent patients. In recent years, many public hospitals have converted to other ownership categories—primarily private not-for-profit—because local governments have found it increasingly difficult to fund healthcare services and still provide other necessary public services. In addition, the inability of politically governed organizations to respond quickly to the changing healthcare environment contributed to many conversions as managers tried to create organizations that are more responsive to external change.

Private not-for-profit hospitals are nongovernment entities organized for the sole purpose of providing inpatient healthcare services. Because of the charitable origins of U.S. hospitals and a tradition of community service, roughly 80 percent of all private hospitals (60 percent of all hospitals) are not-for-profit entities. In return for serving a charitable purpose, these hospitals receive numerous benefits, including exemption from federal and state income taxes, exemption from property and sales taxes, eligibility to receive tax-deductible charitable contributions, favorable postal rates, favorable tax-exempt financing, and tax-favored annuities for employees.

The remaining 20 percent of private hospitals (15 percent of all hospitals) are *investor owned*. This means that they have owners (typically shareholders) that benefit directly from the profits generated by the business. Historically, most investor-owned hospitals were owned by physicians, but now most are owned by large corporations such as HCA, which owns about 170 hospitals; Tenet Healthcare, which owns about 70 hospitals; and Hospital Management Associates (HMA), which owns about 60 hospitals. Unlike not-for-profit hospitals, investor-owned hospitals pay taxes and forgo the other benefits of not-for-profit status. However, investor-owned hospitals typically do not embrace the charitable mission of not-for-profit hospitals. Despite the expressed differences in mission between investor-owned and not-for-profit hospitals, not-for-profit hospitals are being forced to place greater emphasis on the financial implications of operating decisions than in the past. This trend has raised concerns in some quarters that many not-for-profit hospitals are now failing to meet their charitable mission. As this perception grows, some people argue that these hospitals should lose some, if not all, of the benefits associated with their not-for-profit status.

Hospitals are labor-intensive because of their need to provide continuous nursing supervision to patients, in addition to the other services they provide through professional and semiprofessional staffs. Physicians petition for privileges to practice in hospitals. While they admit and provide care to hospitalized patients, physicians, for the most part, are not hospital employees and hence are not directly accountable to hospital management. However, physicians retain a major responsibility for determining which hospital services will be provided to patients and how long patients are hospitalized, so physicians play a critical role in determining a hospital's costs and revenues and hence its financial condition.

Ambulatory (Outpatient) Care

Ambulatory care, also known as *outpatient care*, encompasses services provided to noninstitutionalized patients. Traditional outpatient settings include medical practices, hospital outpatient departments, and emergency rooms. In addition, the 1980s and early 1990s witnessed substantial growth in nontraditional ambulatory care settings such as home health care, ambulatory surgery centers, urgent care centers, diagnostic imaging centers, rehabilitation/sports medicine centers, and clinical laboratories. In general, the new settings offer patients increased amenities and convenience compared to hospital-based services and, in many situations, provide services at a lower cost than hospitals. For example, urgent care and ambulatory surgery centers are typically less expensive than their hospital counterparts because hospitals have higher overhead costs.

Many factors have contributed to the expansion of ambulatory services, but technology has been a leading factor. Often, patients who once required hospitalization because of the complexity, intensity, invasiveness, or risk associated with certain procedures can now be treated in outpatient settings. In addition, third-party payers have encouraged providers to expand their outpatient services through mandatory authorization for inpatient services and by payment mechanisms that provide incentives to perform services on an outpatient basis. Finally, fewer entry barriers to developing outpatient services relative to institutional care exist. Ordinarily, ambulatory facilities are less costly, less often subject to licensure and certificate-of-need regulations (exceptions are hospital outpatient units and ambulatory surgery centers), and generally are not accredited. (Licensure and certificate-of-need regulation are discussed in detail in the next major section.)

As outpatient care consumes an increasing portion of the healthcare dollar, and efforts to control outpatient spending are enhanced, the traditional role of the ambulatory care manager is changing. Ambulatory care managers historically have focused on such routine management tasks as billing, collections, staffing, scheduling, and patient relations, while the owners, often physicians, have tended to make the more important business decisions. However, reimbursement changes, including a new Medicare payment system and increased managed care affiliations, are requiring a higher level of management expertise. This increasing environmental complexity, along with increasing competition, is forcing managers of ambulatory care facilities to become more sophisticated in making business decisions, including finance decisions.

Long-Term Care

Long-term care entails the provision of healthcare services, as well as some personal services, to individuals who lack some degree of functional ability. It usually covers an extended period of time and includes both inpatient and outpatient services, which often focus on mental health, rehabilitation, and nursing home care. Although the greatest use is among the elderly, long-term care services are used by individuals of all ages.

Long-term care is concerned with levels of independent functioning, specifically activities of daily living such as eating, bathing, and locomotion. Individuals become candidates for long-term care when they become too mentally or physically incapacitated to perform necessary tasks and when their family members are unable to provide needed services. Long-term care is a hybrid of healthcare services and social services, and *nursing homes* are a major source of such care.

Three levels of nursing home care exist: (1) skilled nursing facilities, (2) intermediate care facilities, and (3) residential care facilities. *Skilled nursing facilities (SNFs)* provide the level of care closest to hospital care. Services must be under the supervision of a physician and must include 24-hour daily nursing care. *Intermediate care facilities (ICFs)* are intended for individuals who do not require hospital or SNF care but whose mental or physical conditions require daily continuity of one or more medical services. *Residential care* facilities are sheltered environments that do not provide professional healthcare services and thus for which most health insurance programs do not provide coverage.

Nursing homes are more abundant than hospitals and are also smaller, with an average bed size of about 100 beds, compared with about 170 beds for hospitals. Nursing homes are licensed by states, and nursing home administrators are licensed as well. Although the Joint Commission accredits nursing homes, only a small percentage participate because accreditation is not required for reimbursement, and the standards to achieve accreditation are much higher than licensure requirements.

The long-term care industry has experienced tremendous growth in the past three decades. Long-term care accounted for only 1 percent of healthcare expenditures in 1960, but by 2006 it accounted for more than 6 percent of expenditures. Further demand increases are anticipated, as the percentage of the U.S. population age 65 and older increases, from less than 16 percent in 2000 to a forecasted 20 percent in 2030. The elderly are disproportionately high users of healthcare services and are major users of long-term care.

Although long-term care is often perceived as nursing home care, many new services are developing to meet society's needs in less-institutional surroundings such as adult day care, life care centers, and hospice programs. These services tend to offer a higher quality of life, although they are not necessarily less expensive than institutional care. Home health care, provided for an extended time period, can be an alternative to nursing home care for many patients, but it is not as readily available as nursing home care in many rural areas. Furthermore, third-party payers, especially Medicare, have sent mixed signals about their willingness to adequately pay for home health care. In fact, many home health care businesses have been forced to close in recent years as a result of a new, and less generous, Medicare payment system.

Integrated Delivery Systems

Many healthcare experts have extolled the benefits of providing hospital care, ambulatory care, long-term care, and business support services through a single entity called an *integrated delivery system*. The hypothesized benefits of such systems include the following:

- Patients are kept in the corporate network of services (*patient capture*).
- Providers have access to managerial and functional specialists (for example, reimbursement and marketing professionals).
- Information systems that track all aspects of patient care, as well as insurance and other data, can be developed more easily, and the costs to develop them are shared.
- Linked organizations have better access to capital.
- The ability to recruit and retain management and professional staff is enhanced.
- Integrated delivery systems are able to offer payers a complete package of services ("one-stop shopping").
- Integrated delivery systems are better able to plan for and deliver a full range of healthcare services to meet the needs of a defined population, including chronic disease management and health status improvement programs. Many of these population-based efforts typically are not offered by stand-alone providers.

- Incentives that encourage all providers in the system to work together for the common good of the system can be created, which has the potential to both improve quality and control costs.

Although integrated delivery systems can be structured in many different ways, the defining characteristic of such systems is that the organization has the ability to assume full clinical responsibility for the healthcare needs of a defined population. Because of current state laws, which typically mandate that the insurance function can be assumed only by licensed insurers, integrated delivery systems typically contract with insurers rather than directly with employers. Sometimes, the insurer, often a managed care plan, is owned by the integrated delivery system itself, but generally it is separately owned. In contracts with managed care plans, the integrated delivery system often receives a fixed payment per plan member and hence assumes both the financial and clinical risks associated with providing healthcare services.

To be an effective competitor, integrated delivery systems must minimize the provision of unnecessary services because additional services create added costs but do not necessarily result in additional revenues. Thus, the objective of integrated delivery systems is to provide all needed services to its member population in the lowest cost setting. To achieve this goal, integrated delivery systems invest heavily in primary care services, especially prevention, early intervention, and wellness programs. The primary care gatekeeper concept is frequently used to control utilization and hence costs. While hospitals continue to be centers of technology, integrated delivery systems have the incentive to shift patients toward lower cost settings. Thus, clinical integration among the various providers and components of care is essential to achieving quality, cost efficiency, and patient satisfaction.

One of the most common types of integrated delivery system is the *physician hospital organization (PHO)*, which is a separate organization formed by a hospital and a physician group to provide contracted healthcare services to managed care plans and, when permitted, directly to employers. The PHO must provide utilization and quality management, physician credentialing, claims processing, marketing, and revenue distribution for the system. Another common type is the *management service organization (MSO)*, which is a hospital-based organization that provides physician billing and medical group management services. Some of the larger integrated systems are a combination of PHOs, MSOs, and managed care organizations, which can provide all clinical services as well as the insurance function. Most of these large systems were developed by hospitals, but others were started by health plans or by large physician group practices.

In spite of the hypothesized benefits of integration, executives of healthcare systems have found it more difficult than they originally envisioned to manage large, diverse enterprises. This difficulty has been especially true when hospitals or health systems have acquired physician practices. In many cases, the financial and patient care gains predicted were not realized, and some of the integrated delivery systems that were formed in the 1990s have broken up. Today, it is not clear whether large integrated health systems are better suited for success than are smaller, more-focused organizations. Only time will tell.

1. What are some different types of hospitals, and what trends are occurring in the hospital industry?
2. What trends are occurring in outpatient and long-term care?
3. What is an integrated delivery system?
4. Do you think that integrated delivery systems will be more or less prevalent in the future? Explain your answer.

Self-Test Questions

Regulatory and Legal Issues

Entry into the health services industry is heavily regulated. Examples of such regulation include licensure, certificate of need, rate setting, and review programs. In addition, legal issues, especially malpractice, are prominent in discussions of healthcare cost control.

States require *licensure* of certain healthcare providers in an effort to protect the health, safety, and welfare of the public. Licensure regulations establish minimum standards that must be met to provide a service. Many types of providers are licensed, including whole facilities, such as hospitals and nursing homes, as well as individuals, such as physicians, dentists, and nurses. Facilities that are licensed must submit to periodic inspections and review activities. Such reviews have focused more on physical features and safety and less on patient care and outcomes, although some progress is being made in these areas. Thus, licensure has not necessarily ensured that the public will receive quality services. Critics of licensure contend that it is designed more to protect providers than to protect consumers. For example, licensed paramedical professionals are required to work under the supervision of a physician or dentist, and thus it is impossible for the paramedical professions to compete with physicians or dentists. Despite the limitations of licensure, it is probably here to stay.

Certificate of need (CON) legislation was enacted by Congress in 1974 in an effort to control increasing healthcare costs. States were required to conduct healthcare planning, and a logical extension of this planning was to require providers to obtain approval based on community need for construction and renovation projects that either relate to specific services or exceed a defined cost threshold. This attempt to control capital expenditures by controlling expansion and preventing duplication of services lasted less than a decade before the Reagan administration began to downplay CON regulation and to promote cost controls through competition, although CON regulation still exists in most states.

Critics of CON regulation argue that it does not provide as much control over capital expenditures as originally envisioned and it increases healthcare costs by forcing providers to incur additional administrative costs when new facilities are needed. Perhaps the biggest criticism of CON regulation is that it creates a territorial franchise for services that it covers; that is, it makes it difficult for new entities to enter markets, even though the new businesses may be more cost efficient and offer better patient care than the existing ones.

In addition to CON regulation, *cost containment programs* were enacted in many states at the time when most health services reimbursement was based on costs. By the late 1970s, nine states had mandatory cost containment programs, and many other states had voluntary programs or programs that did not mandate compliance. The primary tool for cost containment programs is the *rate review* system. Three types of systems have been used: (1) detailed budget reviews with approval or setting of rates; (2) formula methods, which use inflation formulas to set target rates; and (3) negotiated rates involving joint decision making between the provider and the rate setter. Some states that use rate review systems have reduced the rate of increase in healthcare costs below the national average, while others have failed. However, rate review, as a sole means of cost containment, has been criticized because it does not address the issue of demand for healthcare services.

Healthcare services are subject to many other forms of regulation. For example, pharmacy services are regulated by state and federal laws, and radiology services are highly regulated because of the handling and disposal of radioactive materials. The costs of complying with regulation are not trivial. The CEO of a 430-bed hospital estimated that the cost of dealing with regulatory agencies, including third-party payers, is about $8 million annually, requiring a staff of 140 full-time workers to handle the process.

The primary legal concern of health services providers is *professional liability*. Malpractice suits are the oldest forms of quality assurance in the U.S. healthcare system, and such suits now are used to an extreme extent. Many people believe that the United States is facing a malpractice insurance crisis. Total malpractice premiums, which have doubled in the last ten years, have been passed on to healthcare purchasers. Some specialist physicians pay malpractice premiums of more than $100,000 per year, and each month U.S. courts manage approximately 20,000 new malpractice suits, with awards averaging $300,000 for cases that go to trial. Although providers have been successful in achieving some tort reforms, malpractice litigation continues to be perceived as inefficient because it diverts resources to lawyers and courts and creates disincentives for physicians to practice high-risk specialties and for hospitals to offer high-risk services. In addition, such litigation encourages the practice of defensive medicine in which physicians overutilize diagnostic services in an effort to protect themselves.

Although professional liability is the most visible legal concern in health services, the industry is subject to many other legal issues, including those typical of other industries, such as general liability and antitrust issues. Finally, healthcare providers are confronted with unique ethical issues, such as the right to die or to prolong life, which are often resolved through the legal system.

1. What are some forms of regulation used in the health services industry? 2. What is the most pressing legal issue facing healthcare providers today?	**Self-Test Questions**

Current Challenges

In 2006 two articles were published that list the current concerns of healthcare managers.[1] The first article focused on issues of concern among hospital CEOs surveyed by the American College of Healthcare Executives (ACHE). The CEOs' top concern was financial challenges, by almost a two to one margin over the second-ranking concern (personnel shortages). In fact, financial concerns have headed the list of challenges on every survey conducted since the survey began in 2002. Tom Dolan, ACHE president and CEO, said: "This year's survey results are a continuation of previous concerns. First and foremost is finance." When asked to rank their specific financial concerns, CEOs put reimbursement at the forefront, with Medicaid, Medicare, and bad debt losses also near the top of the list. (Reimbursement will be discussed in Chapter 2.) Clearly, the ability of government payers to adequately reimburse providers leads the list of concerns.

The second article focused on issues of concern to CFOs. Their most pressing issue was balancing clinical and financial issues—in essence, how can financial performance be improved without having a negative impact on clinical performance? Other issues of concern included improving the revenue cycle (billing and collecting on a timely basis) and developing different ways to access (raise) capital.

Taken together, these articles confirm the fact that finance is of primary importance to today's healthcare managers. The remainder of this book is dedicated to helping you confront and solve these issues.

1. What are some important issues facing healthcare managers today?	**Self-Test Question**

Organization of the Book

In *Alice in Wonderland*, Lewis Carroll wrote: "Any road will do if you don't know where you are going." Because not just any road will ensure that this book meets its goals, the destination has been carefully charted: to provide an introduction to healthcare finance. Furthermore, the book is organized to pave the road to this destination.

Part I (The Healthcare Environment) contains fundamental background materials essential to the practice of healthcare finance. Chapter 1 introduces the book, while Chapter 2 provides additional insights into the uniqueness of the health services industry. Healthcare finance cannot be studied in a vacuum because the practice of finance is profoundly influenced by the economic and social environment of the industry, including alternative types of ownership, taxes, and reimbursement methods.

Part II (Financial Accounting) begins the actual discussion of healthcare finance principles and practices. Financial accounting, which involves the creation of statements that summarize a business's financial status, is most useful for managing at the organizational (aggregate) level. In Chapter 3, financial accounting concepts and the income statement are discussed, while in Chapter 4 the balance sheet and statement of cash flows are reviewed.

Part III (Managerial Accounting), which consists of Chapters 5 through 8, focuses on the creation of data used in the day-to-day management and control of a business. Here, the focus changes from the aggregate organization to sub-unit (department) level management. The key topics in Part III include cost behavior, profit planning, cost allocation, pricing and service decisions, and planning and budgeting.

In Part IV (Basic Financial Management Concepts), the focus moves from accounting to financial management. Chapter 9 covers time value analysis, which provides techniques for valuing future cash flows, and Chapter 10 presents financial risk and required return—two of the most important concepts in financial decision making.

Part V (Long-Term Financing) turns to the capital acquisition process. Businesses need capital, or funds, to purchase assets, and in Chapters 11 and 12 the two primary types of financing—long-term debt and equity—are examined. These chapters not only provide descriptive information about securities and the markets in which they are traded but also discuss security valuation. Chapter 13 provides the framework for analyzing the appropriate mix of capital financing and assessing its cost to the business.

In Part VI (Capital Investment Decisions), the vital topic of how businesses analyze new capital investment opportunities (or capital budgeting) is considered. Because major capital projects take years to plan and execute, and because these decisions generally are not easily reversed and will affect operations for many years, their impact on the future of an organization is profound. Chapter 14 focuses on basic concepts, while Chapter 15 discusses risk assessment and incorporation.

Part VII (Other Topics) contains three chapters. In Chapter 16, the management of short-term assets is reviewed, including cash, receivables, and inventories as well as how such assets are financed. The techniques used to analyze a business's financial and operating condition are discussed in Chapter 17. Health services managers must be able to assess the current financial condition of their organizations. Even more important, managers must be able to monitor and control current operations and to assess ways in which alternative courses of action will affect the organization's future financial condition. Finally, Chapter 18 covers two unrelated topics: lease financing and business valuation.

In addition to the printed text, there are two chapters available from the publisher's website for this book. Chapter 19 (Distributions to Owners: Bonuses, Dividends, and Repurchases) discusses how profits in investor-owned businesses are returned to owners, and Chapter 20 (Capitation, Rate Setting, and Risk Sharing) provides the details of capitation reimbursement and how insurers set premium rates. To access these chapters, see ache.org /books/HCFinance4.

1. Briefly, what is the organization of this book?	**Self-Test Question**

How to Use this Book

As mentioned earlier, the overriding goal in creating this book is to provide an easy-to-read, content-filled introductory text on healthcare finance. The book contains several features designed to assist in learning the material.

First, pay particular attention to the *LEARNING OBJECTIVES* listed at the beginning of each chapter. These objectives provide a feel for the most important topics in each chapter and what readers should set as learning goals for the chapter. After each major section, except the Introduction, one or more *SELF-TEST QUESTIONS* are included. As you finish reading each major section, try to provide reasonable answers to these questions. Your responses do not have to be perfect, but if you are not satisfied with your answer, it would be best to reread the section before proceeding. Answers are not provided for the self-test questions, so a review of the section is indicated if you are in doubt about whether your answers are satisfactory.

Within the book, italics and boldface are used to indicate importance. *Italics* are used whenever a key term is introduced; thus, italics alert readers that a new and important concept is being presented. **Boldface** is solely used for emphasis; thus, the meaning of a boldfaced word or phrase has particular significance to the point under discussion.

In addition to in-chapter learning aids, materials designed to help readers learn healthcare finance are included at the end of each chapter. First, each chapter ends with a summary section titled *KEY CONCEPTS*, which very briefly summarizes the most important principles and practices covered in that chapter. If the meaning of a key concept is not apparent, you may find it useful to review the applicable section. Each chapter also contains a series of *QUESTIONS* designed to assess your understanding of the qualitative material in the chapter. The questions are followed by a set of *PROBLEMS* designed to assess your understanding of the quantitative material.

Finally, each chapter ends with a set of *REFERENCES*. The books and articles cited can provide a more in-depth understanding of the material covered in the chapter. Taken together, the pedagogic structure of the book is designed to make the learning of healthcare finance as easy and enjoyable as possible.

Key Concepts

This chapter provided an introduction to healthcare finance. The key concepts of this chapter are:

* The term *healthcare finance*, as it is used in this book, means the accounting and financial management principles and practices used within health services organizations to ensure the financial well-being of the enterprise.
* The *primary role of finance* in health services organizations, as in all businesses, is to plan for, acquire, and use resources to maximize the efficiency and value of the enterprise.
* Finance activities generally include the following: (1) *planning and budgeting*, (2) *financial reporting*, (3) *capital investment decisions*, (4) *financing decisions*, (5) *working capital management*, (6) *contract management*, and (7) *financial risk management*. These activities can be summarized by the "four Cs": costs, cash, capital, and control.
* The size and structure of the finance department within health services organizations depend on the type of provider and its size. Still, the finance department within larger provider organizations generally consists of a *chief financial officer (CFO)*, who typically reports directly to the *chief executive officer (CEO)* and is responsible for all finance activities within the organization. Reporting to the CFO are the *comptroller*, who is responsible for accounting and reporting activities, and the *treasurer*, who is responsible for the acquisition and management of capital (funds).
* In larger organizations, the comptroller and treasurer direct managers who have responsibility for specific functions, such as the *patient accounts manager*, who reports to the comptroller, and the *cash manager*, who reports to the treasurer.
* In very small health services organizations, the finance responsibilities are combined and assigned to one individual, often called the *business (practice) manager*.
* All business decisions have *financial implications*, so all managers—whether in operations, marketing, personnel, or facilities—must know enough about finance to incorporate its implications into their own specialized decision processes.
* Healthcare services are provided in numerous settings, including hospitals, ambulatory care facilities, long-term care facilities, and even at home.

- *Hospitals* differ in function (*general acute care* versus *specialty*), patient length of stay, size, and ownership (*governmental* versus *private* and, within the private sector, *for-profit* versus *not-for-profit*).
- *Ambulatory care*, also known as *outpatient care*, encompasses services provided to noninstitutionalized patients. Outpatient settings include medical practices, hospital outpatient departments, ambulatory surgery centers, urgent care centers, diagnostic imaging centers, rehabilitation/sports medicine centers, and clinical laboratories.
- *Home health care* brings many of the same services provided in ambulatory care settings into the patient's home.
- *Long-term care* entails healthcare services that cover an extended period of time, including inpatient, outpatient, and home health care, often with a focus on mental health, rehabilitation, or nursing home care.
- The defining characteristic of an *integrated delivery system* is that the organization assumes full clinical, and in certain cases financial, responsibility for the healthcare needs of the covered population.
- Entry into the health services industry has been heavily regulated. Examples of regulation include *licensure*, *certificate of need*, and *rate setting and review* programs.
- Legal issues, such as *malpractice*, are prominent in discussions about controlling healthcare costs.
- Two recent surveys of health services executives confirm the fact that healthcare managers view financial concerns as the most important current issue.

In the next chapter, the discussion of the healthcare environment is continued, moving to more finance-related topics such as forms of organization, reimbursement, and taxes.

Questions

1.1 a. What are some of the industries in the healthcare sector?
    b. What is meant by the term *healthcare finance* as used in this book?
    c. What are the two broad areas of healthcare finance?
    d. Why is it necessary to have a book on healthcare finance as opposed to a generic finance book?
1.2 a. Briefly discuss the role of finance in the health services industry.
    b. Has this role increased or decreased in importance in recent years?
1.3 a. Briefly describe the following health services settings:
       • Hospitals
       • Ambulatory care
       • Home health care
       • Long-term care
       • Integrated delivery systems

b. What are the benefits attributed to integrated delivery systems?

1.4 What role does regulation play in the health services industry?

1.5 What is the structure of the finance function within health services organizations?

1.6 What is the primary legal issue facing providers today?

1.7 Describe the organization of this book and the learning tools embedded in each chapter.

Note

1. See Melanie Evans, "What Really Matters Most," *Modern Healthcare*, January 9, 2006, and Margaret S. Veach, "What's On Your Plate? Ten Top Issues for 2006," *Healthcare Financial Management*, January 2006.

References

For a general introduction to the healthcare system in the United States, see

Barton, P. L. 2006. *Understanding the U.S. Health Services System*. Chicago: Health Administration Press.

Lee, P. R., and C. L. Estes. 2003. *The Nation's Health*. Sudbury, MA: Jones and Bartlett.

Williams, S. J., and P. R. Torrens. 2008. *Introduction to Health Services*. Albany, NY: Delmar Publishers.

For the latest information on events that affect health services organizations, see
Modern Healthcare, published weekly by Crain Communications Inc., Chicago.

For ideas on the future of healthcare in the United States and other pertinent information, see

Darling, H. 2005. "Healthcare Cost Crisis and Quality Gap: Our National Dilemma." *Healthcare Financial Management* (May): 64–68.

Goldsmith, J. 2000. "How Will the Internet Change Our Health Care System." *Health Affairs* (January/February): 148–156.

Halvorson, G. C. 2005. "Healthcare Tipping Points." *Healthcare Financial Management* (March): 74–80.

Healthcare Financial Management Association. 2005. "The Uninsured." *Healthcare Financial Management* (March): Issue Focus.

Kajander, J., and M. Samuels. 1996. "Future Trends in the Health Care Economy." *Journal of Health Care Finance* (Fall): 17–22.

Kaufman, K. 2007. "Taking Care of Your Organization's Financial Health." *Healthcare Executive* (January/February): 15–20.

Morrison, I. 1999. *Health Care in the New Millennium*. New York: Joseph Wiley & Sons.

National Coalition on Health Care. 1997. "How Americans Perceive the Health Care System: A Report on a National Survey." *Journal of Health Care Finance* (Summer): 12–20.

Nauert, R. C. 2000. "The New Millennium: Health Care Evolution in the 21st Century." *Journal of Health Care Finance* (Spring): 1–14.

Sullivan, J. M. 1992. "Health Care Reform: Towards a Healthier Society." *Hospital & Health Services Administration* (Winter): 519–532.

Taylor, R., and L. Lessin. 1996. "Restructuring the Health Care Delivery System in the United States." *Journal of Health Care Finance* (Summer): 33–60.

THE FINANCIAL ENVIRONMENT

Learning Objectives

After studying this chapter, readers will be able to:

- Describe the alternative forms of business organization and ownership.
- Explain why taxes are important to healthcare finance.
- Briefly describe the third-party-payer system.
- Explain the different types of payment methods used by payers.
- Describe the incentives created by the different payment methods and their impact on provider risk.

Introduction

Fortunately, most of the basic concepts of healthcare finance are independent of the specific industry (for example, hospital versus long-term care versus medical practice) and organizational setting. However, some aspects of healthcare finance are influenced by industry setting, while the unique ownership structure of healthcare providers influences specific applications of finance concepts. In this chapter, some background material is presented that creates the context in which finance is practiced in health services organizations.

The fact that many healthcare businesses are organized as not-for-profit corporations has a significant impact on the practice of finance. Thus, the chapter begins with a discussion of alternative forms of business organization and ownership. Because ownership affects taxes, tax laws also are briefly introduced. The chapter ends with a discussion of third-party payers and the reimbursement methods that they use.

Alternative Forms of Business Organization

Throughout this book, the focus is on business finance—that is, the practice of accounting and financial management within business organizations. There are three primary forms of *business organization*: proprietorship, partnership, and corporation. In addition, there are several hybrid forms. Because most health services managers work for corporations and because not-for-profit businesses are organized as corporations, this form of organization is emphasized. However, many individual medical practices are organized as proprietorships, and partnerships are common in group practices and joint ventures, so health services managers must be familiar with all forms of business organization.

Proprietorships and Partnerships

A *proprietorship*, sometimes called a *sole proprietorship*, is a business owned by one individual. Going into business as a proprietor is easy—the owner merely begins business operations. However, most cities require even the smallest businesses to be licensed, and state licensure is required for most healthcare professionals.

The proprietorship form of organization is easily and inexpensively formed, is subject to few governmental regulations, and pays no corporate income taxes. All earnings of the business, whether reinvested in the business or withdrawn by the owner, are taxed as personal income to the proprietor. In general, a sole proprietorship will pay lower total taxes than a comparable, taxable corporation because corporate profits are taxed twice—once at the corporate level and again by stockholders at the personal level when profits are distributed as dividends and when the stock is sold.

A *partnership* is formed when two or more persons associate to conduct a non-incorporated business. Partnerships may operate under different degrees of formality, ranging from informal oral understandings to formal agreements filed with the state in which the partnership does business. Like a proprietorship, the major advantage of the partnership form of organization is its low cost and ease of formation. In addition, the tax treatment of a partnership is similar to that of a proprietorship: the partnership's earnings are allocated to the partners and taxed as personal income regardless of whether the earnings are actually paid out to the partners or retained in the business.[1]

Proprietorships and partnerships have several disadvantages, including the following:

- Selling their interest in the business is difficult for owners.
- The owners have unlimited personal liability for the debts of the business, which can result in losses greater than the amount invested in the business. In a proprietorship, unlimited liability means that the owner is personally responsible for the debts of the business. In a partnership, it means that if any partner is unable to meet his or her pro rata obligation in the event of bankruptcy, the remaining partners are responsible for the unsatisfied claims and must draw on their personal assets if necessary.
- The life of the business is limited to the life of the owners.

For these reasons, proprietorships and most partnerships are restricted to small businesses.[2]

The three disadvantages listed above lead to the fourth, and perhaps the most important, disadvantage from a finance perspective: the difficulty that proprietorships and partnerships have in attracting substantial amounts of capital. This is no particular problem for a very small business or when the owners are very wealthy, but the difficulty of attracting capital becomes a real handicap if the business needs to grow substantially to take advantage of market opportunities. Thus, many companies start out as sole proprietorships or partnerships but then ultimately convert to the corporate form of organization.

Corporation

A *corporation* is a legal entity that is separate and distinct from its owners and managers. The creation of a separate business entity gives these primary advantages:

- A corporation has unlimited life and can continue in existence after its original owners and managers have died or left the company.
- It is easy to transfer ownership in a corporation because ownership is divided into shares of stock that can be easily sold.
- Owners of a corporation have limited liability.

To illustrate limited liability, suppose that an individual made an investment of $10,000 in a partnership that subsequently went bankrupt, owing $100,000. Because the partners are liable for the debts of the partnership, that partner could be assessed for a share of the partnership's debt in addition to the loss of his or her initial $10,000 contribution. In fact, if the other partners were unable to pay their shares of the indebtedness, one partner would be held liable for the entire $100,000. However, if the $10,000 had been invested in a corporation that went bankrupt, the potential loss for the investor would be limited to the $10,000 investment. (However, in the case of small, financially weak corporations, the limited liability feature of ownership is often fictitious because bankers and other lenders will require personal guarantees from the stockholders.) With these three factors—unlimited life, ease of ownership transfer, and limited liability—corporations can more easily raise money in the financial markets than can sole proprietorships or partnerships.[3]

The corporate form of organization has two primary disadvantages. First, corporate earnings of taxable entities are subject to double taxation— once at the corporate level and then again at the personal level. Second, setting up a corporation, and then filing the required periodic state and federal reports, is more costly and time consuming than what is required to establish a proprietorship or partnership.

Although a proprietorship or partnership can begin operations without much legal paperwork, setting up a corporation requires that the founders, or their attorney, prepare a charter and a set of bylaws. Today, attorneys have standard forms for charters and bylaws on their computers, so they can set up a "no frills" corporation with modest effort. However, setting up a corporation remains relatively difficult when compared to a proprietorship or partnership, and it is still more difficult if the corporation has nonstandard features.

The corporate *charter* includes the name of the business, its proposed activities, the amount of stock to be issued (if investor owned), and the number and names of the initial set of directors. The charter is filed with the appropriate official of the state in which the business will be incorporated, and when it is approved, the corporation is officially in existence.[4] After the corporation has been officially formed, it must file quarterly and annual reports with various governmental agencies.

The *bylaws* are a set of rules drawn up by the founders to provide guidance for the governing and internal management of the corporation. Bylaws include features such as how directors are to be elected, whether existing shareholders have the first right to buy any new shares that the firm issues, and the procedures for changing the charter or bylaws.

The value of any investor-owned business, other than a very small one, generally will be maximized if it is organized as a corporation, for the following reasons:

- Limited liability reduces the risks borne by equity investors (the owners); with all else the same, the lower the risk, the higher the value of the investment.
- A business's value is dependent on growth opportunities, which in turn are dependent on the business's ability to attract capital. Because corporations can obtain capital more easily than other forms of business can, they are better able to take advantage of growth opportunities.
- The value of any investment depends on its *liquidity*, which means the ease at which it can be sold for a fair price. Because an equity investment in a corporation is much more liquid than a similar investment in a proprietorship or partnership, the corporate form of organization creates more value for its owners.

Hybrid Forms of Organization

Although the three basic forms of organization—proprietorship, partnership, and corporation—dominate the overall business scene, several hybrid forms of organization also are used by businesses. Some of these forms are found in the health services industry.

Several specialized types of partnerships have characteristics somewhat different from a standard form of partnership. First, limiting some of the partners' liabilities is possible by establishing a *limited partnership*, wherein certain partners are designated *general partners* and others *limited partners*. The limited partners, like the owners of a corporation, are liable only for the amount of their initial investment in the partnership, while the general partners have unlimited liability. However, the limited partners typically have no control, which rests solely with the general partners. Limited partnerships are quite common in real estate and mineral investments; they are not as common in the health services industry because finding one partner that is willing to accept all of the business's risk and a second partner that is willing to relinquish control is difficult.

The *limited liability partnership (LLP)* is a relatively new type of partnership that is available in many states. In a limited liability partnership, the partners have joint liability for all actions of the partnership, including personal injuries and indebtedness. However, all partners enjoy limited liability regarding professional malpractice because partners are only liable for their own individual malpractice actions, not those of the other partners. In spite of limited malpractice liability, the partners are jointly liable for the partnership's debts.

The *limited liability company (LLC)* is another new type of business organization. It has some characteristics of both a partnership and a corporation. The owners of an LLC are called *members*, and they are taxed as if they are partners in a partnership. However, a member's liability is like that of a stockholder of a corporation because liability is limited to the member's initial contribution in the business. Personal assets are only at risk if the member assumes specific liability, such as by signing a personal loan guarantee. Both the LLP and LLC are relatively new and complex forms of organizations, so setting them up can be time consuming and costly.

The *professional corporation (PC)*, which is called a *professional association (PA)* in some states, is a form of organization that is common among physicians and other individual and group practice healthcare professionals. All 50 states have statutes that prescribe the requirements for such organizations, which provide the usual benefits of incorporation but do not relieve the participants of professional liability. Indeed, the primary motivation behind the professional corporation, which is a relatively old business form compared to the LLP and LLC, was to provide a way for professionals to incorporate yet still be held liable for professional malpractice.

For tax purposes, standard for-profit corporations are called *C corporations*. If certain requirements are met, either one or a few individuals can incorporate but, for tax purposes only, elect to be treated as if the business were a proprietorship or partnership. Such corporations, which differ only in how the owners are taxed, are called *S corporations*. Although S corporations are similar to LLPs and LLCs regarding taxes, LLPs and LLCs provide more flexibility and benefits to owners. Many businesses, especially group practices, are therefore converting to the newer forms.

Self-Test Questions

1. What are the three primary forms of business organization, and how do they differ?
2. What are some different types of partnerships?
3. What are some different types of corporations?

Alternative Forms of Ownership

Unlike other sectors in the economy, not-for-profit corporations play a major role in the healthcare sector, especially among providers. As we discussed in Chapter 1, about 60 percent of the hospitals in the United States are private not-for-profit hospitals. Only 15 percent of all hospitals are investor owned; the remaining 25 percent are governmental. Furthermore, not-for-profit ownership is common in the nursing home, home health care, and health insurance industries.

Investor-Owned Corporations

When the average person thinks of a corporation, he or she probably thinks of an *investor-owned*, or *for-profit, corporation*. Larger businesses (e.g., Ford, IBM, and General Electric) are investor-owned corporations.

Investors become owners of such businesses by buying shares of *common stock* in the company. Investors may buy common stock when it is put up for sale by a company in what is called a *primary market transaction*. In such a transaction, the funds raised from the sale go to the corporation.[5] After the shares have been sold by the corporation, they are traded in the *secondary market*. These sales typically take place on *exchanges,* such as the New York Stock Exchange (NYSE) and the American Stock Exchange (AMEX), or in the *over-the-counter (OTC) market*, which is composed of a large number of dealers/brokers connected by a sophisticated electronic trading system.[6] When shares are bought and sold in the secondary market, the corporations whose stocks are traded receive no funds from the trades (corporations receive funds only when shares are first sold to investors).

Investor-owned corporations may be either publicly held or privately held. The shares of *publicly held* companies are owned by a large number of investors and are widely traded. For example, Health Management Associates (HMA), which owns and operates roughly 60 hospitals, has about 240 million shares outstanding that are owned by some 30,000 individual and institutional stockholders. Another example is Manor Care, which owns and operates about 350 nursing homes and has about 75 million shares outstanding that are owned by some 8,000 stockholders. Drug companies such as Merck and Pfizer, and medical equipment manufacturers such as St. Jude Medical, which makes heart valves, are all publicly held corporations.

Conversely, the shares of *privately held* (also called *closely held*) companies are owned by just a handful of investors and are not publicly traded. In general, the managers of privately held companies are major stockholders. For example, HCA, the nation's largest for-profit hospital chain with more than 200 hospitals, was a publicly held company until late 2006. At that time, the outstanding stock of the company was purchased by a small group of investors, taking the company private. With regard to ownership and control, privately held companies are more similar to partnerships than to publicly held companies. Often, the privately held corporation is a transitional form of organization that exists for a short time between a proprietorship or partnership and a publicly owned corporation in which the motivation to sell shares to the public is driven by capital needs. In the case of HCA, the expectation is that the new investors will sell off poorly performing hospitals, improve the operations of the remaining hospitals, and then in several years "go public" again to "cash out" on their investment.

The *stockholders* (also called *shareholders*) are the owners of investor-owned companies. As owners, they have these basic rights:

- **The right of control.** Common stockholders have the right to vote for the corporation's *board of directors*, which oversees the management of the company. Each year, a company's stockholders receive a *proxy* ballot, which they use to vote for directors and to vote on other issues that are proposed by management or stockholders. In this way, stockholders exercise control. In the voting process, stockholders cast one vote for each common share held.
- **A claim on the residual earnings of the firm.** A corporation sells products or services and realizes revenues from the sales. To produce these revenues, the corporation must incur expenses for materials, labor, insurance, debt capital, and so on. Any excess of revenues over expenses—the *residual earnings*—belong to the shareholders of the business. Often, a portion of these earnings are paid out in the form of *dividends*, which are merely cash payments to stockholders, or *stock repurchases*, in which the company buys back shares held by stockholders. However, management typically elects to reinvest some (or all) of the residual earnings in the business, which presumably will produce even higher payouts to stockholders in the future. (See Chapter 19, which is available online, for more information about how corporate earnings are distributed to shareholders.)
- **A claim on liquidation proceeds.** In the event of bankruptcy and liquidation, shareholders are entitled to any proceeds that remain after all other claimants have been satisfied.

In summary, there are three key features of investor-owned corporations. First, the owners (the stockholders) of the business are well defined and they exercise control of the firm by voting for directors. Second, the residual earnings of the business belong to the owners, so management is responsible only to the stockholders for the profitability of the firm. Finally, investor-owned corporations are subject to taxation at the local, state, and federal levels.

Not-for-Profit Corporations

If an organization meets a set of stringent requirements, it can qualify for incorporation as a *tax-exempt*, or *not-for-profit, corporation*. Tax-exempt corporations are sometimes called *nonprofit corporations*. Because nonprofit businesses (as opposed to pure charities such as the American Red Cross) need profits to sustain operations, and because it is hard to explain why nonprofit corporations should earn profits, the term "not-for-profit" is more descriptive of such health services corporations.

Tax-exempt status is granted to businesses that meet the tax definition of a charitable corporation as defined by Internal Revenue Service (IRS) Tax Code Section 501(c)(3) or (4). Hence, such corporations are also known as *501(c)(3) or (4) corporations*.[7] The tax code defines a charitable organization as "any corporation, community chest, fund, or foundation that is organized and operated exclusively for religious, charitable, scientific, public safety, literary, or educational purposes." Because the promotion of health is commonly considered a charitable activity, a corporation that provides healthcare services can qualify for tax-exempt status, provided that it meets other requirements.

In addition to the charitable purpose, a not-for-profit corporation must be organized and operated so that it operates exclusively for the public, rather than private, interest. Thus, no profits can be used for private gain and no direct political activity can be conducted. Also, if the corporation is liquidated or sold to an investor-owned business, the proceeds from the liquidation or sale must be used for a charitable purpose. Because individuals cannot benefit from the profits of not-for-profit corporations, such organizations cannot pay dividends. However, prohibition of private gain from profits does not prevent parties, such as managers and physicians, from benefiting through salaries, perquisites, contracts, and so on.

Not-for-profit corporations differ significantly from investor-owned corporations. Because not-for-profit firms have no shareholders, no single body of individuals has ownership rights to the firm's residual earnings or exercises control of the firm. Rather, control is exercised by a *board of trustees* that is not constrained by outside oversight. Also, not-for-profit corporations are generally exempt from taxation, including both property and income taxes, and have the right to issue tax-exempt debt (municipal bonds). Finally, individual contributions to not-for-profit organizations can be deducted from taxable income by the donor, so not-for-profit firms have access to tax-subsidized contribution capital. (The tax benefits enjoyed by not-for-profit corporations are discussed in more detail in a later section on tax laws.)

The financial problems facing most federal, state, and local governments have caused politicians to take a closer look at the tax subsidies provided to not-for-profit hospitals. For example, several bills that require hospitals to meet minimum levels of care to the indigent to retain tax-exempt status have been introduced in Congress. Such efforts by Congress prompted the American Hospital Association in 2006 to propose guidelines for charity care that include (1) giving discounts to uninsured patients of "limited means"; (2) establishing a common definition for "community benefits," which encompass the full range of services provided to the population served; and (3) improving "transparency," or the ability of outsiders to understand a business's governance structure and policies, including executive compensation.

In addition to recent congressional action, since 2004 officials in 20 states have proposed legislation that mandates the amount of charity care provided by not-for-profit hospitals and the billing and collections procedures applied to the uninsured. For example, Texas has established minimum requirements for charity care, which in effect hold not-for-profit hospitals accountable to the public for the tax exemptions they receive. The Texas law specifies four tests, and each hospital must meet at least one of them. The test that most hospitals use to comply with the law requires that at least 4 percent of net patient service revenue be spent on charity care. Under a proposed Illinois law, not-for-profit hospitals would be required to devote at least 8 percent of their operating costs to charity care and to establish discounts to the uninsured on the basis of income level.

Finally, money-starved municipalities in several states have attacked the property tax exemption of not-for-profit hospitals that have "neglected" their charitable missions. For example, tax assessors are fighting to remove property tax exemptions from not-for-profit hospitals in several Pennsylvania cities after a recent appellate court ruling supported a school district's authority to tax a local hospital that had strayed too far from its charitable purpose. According to one estimate, if all not-for-profit hospitals had to pay taxes comparable to their investor-owned counterparts, local, state, and federal governments would garner an additional $3.5 billion in tax revenues. This explains why tax authorities in many jurisdictions view not-for-profit hospitals as a potential source of revenue.

The inherent differences between investor-owned and not-for-profit organizations have profound implications for many aspects of healthcare finance, including organizational goals, financing decisions (i.e., the choice between debt and equity financing and the specific types of securities to issue), and capital investment decisions. How ownership affects the application of healthcare finance concepts will be addressed throughout the book.

Self-Test Questions

1. What are the major differences between investor-owned and not-for-profit corporations?
2. What pressures recently have been placed on not-for-profit hospitals to ensure that they meet their charitable mission?

Organizational Goals

Healthcare finance is not practiced in a vacuum; it is practiced with some objective in mind. Finance goals within an organization clearly must be consistent with, as well as supportive of, the overall goals of the business. Thus, by discussing organizational goals, a framework for financial decision making within health services organizations is established.

Small Businesses

In a proprietorship, partnership, or small privately owned corporation, the owners of the business generally are also its managers. In theory, the business can be operated for the exclusive benefit of the owners. If the owners want to work very hard to maximize wealth, they can. On the other hand, if every Wednesday is devoted to golf, no one is hurt by such actions. (Of course, the business still has to satisfy its customers or it will not survive.) It is in large, publicly held corporations, in which owners and managers are separate parties, that organizational goals become very important to finance.

Publicly Held Corporations

From a finance perspective, the primary goal of large investor-owned corporations is generally assumed to be *shareholder wealth maximization*, which translates to stock price maximization. Investor-owned corporations do, of course, have other goals. Managers, who make the actual decisions, are interested in their own personal welfare, in their employees' welfare, and in the good of the community and society at large. Still, the goal of stock price maximization is a reasonable operating objective upon which to build financial decision rules.

The primary obstacle to shareholder wealth maximization as the goal of investor-owned corporations is the *agency problem*. An agency problem exists when one or more individuals (the *principals*) hire another individual or group of individuals (the *agents*) to perform a service on their behalf and then delegate decision-making authority to those agents. Such a problem occurs between stockholders and managers of large investor-owned corporations because the managers typically hold only a very small proportion of the firm's stock, and hence they benefit relatively little from stock price increases. On the other hand, managers benefit substantially from actions such as increasing the size of the firm to justify higher salaries and more fringe benefits; awarding themselves generous retirement plans; and spending too much on office space, personal staff, and travel—actions that are often detrimental to shareholders' wealth. Clearly, many situations can arise in which managers are motivated to take actions that are in their own best interests rather than in the best interests of stockholders.

Shareholders recognize the agency problem and counter it by creating compensation incentives, such as stock options and performance-based bonus plans, that encourage managers to act in shareholders' interests. In addition, other factors, such as the threat of takeover or removal, work to keep managers focused on shareholder wealth maximization.

Clearly, managers of investor-owned corporations can have motivations that are inconsistent with shareholder wealth maximization. Still, sufficient incentives and sanctions are in place to force managers to view shareholder wealth maximization as an important goal. Thus, shareholder wealth maximization is a reasonable goal for financial decision making within investor-owned corporations.

Not-for-Profit Corporations

Not-for-profit corporations consist of a number of classes of *stakeholders*, which include all parties that have an interest, usually of a financial nature, in the organization. For example, a not-for-profit hospital's stakeholders include the board of trustees, managers, employees, physicians, creditors, suppliers, patients, and even potential patients, which may include the entire community. An investor-owned hospital has the same set of stakeholders, plus stockholders, who dictate the goal of shareholder wealth maximization. While managers of investor-owned companies have to please primarily one class of stakeholders—the shareholders—to keep their jobs, managers of not-for-profit firms face a different situation. They have to try to please all of the organization's stakeholders because no single well-defined group exercises control.

Many people argue that managers of not-for-profit corporations do not have to please anyone at all because they tend to dominate the boards of trustees that are supposed to exercise oversight. Others argue that managers of not-for-profit firms have to please all of the firm's stakeholders to a greater or lesser extent because all are necessary to the successful performance of the business. Of course, even managers of investor-owned firms should not attempt to enhance shareholder wealth by treating other stakeholders unfairly because such actions ultimately will be detrimental to shareholders.

Typically, the goal of not-for-profit corporations is stated in terms of a mission statement. For example, here is the current mission statement of Riverside Memorial Hospital, a 450-bed, not-for-profit acute care hospital:

> Riverside Memorial Hospital, along with its medical staff, is a recognized, innovative healthcare leader dedicated to meeting the needs of the community. We strive to be the best comprehensive healthcare provider through our commitment to excellence.

Although this mission statement provides Riverside's managers and employees with a framework for developing specific goals and objectives, it does not provide much insight into the goal of the hospital's finance function. For Riverside to accomplish its mission, its managers have identified the following five financial goals:

1. The hospital must maintain its financial viability.
2. The hospital must generate sufficient profits to continue to provide the current range of healthcare services to the community. This means that current buildings and equipment must be replaced as they become obsolete.
3. The hospital must generate sufficient profits to invest in new medical technologies and services as they are developed and needed.
4. Although the hospital has an aggressive philanthropy program in place, it does not want to rely on this program or government grants to fund its operations.
5. The hospital will strive to provide services to the community as inexpensively as possible, given the above financial requirements.

In effect, Riverside's managers are saying that to achieve the hospital's commitment to excellence as stated in its mission statement, the hospital must remain financially strong and profitable. Financially weak organizations cannot continue to accomplish their stated missions over the long run. What is interesting is that Riverside's five financial goals are probably not much different from the finance goals of Jefferson Regional Medical Center (JRMC), a for-profit competitor. Of course, JRMC has to worry about providing a return to its shareholders, and it receives only a very small amount of contributions and grants. However, to maximize shareholder wealth, JRMC also must retain its financial viability and have the financial resources necessary to offer new services and technologies. Furthermore, competition in the market for hospital services will not permit JRMC to charge appreciably more for services than its not-for-profit competitors.

Self-Test Questions

1. What is the difference in goals between investor-owned and not-for-profit businesses?
2. What is the agency problem, and how does it apply to investor-owned firms?
3. What factors tend to reduce the agency problem?

Tax Laws

The value of any investment—whether the investment is a stock, a bond, or an entire business—depends on the **usable** cash flows that the investment is expected to provide to the owner. Because taxes reduce usable cash flows, both individuals and managers of for-profit businesses must be concerned about taxes.

Tax laws are very complicated and are constantly changing. Consequently, covering even the most basic features of our tax laws in an introductory finance book is impossible. However, what is important is to recognize that individuals must pay *personal (individual) taxes* to federal and state (in most states) authorities that can approach 50 percent of income. Thus, income from proprietorships and partnerships, as well as dividends and capital gains on stock investments, will be reduced when personal taxes are taken into account.[8]

To illustrate the effect of personal taxes, assume that an individual's tax rate is 35 percent and he or she receives $100 in partnership income. Using the letter T to represent tax rate, that person must pay T × $100 = 0.35 × $100 = $35 in taxes on the income, which leaves him or her with only $100 − $35 = $65 on an after-tax basis. This tax analysis leads to the following useful equation:

$$AT = BT - (T \times BT)$$
$$= BT \times (1 - T),$$

where AT = after-tax and BT = before-tax. Thus, the after-tax income amount to the investor is AT = BT × (1 − T) = $100 × (1 − 0.35) = $100 × 0.65 = $65. (This equation can be applied to interest rates as well as dollar amounts. See Problem 2.3 as an example.) Clearly, taxes will influence investment decisions, so any differential tax implications on investment alternatives must be considered in the decision process.

In addition to personal taxes paid by individuals, investor-owned (for-profit) corporations must pay both federal and state *corporate taxes*, which can exceed 40 percent of the corporation's taxable income. Corporate taxes are paid on earnings before dividends are distributed, so corporate income is subject to double taxation—once at the corporate level and again when stockholders receive dividends or capital gains.

Not-for-profit corporations, for the most part, are not subject to income or property taxes. In addition, such organizations benefit from being able to issue (take on) debt with interest payments that are exempt from personal taxes. To illustrate the advantage of being able to issue tax-exempt debt, first consider the bonds issued by Jefferson Regional Medical Center (JRMC), an investor-owned hospital. Its debt carries an interest rate of 10 percent, so bond investors receive 0.10 × $100 = $10 in annual interest for every $100 worth of bonds that they own. For a bond investor that pays 40 percent in federal and state income taxes, each $10 of interest provides the investor with AT = BT × (1 − T) = $10 × (1 − 0.40) = $6 of after-tax interest. However, if the bonds had been issued by Riverside Memorial Hospital, a not-for-profit corporation, the investor would have to pay no taxes on the interest and hence would keep the entire $10. If investors truly require a $6 after-tax return, Riverside can issue debt with an interest rate of only 6 percent and, with all else the same, investors in the 40 percent tax bracket would be as willing to buy these bonds as they are the JRMC 10 percent bonds. Thus, the interest rate that Riverside must set on its debt issues to sell them to investors is lower than the rate that JRMC must set because of the tax exemption on debt issued by not-for-profit corporations.

Finally, contributions that individuals make to not-for-profit corporations are tax deductible to the donor. If John Brooks is in the 40 percent tax bracket and he donates $1,000 to Riverside Memorial Hospital, his taxable income would be reduced by $1,000. A reduction in taxable income of this amount would save John $T \times \$1,000 = 0.40 \times \$1,000 = \$400$ in taxes. Thus, the effective cost of his contribution would only be $600. In effect, the government will pay John 40 cents for every dollar he contributes. Thus, not-for-profit corporations have access to a source of financing that, for all practical purposes, is not available to investor-owned businesses.

Because of the impact that taxes have on usable earnings of investor-owned businesses and because not-for-profit ownership has important tax consequences, tax implications are highlighted and explained as necessary throughout the book. Still, what is most important now is to recognize that taxes will play a critical role in many topics to be discussed.

Self-Test Questions

1. Why does a finance book have to consider taxes?
2. Why is the ability to issue tax-exempt debt an advantage for not-for-profit corporations?
3. What advantage accrues to businesses that qualify for tax-exempt contributions?

Third-Party Payers

Up to this point in the chapter, basic concepts about the form and ownership of healthcare businesses have been considered. A large proportion of the health services industry receives its revenues not directly from the users of their services—the patients—but from insurers known collectively as *third-party payers*. Because an organization's revenues are key to its financial viability, this section contains a brief examination of the sources of most revenues in the health services industry. In the next section, the types of reimbursement methods employed by these payers are reviewed in more detail.

Health insurance originated in Europe in the early 1800s when mutual benefit societies were formed to reduce the financial burden associated with illness or injury. Today, health insurers fall into two broad categories: private insurers and public programs.

Private Insurers

In the United States, the concept of public, or government, health insurance is relatively new, while private health insurance has been in existence since the early 1900s. In this section, the major private insurers are discussed: Blue Cross/Blue Shield, commercial insurers, and self-insurers.

Blue Cross/Blue Shield organizations trace their roots to the Great Depression, when both hospitals and physicians were concerned about their patients' abilities to pay healthcare bills.

Blue Cross/Blue Shield

 Blue Cross originated as a number of separate insurance programs offered by individual hospitals. At that time, many patients were unable to pay their hospital bills, but most people, except the very poorest, could afford to purchase some type of hospitalization insurance. Thus, the programs were initially designed to benefit hospitals as well as patients. The programs were all similar in structure: Hospitals agreed to provide a certain amount of services to program members who made periodic payments of fixed amounts to the hospitals whether services were used or not. In a short time, these programs were expanded from single hospital programs to communitywide, multihospital plans that were called *hospital service plans.* The American Hospital Association (AHA) recognized the benefits of such plans to hospitals, so a close relationship was formed between the AHA and the organizations that offered hospital service plans.

 In the early years, several states ruled that the sale of hospital services by prepayment did not constitute insurance, so the plans were exempt from regulations governing insurance companies. However, the legal status of hospital service plans clearly would be subject to future scrutiny unless their status was formalized. The states, one by one, passed enabling legislation that provided for the founding of not-for-profit hospital service corporations that were exempt both from taxes and from the capital requirements mandated for other insurers. However, state insurance departments had—and continue to have—oversight over most aspects of the plans' operations. The Blue Cross name was officially adopted by most of these plans in 1939.

 Blue Shield plans developed in a manner similar to Blue Cross plans, except that the providers were physicians instead of hospitals and the professional organization was the American Medical Association (AMA) instead of the AHA. Today, 38 Blue Cross/Blue Shield (the "Blues") organizations exist, some of which offer only one of the two plans but most offer both plans. The Blues are organized as independent corporations, but all belong to a single national association that sets standards that must be met to use the Blue Cross/Blue Shield name. Collectively, the Blues provide healthcare coverage for more than 94 million people in all 50 states, the District of Columbia, and Puerto Rico. Historically, the Blues were not-for-profit corporations that enjoyed the full benefits accorded to that status, including freedom from taxes. In 1986, however, Congress eliminated the Blues' tax exemption on the grounds that they operated commercial-type insurance activities, but the plans were given special deductions that resulted in lower taxes than those paid by commercial insurance companies. In spite of the 1986 change in tax status, the national association continued to require all Blues to operate entirely as not-for-profit corporations, although they could establish for-profit subsidiaries. In 1994, however, the national association lifted its traditional ban on member plans becoming investor-owned companies, and four Blue Cross/Blue Shield corporations have since converted to for-profit status.

In spite of these conversions, it is unlikely that many more Blues will convert to for-profit status because of the legal problems inherent in conversion and because they already have the ability to create for-profit subsidiaries. The primary rationale for converting or creating for-profit subsidiaries is having access to investor-supplied equity capital, which many experts believe to be necessary for insurers to be competitive in today's healthcare market.

Commercial Insurers *Commercial health insurance* is issued by life insurance companies, by casualty insurance companies, and by companies that were formed exclusively to write health insurance. Examples of commercial insurers include Aetna, Humana, and UnitedHealth Group. Commercial insurance companies can be organized either as stock companies or as mutual companies. *Stock companies* are shareholder owned and can raise capital by selling shares of stock just like any other for-profit company. Furthermore, the stockholders assume the risks and responsibilities of ownership and management. A *mutual company* has no shareholders; its management is controlled by a board of directors elected by the company's policyholders. Regardless of the form of ownership, commercial insurance companies are taxable entities.

Commercial insurers moved strongly into health insurance following World War II. At that time, the United Auto Workers (UAW) negotiated the first contract with employers in which fringe benefits were a major part of the contract. Like the Blues, the majority of individuals with commercial health insurance are covered under *group policies* with employee groups, professional and other associations, and labor unions.

Self-Insurers The third major form of private insurance is *self-insurance*. An argument can be made that all individuals who do not have some form of health insurance are self-insurers, but this is not technically correct. Self-insurers make a conscious decision to bear the risks associated with healthcare costs and then set aside (or have available) funds to pay future costs as they occur. Individuals, except the very wealthy, are not good candidates for self-insurance because they face too much uncertainty concerning healthcare expenses. On the other hand, large groups, especially employers, are good candidates for self-insurance. Today, most large groups are self-insured. For example, employees of the State of Florida are covered by health insurance whose costs are paid directly by the state. Blue Cross/Blue Shield is paid a fee to administer the plan, but the state bears all risks associated with cost and utilization uncertainty.

Many firms today are even going one or two steps further in their self-insurance programs. For example, Digital Equipment Corporation, a major computer maker, negotiates discounts directly with hospitals and physicians and self-administers its program. Others, such as Deere & Company, a farm-implements manufacturer, have set up company-owned subsidiaries to provide healthcare services to their employees. These companies believe that they can lower healthcare costs by applying the kind of management attention to healthcare that they do to their core businesses.

Public Insurers

Government is a major insurer as well as a direct provider of healthcare services. For example, the government provides healthcare services directly to qualifying individuals through the Department of Veterans Affairs (VA), Department of Defense (DOD), and Public Health Service (PHS) medical facilities. In addition, the government either provides or mandates a variety of insurance programs, such as worker's compensation and TRICARE (health insurance for uniformed service members and families). In this section, however, the focus is on the two major government insurance programs: Medicare and Medicaid.

Medicare was established by the federal government in 1966 to provide medical benefits to individuals age 65 and older. Medicare consists of three separate coverages: (1) *Part A*, which provides hospital and some skilled nursing home coverage; (2) *Part B*, which covers physician services, ambulatory surgical services, outpatient services, and certain other miscellaneous services; and (3) *Part D*, which covers prescription drugs. Part A coverage is free to all individuals eligible for social security benefits. Individuals who are not eligible for social security benefits can obtain Part A medical benefits by paying premiums of $410 per month (for 2007). Part B is optional to all individuals who have Part A coverage, and it requires a monthly premium for most enrollees of $93.50 (for 2007). (Starting in 2007, high-income enrollees will pay more than $93.50 for Part B coverage.) About 97 percent of Part A participants purchase Part B coverage. Part D, which began on January 1, 2006, offers prescription drug coverage through plans offered by more than 70 private companies. Each plan offers somewhat different coverage, so the cost of Part D coverage varies widely.

The Medicare program falls under the *Department of Health and Human Services (DHHS)*, which creates the specific rules of the program on the basis of enabling legislation. Medicare is administered by an agency in DHHS called the *Centers for Medicare and Medicaid Services (CMS)*. CMS has eight regional offices that oversee the Medicare program and ensure that regulations

Medicare

are followed. Medicare payments to providers are not made directly by CMS but by contractors at the state or local level called *intermediaries* for Part A payments and *carriers* for Part B payments.

Medicaid   *Medicaid* began in 1966 as a modest program to be jointly funded and operated by the states and the federal government that would provide a medical safety net for low-income mothers and children and for elderly, blind, and disabled individuals who receive benefits from the Supplemental Security Income (SSI) program. Congress mandated that Medicaid cover hospital and physician care, but states were encouraged to expand on the basic package of benefits either by increasing the range of benefits or extending the program to cover more people. States with large tax bases were quick to expand coverage to many groups, while states with limited abilities to raise funds for Medicaid were forced to construct more limited programs. A mandatory nursing home benefit was added in 1972.

Over the years, Medicaid has provided access to healthcare services for many low-income individuals who otherwise would have no insurance coverage. Furthermore, Medicaid has become an important source of revenue for healthcare providers, especially for nursing homes and other providers that treat large numbers of indigent patients. However, Medicaid expenditures have been growing at an alarming rate, which has forced both federal and state policymakers to search for more effective ways to improve the program's access, quality, and cost.

Self-Test Questions
1. What are some different types of private insurers?
2. Briefly, what are the origins and purpose of Medicare?
3. What is Medicaid, and how is it administered?

Managed Care Plans

Managed care plans strive to combine the provision of healthcare services and the insurance function into a single entity. Traditionally, such plans have been created by insurers who either directly own a provider network or create one through contractual arrangements with independent providers. Recently, however, providers in some areas have banded together to form *integrated delivery systems* (*IDSs*) that are capable of offering both insurance and healthcare services.

One type of managed care plan is the *health maintenance organization* (*HMO*). HMOs are based on the premise that the traditional insurer/provider relationship creates perverse incentives that reward providers for treating patients' illnesses while offering little incentive for providing prevention and rehabilitation services. By combining the financing and delivery of comprehensive healthcare services into a single system, HMOs theoretically have as strong an incentive to prevent as to treat illnesses.

Because of the many types of organizational structures, ownership, and financial incentives provided, HMOs vary widely in cost and quality. HMOs use a variety of methods to control costs. These include limiting patients to particular providers by using *gatekeeper* physicians who must authorize any specialized or referral services, using *utilization review* to ensure that services rendered are appropriate and needed, using *discounted rate schedules* for providers, and using payment methods that transfer some risk to providers. In general, services are not covered if beneficiaries bypass their gatekeeper physician or use providers that are not part of the HMO.

The federal Health Maintenance Act of 1973 encouraged the development of HMOs and created a great deal of interest in the concept by providing federal funds for HMO-operating grants and loans. In addition, the Act required larger employers that offer healthcare benefits to their employees to include a federally qualified HMO as a healthcare alternative, if one was available, in addition to traditional insurance plans.

Another type of managed care plan, the *preferred provider organization (PPO)*, evolved during the early 1980s. PPOs are a hybrid of HMOs and traditional health insurance plans that use many of the cost-saving strategies developed by HMOs. PPOs do not mandate that beneficiaries use specific providers, although financial incentives are created that encourage members to use those providers that are part of the *provider panel*, which are those providers that have contracts (usually at discounted prices) with the PPO. Unlike HMOs, PPOs do not require beneficiaries to use pre-selected gatekeeper physicians who serve as the initial contact and authorize all services received. In general, PPOs are less likely than HMOs to provide preventive services and do not assume any responsibility for quality assurance because enrollees are not constrained to use only the PPO panel of providers.

HMOs and PPOs grew rapidly in number and size during the 1980s and 1990s; however, both the number of HMOs and the number of enrollees have fallen significantly since 2000. Still, hybrids of HMOs and PPOs continue to develop. For example, *exclusive provider organizations (EPOs)* are PPO-like plans that require members to use only participating providers but do not designate a specific gatekeeper. Also, *point of service (POS) plans* permit enrollees to obtain services either from within the HMO panel or to bear higher out-of-pocket costs to obtain services outside the panel.

In an effort to achieve the potential cost savings of managed care plans, insurance companies have started to apply managed care strategies to their conventional plans. Such plans, which are called *managed fee-for-service plans*, are using pre-admission certification, utilization review, and second surgical opinions to control inappropriate utilization. Although the distinctions between managed care and conventional plans were once quite apparent, considerable overlap now exists in the strategies and incentives employed. Thus, the term *managed care* now describes a continuum of plans, which can vary significantly in their approaches to providing combined insurance and healthcare services. The common feature in managed care plans is that the insurer has a mechanism by which it controls, or at least influences, patients' utilization of healthcare services.

Self-Test Questions

1. What is meant by the term *managed care*?
2. What are some different types of managed care plans?

Alternative Reimbursement Methods

Regardless of the payer for a particular healthcare service, only a limited number of payment methods are used to reimburse providers. Payment methods fall into two broad classifications: fee-for-service and capitation. In *fee-for-service* payment methods, of which many variations exist, the greater the amount of services provided, the higher the amount of reimbursement. Under *capitation*, a fixed payment is made to providers for each *covered life*, or *enrollee*, that is independent of the amount of services provided. In this section, we discuss the mechanics, incentives created, and risk implications of alternative reimbursement methods.

Fee-for-Service Methods

The three primary fee-for-service methods of reimbursement are cost based, charge based, and prospective payment.

Cost-Based Reimbursement

Under *cost-based reimbursement*, the payer agrees to reimburse the provider for the costs incurred in providing services to the insured population. Reimbursement is limited to *allowable costs*, usually defined as those costs directly related to the provision of healthcare services. Nevertheless, for all practical purposes, cost-based reimbursement guarantees that a provider's costs will be covered by payments from the payer. Typically, the payer makes *periodic interim payments (PIPs)* to the provider, and a final reconciliation is made after the contract period expires and all costs have been processed through the provider's managerial (cost) accounting system. During its early years (1966–1982), Medicare reimbursed hospitals on the basis of costs incurred.

Charge-Based Reimbursement

When payers pay *billed charges*, or just *charges*, they pay according to a rate schedule established by the provider, called a *chargemaster*. To a certain extent, this reimbursement system places payers at the mercy of providers in regards to the cost of healthcare services, especially in markets where competition is limited. In the very early days of health insurance, all payers reimbursed providers on the basis of billed charges. Some insurers still reimburse providers according to billed charges, but the trend for payers is toward other, less-generous reimbursement methods. If this trend continues, the only payers that will be expected to pay billed charges are self-pay, or private-pay, patients. Even then, low-income patients often are billed at rates less than charges.

Some payers that historically have reimbursed providers on the basis of billed charges now pay by *negotiated*, or *discounted*, *charges*. This is especially true for insurers that have established managed care plans such as HMOs and PPOs. HMOs and PPOs, as well as some conventional insurers, often have bargaining power because of the large number of patients that they bring to a provider, so they can negotiate discounts from billed charges. Such discounts generally range from 20 to 50 percent, or even more, of billed charges. The effect of these discounts is to create a system very similar to hotel or airline pricing, where there are listed rates (rack rates or full fares) that very few people pay.

In a *prospective payment system*, the rates paid by payers are determined **by the payer** before the services are provided. Furthermore, payments are not directly related to either reimbursable costs or chargemaster rates. Here are some common units of payment used in prospective payment systems: **Prospective Payment**

- **Per procedure.** Under *per procedure* reimbursement, a separate payment is made for each procedure performed on a patient. Because of the high administrative costs associated with this method when applied to complex diagnoses, per procedure reimbursement is more commonly used in outpatient than in inpatient settings.
- **Per diagnosis.** In the *per diagnosis* reimbursement method, the provider is paid a rate that depends on the patient's diagnosis. Diagnoses that require higher resource utilization, and hence are more costly to treat, have higher reimbursement rates. Medicare pioneered this basis of payment in its *diagnosis related group (DRG)* system, which it first used for hospital inpatient reimbursement in 1983.
- **Per day (per diem).** If reimbursement is based on a *per diem* rate, the provider is paid a fixed amount for each day that service is provided, regardless of the nature of the services. Note that per diem rates, which are applicable only to inpatient settings, can be *stratified*. For example, a hospital may be paid one rate for a medical/surgical day, a higher rate for a critical care unit day, and yet a different rate for an obstetrical day. Stratified per diems recognize that providers incur widely different daily costs for providing different types of care.
- **Global pricing.** Under *global pricing*, payers pay a single prospective payment that covers all services delivered in a single episode, whether the services are rendered by a single or by multiple

providers. For example, a global fee may be set for all obstetric services associated with a pregnancy provided by a single physician, including all prenatal and postnatal visits, as well as the delivery. For another example, a global price may be paid for all physician and hospital services associated with a cardiac bypass operation.

Capitation Method

Up to this point, the prospective payment methods presented have been fee-for-service methods—that is, providers are reimbursed on the basis of the amount of services provided. The service may be defined as a visit, a diagnosis, a hospital day, or in some other manner, but the key feature is that the more services that are performed, the greater the reimbursement amount. *Capitation*, although a form of prospective payment, is an entirely different approach to reimbursement and hence deserves to be treated as a separate category. Under capitated reimbursement, the provider is paid a fixed amount per covered life per period (usually a month) regardless of the amount of services provided. For example, a primary care physician might be paid $15 per member per month for handling 100 members of an HMO plan.

Capitation payment, which is used primarily by managed care plans, dramatically changes the financial environment of healthcare providers. It has implications for financial accounting, managerial accounting, and financial management. A discussion of how capitation, as opposed to fee-for-service reimbursement, affects healthcare finance is provided throughout the remainder of this book. (See Chapter 20, which is available online, for more information about capitation.)

Provider Incentives

Providers, like individuals and businesses, react to the incentives created by the financial environment. For example, individuals can deduct mortgage interest from income for tax purposes, but they cannot deduct interest payments on personal loans. Loan companies have responded by offering home equity loans that are a type of second mortgage. The intent is not that such loans would be used to finance home ownership, as the tax laws assumed, but that the funds would be used for other purposes, including paying for vacations and purchasing cars or appliances. In this situation, tax laws created incentives for consumers to have mortgage debt rather than personal debt, and the mortgage loan industry responded accordingly.

In the same vein, it is interesting to examine the incentives that alternative reimbursement methods have on provider behavior. Under cost-based reimbursement, providers are given a "blank check" in regards to acquiring facilities and equipment and incurring operating costs. If payers reimburse providers for all costs, the incentive is to incur costs. Facilities will be lavish and conveniently located, and staff will be available to ensure that patients are given "deluxe" treatment. Furthermore, as in billed charges reimbursement, services that may not truly be required will be provided because more services lead to higher costs, which leads to higher revenues.

Under charge-based reimbursement, providers have the incentive to set high charge rates, which leads to high revenues. However, in competitive markets, there will be a constraint on how high providers can go. But, to the extent that insurers, rather than patients, are footing the bill, there is often considerable leeway in setting charges. Because billed charges is a fee-for-service type of reimbursement in which more services result in higher revenue, a strong incentive exists to provide the highest possible amount of services. In essence, providers can increase utilization, and hence revenues, by *churning*—creating more visits, ordering more tests, extending inpatient stays, and so on. Although charge-based reimbursement does encourage providers to contain costs, the incentive is weak because charges can be increased more easily than costs can be reduced. Note, however, that discounted charge reimbursement places additional pressure on profitability and hence increases the incentive for providers to lower costs.

Under prospective payment reimbursement, provider incentives are altered. First, under per procedure reimbursement, the profitability of individual procedures will vary depending on the relationship between the actual costs incurred and the payment for that procedure. Providers, usually physicians, have the incentive to perform procedures that have the highest profit potential. Furthermore, the more procedures the better because each procedure typically generates additional profit. The incentives under per diagnosis reimbursement are similar. Providers, usually hospitals, will seek patients with those diagnoses that have the greatest profit potential and discourage (or even discontinue) those services that have the least potential. Furthermore, to the extent that providers have some flexibility in selecting procedures (or assigning diagnoses) to patients, an incentive exists to *upcode* procedures (or diagnoses) to ones that provide the greatest reimbursement.

In all prospective payment methods, providers have the incentive to reduce costs because the amount of reimbursement is fixed and independent of the costs actually incurred. For example, when hospitals are paid under per diagnosis reimbursement, they have the incentive to reduce length of stay and hence costs. Note, however, when per diem reimbursement is used, hospitals have an incentive to increase length of stay. Because the early days of a hospitalization typically are more costly than the later days, the later days are more profitable. However, as mentioned previously, hospitals have the incentive to reduce costs during each day of a patient stay.

Under global pricing, providers do not have the opportunity to be reimbursed for a series of separate services, which is called *unbundling*. For example, a physician's treatment of a fracture could be bundled, and hence billed as one episode, or it could be unbundled with separate bills submitted for diagnosis, x-rays, setting the fracture, removing the cast, and so on. The rationale for unbundling is usually to provide more detailed records of treatments rendered, but often the result is higher total charges for the parts than would be charged for the entire package. Also, global pricing, when applied to multiple providers for a single episode of care, forces involved providers (e.g., physicians and a hospital) to jointly offer the most cost-effective treatment. Such a joint view of cost containment may be more effective than each provider separately attempting to minimize its treatment costs because lowering costs in one phase of treatment could increase costs in another.

Finally, capitation reimbursement totally changes the playing field by completely reversing the actions that providers must take to ensure financial success. Under all fee-for-service methods, the key to provider success is to work harder, increase utilization, and hence increase profits; under capitation, the key to profitability is to work smarter and decrease utilization. As with prospective payment, capitated providers have the incentive to reduce costs, but now they also have the incentive to reduce utilization. Thus, only those procedures that are truly medically necessary should be performed, and treatment should take place in the lowest cost setting that can provide the appropriate quality of care. Furthermore, providers have the incentive to promote health, rather than just treat illness and injury, because a healthier population consumes fewer healthcare services.

Financial Risks to Providers

A key issue facing providers is the impact of various reimbursement methods on financial risk. For now, think of financial risk in terms of the effect that the reimbursement methods have on profit uncertainty—the greater the chance of losing money, the higher the risk. (Financial risk is discussed in detail in Chapter 10.)

Cost- and charge-based reimbursement are the least risky for providers because payers more or less ensure that costs will be covered, and hence profits will be earned. In cost-based systems, costs are automatically covered, and a profit component typically is added. In charge-based systems, providers typically can set charges high enough to ensure that costs are covered, although discounts introduce uncertainty into the reimbursement process.

In all reimbursement methods except cost-based, providers bear the cost-of-service risk in the sense that costs can exceed revenues. However, a primary difference among the reimbursement types is the ability of the provider to influence the revenue–cost relationship. If providers set charge rates for each type of service provided, they can most easily ensure that revenues exceed costs. Furthermore, if providers have the power to set rates above those that would exist in a truly competitive market, charge-based reimbursement could result in higher profits than cost-based reimbursement.

Prospective payment adds a second dimension of risk to reimbursement contracts because the bundle of services needed to treat a particular patient may be more extensive than that assumed in the payment. However, when the prospective payment is made on a per procedure basis, risk is minimal because each procedure will produce its own revenue. When prospective payment is made on a per diagnosis basis, provider risk is increased. If, on average, patients require more intensive treatments, and for inpatients a longer length of stay (LOS), than assumed in the prospective payment amount, the provider must bear the added costs.[9]

When prospective payment is made on a per diem basis, even when stratified, one daily rate usually covers a large number of diagnoses. Because the nature of the services provided could vary widely, both because of varying diagnoses as well as intensity differences within a single diagnosis, the provider bears the risk that costs associated with the services provided on any day exceed the per diem rate. However, patients with complex diagnoses and greater intensity tend to remain hospitalized longer, and per diem reimbursement does differentiate among different LOSs, but the additional days of stay may be insufficient to make up for the increased resources consumed. In addition, providers bear the risk that the payer, through the utilization review process, will constrain LOS and hence increase intensity during the days that a patient is hospitalized. Thus, under per diem, compression of services and shortened LOS can put significant pressure on providers' profitability.

Under global pricing, a more inclusive set of procedures, or providers, are included in one fixed payment. Clearly, the more services that must be rendered for a single payment—or the more providers that have to share a single payment—the more providers are at risk for intensity of services.

Finally, under capitation, providers assume utilization risk along with the risks assumed under the other reimbursement methods. The assumption of *utilization risk* has traditionally been an insurance, rather than a provider, function. In the traditional fee-for-service system, the financial risk of providing healthcare is shared between purchasers and insurers. Hospitals, physicians, and other providers bear negligible risk because they are paid on the basis of the amount of services provided. Insurers bear short-term risk in that payments to providers in any year can exceed the amount of premiums collected. However, poor profitability by insurers in one year usually can be offset by premium increases to purchasers the next year, so the long-term risk of financing the healthcare system is borne by purchasers. Capitation, however, places the burden of short-term utilization risk on providers.

When provider risk under different reimbursement methods is discussed in this descriptive fashion, an easy conclusion to make is that capitation is by far the riskiest to providers, while cost- and charge-based reimbursement are by far the least risky. Although this conclusion is not a bad starting point for analysis, financial risk is a complex subject, and its surface has just been scratched. One of the key issues throughout the remainder of this book is financial risk, so readers will see this topic over and over. For now, keep in mind that different payers use different reimbursement methods. Thus, providers can face conflicting incentives and differing risk, depending on the predominant method of reimbursement.

In closing, note that all prospective payment methods involve a transfer of risk from insurers to providers that increases as the payment unit moves from per procedure to capitation. The added risk does not mean that providers should avoid such reimbursement methods; indeed, refusing to accept contracts with prospective payment provisions would be tantamount to organizational suicide for most providers. However, providers must understand the risks involved in prospective payment arrangements, especially the effect on profitability, and make every effort to negotiate a level of payment that is consistent with the risk incurred.

Self-Test Questions

1. Briefly explain the following payment methods:
   - Cost-based
   - Charge-based and discounted charges
   - Per procedure
   - Per diagnosis
   - Per diem
   - Global
   - Capitation
2. What is the major difference between fee-for-service reimbursement and capitation?
3. What provider incentives are created under each of the payment methods previously listed?
4. Which of these payment methods carries the least risk for providers? The most risk? Explain your answer.

Key Concepts

In this chapter, important background material was presented that will be used throughout the remainder of the book. The key concepts of this chapter are:

- The three main forms of business organization are the *proprietorship*, *partnership*, and *corporation*. Although each form of organization has its own unique advantages and disadvantages, most large organizations, and all not-for-profit entities, are organized as *corporations*.
- *Investor-owned corporations* have *stockholders* who are the owners of the corporation. Stockholders exercise control through the *proxy* process in which they elect the corporation's *board of directors* and vote on matters of major consequence to the firm. As owners, stockholders have claim on the *residual earnings* of the corporation. Investor-owned corporations are fully taxable.
- Charitable organizations that meet certain criteria can be organized as *not-for-profit corporations*. Rather than having a well-defined set of owners, such organizations have a large number of *stakeholders* who have an interest in the organization. Not-for-profit corporations do not pay taxes;

they can accept tax-deductible contributions, and they can issue tax-exempt debt.

- From a financial management perspective, the primary goal of investor-owned corporations is *shareholder wealth maximization*, which translates to stock price maximization. For not-for-profit corporations, a reasonable goal for financial management is to ensure that the organization can fulfill its mission, which translates to *maintaining financial viability.*
- An *agency problem* is a conflict of interests that can arise between principals and agents. One type of agency problem that is relevant to healthcare finance is the conflict between the owners of a large for-profit corporation and its managers.
- The value of any income stream depends on the amount of *usable,* or *after-tax, income.* Thus, tax laws play an important role in financial management decisions.
- Most provider revenue is not obtained directly from patients but from healthcare insurers that are known collectively as *third-party payers.*
- Third-party payers are classified as *private insurers* (Blue Cross/Blue Shield, commercial, and self-insurers) and *public insurers* (Medicare and Medicaid).
- *Managed care plans,* such as *health maintenance organizations (HMOs),* strive to combine both the insurance function and the provision of healthcare services.
- Third-party payers use many different payment methods that fall into two broad classifications: *fee-for-service* and *capitation.* Each payment method creates a unique set of incentives and risk for providers.

Because the managers of health services organizations must make financial decisions within the constraints imposed by the economic environment, these background concepts will be used over and over throughout the remainder of the book.

Questions

2.1 What are the three primary forms of business organization? Describe their advantages and disadvantages.

2.2 What are the primary differences between investor-owned and not-for-profit corporations?

2.3 a. What is the primary goal of investor-owned corporations?
b. What is the primary goal of most not-for-profit healthcare corporations?
c. Are there substantial differences between the finance goals of investor-owned and not-for-profit corporations? Explain.
d. What is the agency problem?

2.4 a. Why are tax laws important to healthcare finance?

    b. What three major advantages do tax laws give to not-for-profit corporations?

2.5 Briefly describe the major third-party payers.

2.6 a. What are the primary characteristics of managed care plans?

    b. Describe different types of managed care plans.

2.7 What is the difference between fee-for-service reimbursement and capitation?

2.8 Describe provider incentives and risks under each of the following reimbursement methods:

    a. Cost-based

    b. Charge-based (including discounted charges)

    c. Per procedure

    d. Per diagnosis

    e. Per diem

    f. Global pricing

    g. Capitation

Problems

2.1 Assume that Provident Health System, a for-profit hospital, has $1 million in taxable income for 2007, and its tax rate is 30 percent.

    a. Given this information, what is the firm's net income? (Hint: net income is what remains after taxes have been paid.)

    b. Suppose the hospital pays out $300,000 in dividends. A stockholder receives $10,000. If the stockholder's tax rate on dividends is 15 percent, what is the after-tax dividend?

2.2 A firm that owns the stock of another corporation does not have to pay taxes on the entire amount of dividends received. In general, only 30 percent of the dividends received by one corporation from another are taxable. The reason for this tax law feature is to mitigate the effect of triple taxation, which occurs when earnings are first taxed at one firm, then its dividends paid to a second firm are taxed again, and finally the dividends paid to stockholders by the second firm are taxed yet again. Assume that a firm with a 35 percent tax rate receives $100,000 in dividends from another corporation. What taxes must be paid on this dividend, and what is the after-tax amount of the dividend?

2.3 John Doe is in the 40 percent personal tax bracket. He is considering investing in HCA bonds that carry a 12 percent interest rate.

    a. What is his after-tax yield (interest rate) on the bonds?

    b. Suppose Twin Cities Memorial Hospital has issued tax-exempt bonds that have an interest rate of 6 percent. With all else the same, should John buy the HCA or the Twin Cities bonds?

    c. With all else the same, what interest rate on the tax-exempt Twin

Cities bonds would make John indifferent between these bonds and the HCA bonds?

2.4 Jane Smith currently holds tax-exempt bonds of Good Samaritan Healthcare that pay 7 percent interest. She is in the 40 percent tax bracket. Her broker wants her to buy some Beverly Enterprises taxable bonds that will be issued next week. With all else the same, what rate must be set on the Beverly bonds to make Jane interested in making a switch?

2.5 George and Margaret Wealthy are in the 48 percent tax bracket, considering both federal and state personal taxes. Norman Briggs, the CEO of Community General Hospital, has been aggressively pursuing the couple to contribute $500,000 to the hospital's soon-to-be-built Cancer Care Center. Without the contribution, the Wealthy's taxable income for 2008 would be $2 million. What impact would the contribution have on the Wealthy's 2008 tax bill?

Notes

1. A tax-exempt corporation can be one partner of a partnership. In this situation, profits allocated to the tax-exempt partner are not taxed, but those allocated to taxable partners are subject to taxation.
2. Although most partnerships are small, there are some very large businesses that are organized as partnerships or as hybrid organizations. Examples include the major public accounting firms and many large law firms.
3. *Financial markets* bring together people and businesses that need money with other people and businesses that have funds to invest. In a developed country such as the United States, a great many financial markets exist. Some markets deal with debt capital and others with equity (ownership) capital, some deal with short-term capital and others with long-term capital, and so on. How financial markets operate and their benefit to health services organizations are discussed throughout the book.
4. More than 60 percent of corporations in the United States are chartered in Delaware, which over the years has provided a favorable governmental and legal environment for corporations. A firm does not have to be headquartered or conduct business operations in its state of incorporation.
5. Stock sales are discussed in much more detail in Chapter 12.
6. The OTC market is also known as *NASDAQ*, which stands for National Association of Securities Dealers Automated Quotation (System).
7. This entire chapter could easily be filled with the details of obtaining and maintaining tax-exempt status, but that is not the purpose of this book. Enough information is provided to show the ways in which not-for-profit status has an impact on financial decisions, but the details concerning tax-exempt status are left to outside readings or other courses.
8. Note that ordinary income, which consists primarily of wages and income distributed from proprietorships and partnerships, is taxed at higher rates

than income from dividends or capital gains that result from corporate stock ownership. (A capital gain is realized when stock is sold at a price greater than the purchase price.) For example, in 2007 an individual investor in the 35 percent tax bracket for ordinary income would pay only 15 percent taxes on income from dividends and capital gains.

9. Most prospective payment systems contain *outlier clauses*, whereby providers receive additional reimbursement when costs are far above average for a particular patient. However, such extra payments typically do not cover the full amount of the cost differential.

References

For the latest information on events that affect the healthcare sector, see
Modern Healthcare, published weekly by Crain Communications Inc., Chicago.

For additional information related to this chapter, access the following chapters on
ache.org/books/HCFinance4:
Chapter 19: Distributions to Owners: Bonuses, Dividends, and Repurchases
Chapter 20: Capitation, Rate Setting, and Risk Sharing

Other references pertaining to this chapter include
Blair, J. D., G. T. Savage, and C. J. Whitehead. 1989. "A Strategic Approach for Negotiating with Hospital Stakeholders." *Health Care Management Review* (Winter): 13–23.
Brock, T. H. 2003. "CMS Investigates Outlier Payments." *Healthcare Financial Management* (February): 70–74.
Clement, J. P., D. G. Smith, and J. R. C. Wheeler. 1994. "What Do We Want and What Do We Get from Not-for-Profit Hospitals?" *Hospital & Health Services Administration* (Summer): 159–178.
Coddington, D. C., D. J. Keene, K. D. Moore, and R. L. Clarke. 1991. "Factors Driving Costs Must Figure into Reform." *Healthcare Financial Management* (July): 44–62.
Corrigan, K., and R. H. Ryan. 2004. "New Reimbursement Models Reward Clinical Excellence." *Healthcare Financial Management* (November): 88–92.
Fallon, R. P. 1991. "Not-For-Profit ≠ No Profit: Profitability Planning in Not-For-Profit Organizations." *Health Care Management Review* (Summer): 47–59.
Fottler, M. D., J. D. Blair, C. J. Whitehead, M. D. Laus, and G. T. Savage. 1989. "Assessing Key Stakeholders: Who Matters to Hospitals and Why?" *Hospital & Health Services Administration* (Winter): 525–546.
Healthcare Financial Management. The July 1997 issue has several articles related to the tax sanctions imposed on not-for-profit corporations when excess benefits accrue to individuals.
Herzlinger, R. E., and W. S. Krasker. 1987. "Who Profits From Nonprofits?" *Harvard Business Review* (January–February): 93–105.
Hill, J. F. 1986. "Third Party Payment Strategies." *Topics in Health Care Financing* (Winter): 1–88.

Keough, C. L. 2003. "Hospitals Await Final Outlier Rule." *Healthcare Financial Management* (June): 30–34.

Lamm, R. D. 1990. "High-Tech Health Care and Society's Ability to Pay." *Healthcare Financial Management* (September): 20–30.

McLean, R. A. 1989. "Agency Costs and Complex Contracts in Health Care Organizations." *Health Care Management Review* (Winter): 65–71.

Nauert, R. C., A. B. Sanborn, II, C. F. MacKelvie, and J. L. Harvitt 1988. "Hospitals Face Loss of Federal Tax-Exempt Status." *Healthcare Financial Management* (September): 48–60.

Pink, G. H., and P. Leatt. 1991. "Are Managers Compensated for Hospital Financial Performance?" *Health Care Management Review* (Summer): 37–45.

Quinn, K. 2004. "Dividing a Trillion-Dollar Pie." *Healthcare Financial Management* (April): 60–68.

Umbdenstock, R. J., W. M. Hageman, and B. Amundson. 1990. "The Five Critical Areas for Effective Governance of Not-for-Profit Hospitals." *Hospital & Health Services Administration* (Winter): 481–492.

Unland, J. J., and J. J. Baker. 2002. "Prospective Payment." *Journal of Healthcare Finance* (Spring): 1–119.

Walker, C. L., and L. W. Humphreys. 1993. "Hospital Control and Decision Making: A Financial Perspective." *Healthcare Financial Management* (June): 90–96.

Wolfson, J., and S. L. Hopes. 1994. "What Makes Tax-Exempt Hospitals Special?" *Healthcare Financial Management* (July): 57–60.

Financial Accounting

Part I discussed the unique background that creates the framework for the practice of healthcare finance. Now, in Part II, we begin the actual coverage of healthcare finance with financial accounting, which involves the preparation of a business's financial statements. The three most important statements are the income statement, balance sheet, and statement of cash flows.

Chapter 3 provides some introductory information about financial accounting and then moves on to discuss, in some detail, the income statement. Chapter 4 covers the balance sheet and statement of cash flows. In total, these chapters should provide you with a sound understanding of the format and content of a business's financial statements. Note that Chapter 17 (Financial Condition Analysis) illustrates various techniques that are applied to financial statement data to gain better insights into a business's financial condition.

FINANCIAL ACCOUNTING BASICS AND THE INCOME STATEMENT

Learning Objectives

After studying this chapter, readers will be able to:

- Explain why financial statements are so important both to managers and to outside parties.
- Describe the standard setting process, under which financial accounting information is created and reported, as well as the underlying principles applied.
- Describe the components of the income statement—revenues, expenses, and net income—and the relationships within and between these components.
- Explain the difference between net income and cash flow.

Introduction

Financial accounting involves identifying, measuring, recording, and communicating in dollar terms the economic events and status of an organization. This information is summarized and presented in *financial statements*—the three most important being the income statement, the balance sheet, and the statement of cash flows. Because these statements communicate financial information about an organization, financial accounting is often called "the language of business." Managers of health services organizations must understand the basics of financial accounting because financial statements are the best way to summarize a business's financial status and performance.

Our coverage of financial accounting extends over several chapters. This chapter begins with an introduction to basic financial accounting concepts and then explains how organizations report financial performance, specifically revenues, costs, and profits. In Chapter 4, the discussion is extended to the reporting of financial status, which includes assets, liabilities, and equity. In addition, Chapter 4 covers the reporting of cash flows. Finally, Chapter 17 again discusses financial statements, but here the focus is on how interested parties use financial statements to assess the financial condition of an organization. That chapter has purposely been placed at the end of the book because the nuances of financial statement analysis can be better understood after learning more about the financial workings of a business. These three chapters will provide you with a basic understanding of how financial statements are created and used to make judgments regarding the financial condition of a health services organization.

Historical Foundations of Financial Accounting

It is all too easy to think of financial statements merely as pieces of paper with numbers written on them, rather than in terms of the economic events and *physical assets*—such as land, buildings, and equipment—that underlie the numbers. However, if readers of financial statements understand how and why financial accounting began and how financial statements are used, they can better visualize what is happening within a business and why financial accounting information is so important.

Thousands of years ago, individuals or families were self-contained in the sense that they gathered their own food, made their own clothes, and built their own shelters. When specialization began, some individuals or families became good at hunting, others at making arrowheads, others at making clothing, and so on. With specialization came trade, initially by bartering one type of goods for another. At first, each producer worked alone, and trade was strictly local. Over time, some people set up production shops that employed workers, simple forms of money were used, and trade expanded beyond the local area. As these simple economies expanded, more formal forms of money developed and a primitive form of banking began, with wealthy merchants lending profits from past dealings to enterprising shop owners and traders who needed money to expand their operations.

When the first loans were made, lenders could physically inspect borrowers' assets and judge the likelihood of repayment. Eventually, though, lending became much more complex. Industrial borrowers were developing large factories, merchants were acquiring fleets of ships and wagons, and loans were being made to finance business activities at distant locations. At that point, lenders could no longer easily inspect the assets that backed their loans, and they needed a practical way of summarizing the value of those assets. Also, certain loans were made on the basis of a share of the profits of the business, so a uniform, widely accepted method for expressing income was required. In addition, owners required reports to see how effectively their own enterprises were being operated, and governments needed information for use in assessing taxes. For all these reasons, a need arose for financial statements, for accountants to prepare the statements, and for auditors to verify the accuracy of the accountants' work.

The economic systems of industrialized countries have grown enormously since the beginning, and financial accounting has become much more complex. However, the original reasons for accounting statements still apply: Bankers and other investors need accounting information to make intelligent investment decisions; managers need it to operate their organizations efficiently; and taxing authorities need it to assess taxes in an equitable manner.

It should be no surprise that problems can arise when translating physical assets and economic events into accounting numbers. Nevertheless, that is what accountants must do when they construct financial statements. To illustrate the translation problem, the numbers shown on the balance sheet to reflect a business's assets and liabilities generally reflect historical costs and prices. However, inventories may be spoiled, obsolete, or even missing; land, buildings, and equipment may have current values that are much higher or lower than their historical costs; and money owed to the business may be uncollectible. Also, some liabilities, such as obligations to make lease payments, may not even show up in the numbers. Similarly, costs reported on an income statement may be understated or overstated, and some costs, such as depreciation, do not even represent current cash expenses. When examining a set of financial statements, it is best to keep in mind the physical reality that underlies the numbers and also to recognize that many problems occur in the translation process.

1. What are the historical foundations of financial accounting statements?
2. Do any problems arise when translating physical assets and economic events into monetary units? Give one or two illustrations to support your answer.

Self-Test Questions

The Users of Financial Accounting Information

The predominant users of financial accounting information are those parties who have a *financial interest* in the organization and hence are concerned with its economic status. All organizations, whether not-for-profit or investor owned, have *stakeholders* who have an interest in the business. In a not-for-profit organization, such as a community hospital, the stakeholders include managers, staff physicians, employees, suppliers, creditors, patients, and even the community at large. Investor-owned organizations have essentially the same set of stakeholders, plus owners. Because all stakeholders, by definition, have an interest in the organization, all stakeholders have an interest in its financial condition.

Of all the outside stakeholders, *investors*, who supply the *capital* (funds) needed by businesses, typically have the greatest **financial** interest in health services organizations. Investors fall into two categories: (1) owners (often *stockholders*) who supply equity capital to investor-owned businesses, and (2) *creditors* (or *lenders*) who supply debt capital to both investor-owned and not-for-profit businesses. In general, there is only one category of owners. However, creditors constitute a diverse group of investors that includes banks, suppliers granting trade credit, and bondholders. Because of their direct financial interest in healthcare businesses, investors are the primary outside users of financial accounting information. They use the information to make judgments about whether to make a particular investment as well as to set the return required on the investment. (Investor-supplied capital is covered in greater detail in Chapters 11, 12, and 13.)

Although financial accounting developed primarily to meet the information needs of outside parties, the managers of an organization, including its board of directors (trustees), also are important users of the information. After all, managers are charged with ensuring that the organization has the financial strength to accomplish its mission, whether that mission is to maximize the wealth of its owners or to provide healthcare services to the community at large. Thus, an organization's managers are not only involved with creating financial statements, but they are also important users of the statements, both to assess the current financial condition of the organization and to formulate plans to ensure that the future financial condition of the organization will support its goals.

In summary, investors and managers are the predominant users of financial accounting information as a result of their direct financial interest in the organization. Furthermore, investors are not merely passive users of financial accounting information; they do more than just read and interpret the statements. Often, they create financial targets based on the numbers reported in financial statements that managers must attain or suffer some undesirable consequence. For example, many debt agreements require borrowers to maintain stated financial standards, such as a minimum earnings level, to keep the debt in force. If the standards are not met, the lender can demand that the business immediately repay the full amount of the loan. If the business fails to do so, it may be forced into bankruptcy.

| **Self-Test Questions** | 1. Who are the primary users of financial accounting information? |
| | 2. Are investors passive users of this information? |

Regulation and Standards in Financial Accounting

As a consequence of the Great Depression of the 1930s, which caused many businesses to fail and almost brought down the entire securities industry, the federal government began regulating the form and disclosure of information related to publicly traded securities. The regulation is based on the theory that financial information constructed and presented according to standardized rules allows investors to make the best-informed decisions. The newly formed *Securities and Exchange Commission (SEC)*, an independent regulatory agency of the U.S. government, was given the authority to establish and enforce the form and content of financial statements. Nonconforming companies are prohibited from selling securities to the public, so many businesses comply to gain access to large amounts of capital. In addition, not-for-profit corporations must file financial statements with state authorities that conform to SEC standards. Finally, most for-profit businesses that do not sell securities to the public are willing to follow the SEC-established guidelines to ensure uniformity of presentation of financial data. The end result is that all businesses, except for the very smallest, create SEC-conforming financial statements.

Rather than directly manage the process, the SEC designates other organizations to create and implement the standard system. For the most part, the SEC has delegated the responsibility for establishing standards to the *Financial Accounting Standards Board (FASB)*—a private organization whose mission is to establish and improve standards of financial accounting and reporting for private businesses. Typically, the guidance issued by the FASB, which is promulgated by numbered *statements*, applies across a wide range of industries and, by design, is somewhat general in nature.[1] More specific implementation guidance, especially when industry-unique circumstances must be addressed, is provided by *Industry Committees* established by the *American Institute of Certified Public Accountants (AICPA)*—the professional association of public (financial) accountants. For example, financial statements in the health services industry are based on the AICPA Audit and Accounting Guide titled *Health Care Organizations*, which was published most recently on May 1, 2006.

When even more specific guidance is required, other professional organizations may participate in the standard-setting process, although such work does not have the same degree of influence as the FASB or the AICPA. For example, the Healthcare Financial Management Association (HFMA) has established a *Principles and Practices Board*, which develops position statements on issues that require further guidance—for example, its November 7, 2006 statement regarding the valuation and financial statement presentation of charity care and bad-debt losses.

When taken together, all the guidance issued by FASB and the other organizations constitute a set of guidelines called *generally accepted accounting principles (GAAP)*. GAAP can be thought of as a set of objectives, conventions, and principles that have evolved through the years to guide the preparation and presentation of financial statements. In essence, GAAP set the rules for the financial statement preparation game. Note, however, that GAAP apply only to the area of financial accounting, as distinct from other areas of accounting, such as managerial accounting (discussed in later chapters) and tax accounting.

For large organizations, the final link in the financial statement quality assurance process is the *external audit*, which is performed by an independent (outside) *auditor*—usually one of the major accounting firms. The results of the external audit are reported in the *auditor's opinion*, which is a letter attached to the financial statements stating whether or not the statements are a fair presentation of the business's operations, cash flows, and financial position as specified by GAAP.

There are several categories of opinions given by auditors. The most favorable, which is essentially a "clean bill of health," is called an *unqualified opinion*. Such an opinion means that, in the auditor's opinion, the financial statements conform to GAAP, are presented fairly and consistently, and contain all necessary disclosures. A *qualified opinion* means that the auditor has some reservations about the statements, while an *adverse opinion* means that the auditor believes that the statements do not present a fair picture of the financial status of the business. The entire audit process, which is performed both by the organization's internal auditors and the external auditor, is a means of verifying and validating the organization's financial statements.[2] Of course, an unqualified opinion gives users, especially those external to the organization, more confidence that the statements truly represent the business's current financial condition.

Although one would think that the guidance given under GAAP, along with auditing rules, would be sufficient to prevent fraudulent financial statements, in the early 2000s several large companies, including HEALTH-SOUTH, were found to be "cooking the books." Because our financial system is so dependent on the reliability of financial statements, on July 30, 2002, President Bush signed the Sarbanes-Oxley Act, which mandated many changes to the financial statement management and auditing process. Here are some of the more important provisions of the Act:

- An independent Public Accounting Oversight Board was created to oversee the entire audit process.
- Auditors can no longer provide nonaudit (consulting) services to the companies that they audit.
- The lead partners of the audit team for any company must rotate off the team every five years (or more often).
- Senior managers involved in the audits of their companies cannot have been employed by the auditing firm during the one-year period preceding the audit.
- Each member of the audit committee shall be a member of the company's board of directors and shall otherwise be independent of the audit function.
- The chief executive officer (CEO) and chief financial officer (CFO) shall personally certify the "appropriateness and fairness" of the business's financial statements.

It is hoped that these provisions, along with others in the Act, will deter future fraudulent behavior by managers and auditors. So far, so good.

It should be of no surprise that the field of financial accounting is typically classified as a social science rather than a physical science. Financial accounting is as much an art as a science, and the end result represents negotiation, compromise, and interpretation. The organizations involved in setting standards are continuously reviewing and revising the GAAP to ensure the best possible development and presentation of financial data. This task, which is essential to economic prosperity, is motivated by the fact that the U.S. economy is constantly evolving, with new types of business arrangements and securities being created almost daily.[3]

Self-Test Questions

1. Why are widely accepted principles important for the measurement and recording of economic events?
2. What entities are involved in regulating the development and presentation of financial statements?
3. What do GAAP stand for, and what is their primary purpose?
4. What is the purpose of the auditor's opinion?

Basic Concepts of Financial Accounting

Because the actual preparation of financial statements is done by accountants, a detailed presentation of accounting theory is not required in this book. However, to better understand the content of financial statements, it is useful to discuss some of the basic concepts that accountants apply when they develop financial accounting data and prepare an organization's financial statements.[4]

Accounting Entity

The first step in the preparation of financial statements is to define the *accounting entity*. This step is important for two reasons. First, for investor-owned businesses, financial accounting data must be pertinent to the business activity as opposed to the personal affairs of the owners. Second, within any business, the accounting entity defines the specific areas of the business to be included in the statements. For example, a healthcare system may create one set of financial statements for the system as a whole as well as separate statements for its subsidiary hospitals. In effect, the accounting-entity specification establishes boundaries that tell accountants what data must be included as well as inform readers what business (or businesses) is being reported.

Going Concern

It is assumed that the accounting entity will operate as a *going concern* and will have an indefinite life. This means that most assets should be valued on the basis of their value to the ongoing business as opposed to their current market (liquidation) value. For example, the land, buildings, and equipment of a hospital may have a value of $50 million when used to provide patient services, but if they are sold to an outside party for other purposes, the value of these assets might only be $20 million. Furthermore, short-term events should not be allowed to unduly influence the data presented in financial statements. The going concern assumption, coupled with the fact that financial statements must be prepared for relatively short periods (as explained next), means that financial accounting data are not exact but represent logical and systematic approaches applied to complex measurement problems.

Accounting Period

Because it is assumed that accounting entities have an indefinite life, but users of financial statements require the information that they convey on a frequent basis, it is common to report financial results on a regular basis. The period covered by such statements, which is called an *accounting period*, can be any length of time over which an organization's managers, or outside parties, want to evaluate operational results. Most health services organizations use calendar periods—months, quarters, and years—as their accounting periods. However, occasionally an organization will use a *fiscal year* (financial year) that does not coincide with the calendar year. For example, Access Health, a provider of management services for health maintenance organizations, has a fiscal year that runs from October 1 to September 30. In this book, an annual accounting period is used in the illustrations. However, financial statement information typically is also prepared for periods shorter than one year.[5]

Objectivity and Reliability

The conversion of economic events to financial accounting data is not an easy task. One of the cornerstones of measurement is *objectivity*; that is, the information reported in financial statements must, to the extent possible, be based on objective, verifiable supporting data. Thus, rather than pull data "out of the air," financial statement preparers should base their data on supporting documentation such as invoices and contracts.

In addition, financial accounting information should be *reliable*, which means that users can depend on it to be reasonably free of error and bias and hence can assume that the information fairly represents the economic events being portrayed. In general, reliability is ensured when independent measurers (auditors), following identical guidelines, reach the same conclusions regarding the values in the financial statements as do the in-house preparers.

Monetary Unit

The *monetary unit* provides the common basis by which economic events are measured. In the United States, this unit is the dollar. Thus, all transactions and events must be expressed in dollar terms. Although this concept is simple enough, a major problem arises in implementation. In essence, the assumption is made that the monetary unit has constant purchasing power over time. In other words, financial statements ignore inflation. Thus, a dollar of revenue today is treated the same as a dollar of revenue earned ten years ago, although today's dollar is worth less (has less purchasing power) than the dollar received years ago. Similarly, a clinic today that could be built for $10 million might have been built for $5 million ten years ago. The accounting profession has grappled with the inflation impact problem for years but has not yet developed a feasible solution.

Relevance

Financial statements must be *relevant* to their users, which means that the information must make a difference in decisions that are being made. Thus, financial statements must include sufficient information upon which to base decisions but not so much information that decision making becomes bogged down by nonessential detail. In general, information that is not relevant makes decision making harder rather than easier. However, the concept of relevance is complicated by the fact that different information often is relevant to different users and when different decisions are being made by the same user. Thus, financial accountants would rather err on the side of providing too much information rather than too little.

Full Disclosure

Financial statements must contain a complete picture of the economic events of the business. Anything less would be misleading by omission. Furthermore, because financial statements must be relevant to a diversity of users, full disclosure, like relevance, pushes financial accountants to include more, rather than less, information in financial statements.

Materiality

If the financial statements contained all possible information, they would be so long and detailed that making inferences about the organization's economic status would be very difficult without a great deal of analysis. Thus, to keep the statements manageable, only entries that are *material* to the financial condition of an organization need to be separately categorized.

In general, the materiality principle affects the presentation of the financial statements rather than their aggregate financial content (i.e., the final numbers). For example, medical equipment manufacturers carry large inventories of materials that are both substantial in dollar value relative to other assets and instrumental to their core business, so such businesses report inventories as a separate asset item on the balance sheet. Hospitals, on the other hand, carry a relatively small amount of inventories. Thus, many hospitals, and other healthcare providers, do not report inventories separately but combine them with other assets. Clearly, leeway exists for interpretation as to what is and is not material, so some differences are likely to occur.

Conservatism

Although financial accountants try their best to paint a fair picture of a business's financial status, if uncertainty in the data or GAAP permit alternative interpretations, the *conservatism* concept says to choose the approach that is least likely to overstate the business's financial condition. This does not mean that financial statements should deliberately understate a business's position, but that, when in doubt, it is best to choose the path that will least likely overstate the position.

Consistency and Comparability

Consistency involves the application of like guidelines to a single accounting entity over time. When a business's financial statements are compared over extended periods—say, annual statements for the past ten years—users must feel confident that they are comparing "apples to apples" and not "apples to oranges." Consistency does not mean that a business, when there is a choice, must stick with the convention chosen forever. However, any change that would create inconsistent data must be disclosed, along with the impact of that change.

Comparability is similar to consistency, except that the concept applies across businesses and to different accounting periods. When users look at quarterly and annual financial statements of the same business, they must feel confident that the data are comparable. Furthermore, when the statements of one business are compared with the statements of another, but similar business—say, two hospitals—the data must be comparable.

Self-Test Question

1. Briefly explain the following basic concepts as they apply to the preparation of financial statements:
   • Accounting entity
   • Going concern
   • Accounting period
   • Objectivity and reliability
   • Monetary unit
   • Relevance
   • Full disclosure
   • Materiality
   • Conservatism
   • Consistency and comparability

Accounting Methods: Cash Versus Accrual

In the implementation of the accounting concepts discussed in the previous section, two different methods have been applied: cash accounting and accrual accounting. Although, as we discuss below, each method has its own set of advantages and disadvantages, GAAP specify that only the accrual method can receive an unqualified auditor's opinion, so accrual accounting dominates the preparation of financial statements. Still, many small businesses that do not require audited financial statements use the cash method, and knowledge of the cash method helps our understanding of the accrual method, so we will discuss both methods here.

Cash Accounting

Under *cash accounting*, often called *cash basis accounting*, economic events are recognized when the financial transaction occurs. For example, suppose Sunnyvale Clinic, a large multispecialty group practice, provided services to a patient in December 2007. At that time, the clinic billed the insurer, Blue Cross/Blue Shield of Florida, the full amount that the insurer is obligated to pay—$700. However, Sunnyvale did not receive payment from the insurer until February 2008. If it used cash accounting, the $700 obligation on the part of the insurer would not appear in Sunnyvale's 2007 financial statements. Rather, the revenue would not be recognized until the cash was actually received in February 2008. The core argument in favor of cash accounting is that the most important event to record is the receipt of cash, not the provision of the service (i.e., the obligation to pay). Similarly, Sunnyvale's expenditures would be recognized as the cash is physically paid out: inventory costs would be recognized as supplies are purchased, labor costs would be recognized when employees are paid, new equipment purchases would be recognized when the invoices are paid, and so on. To put it simply, cash accounting records the actual flow of money into and out of a business.

There are two advantages to cash accounting. First, it is simple and easy to understand. No complex accounting rules are required for the preparation of financial statements. Second, cash accounting is closely aligned to accounting for tax purposes, and hence it is very easy to translate cash accounting statements into income tax filing data. Because of these advantages, about 80 percent of all medical practices, typically the smaller ones, use cash accounting. However, cash accounting has its disadvantages, primarily the fact that in its pure form it does not present information on revenues owed to a business by payers or the business's existing payment obligations.

Before closing our discussion of cash accounting, we should note that most businesses that use cash accounting do not use the "pure" method described earlier but use a modified method. The modified statements combine some features of cash accounting, usually to report revenues and expenses, with some features of accrual accounting, usually to report assets and liabilities. Still, the cash method presents an incomplete picture of the financial status of a business and hence the preference by GAAP for accrual accounting.

Accrual Accounting

Under *accrual accounting*, often called *accrual basis accounting*, the economic event that creates the financial transaction, rather than the transaction itself, provides the basis for the accounting entry. When applied to revenues, the accrual concept implies that revenue earned does not necessarily correspond to the receipt of cash. Why? Earned revenue is recognized in financial statements when a service has been provided **that creates a payment obligation** on the part of the purchaser, rather than when the payment is actually received. For healthcare providers, the payment obligation typically falls on the patient, a third-party payer, or both. If the obligation is satisfied immediately, such as when a patient makes full payment at the time the service is rendered, the revenue is in the form of cash. Thus, the revenue is recorded for financial accounting purposes whether cash or accrual accounting is used.

However, in most cases, the bulk of the payment for services is not received until later, perhaps several months after the service is provided. In this situation, the revenue created by the service does not create an immediate cash payment. If the payment is received within an accounting period—one year, for our purposes—the conversion of revenues to cash will be completed, and as far as the financial statements are concerned, the reported revenue is cash. However, when the revenue is recorded (i.e., services are provided) in one accounting period and payment does not occur until the next period, the revenue reported has not yet been collected, and hence no cash has been received.

Consider the Sunnyvale Clinic example discussed earlier. Although the services were provided in December 2007, the clinic did not receive its $700 payment until February 2008. Because Sunnyvale's accounting year ended on December 31, and the clinic actually uses accrual accounting, the clinic's books were closed after the revenue had been recorded but before the cash was received. Thus, Sunnyvale reported this $700 of revenue on its 2007 financial statements, even though no cash was collected. When accrual accounting is used, the amount of revenues not collected is listed in the financial statements, so users will know that not all revenues represent cash receipts.

The accrual accounting concept also applies to expenses. To illustrate, assume that Sunnyvale had payroll obligations of $50,000 for employees' work during the last week of 2007 that would not be paid until the first payday in 2008. Because the employees actually performed the work, the obligation to pay the salaries was created in 2007. However, because the payment will not be made until the next accounting period, an expense will be recorded even though no cash payment was made. (Under the cash basis of accounting, Sunnyvale would not recognize the expense until it was paid, in this case in 2008.) Under accrual accounting, the $50,000 will be shown as an expense on the financial statements in 2007, and, at the same time, the statements will indicate that a $50,000 liability, or obligation to pay employees, exists.

There are two principles that are key components of accrual accounting: revenue recognition and matching.

The Revenue Recognition Principle   The *revenue recognition principle* requires that revenues be recognized in the period when they are realizable and earned. Generally, this is the period in which the service is rendered, because at that point the price is known (realizable) and the service has been provided (earned). However, in some instances, difficulties in revenue recognition arise, primarily when there are uncertainties surrounding the price or the completion of the service.

The *matching principle* requires that an organization's expenses be matched, to the extent possible, with the revenues to which they are related. In essence, after the revenues have been allocated to a particular accounting period, all expenses associated with producing those revenues should be matched to the same period.

The Matching Principle

Although the concept is straightforward, implementation of the matching principle creates many problems. One such problem occurs with long-lived assets such as buildings and equipment. Because such assets—for example, a hospital ward—provide revenues for many years, the matching principle dictates that its costs should be spread over those same years. However, there are many alternative ways to do this, and no single method is clearly best. For another example of the matching principle, consider a clinic that is paid under capitation. Its revenues are received up-front, while much of the expense associated with providing services to the covered population occurs later, perhaps much later. To adhere to the matching principle, the clinic must forecast the costs associated with the revenues collected and record them in the same accounting period that the revenues are reported. Obviously, this is no easy task.

1. Briefly explain the differences between cash and accrual accounting.
2. Why do GAAP favor accrual over cash accounting?
3. What is the revenue recognition principle? The matching principle?
4. Explain two problems that can occur when the matching principle is implemented.

Self-Test Questions

Recording and Compiling Accounting Data

The ultimate goal of a business's financial accounting system is to produce financial statements. However, the road from the recording of basic accounting data to the completion of the financial statements is long and arduous, especially for large, complex organizations. The starting point for the identification and recording of financial accounting information is a *transaction*, which is defined as an exchange of goods or services from one individual or enterprise to another. To satisfy the objectivity concept, each transaction must be supported by relevant documentation, which is retained for some required length of time.

Once a transaction is identified, it must be recorded, or *posted*, to an *account*, which is a record of transactions for one uniquely identified activity. For example, under the general heading of cash, separate accounts might be established for till cash, payroll checks, vendor checks, other checks, and the like. A large business can easily have hundreds, or even thousands, of separate *primary accounts*, which are combined to form the *general ledger*, plus *subsidiary accounts* that support the primary accounts. The subsidiary accounts, which pertain to very specific assets or liabilities or to individual patients or vendors, are aggregated to create data for a primary (general ledger) account. For example, individual patient charges, which are carried in subsidiary accounts, are aggregated into one or more general ledger revenue accounts.

To help manage the large number of accounts, businesses have a document called a *chart of accounts*, which assigns a unique numeric code to each account. For example, the till cash account might have the code 1–1000-00 while the payroll checks account might have the code 1–1100-00. The first 1 indicates that the account is an asset account; the second 1 indicates a cash account; and the next digit, 0 or 1, indicates the specific cash account. Further numbers are available should the organization decide to subdivide either the till cash or the payroll checks accounts into subsidiary accounts. Because everyone who deals with the accounts is familiar with the business's chart of accounts, transactions can be easily sorted by account code to ensure that transactions are posted to the correct account.

Within the system of primary and subsidiary accounts, accounts are further classified as follows:

- *Permanent accounts* include items that must be carried from one accounting period to another. Thus, permanent accounts remain active until the items in the account are no longer "on the books" of the business. For example, an account might be created, or *opened*, to contain all transactions related to a five-year bank loan. The account would remain open to record transactions relating to the loan—say, annual interest payments—until the loan was paid off in five years, at which time the account would be closed.
- *Temporary accounts* are for those items that will automatically be closed at the end of each accounting period. For example, a business's revenue and expense accounts typically are closed at the end of the accounting period, and then new accounts are opened, with a zero balance, at the beginning of the next period.
- *Contra accounts* are special accounts that convert the gross value of some other account into a net value. As you will see in the next chapter, there is a contra account associated with depreciation expense.

Each transaction is recorded in an account by a *journal entry*. The system used in making journal entries is called the *double entry system* because each transaction must be entered in at least two different accounts—once as a *debit* and once as a *credit*. (We will not explore debits and credits further, because their definitions depend on the specific account in which the entry is made.) Because accounts have both debit and credit entries, they traditionally have been set up in a "T" format, and hence are called *T accounts*, with debits entered on the left side of the vertical line and credits entered on the right side. To illustrate the double entry system, assume that Sunnyvale Clinic receives $100 in cash from a self-pay patient at the time of the visit. A debit entry would be made in the cash account indicating a $100 receipt, while a credit entry would be made in the equity account indicating that the business's value has increased by the amount of the cash revenue. The double entry system ensures consistency among the financial statements.

Ultimately, after the journal entries are verified, consolidated, and reconciled, they are formatted into the business's financial statements, which include the income statement, the balance sheet, and the statement of cash flows.[6] Often, the primary means for disseminating this information to outsiders is the business's *annual report*. It typically begins with a verbal section that discusses in general terms the organization's operating results over the past year as well as developments that are expected to affect future operations. The verbal section is followed by the business's financial statements.

Because the financial statements cannot possibly contain all relevant information, additional information is provided in *footnotes*. For health services organizations, these notes contain information on such topics as inventory accounting practices, the composition of long-term debt, pension plan status, amount of charity care provided, and the cost of malpractice insurance. Because the footnotes contain a great deal of information essential to a good understanding of the financial statements, a thorough examination always considers the footnotes.

This chapter provides a detailed discussion of the contents and logic behind the income statement. In Chapter 4, the remaining two statements—the balance sheet and the statement of cash flows—are discussed.

Self-Test Questions

1. Briefly explain the following terms used in the recording and compiling of accounting data:
   - Transaction
   - Account
   - Posting
   - Chart of accounts
   - General ledger
   - T account
   - Double entry system
2. What are the three primary financial statements?
3. Why are the footnotes to the financial statements important?

Income Statement Basics

The purpose of our financial accounting discussion is to provide readers with a basic understanding of the preparation, content, and interpretation of a business's financial statements. Unfortunately, the financial statements of large organizations can be long and complex, and there is significant leeway regarding the format used, even within health services organizations. Thus, in our discussion of the statements, we will use simplified illustrations and focus on the key issues. This is the best way to learn the basics; the nuances must be left to other books that focus exclusively on accounting issues.

Perhaps the most frequently asked, and the most important, question about a business is this: Is the business making money? The *income statement* summarizes the operations (i.e., the activities) of an organization with a focus on its revenues, expenses, and profitability. Thus, the income statement is also called the *statement of operations* or the *statement of activities*.

The income statements of Sunnyvale Clinic are presented in Table 3.1. Most financial statements contain two years of data, with the most recent year presented first. The *title section* tells us that these are annual income statements, ending on December 31, for the years 2007 and 2006. Whereas the balance sheet, which is covered in Chapter 4, reports a business's financial position at a single point in time, the income statement contains operational results **over a specified period of time**. Because these income statements are part of Sunnyvale's annual report, the time period is one year. Also, the dollar amounts reported are listed in **thousands** of dollars, so the $169,013 reported as net patient service revenue for 2007 is actually $169,013,000.

The core components of the income statement are straightforward: revenues, expenses, and profitability (i.e., net income). *Revenues*, as discussed previously in the section on cash versus accrual accounting, represent both the cash received to date and the unpaid obligations of payers for services provided during the period. For healthcare providers, the revenues result mostly from the provision of patient services.

To produce revenues, organizations must incur *costs*, or *expenses*, which are classified as *operating* or *capital* (*financial*). Although not separately broken out on the income statement, *operating costs* consist of salaries, supplies, insurance, and other costs directly related to providing services. *Capital costs* are the costs associated with the buildings and equipment used by the organization, such as depreciation, lease, and interest expenses. Expenses decrease the profitability of a business, so expenses are subtracted from revenues to determine an organization's profitability:

$$\text{Revenues} - \text{Expenses} = \text{Net income.}$$

Note that net income may be positive or negative. When revenues exceed expenses, the result is called *net income*. When expenses exceed revenues, a *net loss* (negative net income) results.

	2007	2006
Revenues:		
Net patient service revenue	$ 169,013	$ 140,896
Other revenue	7,079	5,704
Total revenues	$ 176,092	$ 146,600
Expenses:		
Salaries and benefits	$ 126,223	$ 102,334
Supplies	20,568	18,673
Insurance	4,518	3,710
Lease	3,189	2,603
Depreciation	6,405	5,798
Provision for bad debts	2,000	1,800
Interest	5,329	3,476
Total expenses	$ 168,232	$ 138,394
Net income	$ 7,860	$ 8,206

TABLE 3.1
Sunnyvale
Clinic: Income
Statements
Years Ended
December 31,
2007 and 2006
(in thousands)

Net income is an important measure of a business's profitability. (Several other measures of profitability are discussed in later chapters.) The greater the net income, the greater the accounting profitability of the business and, with all else the same, the better its financial position.

The income statement, then, summarizes the ability of an organization to generate profits. Basically, it lists the organization's income (revenues), the costs that must be incurred to produce the income (expenses), and the difference between the two (net income). In the following sections, the major components of the income statement are discussed in detail.

1. What is the primary purpose of the income statement?
2. In regards to time, how do the income statement and balance sheet differ?
3. What are the major components of the income statement?

Self-Test Questions

Revenues

Revenues can be shown on the income statement in several different formats. In fact, there is more latitude in the construction of the income statement than there is in the balance sheet, so the income statements for different types of healthcare providers tend to differ more in presentation than do their balance sheets. (See Problems 3.2 and 3.3, as well Table 17.1, for examples of income statements from other types of providers.)

Sunnyvale reported *net patient service revenue* of $169,013,000 for 2007. The key terms here are *net* and *patient service*. This line contains revenues that stem solely from patient services, as opposed to revenues that stem from other sources, such as charitable contributions or interest earned on securities investments. The term *net* signifies that the amount shown is less than the clinic's gross charges for the services provided. Sunnyvale, like all healthcare providers, has a *charge description master* file, or *charge master*, that contains the charge code and gross price for each service that it provides. However, the charge master price does not always represent the amount the clinic expects to be paid for a particular service. For example, the price for a particular service might be $80, while the contract with a particular payer might specify a reimbursement amount of $50. This agreed-upon payment, which is less than the charge master price, results from a $30 *discount* from charges. For services provided at a discount, the clinic expects to be paid less than the amount shown on the charge master, so the amount to be paid is the listed charge less the negotiated discount. Such discounts are incorporated **before** the revenue is recorded on the net patient service revenue line, so the patient service revenue amounts shown on the income statement are **net of discounts**. In this example, the amount of net patient service revenue reported would be $50.

Furthermore, some services have been provided as *charity care* to indigent patients. (*Indigent patients* are those who presumably are willing to pay for services provided but do not have the ability to do so.) Sunnyvale has no expectation of ever collecting for these services, so, like discounts, charges for charity care services are **not** reflected in the $169,013,000 net patient service revenue reported for 2007. Finally, some revenues that are expected to be collected, and hence reported, will never be realized and ultimately will become *bad debt losses*. To recognize that Sunnyvale does not really expect to collect the entire $169,013,000 net patient service revenue reported, the clinic lists as an expense for 2007 a $2,000,000 provision for bad debts. (This expense item is discussed in more detail in the next section.)

Note the distinction between charity care and bad debt losses. Charity care represents services that are provided to patients that **do not have** the capacity to pay. Bad debt losses result from the failure to collect for services provided to patients or third-party payers that **do have** the capacity to pay.

A description of policies regarding discounts and charity care will often appear in the footnotes to the financial statements. To illustrate, Sunnyvale's financial statements include the following two footnotes:

> **Revenues.** Sunnyvale has entered into agreements with third-party payers, including government programs and managed care plans, under which it is paid for services on the basis of established charges, the cost of providing services, predetermined rates per diagnosis, or discounts from established charges. Revenues are recorded at estimated amounts due from patients and third-party payers for the services provided. Settlements under reimbursement agreements

with third-party payers are estimated and recorded in the period the related services are rendered and are adjusted in future periods, as final settlements are determined. The adjustments to estimated settlements for prior years are not considered material and thus are not shown in the financial statements or footnotes.

Charity care. Sunnyvale has a policy of providing charity care to indigent patients in emergency situations. These services, which are subtracted from gross revenues, amounted to $67,541 in 2007 and $51,344 in 2006.

Even though Sunnyvale ultimately expects to collect all of its reported net patient service revenue not yet received, less realized bad debt losses, the clinic did not actually receive $169,013,000 in cash payments in 2007. Rather, some of the revenue has not yet been collected. As readers will learn in Chapter 4, the yet-to-be-collected portion of the net patient service revenue, $28,509,000, appears on the balance sheet (Table 4.1) as net patient accounts receivable.

In a fee-for-service environment, providers offer healthcare services that are paid for on the basis of utilization (i.e., the volume of services provided); that is, revenues stem from reimbursement made on a per diem, per test, per visit, per procedure, or per ancillary service basis, and so on, so revenues are tied to the amount of services provided. Sunnyvale operates primarily as a fee-for-service provider, so its patient service revenue is reported as shown in Table 3.1.

Revenue associated with capitation contracts is often called *premium revenue* when reported on the income statement. If the provider has almost all capitated revenue, it may replace the patient service revenue category as reported by Sunnyvale with the premium revenue category. Other providers, with significant amounts of both fee-for-service and capitation revenue, may report both patient service revenue and premium revenue on the income statement. The key difference is that patient service revenue is reported when services are provided, but premium revenue is reported at the start of each contract payment period—typically the beginning of each month. Thus, premium revenue implies an obligation on the part of the reporting organization to provide future services, while patient service revenue represents an obligation on the part of payers to pay the reporting organization for services already provided. Also, different types of providers may use different terminology for revenues; for example, some nursing homes report *resident service revenue*.

Most health services organizations have revenue besides that arising from patient services, and Sunnyvale is no exception. In 2007, Sunnyvale reported *other revenue* of $7,079,000. One major source of other revenue is *interest earned* on securities investments. Although not shown directly on the income statement, the footnotes to the financial statements indicated that the clinic earned $3,543,000 in interest income during 2007.

Unrestricted charitable contributions represent the second major component of the other revenue category. Some not-for-profit organizations, especially those with large, well-endowed foundations, rely heavily on charitable contributions, as well as earnings on securities investments, as a revenue source. However, health services managers must recognize that such revenue is not central to the core business, which is providing healthcare services. Over-reliance on other revenues could mask serious operational inefficiencies that, if not corrected, could lead to future financial problems.

Additional sources of other revenues include parking garages; nonpatient food services (cafeteria); office and concession rentals; and sales of pharmaceuticals to employees, staff, and visitors. A unique problem facing not-for-profit providers is that a large amount of revenue associated with tangential activities, which is good financially, may be perceived by others, especially tax authorities, as evidence that the provider has strayed from its charitable purpose. This could lead to either explicit or implicit taxation. An interesting example of this problem involved a not-for-profit hospital in Buffalo, New York, that generated substantial revenue from a yacht cruise business on Lake Erie. The Internal Revenue Service (IRS), which does not take such activities lightly, revoked the hospital's not-for-profit status. In hindsight, the hospital would have been much better off had it created a for-profit subsidiary for the cruise business and paid taxes on these revenues like any other cruise operator. By doing so, it would have protected the tax-exempt status for its patient service revenue.

At this point, it is worthwhile to spend some time on historical perspective. Until 1996, healthcare providers reported *gross patient service revenue* based on the charge master, deductions for contractual allowances and charity care, and net patient service revenue directly on the income statement. This made the income statements of healthcare providers different from businesses in virtually every other industry. For example, airlines have a set of full fares such as $1,500 for a round-trip coach ticket from New York to Chicago. Most travelers in coach do not pay this fare, however. Rather, they pay restricted excursion fares that could be as low as $400, or even less. When an airline prepares its income statement, it does not list revenues at full fares and then subtract an allowance for discount fares. What it shows on the income statement are those revenues that it actually expects to collect. Thus, the "rest of the world" reports only those revenues that businesses truly expect to receive, except for bad debt losses, which are accounted for by other means. Thus, healthcare providers were forced to report revenues the same way as everyone else—net of allowances (discounts).

Under the old guidelines, the charity care given by a healthcare provider was reported as a deduction to gross patient service revenue directly on the income statement; that is, if $500 worth of charity services were provided, the income statement included this $500 in gross patient service revenue, then deducted the $500 as charity care, resulting in $0 net patient service revenue for those services. This accounting treatment allowed providers, particularly those with not-for-profit status, to highlight the amount of charity care provided. However, it also created measurement problems because there is no widely accepted methodology for setting the value of charity care that should be reported as revenue. Is it the charge on the provider's charge master, the charge less some discount, the provider's cost of providing the service, the societal value for the service, or some other amount? Because of the measurement problem, reporting charity care directly on the income statement made it more difficult to compare one provider's income statement to another's. Now, a broad description of the organization's charity care policy, along with the volume and an estimate of the value of such care provided, is contained in the footnotes to the financial statements.

Self-Test Questions

1. What categories of revenue are reported on the income statement?
2. Briefly, what is the difference between gross patient service revenue and net patient service revenue?
3. Describe how the following types of revenue are reported on the income statement:
   - Discounts from charges
   - Charity care
   - Bad debt losses

Expenses

Expenses are the costs of doing business. As shown in Table 3.1, Sunnyvale reports its expenses in categories such as salaries and benefits, medical supplies, insurance, and so on. According to GAAP, expenses may be reported using either a *natural classification*, which classifies expenses by the nature of the expense, as Sunnyvale does, or a *functional classification*, which classifies expenses by purpose, such as inpatient services, outpatient services, and administrative. The number and nature of expense items reported on the income statement, which depends on the nature and complexity of the organization, can vary widely. For example, some businesses, typically smaller ones, may report only two categories of expenses: health services and administrative. Others may report a whole host of categories. Sunnyvale takes a middle-of-the-road approach to the number of expense categories. Most users of financial statements would prefer more, as well as a mixing of classifications, rather than less because more insights can be gleaned if an organization reports revenues and expenses both by service breakdown (e.g., inpatient versus outpatient) and by type (e.g., salaries versus supplies).

Sunnyvale is typical of most healthcare providers in that the dominant portion of its cost structure is related to labor. The clinic reported *salaries and benefits* of $126,223,000 for 2007. The detail of how these costs are broken down by department or contract, or the relationship of these expenses to volume, is not part of the financial accounting information system. However, such information, which is very important to managers, is provided by Sunnyvale's managerial accounting system. Chapters 5 through 8 focus on managerial accounting matters.

The expense item titled *supplies* represents the cost of supplies (primarily medical) used in providing patient services. Sunnyvale does not order and pay for supplies when a particular patient service requires them. Rather, the clinic's managers estimate the usage of individual supply items, order them beforehand, and then maintain a medical supplies inventory. As readers will see in Chapter 4, the amount of supplies on hand is reported on the balance sheet. The income statement expense reported by Sunnyvale represents the cost of the supplies **actually consumed** in providing patient services. Thus, the expense reported for supplies does **not** reflect the actual cash spent by Sunnyvale on supplies purchases. In theory, Sunnyvale could have several years' worth of supplies in its inventories at the beginning of 2007, could have used some of these supplies without replenishing the stocks, and hence might not have actually spent one dime of cash on supplies during that year.

Sunnyvale uses commercial insurance to protect against many risks, including both property risks, such as fire and damaging weather, and liability risks, such as managerial malfeasance and professional (medical) liability. The cost of this protection is reported on the income statement as *insurance* expense. Sunnyvale owns all of its land and buildings but *leases* (rents) much of its diagnostic equipment. The total amount of lease payments, $3,189,000 for 2007, is reported as an expense on the income statement.

The next expense category, *depreciation*, requires closer examination. Businesses require *fixed assets* (i.e., long-term assets such as buildings and equipment) to provide goods and services. Although some of these assets are leased, Sunnyvale owns most of the fixed assets necessary to support its mission. When the fixed assets were initially purchased, Sunnyvale did not report their purchase price as an expense on the income statement, but the fixed assets were listed on the balance sheet as property owned by the clinic. The logic of not reporting the cost of such assets when purchased is that it would be improper to allocate fixed asset acquisition costs to a single accounting period because these assets are used to produce revenues over a much longer time. A more pragmatic reason for not reporting the costs of fixed assets when they are acquired is that such outlays would have a severe impact on reported profitability in years when large amounts are purchased. Furthermore, reported earnings would fluctuate widely from year to year on the basis of the amount of fixed assets acquired.

To match the cost of fixed assets to the revenues produced by such long-lived assets, accountants use the concept of *depreciation expense*, which spreads the cost of a fixed asset over many years. Note that most people use the terms "cost" and "expense" interchangeably. To accountants, however, the terms can have different meanings. Depreciation expense is a good example. Here, the term "cost" is applied to the actual cash outlay for a fixed asset, while the term "expense" is used to describe the allocation of that cost over time.

The calculation of depreciation expense is somewhat arbitrary, so the amount of depreciation expense applied to a fixed asset in any year generally is not closely related to the actual usage of the asset or its loss in market value. To illustrate, Sunnyvale owns a piece of diagnostic equipment that it uses infrequently. In 2006 it was used 23 times, while in 2007 it was used only nine times. Still, the depreciation expense associated with this equipment was the same, $7,725, in both years. Also, the clinic owns another piece of equipment that could be sold today for about the same price that Sunnyvale paid for it four years ago, yet each year the clinic reports a depreciation expense for that equipment, which implies loss of value.

Depreciation expense, like all other financial statement entries, is calculated in accordance with GAAP.[7] The calculation typically uses the *straight-line method*—that is, the depreciation expense is obtained by dividing the historical cost of the asset, less its estimated salvage value, by the number of years of its estimated useful life. (*Salvage value* is the amount, if any, expected to be received when final disposition occurs at the end of an asset's useful life.) The result is the asset's annual depreciation expense, which is the charge that is reflected in each year's income statement over the estimated life of the asset and, as readers will discover in Chapter 4, accumulated over time on the organization's balance sheet. (The term *straight-line* stems from the fact that the depreciation expense is constant in each year, and hence the implied value of the asset declines evenly—like a straight line—over time.)

The next expense category on Sunnyvale's income statement is *provision for bad debts*. As discussed previously, the clinic reports as revenue in each year the charges for services provided minus discounts and charity care. Thus, it either collected, or expects to collect, a total of $169,013,000 for patient services provided in 2007. However, past experience indicates that the clinic will not collect every dollar that it expects to collect, even though the payers are assumed to have the ability to pay. Of the reported $169,013,000 in net patient service revenue, Sunnyvale expects that $2,000,000 will never be collected. Thus, the clinic either has already collected, or expects to collect, $167,013,000 for patient services provided in 2007. With bad debt losses running at about $2,000 / $169,013 = 0.012 = 1.2% of patient service revenue, Sunnyvale is not losing a high percentage to deadbeat payers. Still, $2,000,000 is a great deal of money, and managers should review the clinic's collection policy to ensure that its collection efforts are effective. Finally, accountants must reconcile actual realized bad debt losses (which will not be known for some time) with past estimates.

The final expense line reports *interest expense*. Sunnyvale owes or paid its lenders $5,329,000 in interest expense for debt capital supplied during

2007. Not all of the interest expense reported has been paid because Sunnyvale typically pays interest monthly or semiannually, and hence interest has accrued on some loans that will not be paid until 2008. The amount of interest expense reported by an organization is influenced primarily by its *capital structure*, which reflects the amount of debt that it uses. Also, interest expense is affected by the borrower's creditworthiness, its mix of long-term versus short-term debt, and the general level of interest rates. (These factors are discussed in detail at different points in later chapters.)

In closing our discussion of expenses, note that many income statements contain a catchall category labeled "other." Listed here are general and administrative expenses that individually are too small to list separately, including items such as marketing expenses and external auditor's fees. Although organizations cannot possibly report every expense item separately, it is frustrating for users of financial statement information to come across a large, unexplained expense item. Thus, income statements that include the "other" category often add a footnote that provides additional detail regarding these expenses.

Self-Test Questions	1. What is an expense?
	2. Briefly, what are some of the commonly reported expense categories?
	3. What is the logic behind depreciation expense?
	4. What is the logic behind the provision for bad losses?

Net Income

Although the reporting of revenues and expenses is clearly important, the most important single piece of information on the income statement is profitability, as captured in Table 3.1 by the line titled *net income*. As discussed earlier, net income is merely the difference between total revenues and total expenses. To illustrate, Sunnyvale reported net income of $7,860,000 for 2007: $176,092,000 − $168,232,000 = $7,860,000.

Because of its location on the income statement and its importance, net income is referred to as the *bottom line*. The income statements of not-for-profit organizations often call the profit line *revenues over expenses, excess of revenues over expenses, change in net assets*, or something else. Regardless of the terminology used, not-for-profit organizations are required by GAAP to include a *performance indicator* on their income statements that reports the financial results (profitability) of the organization. Throughout this book, we will refer to this performance indicator as net income because this terminology, which is used on for-profit income statements, has universal recognition.

In spite of the fact that Sunnyvale is a not-for-profit organization, **it still must make a profit**. If the clinic is to offer new services in the future, it must earn a profit today to produce the funds needed for new assets. Because of inflation, the clinic could not even replace its current fixed asset base as needed without the funds generated by profitable operations. Thus, turning a profit is essential for all businesses, including those having not-for-profit status.

What happens to an organization's net income? For the most part, it is reinvested in the organization. Not-for-profit businesses **must** reinvest all earnings in the business. An investor-owned business, on the other hand, may return a portion or all of its net income to owners in the form of *dividend payments*. The amount of profits reinvested in an investor-owned business, therefore, is net income minus the amount paid out as dividends.

The proportion of net income paid out to owners is called the *payout ratio*, while the proportion retained within the business is called the *retention ratio*. Thus, if Sunnyvale **were an investor-owned clinic**, and if it paid $2,000,000 in dividends in 2007, its payout ratio would be $2,000 / $7,860 = 0.254 = 25.4\%$ and its retention ratio would be $(\$7,860 - \$2,000) / \$7,860 = \$5,860 / \$7,860 = 0.746 = 74.6\%$. Note that net income only has two places to go—to owners as dividends or to the business as retained earnings—so Retention ratio = 1 − Payout ratio and Payout ratio = 1 − Retention ratio.

Net income measures profitability **as defined by GAAP**. In establishing GAAP, accountants have created guidelines that attempt to measure the *economic income* of a business, which, in all honesty, is a very difficult task because economic gains and losses often are not tied to easily identifiable events. Furthermore, because of accrual accounting and the matching principle, the fact that Sunnyvale reported net income of $7,860,000 for 2007 does not mean that the clinic, on net, experienced a cash inflow of that amount. This point is discussed in greater detail in the next section.

Before moving on, note that some not-for-profit income statements contain a section below the net income entry that reconciles the reported net income with the net assets (i.e., equity) reported on the balance sheet. In essence, the entire amount of net income of not-for-profit organizations must be reinvested in the business, so the amount of net assets reported on the balance sheet, after various adjustments, must increase over the year by the amount of net income. The important relationships between the income statement and the balance sheet are considered in more depth in Chapter 4.

1. How is net income calculated?
2. Why is net income called the bottom line?
3. What happens to net income?
4. What is the payout ratio? The retention ratio?
5. What are the payout and retention ratios of a not-for-profit organization?

Self-Test Questions

Net Income Versus Cash Flow

As stated previously, the income statement reports profitability as net income, which is determined in accordance with GAAP. Although net income is an important measure of profitability, an organization's financial condition, at least in the short run, depends more on the actual cash that flows into and out of the business than it does on reported net income. Thus, occasionally a business will go bankrupt even though its net income has historically been positive. More commonly, many businesses that have reported negative net incomes (i.e., net losses) have survived with little or no financial damage. How can these things happen?

The problem is that the income statement is like a mixture of apples and oranges. Consider Table 3.1. Sunnyvale reported total revenues of $176,092,000 for 2007. Yet, even if we assume no bad debt losses, this is not the amount of cash that was actually collected during the year, because some of these revenues will not be collected until 2008. Furthermore, some revenues reported for 2006 were actually collected in 2007, but these don't appear on the 2007 income statement. Thus, because of accrual accounting, reported revenue is not the same as cash revenue. The same logic applies to expenses; few of the values reported as expenses on the income statement are the same as the actual cash outflows. To make matters even worse, not one cent of depreciation expense was paid out as cash. Depreciation expense is an accounting reflection of the cost of fixed assets, but Sunnyvale did not actually pay out $6,405,000 in cash to someone called the "collector of depreciation." According to the balance sheet (Table 4.1), Sunnyvale actually paid out $88,549,000 sometime in the past to purchase the clinic's total fixed assets, of which $6,405,000 was recognized in 2007 as a cost of doing business, just as salaries and fringe benefits are a cost of doing business.

Can net income be converted to *cash flow*—the actual amount of cash generated during the year? As a **rough estimate**, cash flow can be thought of as net income plus *noncash expenses*. Thus, the cash flow generated by Sunnyvale in 2007 is not merely the $7,860,000 reported net income, but this amount plus the $6,405,000 shown for depreciation, for a total of $14,265,000. Depreciation expense must be added back to net income to get cash flow because it initially was subtracted from revenues to obtain net income even though there was no associated cash outlay.

Here is another way of looking at cash flow versus accounting income: If Sunnyvale showed no net income for 2007, it would still be generating cash of $6,405,000 because that amount was listed as an expense but not actually paid out in cash. The idea behind the income statement treatment is that Sunnyvale would be able to set aside the depreciation amount, which is above and beyond its operating expenses, this year and in future years. Eventually, the accumulated total of *depreciation cash flow* would be used by

Sunnyvale to replace its fixed assets as they wear out or become obsolete. Thus, the incorporation of depreciation expense into the cost and, ultimately, the price structure of services provided is designed to ensure the ability of an organization to replace its fixed assets as needed, assuming that the assets could be purchased at their historical cost. To be more realistic, businesses must plan to generate net income, in addition to the accumulated depreciation funds, sufficient to replace existing fixed assets in the future at inflated costs or even to expand the asset base. It appears that Sunnyvale does have such capabilities, as reflected in its $7,860,000 net income and $14,265,000 cash flow for 2007.

It is important to understand that the $14,265,000 cash flow calculated here is only an **estimate** of actual cash flow for 2007, because almost every item of revenues and expenses listed on the income statement does not equal its cash flow counterpart. The greater the difference between the reported values and cash values, the less reliable is the rough estimate of cash flow defined here. The value of knowing the precise amount of cash generated or lost has not gone unnoticed by accountants. In Chapter 4, readers will learn about the statement of cash flows, which can be thought of as an income statement that is recast to focus on cash flow.

1. What is the difference between net income and cash flow? 2. How can income statement data be used to estimate cash flow? 3. Why do not-for-profit businesses need to make profits?	**Self-Test Questions**

Income Statements of Investor-Owned Firms

Our income statement discussion focused on a not-for-profit organization: Sunnyvale Clinic. What do the income statements for investor-owned firms such as Health Management Associates and Manor Care look like? The financial statements of investor-owned firms and not-for-profit businesses are generally similar except for transactions, such as tax payments, that are applicable only to one form of ownership. Because the transactions of all health services organizations in the same core business are similar, ownership plays only a minor role in the presentation of financial statement data. In reality, more differences exist in financial statements because of lines of business (e.g., hospitals versus nursing homes versus managed care plans) than differences because of ownership.

1. Are there appreciable differences in the income statements of not-for-profit businesses and investor-owned businesses?	**Self-Test Question**

A Look Ahead: Using Income Statement Data in Financial Statement Analysis

Chapter 17 discusses in some detail the techniques used to analyze financial statements to gain insights into a business's financial condition. At this point, however, it would be worthwhile to introduce *financial ratio analysis*—one of the techniques used in financial condition analysis. In financial ratio analysis, values found on the financial statements are combined to form ratios that have economic meaning and hence that help managers and investors interpret the numbers.

To illustrate, *total profit margin*, usually just called *total margin*, is defined as net income divided by total revenues. For Sunnyvale Clinic, the total margin for 2007 was $7,860,000 / $176,092,000 = 0.045 = 4.5%. Thus, each dollar of revenues generated by the clinic produced 4.5 cents of profit (i.e., net income). By implication, each dollar of revenues required 95.5 cents of expenses. The total margin is a measure of expense control; for a given amount of revenues, the higher the net income, and hence total margin, the lower the expenses. If the total margin for other clinics were known, judgments about how well Sunnyvale is doing in the area of expense control, relative to its peers, could be made.

Sunnyvale's total margin for 2006 was $8,206,000 / $146,600,000 = 0.060 = 6.0%, so the clinic's total margin slipped from 2006 to 2007. This finding should alert managers to examine carefully the increase in expenses in 2007. In effect, Sunnyvale's expenses increased faster than its revenues, which resulted in falling profitability as measured by the total margin. If this trend continues, it would not take long for the clinic to be operating in the red (i.e., losing money).

A complete discussion of financial ratio analysis can be found in Chapter 17. The discussion here, along with a brief visit in Chapter 4, is merely intended to give readers a preview of how financial statement data can be used to make judgments about a business's financial condition.

Self-Test Questions

1. Explain how ratio analysis can be used to help interpret income statement data.
2. What is the total profit margin, and what does it measure?

Key Concepts

Financial accounting information is the result of a process of identifying, measuring, recording, and communicating the economic events and status of an organization to interested parties. This information is summarized and presented in three primary financial statements: the income statement, the balance sheet, and the statement of cash flows. The key concepts of this chapter are:

- The predominant *users of financial accounting information* are parties who have a direct financial interest in the economic status of a business—primarily its managers and investors.
- *Generally accepted accounting principles (GAAP)* establish the standards for financial accounting measurement and reporting. These principles have been sanctioned by the *Securities and Exchange Commission (SEC)*, developed by the *Financial Accounting Standards Board (FASB)*, and refined by the *American Institute of Certified Public Accountants (AICPA)* and other organizations.
- The preparation and presentation of financial accounting data is based on a set of principles, the most important of which are (1) *accounting entity*, (2) *going concern*, (3) *accounting period*, (4) *objectivity*, (5) *reliability*, (6) *monetary unit*, (7) *relevance*, (8) *full disclosure*, (9) *materiality*, (10) *conservatism*, (11) *consistency*, and (12) *comparability*.
- Under *cash accounting*, economic events are recognized when the financial transaction occurs. Under *accrual accounting*, economic events are recognized when the obligation to make payment occurs. GAAP require that businesses use accrual accounting because it provides a better picture of a business's true financial status.
- Two important concepts that underlie accrual accounting are the *revenue recognition* and *matching principles*.
- The collection and recording of financial accounting data uses the following concepts: (1) *transaction*, (2) *posting*, (3) *chart of accounts*, (4) *general ledger*, (5) *double entry*, and (6) *T account*.
- The *income statement* reports on an organization's operations over a period of time. Its basic structure consists of *revenues, expenses,* and *profit* (i.e., *net income*), which equals revenues minus expenses.
- *Revenues* are monies collected or expected to be collected by the business. Revenues are broken down into categories such as *net patient service revenue, premium revenue,* and *other revenue.*
- *Expenses* are the economic costs associated with the provision of services.
- *Net income* represents the economic profitability of a business as defined by GAAP.
- Because the income statement is constructed using accrual accounting, net income does not represent the actual amount of cash that has been earned or lost during the reporting period. To estimate *cash flow*, noncash expenses (primarily depreciation) must be added back to net income.
- The income statements of investor-owned and not-for-profit businesses tend to look very much alike. However, the income statements of health services organizations in different lines of business can vary. The good news is that all income statements have essentially the same economic content.
- *Financial ratio analysis,* which combines values that are found in the financial statements, helps managers and investors interpret the data with

the goal of making judgments about the financial condition of the business.

In this chapter, we focused on financial accounting basics and the income statement. In Chapter 4, the discussion of financial accounting continues with the remaining two statements: the balance sheet and statement of cash flows.

Questions

3.1 a. What is a stakeholder?
   b. What stakeholders are most interested in the financial condition of a healthcare provider?

3.2 a. What are generally accepted accounting principles (GAAP)?
   b. What is the purpose of GAAP?
   c. What organizations are involved in establishing GAAP?

3.3 Briefly describe the following concepts as they apply to the preparation of financial statements:
   a. Accounting entity
   b. Going concern
   c. Accounting period
   d. Objectivity and reliability
   e. Monetary unit
   f. Relevance
   g. Full disclosure
   h. Materiality
   i. Conservatism
   j. Consistency and comparability

3.4 Explain the difference between cash and accrual accounting. Be sure to include a discussion of the revenue recognition and matching principles.

3.5 Briefly describe the format of the income statement.

3.6 a. What is the difference between gross revenues and net revenues? (Hint: Think about discounts and charity care.)
   b. What is the difference between patient service revenue and other revenue?
   c. What is the difference between charity care and bad debt losses? How is each handled on the income statement?

3.7 a. What is meant by the term *expense*?
   b. What is depreciation expense, and what is its purpose?
   c. What are some other categories of expenses?

3.8 a. What is net income?
   b. Why is net income called the bottom line?
   c. What is the difference between net income and cash flow?
   d. Is financial condition more closely related to net income or to cash flow?

Problems

3.1 Entries for the Warren Clinic 2007 income statement are listed below in alphabetical order. Reorder the data in proper format.

Bad debt expense	$ 40,000
Depreciation expense	90,000
General/administrative expenses	70,000
Interest expense	20,000
Interest income	40,000
Net income	30,000
Other revenue	10,000
Patient service revenue	440,000
Purchased clinic services	90,000
Salaries and benefits	150,000
Total revenues	490,000
Total expenses	460,000

3.2 Consider the following income statement:

BestCare HMO
Statement of Operations
Year Ended June 30, 2007
(in thousands)

Revenue:	
Premiums earned	$26,682
Coinsurance	1,689
Interest and other income	242
Total revenues	$28,613
Expenses:	
Salaries and benefits	$15,154
Medical supplies and drugs	7,507
Insurance	3,963
Provision for bad debts	19
Depreciation	367
Interest	385
Total expenses	$27,395
Net income	$ 1,218

a. How does this income statement differ from the one presented in Table 3.1?

b. Did BestCare spend $367,000 on new fixed assets during fiscal year 2007? If not, what is the economic rationale behind its reported depreciation expense?

c. Explain the provision for bad debts entry.

d. What is BestCare's total profit margin? How can it be interpreted?

3.3 Consider this income statement:

Green Valley Nursing Home, Inc.
Statement of Income
Year Ended December 31, 2007

Revenue:	
Net patient service revenue	$3,163,258
Other revenue	106,146
Total revenues	$3,269,404
Expenses:	
Salaries and benefits	$1,515,438
Medical supplies and drugs	966,781
Insurance and other	296,357
Provision for bad debts	110,000
Depreciation	85,000
Interest	206,780
Total expenses	$3,180,356
Operating income	$ 89,048
Provision for income taxes	31,167
Net income	$ 57,881

a. How does this income statement differ from the ones presented in Table 3.1 and Problem 3.2?

b. Why does Green Valley show a provision for income taxes while the other two income statements did not?

c. What is Green Valley's total profit margin? How does this value compare with the values for Sunnyvale Clinic and BestCare?

d. The before-tax profit margin for Green Valley is operating income divided by total revenues. Calculate Green Valley's before-tax profit margin. Why may this be a better measure of expense control when comparing an investor-owned business with a not-for-profit business?

3.4 Great Forks Hospital reported net income for 2007 of $2.4 million on total revenues of $30 million. Depreciation expense totaled $1 million.

a. What were total expenses for 2007?

b. What were total cash expenses for 2007? (Hint: Assume that all expenses, except depreciation, were cash expenses.)

c. What was the hospital's 2007 cash flow?

3.5 Brandywine Homecare, a not-for-profit business, had revenues of $12 million in 2007. Expenses other than depreciation totaled 75 percent of revenues, and depreciation expense was $1.5 million. All revenues were collected in cash during the year and all expenses other than depreciation were paid in cash.

  a. Construct Brandywine's 2007 income statement.
  b. What were Brandywine's net income, total profit margin, and cash flow?
  c. Now, suppose the company changed its depreciation calculation procedures (still within GAAP) such that its depreciation expense doubled. How would this change affect Brandywine's net income, total profit margin, and cash flow?
  d. Suppose the change had halved, rather than doubled, the firm's depreciation expense. Now, what would be the impact on net income, total profit margin, and cash flow?

3.6 Assume that Mainline Homecare, a for-profit corporation, had exactly the same situation as reported in Problem 3.5. However, Mainline must pay taxes at a rate of 40 percent of pretax income. Assuming that the same revenues and expenses reported for financial accounting purposes would be reported for tax purposes, redo Problem 3.5 for Mainline.

Notes

1. The *Government Accounting Standards Board (GASB)* has the identical responsibility for businesses that are partially or totally funded by a government entity. Also, note that the predecessor organization to FASB was called the *Accounting Principles Board (APB)*, which provided guidance in the form of *opinions*.

2. Historically, external auditors were mostly concerned with the letter of the law. Their work was relatively narrow in scope, primarily ensuring that financial statements were prepared and presented in accordance with GAAP. However, this approach seldom identified problems, especially fraud, which affected the organization's financial condition. After several large lawsuits found major accounting firms negligent in failing to identify problem areas, auditors are now paying much more attention to the activities behind the numbers.

3. Each year, the FASB must deal with very difficult and controversial matters. As this edition is being written, the FASB is grappling with how to better report the acquisition of one business by another, including acquisitions by not-for-profit businessses.

4. As the globalization of business continues, it becomes more and more important for accounting standards to be uniform across countries. At this time, FASB and the International Accounting Standards Board (IASB) are working jointly to develop a common conceptual framework for financial statement preparation that is both complete and consistent.

5. Investor-owned health services organizations with publicly traded securities are required by the Securities and Exchange Commission (SEC) to file both annual and quarterly financial statements. Many of these statements, along with annual reports, are available for free at various sites on the Internet. For example, see www.sec.gov (then click on Filings & Forms) and www.annualreports.com.

6. Although there are four basic financial statements, this book covers only the three statements that are most important. The fourth statement, titled the *statement of changes in net assets* or the *statement of changes in equity*, focuses on changes in the equity position from one year to the next. Because this statement is relatively short, not-for-profit organizations have the option to include it at the end of the income statement.

7. In addition to depreciation calculated for financial statement purposes, which is called *book depreciation*, for-profit businesses must calculate depreciation for tax purposes. *Tax depreciation* is calculated in accordance with IRS regulations as opposed to GAAP. Also, note that land is not depreciated for either financial reporting or tax purposes.

References

American Institute of Certified Public Accountants (AICPA). 2003. *Audit and Accounting Guide*. New York: AICPA.

———. 2003. *Checklists and Illustrative Financial Statements for Health Care Organizations*. New York: AICPA.

Bitter, M. E., and J. Cassidy. 1992. "Perceptions of New AICPA Audit Guide." *Healthcare Financial Management* (November): 38–48.

Center for Research in Ambulatory Health Care Administration (CRAHCA). 1996. *Medical Group Practice Chart of Accounts*. Englewood, CO: CRAHCA.

Duis, T. E. 1993. "The Need for Consistency in Healthcare Reporting." *Healthcare Financial Management* (July): 40–44.

———. 1994. "Unravelling the Confusion Caused by GASB, FASB Accounting Rules." *Healthcare Financial Management* (November): 66–69.

Healthcare Financial Management Association (HFMA). 2007. "P&P Board Statement 15: Valuation and Financial Statement Presentation of Charity Care and Bad Debts by Institutional Healthcare Providers." *Healthcare Financial Management* (January): 94–103.

Maco, P. S., and S. J. Weinstein. 2000. "Accounting and Accountability: Observations on the AHERF Settlements." *Healthcare Financial Management* (October): 41–46.

Peregrine, M. W., and J. R. Schwartz. 2002. "What CFOs Should Know—And Do—About Corporate Responsibility." *Healthcare Financial Management* (December): 60–63.

Robbins, W. A., and R. Turpin. 1993. "Accounting Practice Diversity in the Healthcare Industry." *Healthcare Financial Management* (May): 111–114.

Seawell, L. V. 1999. *Chart of Accounts for Hospitals*. Chicago: Probus Publishing.

Valetta, R. M. 2005. "Clear as Glass: Transparent Financial Reporting." *Healthcare Financial Management* (August): 59–66.

THE BALANCE SHEET AND STATEMENT OF CASH FLOWS

Learning Objectives

After studying this chapter, readers will be able to:

- Explain the purpose of the balance sheet.
- Describe the contents of the balance sheet and its interrelationship with the income statement.
- Explain the purpose of the statement of cash flows.
- Describe the contents of the statement of cash flows and how it differs from the income statement.
- Describe how a business's transactions affect its income statement and balance sheet.

Introduction

Although the income statement, which was covered in Chapter 3, contains information about an organization's operations, it does not provide information about the resources needed to produce the revenues or how those resources were financed. Another financial statement, the *balance sheet*, contains information about an organization's assets and the financing used to acquire those assets.

In addition to the need to disclose resources and financing, accountants and managers have, over time, become increasingly aware that net income is not the only determinant of financial condition. Although net income, which reflects an organization's long-run economic profitability as defined by GAAP, is an important profitability measure, financial condition, especially in the short run, is also related to the actual flow of cash into and out of a business. The second financial statement discussed in this chapter, the *statement of cash flows*, focuses on this important determinant of financial condition.

Although understanding the composition of the financial statements is essential, it is also very important that managers understand the relationships among the financial statements. Thus, emphasis is placed on the interrelationships among the statements throughout the chapter. Finally, the end of the chapter contains a brief introduction to how actual business transactions work their way into an organization's financial statements. Our purpose here is to provide readers with a feel for how financial statements are actually created.

Balance Sheet Basics

Whereas the income statement reports the results of operations **over a period of time**, the *balance sheet* presents a snapshot of the financial position of an organization **at a given point in time**. For this reason, the balance sheet is also called the *statement of financial position*. The balance sheet changes every day as a business increases or decreases its assets or changes the composition of its financing. The important point is that the balance sheet, unlike the income statement, reflects a business's financial position as of a given date, and the data in it typically become invalid one day later, even when both dates are in the same accounting period. Healthcare providers with seasonal demand, such as a walk-in clinic in Fort Lauderdale, Florida, have especially large changes in their balance sheets during the year. For such businesses, a balance sheet constructed in February can look quite different from one prepared in August. Also, businesses that are growing very rapidly will have significant changes in their balance sheets over relatively short periods of time.

The balance sheet lists, as of the end of the reporting period, the resources of an organization and the claims against those resources. In other words, the balance sheet reports the assets of an organization and how those assets were financed. The balance sheet has the following basic structure:

Assets	Liabilities and Equity
Current assets	Current liabilities
Long-term assets	Long-term liabilities
	Equity
Total assets	Total liabilities and equity

The *assets* side (left side) of the balance sheet lists all the resources, or assets, owned by the organization in dollar terms. In general, assets are broken down into categories that distinguish short-lived assets from long-lived assets. The *liabilities and equity* side (claims side or right side) lists the claims against these resources, again in dollar terms. In essence, the right side reports the sources of financing (capital) used to acquire the assets listed on the left side. The sources of capital are divided into two broad categories: liabilities, which are claims fixed by contract, and equity, which is a residual claim that depends on asset values and the amount of liabilities. As with assets, liabilities are listed by maturity (short-term versus long-term).

Perhaps the most important characteristic of the balance sheet is simply that it must balance—that is, the left side must equal the right side. This relationship, which is called the *accounting identity* or *basic accounting equation*, is expressed in equation form as follows:

$$A = L + E,$$

where A = Total assets, L = Total liabilities, and E = Equity. Because creditor claims are paid before equity claims if a healthcare organization is liquidated, liabilities are shown before equity both on the balance sheet and in the basic accounting equation.

Note that the accounting identity can be rearranged as follows:

$$E = A - L.$$

This format reinforces the concept that equity represents a residual claim against the total assets of the business and also the fact that equity can be negative. If a business writes down (decreases) the value of its assets, its liabilities are unaffected because these amounts are still owed to creditors and others. If total assets are written down so much that their value drops below that of total liabilities, then the equity reported on the balance sheet becomes a negative amount.

Table 4.1 contains Sunnyvale's balance sheet, which follows the basic structure explained above. The title of the balance sheet reinforces the fact that the data are presented for the entire clinic. The balance sheet is not going to provide much information, if any, about the subparts of an organization such as departments or service lines. Rather, the balance sheet will provide an overview of the economic position of the organization as a whole. The timing of the balance sheet is also apparent in the title. The data are reported for 2007 and 2006 as of December 31. Whereas Sunnyvale's income statement indicates the data were for the **years ended** on December 31, the balance sheet merely indicates a closing date. This minor difference in terminology reinforces the point that the income statement reports operational results **over a period** of time, while the balance sheet reports financial position at **a single point** in time. Finally, the amounts reported on Sunnyvale's balance sheet, just as on its income statement, are expressed in thousands of dollars.

The format of the balance sheet emphasizes the basic accounting equation. For example, as of December 31, 2007, Sunnyvale had a total of $154,815,000 in assets that were financed by a total of $154,815,000 in liabilities and equity. Besides this obvious confirmation that the balance sheet balances, this statement indicates that the total assets of Sunnyvale were valued, according to GAAP, at $154,815,000. Liabilities and equity represent claims against the assets of the business by various classes of creditors, other claimants with fixed claims, and "owners." Creditors and other claimants have first priority in claims for $100,747,000, and "owners" follow with a residual claim of $54,068,000. The right side of the balance sheet (liabilities and equity, which are in the bottom section of Table 4.1) reflects the manner in which Sunnyvale raised the capital needed to acquire its assets.

TABLE 4.1
Sunnyvale
Clinic: Balance
Sheet
December 31,
2007 and 2006
(in thousands)

ASSETS	2007	2006
Current Assets:		
Cash	$ 12,102	$ 6,486
Short-term investments	10,000	5,000
Net patient accounts receivable	28,509	25,927
Inventories	3,695	2,302
Total current assets	$ 54,306	$ 39,715
Long-term investments	$ 48,059	$ 25,837
Property and Equipment (Fixed Assets):		
Land	$ 2,954	$ 2,035
Buildings and equipment	85,595	77,208
Gross fixed assets	$ 88,549	$ 79,243
Less: Accumulated depreciation	36,099	29,694
Net fixed assets	$ 52,450	$ 49,549
Total assets	$ 154,815	$ 115,101

LIABILITIES AND EQUITY	2007	2006
Current Liabilities:		
Notes payable	4,334	3,345
Accounts payable	5,022	6,933
Accrued expenses:	6,069	5,037
Total current liabilities	$ 15,425	$ 15,315
Long-term debt	$ 85,322	$ 53,578
Total liabilities	$100,747	$ 68,893
Net assets (Equity)	$ 54,068	$ 46,208
Total liabilities and equity	$ 154,815	$ 115,101

Self-Test Questions

1. What is the purpose of the balance sheet?
2. What are the three major sections of the balance sheet?
3. What is the accounting identity, and what information does it provide?

Assets

Assets either possess or create economic benefit for the organization. Table 4.1 contains three major categories of assets: current assets, long-term investments, and property and equipment (fixed assets). The following sections describe each asset category in detail.

Current Assets

Current assets include cash and other assets that are expected to be converted into cash **within one accounting period**, which in this example is one year. For Sunnyvale, current assets total $54,306,000 at the end of 2007. Suppose that the short-term investments on the books at that time were converted into cash as they matured; the receivables were collected; and the inventories were used, billed to patients, and collected; all at the values stated on the balance sheet. With all else the same, Sunnyvale would have $54,306,000 in cash at the end of 2008. Of course, all else will not be the same, so Sunnyvale's 2008 reported cash balance will undoubtedly be different from $54,306,000. Still, this little exercise reinforces the concept behind the current asset category: the **assumption** that these assets will be converted into cash during the next accounting period.

The conversion of current assets into cash is expected to provide all or part of the funds that will be needed to pay off the $15,425,000 in current liabilities outstanding at the end of 2007 as they become due in 2008. Thus, current assets are one factor that makes up the *liquidity* of the organization. A business is *liquid* if it has the cash available to pay its bills as they become due. The difference between total current assets and total current liabilities is called *net working capital*. Thus, at the end of 2007, Sunnyvale had net working capital of $54,306,000 − $15,425,000 = $38,881,000. From a pure liquidity standpoint, the greater an organization's net working capital, the better. However, as will be pointed out in this and subsequent chapters, there are costs to carrying current assets, so health services organizations have to balance the need for liquidity against the associated costs of maintaining liquidity. Also, as we will discuss elsewhere, there are other factors, such as expected cash inflows, that contribute to a business's overall liquidity.

Within Sunnyvale's current assets, there is $12,102,000 in *cash*—an account that represents actual cash in hand plus money held in commercial checking accounts (demand deposits). There is also $10,000,000 of *short-term investments* (sometimes called *marketable securities*), which represent cash that has been temporarily invested in highly liquid, low-risk securities such as bank savings accounts, money market mutual funds, U.S. Treasury bills, or prime commercial paper.[1] Organizations hold short-term investments because cash and money held in commercial checking accounts do not earn interest. Thus, businesses should hold only enough cash and checking account balances to pay their recurring operating expenses—any funds on hand in excess of immediate needs should be invested in safe, short-term, highly liquid (but interest-bearing) securities. Additionally, short-term investments are built up periodically to meet projected nonoperating cash outlays such as tax payments, investments in property and equipment, and legal judgments. Even though short-term investments pay relatively low interest, any return is better than none, so such investments are preferable to cash holdings.

Short-term investments normally are reported on the balance sheet *at cost*, which is the amount initially paid for the securities. However, because of changing interest rates and other factors, these securities may actually be worth more or less than their purchase price. Still, because short-term investments have maturities of less than one year, it is rare for their market values to be substantially different from their costs. Furthermore, the current market values of the securities are listed in the notes to the financial statements.

Net patient accounts receivable represents money owed to Sunnyvale for services that the clinic has already provided. As discussed in Chapter 2, and reiterated in Chapter 3, third-party payers make most payments for health-care services, and these payments often take weeks or months to be billed, processed, and ultimately paid. The patient accounts receivable amount of $28,509,000 at the end of 2007 is listed on the balance sheet *net* of allowances for discounts, charity care, and bad debt losses. Thus, the presentation on the balance sheet is consistent with the Chapter 3 discussion concerning net patient service revenue.

The $28,509,000 net receivable amount seen on the balance sheet is a subset of the income statement's net patient service revenue of $169,013,000 for 2007 (see Table 3.1 in Chapter 3). The logic is as follows. A total of $169,013,000 was billed to patients and payers during 2007. This is a "net" number as there is some higher gross amount of charges in Sunnyvale's man-agerial accounting system that reflects charges before deductions for discounts and charity care. Of this $169,013,000 of patient service revenue, $2,000,000 is shown as a provision for bad debts on the income statement. This bad debt expense represents Sunnyvale's best estimate, based on past experience, of the total dollar amount of net patient service revenue that will never be collected. Thus, Sunnyvale actually expected to receive $169,013,000 − $2,000,000 = $167,013,000 in cash revenues for services provided during 2007.

The fact that $28,509,000 of this net patient service revenue remains to be collected suggests that the difference between $167,013,000 and $28,509,000, which totals $138,504,000, was collected during 2007. Where is this collected cash? It could be anywhere. Most of it went right out the door to pay operating expenses. Some of the collected cash may have been used to purchase assets (e.g., new equipment) and hence may be sitting in one of the asset accounts on the balance sheet. If the clinic were to close its doors on the last day of 2007, its patient accounts receivable balance of $28,509,000 would fall to zero when the entire amount was eventually collected (except for any errors in the bad debt forecast). However, if Sunnyvale continues as an ongo-ing enterprise, the receivables balance really never falls to zero because while Sunnyvale's collections are lowering it, new services are constantly being pro-vided that create new billings, and hence new receivables, that are added to it.

The final current asset on Table 4.1, *inventories*, primarily reflects Sunnyvale's investment in medical supplies. The value of supplies on hand at the end of 2007 was $3,695,000. As with the cash account, it is not in a business's best interest to hold excessive inventories. There is a certain level of supplies necessary to meet medical needs and to maintain a safety stock to guard against unexpected surges in usage, but any inventories above this level create unnecessary costs. Thus, many health services organizations are limiting their investment in inventories through aggressive inventory management. One technique being used is the *just-in-time* system, in which suppliers are expected to manage the inventory and, as the term suggests, deliver the inventory to providers just before it is needed.

Businesses that hold large amounts of inventories, such as medical supply companies, typically include a footnote that discusses the holdings in some detail. However, most healthcare providers hold relatively small levels of inventories, and hence extensive footnote information often is not provided. In fact, because of the materiality principle discussed in Chapter 2, some providers do not break out inventories as a separate item on their balance sheets, but include the value of inventories in a catchall account called *other current assets*.

It should be obvious that the primary purposes served by the current asset accounts are to support the operations of the organization and to provide liquidity. However, current assets do not generate high returns. For example, cash earns no return, and short-term investments generally earn relatively low returns. The receivables account does not earn interest income nor generate new patient service revenue, and inventories represent dollar amounts invested in items sitting on shelves, which earn no return until patients are billed for their use. Because of the low (or zero) return earned on current assets, businesses try to minimize these accounts yet ensure that the levels on hand are sufficient to support operations and maintain liquidity. (Readers will learn much more about current asset management in Chapter 16.)

Notice that the current assets section of the balance sheet is listed in order of liquidity, or nearness to cash. Cash, as the most liquid asset, is listed first, while the least liquid of current assets, inventories, is listed last. Dollars invested in inventories will first move into patient accounts receivable as the patients are billed for the supplies used. Then, accounts receivable will eventually be converted into cash when they are collected and, perhaps, shifted to securities if the cash is not needed to pay current bills.

The importance of converting current assets into short-term investments as quickly as possible, and hence converting zero-return assets into some-return assets, cannot be overemphasized. Under most reimbursement methods, providers must first build the current assets necessary to provide the services, then actually do the work, and finally, some time later (often 60 days or more), get paid. Providers that operate under capitation have a significant liquidity advantage as compared to those that primarily receive fee-for-service revenue. As discussed in Chapter 2, payment for capitated services occurs up-front, before the services are actually provided. Thus, providers that work in a predominantly capitated environment will have much smaller accounts receivable balances and much larger cash and short-term investments balances than do providers, such as Sunnyvale, that operate in a predominantly fee-for-service environment.

Long-Term Investments

The second major asset category (after current assets) is *long-term investments*, which is the money Sunnyvale has invested in various forms of long-term (maturities that exceed one year) securities. This account represents investments in long-term *financial assets*, as opposed to investments in long-term *real assets*, which are listed next on the balance sheet as property and equipment (fixed assets). The $48,059,000 reported at the end of 2007 represents the amount that Sunnyvale has invested in stocks, bonds, and other investments that have a longer maturity than its short-term investments and that it hopes will provide the clinic with a higher return.

Long-term securities investments are reported on the balance sheet at *fair market value*, rather than initial cost, so changes in market conditions over time will cause the value of this account to change, even if the securities held remain the same. Also, changes in market values of long-term investments result in unrealized gains or losses on the investments, which have additional financial statement implications that are beyond the scope of this book. A footnote will usually reveal the details of the types of security investments held by the organization and the resulting gains and losses. The income earned on both short-term and long-term investments is reported on the income statement as other revenue. As discussed in Chapter 3, Sunnyvale reported other revenue of $7,079,000 for 2007. According to the footnotes, this amount included interest income of $3,543,000.

The discussion of current assets emphasized that businesses try to minimize the amounts held, maintaining only the amounts necessary to support operations. One of the benefits of prudent management of *working capital* (current assets) is that more money can be moved into long-term investments, both financial and real, which generate greater returns than those provided by current assets. The ultimate rewards for minimizing an organization's working capital are both the reduction in carrying costs (current assets cost money because each dollar in assets has to be matched by a dollar of financing) and the increased return available on long-term investments.

Sunnyvale is not in the financial services business; it is in the business of providing healthcare services. Still, not-for-profit organizations typically carry large amounts of long-term securities investments, generally funded from depreciation cash flow and hence often called *funded depreciation*. Eventually, the funds invested in long-term securities investments will be used to purchase real assets that provide new or improved services to Sunnyvale's patients. In contrast, investor-owned businesses usually do not build up such reserves. Any cash flow above the amount needed for near-term reinvestment in the business would likely be returned to the capital suppliers, either by debt repurchases or, more typically, by dividends or stock repurchases. When additional capital is needed for long-term asset investment, an investor-owned business simply accesses the capital markets for additional financing.

Property and Equipment (Fixed Assets)

The third major asset category is *property and equipment,* often called *fixed assets.* Fixed assets, as compared to current assets, and even compared to long-term securities investments, are highly illiquid and are used over long periods of time by the organization. Whereas current assets rise and fall spontaneously with the organization's level of operations, fixed assets (land, buildings, and equipment) are normally maintained at a level sufficient to handle peak patient demand.

Fixed assets are listed at *historical cost* (the purchase price) minus accumulated depreciation as of the date of the balance sheet. *Accumulated depreciation* represents the total dollars of depreciation that have been expensed on the income statement against the historical cost of the organization's fixed assets. Numerically, the amounts of depreciation expense reported on the income statement each year are accumulated over time to create the accumulated depreciation account on the balance sheet.[2] The accumulated depreciation account is an example of a *contra-asset* account because it is a **negative** asset. The greater the value of this account, the smaller an organization's total assets. Contra accounts reduce the value of "parent" accounts; in this case, the parent account is gross fixed assets.

For Sunnyvale, the net balance of property and equipment (*net fixed assets*) is $52,450,000 at the end of 2007. The historical cost of these assets (*gross fixed assets*) is $88,549,000. Some of the fixed assets were purchased in 2007, some in 2006, some in 2005, and some in prior years, but the total purchase price of all the fixed assets being used by Sunnyvale on December 31, 2007, is $88,549,000. The accumulated depreciation on these assets through December 31, 2007, is $36,099,000, which accounts for that portion of the value of the assets that was "spent" in producing income. The difference, or net, of $52,450,000, reflects the remaining *book value* of the clinic's fixed assets. Often, a more detailed explanation of the fixed asset accounts will be found in the footnotes.

As mentioned earlier, the connection of the balance sheet net fixed assets account to the income statement is through depreciation expense. The accumulated depreciation of $36,099,000 reported at the end of 2007 is $6,405,000 greater than the 2006 amount of $29,694,000. This increase in accumulated depreciation on the balance sheet reflects the $6,045,000 in depreciation expense reported on the 2007 income statement.

Depreciation, even though it typically does not reflect the true change in value of a fixed asset over time, at least ensures an orderly recognition of value loss. Occasionally, assets experience a sudden, unexpected loss of value. One example is when changing technology instantly makes a piece of diagnostic equipment obsolete and hence worthless. When this occurs, the asset that has experienced the decline in value is *written off*, which means that its value on the balance sheet is reduced (perhaps to zero) and the amount of the reduction is taken as an expense on the income statement.[3]

In closing our discussion of assets, note that many providers will report a fourth asset category: *other assets*. This is really a catchall category of miscellaneous long-term assets, which may or may not be very significant. Examples include fixed assets not used in the provision of healthcare services and funds that were used to support long-term debt sales that will be expensed over time.

Liabilities

Liabilities and equity, which comprise the right side of the balance sheet, are shown in the lower section of Table 4.1. Together, they represent the *capital* (the money) that has been raised by an organization to acquire the assets shown on the left side. Again, by definition, total capital (the sum of liabilities and equity) must equal total assets. Another way of looking at this is that every dollar of assets on the left side of the balance sheet must be matched by a dollar of liabilities or equity on the right side.

Liabilities represent claims against the assets of an organization that are **fixed by contract**. Some of the liability claims are by workers for unpaid wages and salaries, some are by tax authorities for unpaid taxes, and some are by vendors that grant credit when supplies are purchased. (Even not-for-profit organizations, which do not pay income taxes, typically have unpaid payroll and withholding taxes on their employees.) However, the largest liability claims typically are by *creditors* (lenders) who have supplied debt capital to the business. Most creditors' claims are against the total assets of the organization (unsecured), rather than being tied to specific assets that were used as collateral for the loan. In the event of *default* (nonpayment of interest or principal) by the borrower, creditors have the right to force the business into bankruptcy, with *liquidation* as a possible consequence. If liquidation occurs, the law requires that any proceeds be used first to satisfy liability claims before any funds can be paid to owners or, in the case of not-for-profits, used for charitable purposes. Furthermore, the dollar value of each liability claim is fixed by the amount shown on the balance sheet, while the owners, including the community at large for not-for-profit organizations, have a claim to the residual proceeds of the liquidation rather than to a fixed amount.

Like assets, the balance sheet presentation of liabilities follows a logical format. Current liabilities, which are those liabilities that fall due (must be paid) within one accounting period (one year in this example), are listed first. Long-term debt, distinguished from short-term debt by having maturities greater than one accounting period, is listed second. As shown in Table 4.1, Sunnyvale had total liabilities at the end of 2007 of $100,747,000, which consisted of two parts: total current liabilities of $15,425,000 and total long-term debt of $85,322,000. The following sections describe each liability account in detail.

Current Liabilities

Current liabilities include liabilities that must be paid within one accounting period. Many healthcare businesses use short-term debt—defined as having a maturity of less than one accounting period. Such debt, which often is in the form of bank loans, generally is used to finance seasonal or cyclical working capital (current asset) needs. When listed on the balance sheet, short-term debt typically is called *notes payable*. We see that Sunnyvale had $4,334,000 of short-term debt outstanding at the end of 2007.

Accounts payable, as well as accrued expenses, represent payment obligations that have been incurred as of the balance sheet date but that have not yet been paid. In particular, accounts payable represents amounts due to vendors for supplies purchases. Often, suppliers offer their customers *credit terms*, which allow payment sometime after the purchase is made. For example, one of Sunnyvale's suppliers offers credit terms of 2/10, net 30, which means that if Sunnyvale pays the invoice in ten days, it will receive a 2 percent discount off the list price; otherwise, the total amount of the invoice is due in 30 days. In effect, by allowing Sunnyvale to pay either 10 or 30 days after the supplies have been received, the supplier is acting as a creditor, and the credit being offered is called *trade credit*. The balance sheet tells us that suppliers, at the end of 2007, had extended Sunnyvale $5,022,000 worth of such credit.[4]

Wages and benefits due to employees, interest due on debt financing, accrued utilities expenses, and similar items are included on the balance sheet as *accrued expenses*. Sunnyvale's employees are used to illustrate the logic behind accruals. Sunnyvale's staff earns its wages and benefits on a daily basis as the work is performed. However, the clinic pays its workers every two weeks. Therefore, other than on paydays (assuming no lag), the clinic owes its staff some amount of salaries for work performed. Whenever the obligation to pay wages extends into the next accounting period, an *accrual* is created on the balance sheet. This obligation, as well as taxes due to government authorities and interest due to lenders, appears on Sunnyvale's balance sheet as an accrual.[5]

Long-Term Debt

The *long-term debt* section of the balance sheet represents debt financing to the organization with maturities of more than one accounting period, and hence repayment in this example is not required during the coming year. The long-term debt section lists any debt owed to banks and other creditors (e.g., bondholders) as well as obligations under certain types of lease arrangements. Usually, detailed information relative to the specific characteristics of the long-term debt is disclosed in the footnotes to the financial statements.[6]

Sunnyvale had *total liabilities*, combined current liabilities and long-term debt, of $100,747,000 at the end of 2007. As discussed in the next section, Sunnyvale reported $54,068,000 in equity, for total financing (which must equal total assets) of $154,815,000. Thus, based on the values recorded on the balance sheet, or *book values*, Sunnyvale uses much more debt financing than equity financing. The choice between debt and equity financing is discussed in Chapter 13. Chapter 17 includes coverage of alternative ways to measure the amount of debt financing that an organization uses and its effect on the business's financial condition.

Self-Test Questions
1. What are liabilities?
2. What are some of the accounts that would be classified as current liabilities?
3. Use an example to explain the logic behind accruals.
4. What is the difference between notes payable and long-term debt?

Equity

On the balance sheet, the equity (ownership) claim on an organization's assets is called *net assets* when the organization has not-for-profit status. As the term *net* implies, net assets represent the dollar value of assets remaining when a business's liabilities are stripped out. However, as readers learned in Chapter 2, there is a wide variety of ownership types in the health services industry, which results in an almost bewildering difference in terminology used for the equity portion of the balance sheet. For example, depending on the type of business organization, the equity section of the balance sheet may be called stockholders' equity, owner's net worth, net worth, proprietor's worth, partners' worth, or even something else. To keep things manageable in this book, the term *equity* typically will be used; but the various terms all indicate the same thing: the amount of total assets financed by nonliability capital, or total assets minus total liabilities. To determine what belongs to the owners, whether explicitly recognized in for-profit businesses or implicitly implied in not-for-profit organizations, fixed claims (liabilities) are subtracted from the value of the business's assets. The remainder, the net assets (equity), represents the residual value of the assets of the organization.

The equity section of the balance sheet is extremely important because it, more than anything else in the financial statements, reflects the ownership status of the organization. Because Table 4.1 lists the equity as *net assets*, Sunnyvale is a not-for-profit corporation. Some of the equity capital could have come from charitable contributions and some from government grants, but the vast majority of Sunnyvale's equity capital was obtained by reinvesting earnings within the business. For a not-for-profit organization such as Sunnyvale, **all earnings must be reinvested in the business**.

Sunnyvale's equity increased by $7,860,000 from 2006 to 2007, which is the same amount that Sunnyvale reported as net income for 2007. It is important to recognize that this connection between the bottom line of the income statement and the equity section of the balance sheet is a mathematical necessity. In the case of not-for-profit businesses, there is simply nowhere else for those earnings to go. This highlights a second connection between the balance sheet and the income statement; the first was depreciation.

Sunnyvale's balance sheet balances because the increase in equity of $7,860,000 was matched by a like increase in assets, along with asset increases that resulted from other financing. The asset increases might be in cash, receivables, fixed assets, or in some other account. The key point is that the equity (net asset) balance is **not** a store of cash. As Sunnyvale earned profits over the years that increased the equity account, these funds were invested in supplies, property and equipment, and other assets to provide future services that would likely generate even larger profits in the future. Sunnyvale's total assets grew by $154,815,000 − $115,101,000 = $39,714,000 in 2007, which was supported by an increase in total liabilities of $100,747,000 − $68,893,000 = $31,854,000 and an increase in equity (net assets) of $54,068,000 − $46,208,000 = $7,860,000.

The net assets type of equity section shown in Table 4.1 is typical of not-for-profit organizations such as community or religious hospitals. However, a relatively rare form of not-for-profit organization can sell stock privately, and such organizations may show a limited amount of stock outstanding. This type of stock is not sold in the open market, though, and does not convey ownership rights, as does the stock of investor-owned companies.

Thus far, the discussion of the balance sheet has focused on Sunnyvale, a not-for-profit corporation. In general, the asset and liability sections of the balance sheet are much the same regardless of ownership status. The equity section tends to differ in presentation for different types of ownership because the types have different forms of equity. That is the bad news. The good news is that the economic substance of the equity section remains the same.

Table 4.2 contains the equity section of the balance sheet assuming that Sunnyvale, with a new name (Southeast Healthcare), were an investor-owned (for-profit) corporation. This is the type of presentation that would be seen on the balance sheets of for-profit health services businesses such as HMA, Manor

TABLE 4.2
Southeast
Healthcare:
Balance Sheet
Equity Section
December 31,
2007 and 2006
(in thousands)

	2007	2006
Stockholders' Equity:		
Common stock ($1 par value,	$ 1,000	$ 1,000
1,500,000 shares authorized,		
1,000,000 shares outstanding)		
Capital in excess of par	9,000	9,000
Retained earnings	44,068	36,208
Total equity	$ 54,068	$ 46,208
Total liabilities and equity	$ 154,815	$ 115,101

Care, and UnitedHealthcare. The first major difference is the title of the section, "Stockholders' Equity." This title, or a similar title such as "Shareholders' Equity," provides explicit recognition that stockholders (shareholders) own the business.

The stockholders' equity section of the balance sheet consists of two parts: contributed capital and accumulated earnings. *Contributed capital*, which typically is not identified as such on the balance sheet, is the sum of the common stock and capital in excess of par accounts. This amount represents the dollars of capital contributed directly, or paid out-of-pocket, by stockholders of corporations or by proprietors or partners of unincorporated businesses. The *retained earnings* account represents the accumulated earnings of the organization that have been reinvested in the business. Because not-for-profit organizations cannot pay dividends, all earnings must be retained in the business. However, some portion (or all) of the earnings of for-profit businesses may be distributed to owners by making dividend payments.

Southeast Healthcare was incorporated in 1975, with the bylaws authorizing issuance of 1.5 million shares of common stock. At that time, 1 million shares were sold at a price of $10 per share, so $10 million was collected. However, the stock has a *par value*, which is a somewhat antiquated legal concept that specifies the minimum liability of shareholders in the event of bankruptcy, of $1. Today, par value has limited economic relevance, but accountants continue to separate contributed capital into two separate accounts. Because 1 million shares were sold at a par value of $1, the *common stock* account shows a balance of $1 million. Any proceeds collected from the sale of common stock at a price above par value are listed in the *capital in excess of par* account. Because Southeast Healthcare collected $10 per share, or $9 above par value for each of the 1 million shares sold, this account shows a balance of $9 million.

The *retained earnings* account represents the accumulation of earnings over time that are reinvested in the business. Each year, the amount of net income shown on the income statement, less the amount paid out to stockholders as dividends, is transferred from the income statement to the balance sheet. Suppose that, as with Sunnyvale, Southeast Healthcare had actually earned $7,860,000 in 2007. Because the firm's retained earnings account increased by a like amount, no dividends were paid to stockholders during the year.

Retained earnings, like all equity accounts, represent a claim against assets, and they are not available to buy new equipment, to pay dividends, or for any other purpose. The financing represented by retained earnings has already been used within the business to buy property and equipment; to buy supplies; and, yes, to increase the cash, short-term, and long-term securities investment accounts. Only the portion of retained earnings that is sitting in the cash account is immediately available to the business for use.

Although Table 4.2 shows only the equity section, it is likely that there would be significant differences in the values of other balance sheet accounts between investor-owned and not-for-profit businesses. For example, it is unlikely that a for-profit healthcare business would amass such a large amount of long-term investments (securities), unless the funds were earmarked for a particular use in the next few years. Southeast's stockholders would question why the company had more than $42 million in long-term securities because they would prefer to have all of the business's capital invested in operating assets, which, as indicated earlier, usually earn a higher return than do securities investments. Thus, there would be stockholder pressure on management to return this capital to owners (as dividends or stock repurchases) so that they could themselves make the decision on how to invest these funds. Stockholders have invested in Southeast Healthcare because it is a healthcare provider; if they had wanted to own a bank, they would have bought bank stock. If and when Southeast requires more capital for asset acquisitions, it can always obtain additional debt financing or sell more common stock.

Access to the capital markets is seen as a real economic advantage that for-profit providers—whether they are hospitals, medical practices, or managed care plans—have over not-for-profit providers. The ability to "open the faucet" to acquire more capital has certain advantages in today's highly competitive health services industry, which is reflected in the fact that, in recent years, a number of not-for-profit organizations have converted to for-profit status.[7]

<table>
<tr><td>

1. What is equity (net assets)?
2. What are the differences in the equity sections of not-for-profit and investor-owned providers?
3. What is the relationship between the retained earnings account on the balance sheet and earnings (net income) reported on the income statement?

</td><td>

Self-Test Questions

</td></tr>
</table>

Fund Accounting

One unique feature of many not-for-profit balance sheets is that they classify certain asset and equity (net asset) accounts as being *restricted*. When a not-for-profit organization receives contributions that donors have indicated must be used for a specific purpose, the organization must create multiple funds to account for its assets and equity (net assets). A *fund* is defined as a self-contained pool set up to account for a specific activity or project. Each fund typically has assets, liabilities, and an equity (net asset) balance. Because the balance sheet of an organization that receives restricted contributions is separated into restricted and unrestricted funds, this form of accounting is called *fund accounting*. Only contributions to not-for-profit organizations are tax deductible to the donor, and hence few contributions are made to investor-owned healthcare businesses. Thus, fund accounting is only applicable to not-for-profit organizations.

Restricted contributions and gifts impose legal and fiduciary responsibilities on health services organizations to carry out the written wishes of donors. Thus, numerous rules are associated with fund accounting that go well beyond the scope of this book. The good news is that GAAP encourage organizations that use fund accounting to present outside parties with balance sheets that look roughly like the one in Table 4.1. Thus, with the exception of further breakdown into unrestricted and restricted accounts, such balance sheets have the same economic content as those prepared by nonfund-account health services organizations.

Self-Test Questions
1. What is fund accounting?
2. What type of a health services organization is most likely to use fund accounting?
3. Is there a significant difference in the economic content of balance sheets created by investor-owned and not-for-profit health services organizations?

The Statement of Cash Flows

The balance sheet and income statement are traditional financial statements that have been required for many years. In contrast, the *statement of cash flows* has only been required since 1989 for for-profit businesses and 1995 for not-for-profit businesses.[8] This relatively new financial statement was created by accountants in response to demands by users for better information about a firm's cash inflows and outflows.

While the balance sheet reports the cash balance on hand at the end of the period, it does not provide details on why the cash account is greater or smaller than the previous year's value, nor does the income statement give detailed information on cash flows. In addition to the problems of accrual accounting and noncash expenses discussed in Chapter 3, there may be cash raised by means other than operations that does not even appear on the income statement. For example, Sunnyvale may have raised cash during 2007 by taking on more debt or by selling some fixed assets. Such flows, which are not shown on the income statement, affect a firm's cash balance. Finally, the cash coming into a business does not sit in the cash account forever. Most of it goes to pay operating expenses or to purchase other assets, or for investor-owned firms, some may be paid out as dividends. Thus, the cash account does not increase by the gross amount of cash generated, and it would be useful to know how the difference was spent. The statement of cash flows details where cash resources come from and how they are used.

Two formats for the statement of cash flows are allowed by GAAP. Under the *direct method*, operating cash flow is computed by focusing "directly" on the cash account. Thus, the statement of cash flows contains entries such as "cash received from patients and third-party payers" and "interest received." Under the *indirect method*, the movement of cash into and out of the cash account is imputed by examining both the data on the income statement and changes in balance sheet accounts. Because the indirect method uses financial statement data, while the direct method must pull data from the underlying accounts, most businesses use the indirect method. However, to develop the cash flows for large organizations, many adjustments must be made to the underlying income statement and balance sheet data. These adjustments are often complicated, so it is necessary to be well versed in financial accounting to prepare a complete statement of cash flows.

Sunnyvale's 2007 and 2006 statements are presented in Table 4.3 in the indirect format. To simplify the discussion, the data in the statements have been reduced; they are somewhat shorter and easier to comprehend than most "real world" statements. Nevertheless, an understanding of the composition and presentation of Table 4.3 will give readers an excellent appreciation of the value of the statement of cash flows.

The statement of cash flows is formatted to make it easy to understand why Sunnyvale's cash position increased by $5,616,000 during 2007. In other words, it tells us Sunnyvale's sources of cash and how this cash is used. The statement is divided into three major sections: cash flows from operating activities, cash flows from investing activities, and cash flows from financing activities.

Cash Flows from Operating Activities

The first section, *cash flows from operating activities*, focuses on the sources and uses of cash **tied directly to operations**. Of course, the most important source is net income, so its value for 2007—$7,860,000—is listed first. However, net income does not equal cash flow, so various adjustments must be made. The first adjustment is to add back the noncash expenses that appear on the income statement. As we explained in Chapter 3, as a first approximation, the

TABLE 4.3
Sunnyvale
Clinic:
Statements of
Cash Flows
Years Ended
December 31,
2007 and 2006
(in thousands)

	2007	2006
Cash Flows from Operating Activities:		
Net income	$ 7,860	$ 8,206
Adjustments:		
Depreciation	6,405	5,798
Increase in net patient accounts receivable	(2,582)	(1,423)
Increase in inventories	(1,393)	(673)
Decrease in accounts payable	(1,911)	(966)
Increase in accrued expenses	1,032	865
Net cash from operations	$ 9,411	$ 11,807
Cash Flows from Investing Activities:		
Capital expenditures	($ 9,306)	($ 1,953)
Cash Flows from Financing Activities:		
Increase in short-term investments	($ 5,000)	$ 0
Increase in notes payable	989	0
Increase in long-term investments	(22,222)	(20,667)
Increase in long-term debt	31,744	0
Net cash from financing	$ 5,511	($20,667)
Net increase (decrease) in cash	$ 5,616	($ 10,813)
Cash, beginning of year	$ 6,486	$17,299
Cash, end of year	$ 12,102	$ 6,486

cash flow of a business can be approximated as net income plus depreciation: $7,860,000 + $6,405,000 = $14,265,000.

Adjustments are then made for changes in those balance sheet current asset and liability accounts that are directly affected by operations. For Sunnyvale, this means the net patient accounts receivable, inventories, accounts payable, and accrued expenses accounts. The theory for these adjustments is that these accounts stem directly from operations; hence, any cash that either is generated by, or is used for, these accounts should be included as part of cash flow from operations. In addition, using balance sheet data to calculate operating cash flow recognizes that under accrual accounting not every dollar of revenues or expenses listed on the income statement represents a dollar of cash flow.

Note that short-term investments and notes payable, although they are current accounts, are financing accounts that are not directly tied to operations, and hence these accounts will be handled in the third section of the statement of cash flows. Also, note that the entire statement focuses on the change in cash, so that will be the output of the statement rather than one of its entries.

To illustrate the adjustments to operating cash flow, Sunnyvale's net patient accounts receivable increased from $25,927,000 to $28,509,000, or by $2,582,000, during 2007. Because this amount was included in 2007 revenues and hence reported in net income, but it was added to receivables instead of collected, it is not available as cash flow to Sunnyvale. Thus, it appears as a deduction (negative adjustment) to operating cash flow. To make this point in another way, note that an increase in an asset account requires that the business use cash, so the $2,582,000 increase in receivables reduces the cash flow for other purposes. For another illustration, note that accrued expenses increased by $1,032,000 in 2007. Because an increase in accruals, which is on the right side (liabilities and equity) of the balance sheet, creates financing for the clinic and hence represents a source of cash (as opposed to a use), this change is shown as an addition to operating cash flow.

When all the adjustments are made, Sunnyvale reported $9,411,000 in net cash from operations for 2007. For a business, whether investor-owned or not-for-profit, to be financially sustainable, it must generate a positive cash flow from operations. Thus, at least for 2007 and 2006, Sunnyvale's operations are doing what they should be doing—generating cash. However, the clinic's cash flow from operations has decreased from 2006 to 2007, so its managers should identify why this happened and then take appropriate action. Unlike Sunnyvale's situation, a consistent negative net cash flow from operations would send a warning to managers and investors alike that the business may not be economically sustainable.

Cash Flows from Investing Activities

The second major section on the statement of cash flows is *cash flows from investing activities*. The terminology here can be misleading because the emphasis in this section is on *capital investing*, which is investment in fixed assets (land, buildings, and equipment) as opposed to financial assets (securities). Because depreciation is accounted for in the cash flows from operating activities section, we focus here on the total (gross) investment in fixed assets. As evidenced by the 2006 to 2007 change in gross fixed assets derived from the balance sheets, Sunnyvale spent $9,306,000 to acquire additional plant and equipment. Thus, almost all of the clinic's operating cash flow was spent on new fixed assets. This fact should not be alarming, especially for a not-for-profit business, as long as the investments are prudent. (Chapters 14 and 15 contain a great deal of insights into what makes a prudent capital investment, at least from a financial perspective.)

Cash Flows from Financing Activities

The final major section is *cash flows from financing activities*, which focuses on securities investments and financing. The changes in balance sheet accounts from 2006 to 2007 indicate that the clinic invested $5,000,000 in short-term investments (which requires a use of cash), increased its notes payable by $500,000 (which is a source of cash), invested $22,222,000 in long-term securities (another use), and took on an additional $31,744,000 in long-term debt (another source). On net, Sunnyvale generated a $5,511,000 cash inflow from financing activities. This section shows that Sunnyvale used the vast majority of new debt to purchase securities. In general, new debt would be used to acquire real assets rather than financial assets. However, Sunnyvale is planning to acquire a large group practice in 2008, and the financing activities undertaken in 2007 are in preparation for this purchase.

Net Increase (Decrease) in Cash and Reconciliation

The next line of the statement of cash flows is the *net increase (decrease) in cash*. It is merely the sum of the totals from the three major sections. For Sunnyvale, there is a net increase in cash of $9,411,000 − $9,306,000 + $5,511,000 = $5,616,000 in 2007. Unlike the "bottom line" of the income statement, the change in cash line has limited value in assessing an organization's financial condition because it can be manipulated by financing activities. If an organization is losing cash on operations, but its managers want to report an increase in the cash account, in most cases they simply can borrow the funds necessary to show a net cash increase on the statement of cash flows. Thus, the net cash from operations line is a more important indicator of financial well-being than is the net increase (decrease) in cash line.

The net increase (decrease) in cash line is used to verify the correctness of the entries on the statement of cash flows. As shown in Table 4.3, the $5,616,000 increase in cash reported by Sunnyvale for 2007 is added to the beginning of year cash balance, $6,486,000, to get an end-of-year total of $12,102,000. A check of the end-of-2007 cash balance shown in Table 4.1 confirms the amount calculated on the statement of cash flows.

In summary, the income statement focuses on accounting profitability, while the statement of cash flows focuses on the movement of cash: Where did the money come from and how did the organization use it? While the major concern of the income statement is economic profitability as defined by GAAP, the statement of cash flows is concerned with cash viability. Is the organization generating, and will it continue to generate, sufficient cash to meet both short-term and long-term needs?

Self-Test Questions	1. How does the statement of cash flows differ from the income statement?
	2. Briefly explain the three major categories shown on the statement.
	3. In your view, what is the most important piece of information reported on the statement?

Transactions

As we discussed in the last chapter, the recording of transactions by accountants is the first step in the creation of a business's financial statements. Understanding how transactions ultimately affect the financial statements will help managers better understand and interpret their content.

The transactions that flow to the income statement are relatively apparent. For example, net patient service revenue and related expenses stem directly from the provision of patient services and the expectation of receiving payment. Thus, the provision of services that have a reimbursement amount of $1,000 would increase the net patient services revenue account by $1,000. Similarly, the obligation to pay wages of $150 to an employee for a day's work would increase the salaries expense line by a like amount.

However, the transactions that flow to the balance sheet are less obvious. In this section, ten typical balance sheet transactions are presented. Understanding these transactions will help readers understand how an organization's economic events are transformed into financial statement data. The primary concept behind all balance sheet transactions is that the basic accounting equation must be preserved (i.e., the balance sheet must balance). Thus, each transaction must have a dual effect, either one on the left side and one on the right side, or offsetting effects on the same side.

1. **Investment by owners.** Suppose five radiologists decide to open a diagnostic center that they incorporate as an investor-owned business called Bayshore Radiology Center. They each invest $200,000 cash in the business in exchange for $200,000 of common stock. The transaction results in an equal increase in both assets and equity. In this case, there is an increase in the cash account of $1,000,000 and an increase in the common stock account of $1,000,000. After the transaction, the balance sheet looks like this:

Cash	$1,000,000	Common stock	$1,000,000
Total assets	$1,000,000	Total claims	$1,000,000

2. **Purchase of equipment for cash.** To support operations, the business needs diagnostic equipment. Assume that the first piece of equipment purchased costs $200,000, and it is paid for in cash. This transaction results in an equal increase and decrease in total assets. The composition of assets is changed, however:

Cash	$ 800,000	Common stock	$1,000,000
Gross fixed assets	200,000		
Total assets	$1,000,000	Total claims	$1,000,000

   Total assets and total claims still amount to $1,000,000 because no new capital was acquired by the business.

3. **Purchase of supplies on credit.** Assume that Bayshore purchases medical supplies for $20,000. The supplier's terms give the center 60 days to pay the bill. Assets are increased by this transaction because

of the expected benefit of using these supplies to provide services. Also, liabilities (accounts payable) are increased by the amount due the supplier:

Cash	$ 800,000	Accounts payable	$ 20,000
Supplies	20,000	Common stock	1,000,000
Gross fixed assets	200,000		
Total assets	$1,020,000	Total claims	$1,020,000

4. **Services rendered for credit.** Assume that Bayshore provides $50,000 of services (at net prices) that are billed to third-party payers. This transaction will increase assets (accounts receivable) and the retained earnings portion of equity. The $50,000 would also show up on the income statement as revenue, which, after expenses and dividends are deducted, would ultimately flow through to the balance sheet and hence support the increase in equity:

Cash	$ 800,000	Accounts payable	$ 20,000
Accounts receivable	50,000	Common stock	1,000,000
Supplies	20,000	Retained earnings	50,000
Gross fixed assets	200,000		
Total assets	$1,070,000	Total claims	$1,070,000

Retained earnings (equity) is increased when revenues are earned, even though no cash has been generated. When accounts receivable are collected at a later date, cash will be increased and receivables will be decreased (see Transaction 10).

5. **Purchase of advertising on credit.** Bayshore receives a bill for $10,000 from the *Daily News* for advertising its grand opening, but it does not have to pay the newspaper for 30 days. The transaction results in an increase in liabilities and a decrease in equity; specifically, accounts payable is increased and retained earnings is decreased. The decrease in equity will work its way through the income statement as $10,000 in advertising expense:

Cash	$ 800,000	Accounts payable	$ 30,000
Accounts receivable	50,000	Common stock	1,000,000
Supplies	20,000	Retained earnings	40,000
Gross fixed assets	200,000		
Total assets	$1,070,000	Total claims	$1,070,000

Equity is reduced when expenses are incurred. When payment is made at a later date, both payables and cash will decrease (see Transaction 8). Advertising is an expense, as opposed to an asset (like supplies), because the benefits of the outlay have been immediately realized.

6. **Payment of expenses.** Assume that the center paid $50,000 in cash for rent, salaries, and utilities. These payments result in an equal decrease in cash and equity. The decrease in equity will be matched by a reduction in net income on the income statement:

Cash	$ 750,000	Accounts payable	$ 30,000
Accounts receivable	50,000	Common stock	1,000,000
Supplies	20,000	Retained earnings	(10,000)
Gross fixed assets	200,000		
Total assets	$1,020,000	Total claims	$1,020,000

Note that Bayshore's retained earnings have been driven negative by this transaction. In essence, the equity of the center ($1,020,000 − $30,000 = $990,000) is now worth less than the total capital supplied by the center's stockholders.

7. **Recognition of supplies used.** Assume that $2,000 worth of supplies were used in providing healthcare services to Bayshore's patients. The cost of supplies used is an expense that decreases assets and equity. The expense is also shown on the income statement, and hence net income is reduced by a like amount:

Cash	$ 750,000	Accounts payable	$ 30,000
Accounts receivable	50,000	Common stock	1,000,000
Supplies	18,000	Retained earnings	(12,000)
Gross fixed assets	200,000		
Total assets	$1,018,000	Total claims	$1,018,000

Note, however, that supplies typically are expended in providing services, so revenue would be created that increases assets and equity.

8. **Payment of accounts payable (advertising bill).** Assume that the center paid its $10,000 advertising bill, which was due in 30 days. (The supplies bill is not due for 60 days.) The advertising bill was previously recorded in Transaction 5 as a payable. This payment on an account for an expense already recognized decreases both assets (cash) and liabilities (payables):

Cash	$ 740,000	Accounts payable	$ 20,000
Accounts receivable	50,000	Common stock	1,000,000
Supplies	18,000	Retained earnings	(12,000)
Gross fixed assets	200,000		
Total assets	$1,008,000	Total claims	$1,008,000

Payment of a liability related to an expense that has previously been incurred does not affect equity.

9. **Payment of accounts payable (supplies bill).** One month later, assume that Bayshore paid its $20,000 supplies bill, which decreases cash and accounts payable. Recall that the supplies bill was previously recorded in Transaction 3 as an increase in both assets (supplies) and liabilities (accounts payable). Furthermore, part of the supplies were used and recorded in Transaction 7 as a decrease in assets (supplies) and equity:

Cash	$720,000	Common stock	$1,000,000
Accounts receivable	50,000	Retained earnings	(12,000)
Supplies	18,000		
Gross fixed assets	200,000		
Total assets	$988,000	Total claims	$ 988,000

A payment of a liability related to an asset that has previously been booked does not affect equity. Equity is not affected until the asset has been consumed.

10. **Receipt of cash from a third-party payer.** Assume that $5,000 is received in payment for patient services rendered from one of Bayshore's third-party payers. This transaction does not change Bayshore's total assets or, because of the accounting identity, total claims. It does change the composition of the business's assets by reducing receivables and increasing cash:

Cash	$725,000	Common stock	$1,000,000
Accounts receivable	45,000	Retained earnings	(12,000)
Supplies	18,000		
Gross fixed assets	200,000		
Total assets	$988,000	Total claims	$ 988,000

A collection for services previously billed and recorded does not affect equity. Revenue was already recorded in Transaction 4 and cannot be recorded again.

Of course, an almost limitless number of transactions occur in everyday business activities. The purpose of this section was to give readers a sense of how transactions provide the foundation for a business's financial statements.

Self-Test Questions
1. What condition must be met when entering transactions on the balance sheet?
2. What is the effect on a business's equity account of a payment on a bill that has already been booked (recorded as an accounts payable)?
3. What is the effect of the collection of a receivable on a business's equity account?

Another Look Ahead: Using Balance Sheet Data in Financial Statement Analysis

In Chapter 3, readers were provided an introduction to ratio analysis. In this section, we continue the discussion using balance sheet data. The *debt ratio* (or *debt-to-assets ratio*) is defined as total debt divided by total assets. Total debt can be defined several ways, depending on the use of the ratio, but for purposes here, assume that total debt includes all liabilities (i.e., all non-equity capital). (An alternative would be to include only interest-bearing debt in our definition.) Using Table 4.1 data, Sunnyvale's debt ratio at the end of 2007 was total debt (liabilities) divided by total assets = $100,747,000 / $154,815,000 = 0.65 = 65%. This ratio reveals that each dollar of assets was financed by 65 cents of debt and, by inference, 35 cents of equity.

Sunnyvale's debt ratio at the end of 2006 was $68,893,000 / $115,101,000 = 0.60 = 60%. Thus, the clinic increased its proportional use of debt financing by 5 percentage points in one year. That information is important to Sunnyvale's managers and creditors. (The consequences of increased debt utilization are discussed throughout this book.) Also, it should be clear that judgments about Sunnyvale's capital structure could not be made easily without constructing the debt ratio and other ratios; interpreting the dollar values directly is just too difficult.

Key Concepts

Chapter 3 contained an introduction to financial accounting along with a discussion of the first of three financial statements—the income statement. This chapter extended the discussion to cover the balance sheet and the statement of cash flows, with emphasis on the interrelationships among the three statements. A demonstration of how economic events (transactions) work their way onto the balance sheet was also presented. The key concepts of this chapter are:

- The *balance sheet* may be thought of as a snapshot of the financial position of a business at a given point in time.
- The *accounting identity* specifies that assets must equal liabilities plus equity (total assets must equal total claims). When rearranged, the accounting identity reminds us that a business's equity is really a residual amount that represents the difference between assets and liabilities.
- *Assets* identify the resources owned by a health services organization in dollar terms. Assets are listed *by maturity* (i.e., by order of when the assets are expected to be converted into cash). Current assets are expected to be converted into cash during the next accounting period.
- *Liabilities* are fixed claims by employees, suppliers, tax authorities, and lenders against a business's assets. *Current liabilities*—those obligations that fall due within one accounting period—are listed first. *Long-term*

liabilities (typically debt with maturities greater than one accounting period) are listed second.

- *Equity* is the ownership claim against total assets. Depending on the form of organization and ownership, this claim may be called *net assets, stockholders' equity, proprietor's net worth,* or something else.
- There are two *primary interrelationships* between the balance sheet and the income statement. First, the annual depreciation expense shown on the income statement accumulates on the balance sheet in the accumulated depreciation account. Second, all earnings from the income statement that are reinvested in the business accumulate on the balance sheet in the equity account.
- The structure of the liabilities and equity side of the balance sheet (i.e., the proportions of debt and equity financing) defines the organization's *capital structure.*
- *Fund accounting* is used by organizations that have restricted contributions. This complicates internal accounting procedures and adds additional detail to the balance sheet. However, fund accounting does not alter the basic format of the balance sheet nor its economic interpretation.
- The *statement of cash flows* shows where an organization gets its cash and how it is used. It combines information found on both the income statement and the balance sheet.
- The statement of cash flows has three major sections: *cash flows from operating activities, cash flows from investing activities,* and *cash flows from financing activities.*
- The "bottom line" of the statement of cash flows is the *net increase (decrease) in cash.* Although this amount is useful in verifying the accuracy of the statement, its economic content is not as meaningful as the statement's component amounts.
- *Transactions* are the primary underpinning of the measurement and reporting of financial accounting information. Understanding how transactions affect the financial statements leads to a better understanding of the statements themselves.

This temporarily ends the discussion of financial accounting. The next chapter begins our coverage of managerial accounting. However, the concepts presented in Chapters 3 and 4 are used repeatedly throughout the remainder of the book. In addition, financial accounting concepts are revisited in Chapter 17, which focuses on using the financing statements to assess financial performance.

Questions

4.1 a. What is the difference between the income statement and balance sheet in regards to timing?

   b. What is wrong with this statement: "The clinic's cash balance for

2007 was $150,000, while its net income on December 31, 2007 was $50,000."

4.2 a. What is the accounting identity?

   b. What is the implication of the accounting identity for the numbers on a balance sheet?

   c. What does the accounting identity tell us about a business's equity?

4.3 a. What are assets?

   b. What are the three major categories of assets?

4.4 a. What makes an asset a current asset?

   b. Provide some examples of current assets.

   c. What is net working capital, and what does it measure?

4.5 a. On the balance sheet, what is the difference between long-term investments and property and equipment?

   b. What is the difference between gross fixed assets and net fixed assets?

   c. How does depreciation expense on the income statement relate to accumulated depreciation on the balance sheet?

4.6 a. What is the difference between liabilities and equity?

   b. What makes a liability a current liability?

   c. Give some examples of current liabilities.

   d. What is the difference between long-term debt and notes payable?

4.7 a. Explain the difference between the equity section of a not-for-profit business and an investor-owned business.

   b. What is the relationship between net income on the income statement and the equity section on a balance sheet?

4.8 What is fund accounting, and why is it important to some healthcare providers?

4.9 a. What is the statement of cash flows, and how does it differ from the income statement?

   b. What are the three major sections of the statement of cash flows?

   c. What is the "bottom line" of the statement of cash flows, and how important is it?

Problems

4.1 Middleton Clinic had total assets of $500,000 and an equity balance of $350,000 at the end of 2006. One year later, at the end of 2007, the clinic had $575,000 in assets and $380,000 in equity. What was the clinic's dollar growth in assets during 2007, and how was this growth financed?

4.2 San Mateo Healthcare had an equity balance of $1.38 million at the beginning of the year. At the end of the year, its equity balance was $1.98 million.

   a. Assume that San Mateo is a not-for-profit organization. What was its net income for the period?

b. Now, assume that San Mateo is an investor-owned business.
  • Assuming zero dividends, what was San Mateo's net income?
  • Assuming $200,000 in dividends, what was its net income?
  • Assuming $200,000 in dividends and $300,000 in additional stock sales, what was San Mateo's net income?

4.3 Here is financial statement information on four not-for-profit clinics:

	Pittman	Rose	Beckman	Jaffe
December 31, 2006:				
Assets	$ 80,000	$100,000	g	$150,000
Liabilities	50,000	d	$ 75,000	j
Equity	a	60,000	45,000	90,000
December 31, 2007:				
Assets	b	130,000	180,000	k
Liabilities	55,000	62,000	h	80,000
Equity	45,000	e	110,000	145,000
During 2007:				
Total revenues	c	400,000	i	500,000
Total expenses	330,000	f	360,000	l

Fill in the missing values labeled a through l.

4.4 The following are selected entries for Warren Clinic for December 31, 2007, in alphabetical order. Create Warren Clinic's balance sheet.

Accounts payable	$ 20,000
Accounts receivable, net	60,000
Cash	30,000
Other long-term liabilities	10,000
Long-term debt	120,000
Long-term investments	100,000
Net property and equipment	150,000
Other assets	40,000
Equity	230,000

4.5 Consider the following balance sheet:

BestCare HMO
Balance Sheet
June 30, 2007
(in thousands)

Assets
Current Assets:
  Cash $2,737

Net premiums receivable	821
Supplies	387
Total current assets	$3,945
Net property and equipment	$5,924
Total assets	$9,869

Liabilities and Net Assets

Accounts payable—medical services	$2,145
Accrued expenses	929
Notes payable	382
Total current liabilities	$3,456
Long-term debt	$4,295
Total liabilities	$7,751
Net assets—unrestricted (equity)	$2,118
Total liabilities and net assets	$9,869

a. How does this balance sheet differ from the one presented in Table 4.1 for Sunnyvale?

b. What is BestCare's net working capital for 2007?

c. What is BestCare's debt ratio? How does it compare with Sunnyvale's debt ratio?

4.6 Consider this balance sheet:

Green Valley Nursing Home, Inc.
Balance Sheet
December 31, 2007

Assets

Current Assets:

Cash	$ 105,737
Investments	200,000
Net patient accounts receivable	215,600
Supplies	87,655
Total current assets	$ 608,992
Property and equipment	$2,250,000
Less accumulated depreciation	356,000
Net property and equipment	$1,894,000
Total assets	$2,502,992

Liabilities and Shareholders' Equity

Current Liabilities:

Accounts payable	$ 72,250
Accrued expenses	192,900
Notes payable	180,000
Total current liabilities	$ 445,150
Long-term debt	$1,700,000

Shareholders' Equity:

Common stock, $10 par value	$ 100,000
Retained earnings	257,842
Total shareholders' equity	$ 357,842
Total liabilities and shareholders' equity	$2,502,992

   a. How does this balance sheet differ from the ones presented in Table 4.1 and Problem 4.5?

   b. What is Green Valley's net working capital for 2007?

   c. What is Green Valley's debt ratio? How does it compare with the debt ratios for Sunnyvale and BestCare?

4.7 Refer to the transactions pertaining to Bayshore Radiology Center presented in this chapter. Restate the impact of the transactions on Bayshore's balance sheet using these data:

   a. Transaction 2: The $200,000 equipment purchase is made with long-term borrowings instead of cash.

   b. Transaction 3: The $20,000 in supplies are purchased with cash instead of on trade credit.

   c. Transaction 4: The $50,000 in services provided are immediately paid for by patients instead of billed to third-party payers.

Notes

1. *Money market mutual funds* are mutual funds that invest in safe, short-term securities such as Treasury bills and commercial paper. *Treasury bills* are short-term debt instruments issued by the U.S. government. *Commercial paper* is short-term debt issued by very large and financially strong corporations. All of these securities are relatively safe investments because there is virtually 100 percent assurance that the borrowers (U.S. government and financially strong corporations) will repay the loans when they mature.

2. For-profit firms have to be concerned with both *book depreciation*, which is calculated according to GAAP and reported to stockholders, and *tax depreciation*, which is calculated according to IRS regulations and used to determine the firm's income for tax purposes.

3. Adjustments often must be made to the fixed asset accounts on the balance sheet (and to revenues and costs on the income statement) when assets are sold or lose value. However, such adjustments are beyond the scope of this book.

4. The decision whether or not Sunnyvale should take the extended trade credit (pay in 30 days rather than ten) is discussed in Chapter 16. In essence, the cost of foregoing the discount to gain additional credit (financing) has to be compared to the cost of other financing alternatives.

5. An important current liability account for providers with a high percentage of capitated contracts is *incurred but not reported* (IBNR) *expenses.* This account is not present on Sunnyvale's balance sheet because its payer mix is dominated by fee-for-service reimbursement. Under capitation, providers receive payment before the services are rendered. At the end of an accounting period when the books are closed, there may still be a large number of expenses related to services for the capitated enrollees that have not yet been reported in the accounting system. Many of the expenses will have occurred and been reported, but the costs of services provided near the end of the period may still be in the accounting pipeline. If the provider subcontracts out for some services, these services may have been performed by subcontractors but not yet billed. Even if the services are provided in-house, the episode of care may straddle into the next accounting period, thus resulting in a need to estimate the cost of those services. One of the last accounting entries typically done by capitated providers is to record IBNR expenses both as a current liability on the balance sheet and as an operating expense on the income statement. This procedure properly matches the timing of the costs of services to be provided with the revenue for those services, which was received up-front.

6. Although long-term debt has a maturity of more than one year, many long-term debt issues have provisions mandating that a portion of the borrowed amount (*principal*) be repaid in each year. Furthermore, some long-term debt that was issued in the past may mature in any given year. (The features of long-term debt are discussed in detail in Chapter 11.) The portion of long-term debt that must be paid in the coming year is recorded on the balance sheet as a current liability titled *current maturities of long-term debt.*

7. Conversion of a not-for-profit organization to for-profit status presents a difficult legal challenge because not-for-profit assets must be used for charitable purposes in perpetuity (forever). Thus, the monies received in a conversion must be used to create a foundation that will continue to perform charitable deeds.

8. Prior to the statement of cash flows, a different statement—the statement of changes in financial position—was required. The statement of cash flows presents similar information to the previous statement, but in a much more usable format.

References

American Institute of Certified Public Accountants (AICPA). 2003. *Audit and Accounting Guide.* New York: AICPA.

———. 2003. *Checklists and Illustrative Financial Statements for Health Care Organizations.* New York: AICPA.

Bitter, M. E., and J. Cassidy. 1992. "Perceptions of New AICPA Audit Guide." *Healthcare Financial Management* (November): 38–48.

Doody, D. 2006. "The Balance Sheet: A Snapshot of Your Financial Health." *Healthcare Financial Management* (May): 124–125.

Luecke, R. W., and D. T. Meeting. 1996. "SFAS 124, Accounting for Investments: The Rules Have Changed." *Healthcare Financial Management* (December): 58–63.

Waldron, D. J. 2005. "Technology Strategy and the Balance Sheet: 3 Points to Consider." *Healthcare Financial Management* (May): 70–76.

Managerial Accounting

Thus far, we have concentrated on healthcare finance basics and financial accounting. The next four chapters focus on managerial accounting. In addition to managerial accounting basics, Chapter 5 covers cost behavior and profit analysis—topics that many consider to be the cornerstones of managerial accounting. Then, in Chapters 6 through 8, we look at cost allocation, pricing, planning, and budgeting. After studying these four chapters, you will have a good appreciation of managerial accounting and its value to health services managers.

MANAGERIAL ACCOUNTING BASICS, COST BEHAVIOR, AND PROFIT ANALYSIS

Learning Objectives

After studying this chapter, readers will be able to:

- Explain the differences between financial and managerial accounting.
- Describe how costs are classified according to their relationship with volume.
- Conduct profit analyses to analyze the impact of input value changes on both profitability and breakeven points.
- Explain the primary differences in profit analyses that arise when comparing fee-for-service reimbursement with capitation.

Introduction

Managers of healthcare businesses have many responsibilities. Some of the more important ones are planning and budgeting, establishing policies that control the operations of the organization, and overseeing the day-to-day activities of subordinates. All of these activities require information—to be honest, a great deal of information. Furthermore, this information has to be presented in a format that facilitates analysis, interpretation, and decision making. This is where managerial accounting steps to the fore. Without a timely and effective managerial accounting system, healthcare managers would be left to wander in the dark rather than make decisions on the basis of good information. Of course, accurate information does not ensure good decision making, but without it the chances of making good decisions are almost nil.

The Basics of Managerial Accounting

Whereas financial accounting focuses on organizational-level data for presentation in a business's financial statements, *managerial accounting* focuses mostly on subunit—say, department data used internally for managerial decision making.[1] For example, managerial accounting information is used for routine budgeting processes, allocation of managerial bonuses, and pricing decisions, all of which deal with subunits of an organization. Also, managerial accounting data can be compiled for special projects such as assessing alternative modes of delivery or projecting the profitability of a particular reimbursement contract. In short, the focus of managerial accounting is to develop information to meet the needs of managers within the organization, rather than interested parties (mainly investors) outside the organization. Thus, while financial accounting information is driven primarily by the needs of outsiders, managerial accounting information is driven by the needs of managers.

Managers are more concerned with what will happen in the future than with what has happened in the past. Unlike financial accounting, managerial accounting is for the most part forward-looking. Because the past is known, while most of the future is unknown, managerial accounting information tends to be much less certain than financial accounting data. As managers embark on budgeting and pricing decisions, they often must make many assumptions regarding factors such as utilization (volume), reimbursement, and costs. This requirement for assumptions about the future, combined with the fact that there are no generally agreed-upon rules for developing managerial accounting data, makes it much more flexible than financial accounting data.

In general, financial accounting can be thought of as reporting work, while managerial accounting is best described as decision work. We do not mean to imply that there is little value in financial accounting data. Indeed, as you will see in Chapter 17, financial statements are key to understanding a business's overall financial condition. Still, the managerial decisions that are made on a daily basis that create this condition are influenced much more by managerial accounting data, which focus on individual activities, than by financial accounting data, which focus on the entire business.

A critical part of managerial accounting is the measurement of costs. In fact, the concept of costs is so important that it has spawned its own field of accounting—cost accounting. *Cost accounting* generally is considered to be a subset of managerial accounting, although cost accounting systems also are used to develop the expense data reported on a business's income statement. Therefore, cost accounting bridges both managerial and financial accounting.

Unfortunately, there is no single definition of the term *cost*. Rather, there are different costs for different purposes. As a general rule for healthcare providers, a cost involves a resource use associated with providing or supporting a specific service. However, the cost-per-service identified for pricing purposes can differ from the cost-per-service used for management control purposes. Also, the cost-per-service used for long-range planning purposes may differ from the cost-per-service defined for short-term purposes. Finally, as we discussed in Chapters 3 and 4, costs do not necessarily reflect actual cash outflows.

Costs are classified in two primary ways: by their relationship to the volume (amount) of services provided and by their relationship to the unit (i.e., department) being analyzed. In this chapter, we focus on the first classification method—the relationship of costs to volume. Our discussion of the latter classification method will be deferred until the next chapter.

Cost Classifications: Fixed and Variable

We can define (classify) several types of costs on the basis of their relationship to the amount of services provided, often referred to as *activity, utilization,* or *volume*. However, such cost classifications require the specification of a likely range of volumes. In dealing with the future, there is always volume uncertainty—the number of patient days, number of visits, number of enrollees, number of laboratory tests, and so on. However, managers often have some idea of the potential range of volume over some future time period. For example, the business manager of Northside Clinic, a small walk-in clinic, might estimate that the number of visits next year could range from 12,000 to 14,000 or from about 34 to 40 per day. If there is little likelihood that utilization will fall outside of these bounds, then the range of 12,000 to 14,000 annual visits defines the clinic's *relevant range*. Note that the relevant range pertains to a particular time period—in this case, next year. For other time periods, the relevant range might differ from its estimate for the coming year.

Fixed Costs

Some costs, called *fixed costs*, are more or less known with certainty, regardless of the level of volume **within the relevant range**. For example, Northside Clinic has a labor force of well-trained permanent employees that would be increased or decreased only under unusual circumstances. Thus, as long as volume falls within the relevant range of 12,000 to 14,000 visits, labor costs at the clinic are fixed for the coming year, regardless of the number of patient visits. Other examples of fixed costs include expenditures on facilities, diagnostic equipment, information systems, and the like. After an organization has acquired these assets, it typically is locked into them for some period of time, regardless of volume. Of course, no costs are fixed over the long run. At some point of increasing volume, healthcare businesses must incur additional fixed costs for new property and equipment, additional staffing, and so on. Likewise, if volume decreases by a substantial amount, an organization likely would reduce fixed costs by shedding part of its fixed assets and labor base.

Variable Costs

Whereas some costs are fixed regardless of volume (within the relevant range), other resources are more or less consumed as volume dictates. Costs that are directly related to volume are called *variable costs*. For example, the costs of the clinical supplies (e.g., rubber gloves, tongue depressors, hypodermics, and so on) used by Northside would be classified as variable costs. Also, some of the diagnostic equipment used in the clinic may be leased on a per procedure basis, which would convert the cost of the equipment from a fixed cost to a variable cost. Finally, some health services organizations pay their employees on the basis of the amount of work performed, which would convert labor costs from fixed to variable.

Self-Test Questions

1. Define relevant range.
2. Explain the features and provide examples of fixed and variable costs.
3. How does time period affect the definition of fixed costs?

Cost Behavior

Health services managers are vitally interested in how costs are affected by changes in the organization's activity (volume). The relationship between cost and volume, called *cost behavior* or *underlying cost structure*, is used by managers in planning, control, and decision making. The primary reason for defining an organization's underlying cost structure is to provide healthcare managers with a tool for forecasting costs (and ultimately profits) at different volume levels.

To illustrate the concept of cost behavior, consider the hypothetical cost data presented in Table 5.1 for a hospital's clinical laboratory. The underlying cost structure consists of both fixed and variable costs—that is, some of the costs are expected to be volume sensitive and some are not. This structure of both fixed and variable costs is typical in healthcare businesses as well as most other businesses. To begin our discussion of cost behavior, we **unrealistically** assume that the relevant range is from zero to 20,000 tests.

As noted in Table 5.1, the laboratory has $150,000 in fixed costs that consist primarily of labor, facilities, and equipment costs. These costs will occur even if the laboratory does not perform one test, assuming it is kept open. In addition to the fixed costs, each test, on average, requires $10 in laboratory supplies such as glass slides and reagents. The per unit (per test in this example) variable cost of $10 is defined as the *variable cost rate*. If laboratory volume doubles—for example, from 500 to 1,000 tests— *total variable costs* double from $5,000 to $10,000. However, the variable cost rate of $10 per test remains the same whether the test is the first, the hundredth, or the thousandth. Total variable costs, therefore, increase or decrease proportionately as volume changes, but the variable cost rate remains constant.

Fixed costs, in contrast to total variable costs, remain unchanged as the volume varies. When volume doubles from 500 to 1,000 tests, fixed costs remain at $150,000. Because all costs in this example are either fixed or variable, *total costs* are merely the sum of the two. (In the next section, we

TABLE 5.1
Cost Behavior
Illustration:
Fixed and
Variable Costs

Variable Cost per Test		Fixed Costs per Year	
Laboratory supplies	$10	Labor	$100,000
		Other fixed costs	50,000
			$150,000

Volume	Fixed Costs	Total Variable Costs	Total Costs	Average Cost per Test
0	$150,000	$ 0	$150,000	—
1	150,000	10	150,010	$150,010.00
50	150,000	500	150,500	3,010.00
100	150,000	1,000	151,000	1,510.00
500	150,000	5,000	155,000	310.00
1,000	150,000	10,000	160,000	160.00
5,000	150,000	50,000	200,000	40.00
10,000	150,000	100,000	250,000	25.00
15,000	150,000	150,000	300,000	20.00
20,000	150,000	200,000	350,000	17.50

introduce the concept of semi-fixed costs.) For example, at 5,000 tests, total costs are Fixed costs + Total variable costs = $150,000 + (5,000 × $10) = $150,000 + $50,000 = $200,000. Because variable costs are tied to volume, total variable costs, and hence total costs, increase as the volume increases, even though fixed costs remain constant.

The rightmost column in Table 5.1 contains *average cost* per unit of volume, which in this example is average cost per test. It is calculated by dividing total costs by volume. For example, at 5,000 tests, with total costs of $200,000, the average cost per test is $200,000 / 5,000 = $40. Because fixed costs are spread over more tests as volume increases, the average cost per test declines as volume increases. For example, when volume doubles from 5,000 to 10,000 tests, fixed costs remain at $150,000, but fixed cost per test declines from $150,000 / 5,000 = $30 to $150,000 / 10,000 = $15. With fixed cost per test declining from $30 to $15, the average cost per test declines from $30 + $10 = $40 to $15 + $10 = $25. The fact that higher volume reduces average fixed cost and average cost per unit of activity has important implications regarding the effect of volume changes on profitability. This point will be made clear in a later section.

The cost behavior presented in Table 5.1 in tabular format is presented in graphical format in Figure 5.1. Here, costs are shown on the vertical (Y) axis, and volume (number of tests) is shown on the horizontal (X) axis. Because fixed costs are independent of volume, they are shown as a horizontal dashed line at $150,000. Total variable costs appear as an upward-sloping

FIGURE 5.1

Cost Behavior
Graph

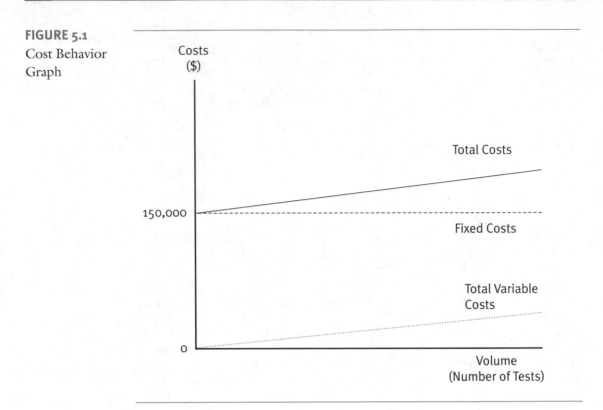

dotted line that starts at the origin (0 tests, $0 costs) and rises at a rate of
$10 for each additional test. Thus, the slope of the total variable costs line
is the variable cost rate. When fixed and total variable costs are combined to
obtain total costs, the result is the upward-sloping solid line parallel to the
total variable costs line but beginning at the Y axis at a value of $150,000 (the
fixed costs amount). In effect, the total costs line is nothing more than the
total variable costs line shifted upward by the amount of fixed costs.

Note that Figure 5.1 is not drawn to scale. Furthermore, the relevant
range is unrealistically large. The intent here is to emphasize the general shape
of a cost behavior graph and not its exact position. Also, note that total variable
costs plot as a straight line (are linear) because the variable cost rate is assumed
to be constant over the relevant range. Although curvilinear total variable costs
can occur in some situations, we assume throughout the book that the variable
cost rate is constant, and hence total variable costs are linear, at least within
the relevant range. Such an assumption is not unreasonable for most health
services organizations in most situations.

**Self-Test
Questions**

1. Construct a simple table like the one in Table 5.1, and discuss its
   elements.
2. Sketch and explain a simple diagram similar to Figure 5.1 to match your
   table.

Cost Classifications: Semi-Fixed

Fixed and variable costs represent two ends of the volume classification spectrum. Here, within the relevant range, the costs are either independent of volume (fixed) or directly related to volume (variable). A third classification, *semi-fixed costs*, falls in between the two extremes.[2] To illustrate, assume that the actual relevant range of volume for the clinical laboratory is 10,000 to 20,000 tests. However, the laboratory's current workforce can only handle up to 15,000 tests per year, so an additional technician, at an annual cost of $35,000, would be required if volume exceeds that level. Now, labor costs are fixed from 10,000 to 15,000 tests, and then again fixed at a higher level from 15,000 to 20,000 tests, but they are not fixed at the same level throughout the entire relevant range of 10,000 to 20,000 tests. Semi-fixed costs are fixed within ranges of volume, but there are multiple ranges of semi-fixed costs within the relevant range. Because a plot of semi-fixed costs versus volume looks like a step function, such costs sometimes are called *step-variable costs*.

Table 5.2 and Figure 5.2 illustrate the cost behavior of the laboratory within the new relevant range and with the addition of semi-fixed costs. As shown in Table 5.2, the inclusion of semi-fixed costs prevents average fixed cost and average cost per test from continuously declining throughout the relevant range. At volumes above 15,000 tests, the laboratory must add an additional technician at a cost of $35,000. This causes a jump in total fixed costs (consisting of fixed and semi-fixed costs), average fixed cost, total costs, and average cost per test. However, once this jump (or step) occurs, average fixed cost and average cost per test again begin to decrease as volume increases.

The jump in total costs is easily identified on the total costs line shown in Figure 5.2. Because of the negative impact of this sudden increase in total costs, the laboratory department head would probably try to avoid hiring an additional technician when volume exceeds 15,000 tests, especially if volume is expected to be only slightly above the jump point or is expected to be

Variable Costs per Test		Fixed Costs per Year		Semi-Fixed Costs	
Laboratory supplies	$10	Labor	$100,000	Increase in labor costs above 15,000 tests	$35,000
		Other fixed costs	50,000		
			$150,000		

Volume	Fixed Costs	Semi-Fixed Costs	Total Fixed Costs	Total Variable Costs	Total Costs	Average Cost per Test
10,000	$150,000	$ 0	$150,000	$100,000	$250,000	$25.00
14,000	150,000	0	150,000	140,000	290,000	20.71
15,000	150,000	0	150,000	150,000	300,000	20.00
16,000	150,000	35,000	185,000	160,000	345,000	21.56
20,000	150,000	35,000	185,000	200,000	385,000	19.25

TABLE 5.2
Cost Behavior Illustration: Fixed, Semi-Fixed, and Variable Costs

FIGURE 5.2
Cost Behavior
Graph

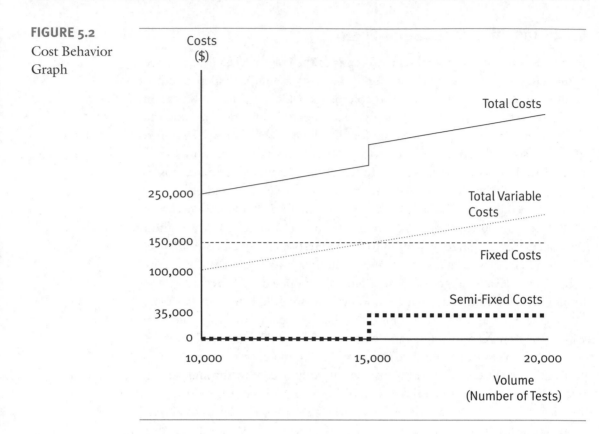

temporary. Perhaps new incentives could be put into place to encourage the current technicians to be more productive. Such an action could lower costs in general and create a situation in which the average cost per test would decline continuously throughout the relevant range.

Although semi-fixed costs are common within health services organizations, they add a level of complexity to profit analysis (the topic covered next) without adding a great deal of additional insight. Thus, the remainder of the examples in this book will assume that an organization's cost structure consists only of fixed and variable costs.

Self-Test Questions

1. What is a semi-fixed cost?
2. How does the addition of semi-fixed costs change a cost behavior graph?
3. What is the impact of semi-fixed costs on per unit average cost?

Profit (CVP) Analysis

Profit analysis is an analytical technique typically used to analyze the effects of volume changes on profit. The same procedures can be used to assess the effects of volume changes on costs, so this type of analysis is often called *cost-volume-profit (CVP) analysis*. CVP analysis allows managers to examine the effects of alternative assumptions regarding costs, volume, and prices. Clearly, such information is useful as managers evaluate future courses of action regarding pricing and the introduction of new services.

Basic Data

Table 5.3 presents the estimated annual costs for Atlanta Clinic, a subsidiary of Atlanta Health Services, for 2008. These costs are based on the clinic's most likely estimate of volume—75,000 visits. The most likely estimate often is called the *base case*, so the data in Table 5.3 represent the clinic's base case cost forecast. Expected total costs for 2008 are $7,080,962. Because these costs support 75,000 visits, the forecasted average cost per visit is $7,080,962 / 75,000 = $94.41.

Focusing solely on total costs does not provide the clinic's managers with much information regarding potential alternative financial outcomes for 2008. In essence, a single (total cost) amount suggests that the clinic's costs will remain constant regardless of the number of patient visits. Similarly, the base case average cost per visit amount of $94.41 implicitly treats all costs as variable costs, suggesting that the cost per visit would be $94.41 regardless of volume. Total cost information is necessary and useful, but the detailed breakdown in Table 5.3 gives the clinic's managers more insight into prospective financial outcomes for 2008 than is possible with a total cost focus.

Table 5.3 categorizes the clinic's total costs of $7,080,962 into two components: total variable costs of $2,113,500 and total fixed costs of $4,967,462. These cost amounts are fundamentally different, both in quantitative and qualitative terms. The total fixed costs of $4,967,462 must be borne by the clinic regardless of the actual volume in 2008. However, total variable costs of $2,113,500 apply only to a volume of 75,000 patient visits. If the actual number of visits realized in 2008 is less than or greater than 75,000,

	Variable Costs	Fixed Costs	Total Costs
Salaries and Benefits:			
Management and supervision	$ 0	$ 928,687	$ 928,687
Coordinators	442,617	598,063	1,040,680
Specialists	0	38,600	38,600
Technicians	681,383	552,670	1,234,053
Clerical/administrative	71,182	58,240	129,422
Social security taxes	89,622	163,188	252,810
Group health insurance	115,924	211,081	327,005
Professional fees	325,489	383,360	708,849
Supplies	313,283	231,184	544,467
Utilities	74,000	45,040	119,040
Allocated costs	0	1,757,349	1,757,349
Total	$2,113,500	$4,967,462	$7,080,962

TABLE 5.3
Atlanta Clinic: Forecasted Cost Data for 2008 (based on 75,000 patient visits)

total variable costs will be less than or greater than $2,133,500. (Of course, this is the primary reason that costs are classified as fixed and variable in the first place.)

The best way to highlight that total variable costs vary with volume is to express variable costs on a per unit (variable cost rate) basis. For Atlanta Clinic, the implied variable cost rate is $2,113,500 / 75,000 visits = $28.18 per visit. Thus, the clinic's total costs at any volume within the relevant range can be calculated as follows:

$$\text{Total costs} = \text{Fixed costs} + \text{Total variable costs}$$
$$= \$4,967,462 + (\$28.18 \times \text{Number of visits}).$$

This equation, the *cost behavior model*, explicitly shows that total costs depend on volume. To illustrate use of the cost behavior model, consider three potential volumes for 2008: 70,000, 75,000, and 80,000 patient visits:

Volume = 70,000:
$$\text{Total costs} = \$4,967,462 + (\$28.18 \times 70,000)$$
$$= \$4,967,462 + \$1,972,600 = \$6,940,062.$$

Volume = 75,000:
$$\text{Total costs} = \$4,967,462 + (\$28.18 \times 75,000)$$
$$= \$4,967,462 + \$2,113,500 = \$7,080,962.$$

Volume = 80,000:
$$\text{Total costs} = \$4,967,462 + (\$28.18 \times 80,000)$$
$$= \$4,967,462 + \$2,254,400 = \$7,221,862.$$

When an organization's costs are expressed in this way, it is easy to see that higher volume leads to higher total costs.

Atlanta Clinic's underlying cost structure is plotted in Figure 5.3. (To simplify the graph, we assume that the relevant range extends to zero visits.) As first illustrated in Figure 5.1, fixed costs are shown as a horizontal dashed line and total costs are shown as an upward-sloping solid line with a slope (rise over run) equal to the variable cost rate—$28.18 per visit. Unlike Figure 5.1, the graphical presentation has been simplified by not showing total variable costs as a separate line starting at the origin. Of course, total variable costs are represented in Figure 5.3 by the vertical distance between the total costs line and the fixed costs line.

Note that Atlanta Clinic does not literally write out a check for $28.18 for each visit, although there may be examples of variable costs in which this is the case. Rather, Atlanta's cost structure indicates that the clinic uses certain resources that its managers have defined as inherently variable, and the best estimate of the value of such resources is $28.18 per visit.

FIGURE 5.3
Atlanta Clinic:
CVP Graphical
Model

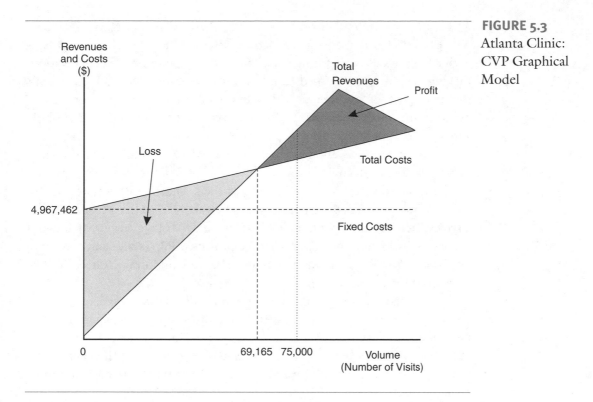

The cost structure shown in Figure 5.3 could be estimated in several ways. One way would be to use time-motion studies and interviews with clinic personnel. However, instead of such an intrusive approach, cost accountants could plot the total costs of the clinic at different volume levels for the past several years and then run a regression on these data. In this case, the beta term (slope) of the regression would be the variable cost rate, $28.18, and the alpha term (intercept) would be fixed costs, $4,967,462.

To complete the CVP model, a revenue component must be added. For 2008, Atlanta Clinic expects revenues, on average, to be $100 per patient visit. Total revenues are plotted on Figure 5.3 as an upward-sloping solid line starting at the origin and having a slope of $100 per visit. If there were no visits, total revenues would be zero; at one visit, total revenues would be $100; at ten visits, total revenues would be $1,000; at 75,000 visits, total revenues would be $7,500,000; and so on. Note that the vertical dashed line is drawn at the point where total revenues equal total costs, and the vertical dotted line is drawn at the base case volume estimate, 75,000 visits. We will examine the significance of these lines in later sections.

The Projected P&L Statement

One of the first steps that Atlanta Clinic's managers could take in terms of the 2008 CVP analysis is to project profit (net income), given the base case assumptions. Such a forecast is called a *projected profit and loss (P&L) statement*. The term *profit and loss statement* distinguishes this statement from

Atlanta Clinic's audited income statement. There are two primary differences between a P&L statement and an income statement. First, P&L statements, as with all managerial accounting data, can be developed to best serve decision-making purposes, as opposed to following GAAP. Second, P&L statements can be created for any subunit within an organization, whereas income statements normally are created only for the overall accounting entity and major subsidiaries.

Atlanta Clinic's 2008 base case projected P&L statement is shown in Table 5.4. The bottom line projects Atlanta's 2008 profit using base case values for costs, volume, and prices. Note that the format of a P&L statement for CVP analysis purposes distinguishes between variable and fixed costs, whereas a typical income statement (and P&L statements for other purposes) does not make this distinction. Also, note that the projected P&L statement contains a line labeled "total contribution margin." This very important concept will be discussed in the next section.

The projected P&L statement used in CVP analysis contains four variables—three of the variables are assumed and the fourth is calculated. In Table 5.4, the assumed variables are expected volume (75,000 visits), expected price ($100 per visit), and expected costs (delineated in terms of the clinic's cost structure). Profit, the fourth variable, is calculated on the basis of the three assumed variables.

The Table 5.4 base case projected P&L statement represents only one point on the Figure 5.3 CVP model. This point is shown by the dotted vertical line at a volume of 75,000 patient visits. Moving up along this dotted line, the distance from the X-axis to the horizontal fixed costs line represents the $4,967,462 fixed costs. The distance from the fixed costs line to the total costs line represents the $2,113,500 total variable costs. The distance between the total costs line and the total revenues line represents the $419,038 profit. As in previous figures, the graph in Figure 5.3 is not drawn to scale because it will not be used to develop numerical data. Rather, it provides the clinic's managers with a pictorial representation of Atlanta's projected financial future.

Contribution Margin

The base case projected P&L statement in Table 5.4 introduces the concept of *contribution margin*, which is defined as the difference between per unit revenue and per unit variable cost (the variable cost rate). In this illustration,

TABLE 5.4
Atlanta Clinic: 2008 Base Case Projected P&L Statement (based on 75,000 patient visits)

Total revenues ($100 × 75,000)	$7,500,000
Total variable costs ($28.18 × 75,000)	2,113,500
Total contribution margin ($71.82 × 75,000)	$5,386,500
Fixed costs	4,967,462
Profit	$ 419,038

the contribution margin is $100.00 - $28.18 = $71.82. What is the inherent meaning of this contribution margin value of $71.82? The contribution margin has the look and feel of profit because it is calculated as revenue minus cost. However, because none of the fixed costs of providing service have been included in the cost amount used in the calculation, it is **not** profit. Rather, because variable costs have been stripped out, the contribution margin is the dollar amount per visit available to cover Atlanta Clinic's fixed costs. Only after fixed costs are fully covered does the contribution margin begin to contribute to profit.

With a contribution margin of $71.82 on each of the clinic's 75,000 visits, the projected base case *total contribution margin* for 2008 is $71.82 × 75,000 = $5,386,500, which is sufficient to cover the clinic's fixed costs of $4,967,462 and then provide a $5,386,500 - $4,967,462 = $419,038 profit. After fixed costs have been covered, any additional visits contribute to the clinic's profit at a rate of $71.82 per visit. Readers will discover that the contribution margin concept is used again and again as our discussion of CVP analysis continues.

<table>
<tr><td>

1. Construct a simple P&L statement like the one in Table 5.4, and discuss its elements.
2. Sketch and explain a simple diagram to match your table.
3. Define and explain the contribution margin.

</td><td>

Self-Test Questions

</td></tr>
</table>

Breakeven Analysis

In healthcare finance, *breakeven analysis* is applied in many different situations, so it is necessary to understand the context to fully understand the meaning of the term *break even*. Generically, breakeven analyses are used to determine a *breakeven point*, which is the value of a given input variable that produces some minimum desired result. In the specific situation at hand, we will use breakeven analysis to determine the volume, called the *breakeven volume*, at which a business or program or service becomes financially self-sufficient. Although the breakeven analysis discussed here is actually part of profit (CVP) analysis, the concept deserves separate consideration.

Note that there are two different definitions of breakeven volume. *Accounting breakeven* is defined as the volume needed to produce zero profit. In other words, the volume that produces revenues equal to accounting costs. Alternatively, *economic breakeven* is defined as the volume needed to produce a target profit level. In other words, the volume that creates revenues equal to accounting costs **plus** the desired profit amount.

As mentioned in the previous section, the P&L statement format used here is a four-variable model. When the focus is profit, the three assumed variables are costs, volume, and price, while profit is calculated. When the focus is volume breakeven, the same four variables are used, but profit is now assumed to be known while volume is the unknown (calculated) value. However, it is also possible to assume a value for volume and price (or costs) and then calculate the breakeven value for costs (or price). A breakeven point can be obtained two ways: algebraically or graphically. To illustrate the algebraic approach, the projected P&L statement presented in Table 5.4 can be expressed algebraically as the following equation:

$$\text{Total revenues} - \text{Total variable costs} - \text{Fixed costs} = \text{Profit}$$
$$(\$100 \times \text{Volume}) - (\$28.18 \times \text{Volume}) - \$4,967,462 = \text{Profit}.$$

By definition, at accounting breakeven the clinic's profit equals zero, so the equation can be rewritten this way:

$$(\$100 \times \text{Volume}) - (\$28.18 \times \text{Volume}) - \$4,967,462 = \$0.$$

Rearranging the terms so that only the terms related to volume appear on the left side produces this equation:

$$(\$100 \times \text{Volume}) - (\$28.18 \times \text{Volume}) = \$4,967,462.$$

Using basic algebra, the two terms on the left side can be combined because volume appears in both. The end result is this:

$$(\$100 - \$28.18) \times \text{Volume} = \$4,967,462$$
$$\$71.82 \times \text{Volume} = \$4,967,462.$$

The left side of the breakeven equation now contains the contribution margin, $71.82, multiplied by volume. Here, the previous conclusion that the clinic will break even when the total contribution margin equals fixed costs is reaffirmed. Solving the equation for volume results in a breakeven point of $4,967,462 / $71.82 = 69,165 visits. Any volume greater than 69,165 visits produces a profit for the clinic, while any volume less than 69,165 results in a loss.

The logic behind the breakeven point is this: Each patient visit brings in $100, of which $28.18 is the variable cost to treat the patient. This leaves a $71.82 contribution margin from each visit. If the clinic sets the contribution margin aside for the first 69,165 visits in 2008, it would have $4,967,430, which is enough (except for a small rounding difference) to cover its fixed costs. Once the clinic exceeds breakeven volume, each visit's contribution margin flows directly to profit. If the clinic achieves its volume estimate of 75,000 visits, the 5,835 visits above the breakeven point result in a total profit of 5,835 × $71.82 = $419,070, which matches the profit (again except for a rounding difference) shown on the clinic's base case projected income statement in Table 5.4.

The second method for determining the breakeven point is by graphical analysis. At accounting breakeven the profit is zero, so total revenues must equal total costs. On a CVP graph such as Figure 5.3, this condition holds at the intersection of the total revenues line and the total costs line. This point is indicated by a vertical dashed line drawn at a volume of 69,165 visits. If a very large sheet of graph paper were used, the lines could be drawn to scale and the breakeven point could be read off of the graph.

The logic of the breakeven point illustrated in Figure 5.3 goes back to the nature of the clinic's fixed and variable cost structure. Before even one patient walks in the door, the clinic has already committed to $4,967,462 in fixed costs. Because the total revenues line is steeper than the total variable costs line, and hence the total costs line, as volume increases total revenues eventually catch up to the clinic's cost structure. Any utilization to the right of the breakeven point, which is shown as a dark-shaded area, produces a profit; any utilization to the left, which is shown as a light-shaded area, results in a loss.

The relationship between breakeven analysis and the projected P&L statement is important to understand. Based on the clinic's base case projection of 75,000 visits, it can anticipate a profit of $419,038. However, management may worry that the clinic will not achieve this projected volume and ask the following question: What is the minimum number of visits that are needed to at least break even? The answer is 69,165 visits.

To verify the breakeven point, Table 5.5 contains a projected P&L statement for 69,165 visits. Except for a small rounding difference, the profit at the breakeven point is $0. (The breakeven point was actually 69,165.1 visits.) As mentioned previously, at breakeven the total contribution margin just covers fixed costs, resulting in zero accounting profit.

This breakeven analysis contains important assumptions. The first assumption is that the price or set of prices for different types of patients and different payers is independent of volume. In other words, volume increases are not attained by lowering prices, and price increases are not met with volume declines. The second assumption is that costs can be reasonably subdivided into fixed and variable components. The third assumption is that both fixed costs and the variable cost rate are independent of volume over the relevant range, so both the total costs line and the total revenues line are linear.

Breakeven analysis is often performed in an iterative manner. After the breakeven volume is calculated, managers must determine whether the resulting volume can realistically be achieved at the price assumed in the analysis.

Total revenues ($100 × 69,165)		$6,916,500
Total variable costs ($28.18 × 69,165)		1,949,070
Total contribution margin		$4,967,430
Fixed costs		4,967,462
Profit		($ 32)

TABLE 5.5
Atlanta Clinic: 2008 Projected P&L Statement (based on 69,165 patient visits)

If the price appears to be unreasonable for the breakeven volume, a new price has to be estimated and the breakeven analysis repeated. Likewise, if the cost structure used for the calculation appears to be unrealistic at the breakeven volume, operational assumptions and hence cost assumptions should be changed and the analysis repeated again.

Instead of asking the number of visits needed for accounting breakeven, Atlanta's managers may ask the number of visits needed to achieve a $100,000 profit or, for that matter, any other profit level. By building a profit target into the breakeven analysis, the focus is now on economic breakeven. The clinic will have a $419,038 profit if it has 75,000 visits, and it will have no profit if it has 69,165 visits. Thus, the number of visits required to achieve a $100,000 profit target (economic breakeven) is somewhere in between 69,165 and 75,000. In fact, the number of visits required is 70,558:

$$\text{Total revenues} - \text{Total variable costs} - \text{Fixed costs} = \text{Profit}$$
$$(\$100 \times \text{Volume}) - (\$28.18 \times \text{Volume}) - \$4,967,462 = \$100,000$$
$$(\$71.82 \times \text{Volume}) - \$4,967,462 = \$100,000$$
$$\$71.82 \times \text{Volume} = \$5,067,462$$
$$\text{Volume} = 70,558.$$

Self-Test Questions
1. What is the purpose of breakeven analysis?
2. What is the equation for volume breakeven?
3. Why is breakeven analysis often conducted in an iterative manner?
4. What is the difference between accounting and economic breakeven?

Operating Leverage

As we have demonstrated, profit analysis is used to examine how changes in volume affect profits and to estimate breakeven points. Assume now that Atlanta Clinic's managers believe that changes in the local market for healthcare services will occur that increase their volume estimate for 2008 to 82,500 visits—an increase of 7,500 visits over the original 75,000 visit base case estimate. Table 5.6 contains the clinic's projected P&L statements at 69,165 (accounting breakeven), 75,000 (base case), and 82,500 visits. The first two columns are the same as previously constructed. The third column, which represents the 82,500 visit estimate, is new.

Now that P&L statements exist at three different volume levels, the consequences of volume changes can be better understood. As the clinic's forecasted volume moves from 75,000 visits to 82,500 visits, its profit increases by $957,688 − $419,038 = $538,650. This increase is equal to the additional 7,500 visits multiplied by the $71.82 contribution margin. When the volume is beyond the accounting breakeven point, any additional visits are

	Number of Visits		
	69,165	75,000	82,500
Total revenues ($100 × volume)	$6,916,500	$7,500,000	$8,250,000
Total variable costs ($28.18 × volume)	1,949,070	2,113,500	2,324,850
Total contribution margin ($71.82 × volume)	$4,967,430	$5,386,500	$5,925,150
Fixed costs	4,967,462	4,967,462	4,967,462
Profit	($ 32)	$ 419,038	$ 957,688

TABLE 5.6

Atlanta Clinic: 2008 Projected P&L Statements (based on 69,165; 75,000; and 82,500 patient visits)

"gravy"—that is, the clinic's fixed costs are now covered, so all contribution margin additions flow directly to profit. Similarly, the outcome is known if the clinic's projected volume dropped from 75,000 to 69,165 visits. In this case, the decrease of 5,835 visits multiplied by the $71.82 contribution margin equals $419,670, which is the loss of profit (except for a rounding difference) that results from the volume decrease.

The movement from 75,000 to 82,500 visits resulted in a (82,500 − 75,000) / 75,000 = 7,500 / 75,000 = 0.10 = 10% increase in volume and thus total revenues. While the top line of the P&L statement—total revenues—increased by 10 percent, the bottom line of the statement—profit—increased by 128.5 percent ($538,650 / $419,038 = 1.285 = 128.5%). This incredible increase in profit occurs because the clinic is reaping the benefit of its cost structure, which includes fixed costs that do not increase with volume.

If a high proportion of a business's total costs are fixed, the business is said to have high *operating leverage*. In physics, leverage implies the use of a lever to raise a heavy object with a small amount of force. In politics, individuals who have leverage can accomplish much with the smallest word or action. In finance, high operating leverage means that a relatively small change in volume results in a large change in profit.

Operating leverage is measured by the *degree of operating leverage (DOL)*, which at any volume is calculated by dividing the total contribution margin by earnings before interest and taxes (EBIT), which for not-for-profit businesses is merely profit plus any interest expense. At a volume of 75,000 visits, Atlanta Clinic's degree of operating leverage is $5,386,500 / $419,038 = 12.85. (We have no information regarding the clinic's interest expense, so we are simply using its expected profit.) The DOL indicates how much profit will change for each 1 percent change in volume. Thus, each 1 percent change in volume produces a 12.85 percent change in profit, so a 10 percent increase in volume results in a 10% × 12.85 = 128.5% increase in profit. Note, however, that the DOL changes with volume, so the 12.85 DOL calculated here is applicable only to a starting volume of 75,000 visits.

Cost structures differ widely among industries and among organizations within a given industry. The DOL is greatest in health services organizations with a large proportion of fixed costs and, consequently, a low proportion of variable costs. The end result is a high contribution margin, which contributes to a high DOL. In economics terminology, high-DOL businesses are said to have *economies of scale* because higher volumes lead to lower per unit total costs. In such businesses, a small increase in revenue produces a relatively large increase in profit. However, high DOL businesses have relatively high breakeven points, which increase the risk of losses. Also, operating leverage is a double-edged sword: High DOL businesses suffer large profit declines, and potentially large losses, if volume falls.

To illustrate the negative effect of a high DOL, consider this question: What would happen to Atlanta Clinic's profit if volume fell by 7.8 percent from the base case level of 75,000 visits? To answer this question, recognize that profit would decline by $7.8\% \times 12.85 \approx 100\%$, so the clinic's profit would fall to zero. The data in Table 5.6 confirm this answer. At a projected volume of 69,165 visits (a decrease of 7.8 percent from 75,000 visits), the clinic's profit is zero. Of course, this volume was previously identified as the breakeven point.

To what extent can managers influence a business's operating leverage? In many respects, operating leverage is determined by the inherent nature of the business. In general, hospitals and other institutional providers must make large investments in fixed assets, and hence they have a high proportion of fixed costs and high operating leverage. Conversely, home health care businesses and other noninstitutional providers need few fixed assets, so they tend to have relatively low operating leverage. Still, managers can somewhat influence operating leverage. For example, organizations can make use of temporary, rather than permanent, employees to handle peak patient loads. Also, assets can be leased on a per use (per procedure) basis, rather than purchased or leased on a fixed rental basis. Actions such as these tend to reduce the proportion of fixed costs in an organization's cost structure, and hence reduce operating leverage.

Self-Test Questions
1. What is operating leverage, and how is it measured?
2. Why is the operating leverage concept important to managers?
3. Can managers influence their firms' operating leverage?
4. How does an organization's cost structure affect its exposure to economies of scale?

Profit Analysis in a Discounted Fee-for-Service Environment

As noted in the previous discussion, profit (CVP) analysis is quite valuable to managers in that it provides information about expected costs and profitability under alternative estimates of volume. To learn more about its usefulness, suppose that one-third (25,000) of Atlanta Clinic's expected 75,000 visits would come from Peachtree HMO, which has proposed that its new contract with the clinic contain a 40 percent discount from charges. Thus, the net price for their patients would be $60 instead of the undiscounted $100. If the clinic refuses, Peachtree has threatened to take its members elsewhere.

At first blush, Peachtree's proposal appears to be unacceptable. Among other reasons, $60 is less than the full cost of providing service, which was determined previously to be $94.41 per visit at a volume of 75,000. Thus, on a full-cost basis, Atlanta would lose $94.41 − $60 = $34.41 per visit on Peachtree's patients. With an estimated 25,000 visits, the discounted contract would result in a total profit loss of 25,000 × $34.41 = $860,250. However, before Atlanta's managers reject Peachtree's proposal, it must be examined more closely.

The Impact of Rejecting the Proposal

If Atlanta's managers reject the proposal, the clinic would lose market share—an estimated 25,000 visits. The projected P&L statement that would result, which is based on 50,000 undiscounted visits, is shown in Table 5.7. At the lower volume, the clinic's total revenues, total variable costs, and total contribution margin decrease proportionately (i.e., by one-third). However, fixed costs are not reduced, so Atlanta would not cover its fixed costs, and hence a loss of $3,591,000 − $4,967,462 = −$1,376,462 would occur. To view the situation another way, the expected volume of 50,000 visits is 19,165 short of the breakeven point, so the clinic would be operating to the left of the breakeven point in Figure 5.3. This shortfall from breakeven of 19,165 visits, when multiplied by the contribution margin of $71.82, produces a loss of $1,376,430, which is the same as shown in Table 5.7 (except for a rounding difference).

Clearly, the major factor behind the projected loss is the clinic's fixed cost structure of $4,967,462. With a projected decrease in volume of 33 percent, perhaps the clinic could reduce its fixed costs. If Atlanta's managers perceive the volume reduction to be permanent, they would begin to reduce the fixed costs currently in place to meet an anticipated volume of 75,000 visits. However, if the clinic's managers believe that the loss of volume is merely a temporary occurrence, they may choose to maintain the current fixed cost structure and absorb the loss expected for next year. It would not make

Total revenues ($100 × 50,000)	$5,000,000
Total variable costs ($28.18 × 50,000)	1,409,000
Total contribution margin ($71.82 × 50,000)	$3,591,000
Fixed costs	4,967,462
Profit	($1,376,462)

TABLE 5.7 Atlanta Clinic: 2008 Projected P&L Statement (based on 50,000 undiscounted patient visits)

Undiscounted revenue ($100 × 50,000)	$5,000,000
Discounted revenue ($60 × 25,000)	1,500,000
Total revenues ($86.67 × 75,000)	$6,500,000
Total variable costs ($28.18 × 75,000)	2,113,500
Total contribution margin ($58.49 × 75,000)	$4,386,500
Fixed costs	4,967,462
Profit	($ 580,962)

sense for them to start selling off equipment and facilities, and firing staff, only to reverse these actions one year later. The critical point, though, is that the loss of volume caused by rejecting Peachtree's proposal can have a significant negative impact on the clinic's profit, which indicates that the clinic's fixed cost structure should be reexamined.

The Impact of Accepting the Proposal

An alternative strategy for the clinic's managers would be to accept Peachtree's proposal. The resulting projected P&L statement is contained in Table 5.8. The average per visit revenue of serving these two different payer groups is $(2/3 \times \$100) + (1/3 \times \$60) = \$86.67$. Total revenues based on this average revenue per visit would be $75,000 \times \$86.67 = \$6,500,250$, which equals the value for total revenues shown in the table (except for a rounding difference). With a lower average revenue per visit, the contribution margin falls to $86.67 − $28.18 = $58.49, which leads to a lower total contribution margin.

The critical point here is that the clinic's total revenues have decreased significantly from the previous situation in which all visits bring in $100 in revenue (see Table 5.4). However, the clinic's total costs remain the same because it is handling the same number of visits—75,000. The impact of the discount is strictly on revenues, and the end result of accepting Peachtree's proposal is a projected loss of $580,962.

Another way of confirming the expected loss at 75,000 visits is to calculate the clinic's accounting breakeven point at the new average per visit revenue of $86.67. The new breakeven point is 84,928 visits, which confirms that the clinic will lose money at 75,000 visits. Because the clinic is projected to be $84,928 − 75,000 = 9,928$ visits below breakeven, and the contribution margin is now $58.49, the projected loss is $9,928 \times \$58.49 = \$580,689$, which is the amount shown in Table 5.8 (except for a rounding difference).

The change in breakeven point that results from accepting Peachtree's proposal is graphed in Figure 5.4, along with the original breakeven point. The new total revenues line (the dot-dashed line) is flatter than the original line, so when it is combined with the existing cost structure, the breakeven point is pushed to the right, to 84,928 visits. However, any cost-control actions taken by Atlanta's managers would either flatten, if variable costs are lowered,

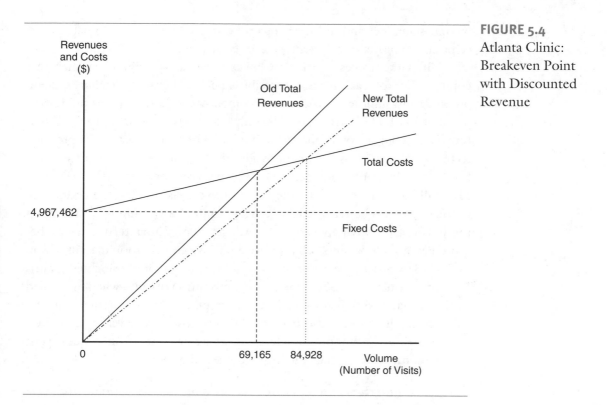

FIGURE 5.4
Atlanta Clinic:
Breakeven Point
with Discounted
Revenue

or lower, if fixed costs are reduced, the total costs line, and hence push the breakeven point back to the left.

Nothing much has changed in terms of core economic underpinnings because of the new discounted-charge environment. The clinic is worse off economically, but the clinic's cost structure, managerial incentives, and solutions to financial problems are essentially the same. To increase profit, more services must be provided. In short, the movement from charges to discounted charges is not that radical with regard to its impact on profit analysis and managerial decision making. The major difference is that the clinic is now under greater financial pressure. However, as we discuss in the next major section, the clinic's entire incentive structure will change if it moves to a capitated environment.

Evaluating the Alternative Strategies

What should Atlanta's managers do? If Peachtree's discount proposal is accepted, the clinic is expected to lose $580,962 rather than make a profit of $419,038 if no discount was demanded. The difference is a swing of $1 million in profit in the wrong direction, hardly an enticing prospect. What happened to the "missing" $1 million? It is now in the hands of Peachtree HMO, which is paying $1 million less to one of its providers (25,000 visits × $40 savings = $1,000,000). This will be reflected as a cost savings on Peachtree's income statement and, if the savings is not passed on to the ultimate payers (typically employers), will result in a profit increase.

If market forces in Atlanta Clinic's service area suggest that making a counter offer to Peachtree is not feasible—perhaps because the clinic is being pitted against another provider—the comparison of a loss of $580,792 to a profit of $419,038 is irrelevant. The only relevant issue at hand for the short-term is the comparison of the $580,792 loss if the clinic accepts the proposal to the $1,376,462 loss if the proposal is rejected and Peachtree's patients are lost to the clinic. Although neither outcome is very appealing, the acceptance of the discount appears to be the lesser of two evils. In fact, the acceptance of the discount is better by $1,376,462 − $580,792 = $795,670. Accepting the discount proposal appears to be Atlanta's best **short-term** strategy because Peachtree's patients still produce a positive contribution margin of $60 − $28.18 = $31.82 per visit, which would be foregone if the clinic rebuffs Peachtree's offer. That $31.82 per visit contribution margin, when multiplied by the expected 25,000 visits on the contract, puts $795,500 on the total contribution margin table that otherwise would be lost. (However, if acceptance of Peachtree's discount proposal leads to similar proposals from other payers, the best **long-term** strategy might be to reject the proposal.)

Marginal Analysis: Short-Term Versus Long-Term Implications

The Atlanta/Peachtree illustration points out one way in which the contribution margin can be used in managerial decision making. To help reinforce the concept, the analysis can be viewed from a different perspective. Suppose the clinic is forecasting a base case volume of only **50,000 visits** for 2008, and Peachtree HMO offers to provide the clinic 25,000 additional visits at $60 revenue per visit. These 25,000 visits are called *marginal*, or *incremental*, *visits*, because they add to the existing base of visits. Should the clinic's managers accept this offer?

Although each marginal visit from the contract brings in only $60 compared with $100 on the clinic's other contracts, the *marginal cost*, which is the cost associated with each additional visit, is the variable cost rate of $28.18. The clinic's $4,967,462 in fixed costs will be incurred whether the offer is accepted or rejected, so these costs are not relevant to the decision. In finance parlance, the clinic's fixed costs are *nonincremental* to the decision. Because the contribution margin of each visit at the margin (the *marginal contribution margin*) is a positive $31.82, each visit contributes positively to Atlanta's recovery of fixed costs and ultimately to profits, so the offer must be seriously considered. Note that this conclusion is based on the assumption that the relevant range of volumes is from 50,000 or fewer visits to at least 75,000 visits, and hence that the current level of fixed costs can support the added volume. If 75,000 visits is beyond the relevant range, then new fixed costs must be incurred and these now become incremental to the decision.

In this situation, the marginal cost consists of the variable cost rate **plus** the incremental fixed cost per additional visit.)

However, Atlanta's managers cannot ignore the long-term implications associated with accepting the proposal. These are not addressed in detail here, but clearly the clinic cannot survive this scenario in the long run because the clinic's revenues are not covering the full costs of providing services. In the meantime, bleeding $580,962 of losses in 2008 may be better than bleeding $1,376,462 until the clinic can adjust to market forces in its service area. This adjustment may be as simple as merely absorbing the losses while the clinic's competitors, perhaps in poorer financial condition, exit the market as they too face the same difficult economic choices. Should this happen, a new equilibrium would be established in the market that would allow the clinic to raise its prices. If the long-term solution is not that simple, Atlanta Clinic must reduce its cost structure or perish.

Another problem associated with accepting the discount offer is that the clinic's other payers will undoubtedly learn about the reduced payments and want to renegotiate their contracts with the same, or even greater, discount. Such a reaction would clearly place the clinic under even more financial pressure, and a draconian change in either volume or operating costs would be required for survival.

1. What is the impact of a discount contract on fixed costs, total variable costs, and the breakeven point?
2. What is meant by marginal analysis?
3. What is meant by the following statement: "Marginal analysis is made more complicated by long-run considerations."

Self-Test Questions

Profit Analysis in a Capitated Environment

As a review of profit analysis, consider how the analysis is changed when a provider operates in a capitated environment. Although capitation is being used less today than it was several years ago, the addition of a capitated payment analysis both provides an excellent review of the concepts presented in previous sections and highlights the basic differences between the two reimbursement methods.

To begin, assume that the purchaser of services from Atlanta Clinic is the Alliance, a local business coalition. As in previous illustrations, assume the Alliance is paying the clinic $7,500,000 to provide services for an expected 75,000 visits, but now the amount is **capitated**. Although projected total revenues remain the same as the previous base case (see Table 5.4), the nature of the capitated revenues is actually quite different. The $7,500,000 that the Alliance is paying is not explicitly related to the amount of services provided by the clinic but to the size of the covered employee group. In essence, Atlanta Clinic is no longer merely selling healthcare services as it had in the fee-for-service or discounted fee-for-service environment. Now the clinic is taking on the insurance function in that it is responsible for the health status (utilization) of the covered population and must bear the attendant risks. If the total costs of services delivered by the clinic exceed the premium revenue (paid monthly on a per member basis), the clinic will suffer the financial consequences. However, if the clinic can efficiently manage the healthcare of the served population, it will be the economic beneficiary.

How might Atlanta's managers evaluate whether or not the $7,500,000 revenue attached to the contract is adequate? To do the analysis, they need two critical pieces of information: cost information and actuarial (utilization) information. The clinic already has the cost accounting information—the full cost per visit is expected to be $94.41 (at a volume of 75,000 visits), with an underlying cost structure of $28.18 per visit in variable costs and $4,967,462 in fixed costs. For its actuarial information, Atlanta's managers estimate that the Alliance will have a covered population of 18,750 members with an expected utilization rate of four visits per member per year. Thus, the total number of visits expected is $18,750 \times 4 = 75,000$. Although this appears to be the same 75,000 visits as in the fee-for-service environment, significant difference exists in the implications of this volume. Because there is no direct linkage between the volume of services provided and revenues, utilization above that expected will bring increased costs with **no corresponding** increase in revenues.

The revenues expected from this contract, $7,500,000, exceed the expected costs of serving this population, which are 75,000 visits multiplied by $94.41 per visit, or $7,080,750. Thus, this contract is expected to generate a profit of $419,250, which, not surprisingly, is the same as the original base case fee-for-service result (except for a rounding difference). (See Table 5.4.)

A Graphical View in Terms of Utilization

Figure 5.5 contains a graphical profit (CVP) analysis for the capitation contract that is constructed similar to the fee-for-service graphs shown in Figures 5.3 and 5.4 in that the horizontal axis shows volume (number of visits), while the vertical axis shows revenues and costs. Also shown is the same underlying cost structure of $4,967,462 in fixed costs coupled with a variable cost rate of $28.18. One very significant difference exists, however. Instead of being upward sloping, the total revenues line is horizontal, which shows that total revenue is $7,500,000 regardless of volume **as measured by the number of visits.**

Several subtle messages are inherent in this flat revenue line. First, it tells managers that revenue is being driven by something other than the volume of services provided. Under capitation, revenue is being driven by the insurance contract (i.e., by the premium payment and the number of covered lives, or

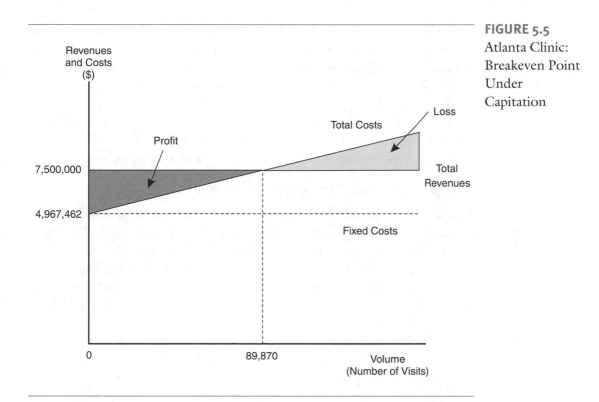

FIGURE 5.5
Atlanta Clinic:
Breakeven Point
Under
Capitation

enrollees). This change in the revenue source is the core of the logic switch from fee-for-service to capitation; the clinic is being rewarded to manage the healthcare of the population served rather than merely to provide services. However, the clinic's costs are still driven by the amount of services provided (the number of visits).

A second critical point about Figure 5.5 is the difference between the flat revenue and the flat fixed-cost base. Atlanta has a spread of $7,500,000 − $4,967,462 = $2,532,538 to work with in the management of the healthcare of this population for the period of the contract. If total variable costs equal $2,532,538, the clinic breaks even; if total variable costs exceed $2,532,538, the clinic loses. Thus, to make a profit, the number of visits must be less than $2,532,538 / $28.18 = 89,870. If everyone in the organization, especially the managers and clinicians, does not understand the inherent utilization risk under capitation, the clinic could find itself in serious financial trouble. On the other hand, if Atlanta's managers and clinicians at all levels understand and manage this utilization risk, a handsome reward may be gained.

A key feature of capitation is the reversal of the profit and loss portions of the graph. To see this, compare Figure 5.5 with Figure 5.3. The idea that profits occur at lower volumes under capitation is contrary to the fee-for-service environment. It is obvious, however, when one recognizes that the contribution margin, on a per visit basis, is $0 − $28.18 = −$28.18. Thus, each additional visit increases costs by $28.18 without bringing in additional revenue. The optimal short-term response to capitation from a purely financial perspective is to take the money and run (provide no services) because zero visits allow the clinic to capture the full spread between total revenues and fixed costs. Of course, the clinic would have trouble renewing the contract in subsequent years, but it will have maximized short-term profit. Obviously, this course of action is neither appropriate nor feasible. Still, its implications are at the heart of concerns expressed by critics of managed care about the incentives to withhold patient care inherent in a capitated environment.

A Graphical View in Terms of Membership

Looking at Figure 5.5 is like being Alice, of *Alice in Wonderland,* peering through the looking glass and finding that everything is reversed. The key to this problem is that the horizontal axis does not measure the volume to which revenues are related—that is, the horizontal axis in Figure 5.5 has number of visits on the horizontal axis, just as if Atlanta Clinic were selling healthcare services. It is not; it is now selling insurance, so the appropriate horizontal axis value is the number of members (enrollees).

Figure 5.6 recognizes that membership, rather than the amount of services provided, drives revenues. With the **number of members** on the horizontal axis, the total revenues line is no longer flat; revenues only look flat when they are considered relative to the number of visits. The revenue earned by the clinic is actually $7,500,000 / 18,750 = $400 per member, which could be broken down to a monthly premium of $400 / 12 = $33.33. Thus, the expected $7,500,000 revenue shown in Figure 5.5 results from an expected enrollee population of 18,750 members. The cost structure can easily be expressed on a membership basis as well. Fixed costs are no problem within the relevant range; they are inherently volume insensitive, whether volume is measured by number of visits or number of members. Thus, Figure 5.6 shows fixed costs as the same flat, dashed line as before. However, the variable cost rate based on number of enrollees is not the same as the variable cost rate based on number of visits. Per member variable cost must be estimated from two other factors: the variable cost rate of $28.18 per visit and the expected utilization of four visits per year. The combination of the two is 4 × $28.18 = $112.72, which is the clinic's expected variable cost per member. Expressed on a per member basis, the contribution margin is now $400 − $112.72 = $287.28, as opposed to the −$28.18 when volume is based on number of visits.

The analysis based on number of members reveals that there are two elements to controlling total variable costs under capitation: the underlying variable cost of the service ($28.18 per visit) and the number of visits per member (four). The two-variable nature of the variable cost rate makes cost control more difficult under capitation. In a fee-for-service environment, cost control entails only minimizing per visit expenses. Utilization is not an issue. If anything, utilization is good because per visit revenue almost always exceeds

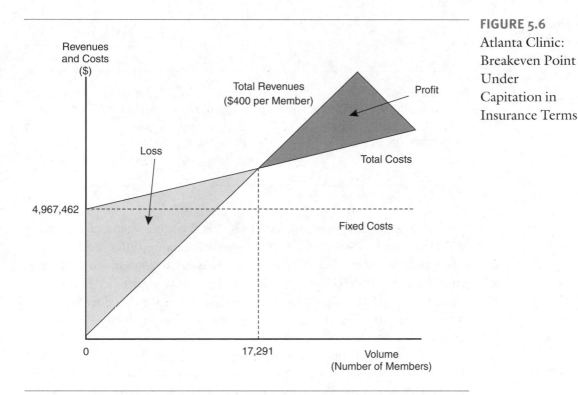

FIGURE 5.6
Atlanta Clinic:
Breakeven Point
Under
Capitation in
Insurance Terms

the variable cost rate. (In other words, there is a positive contribution margin.) Capitation requires a change in management thinking about cost control because utilization is now a component of the variable cost rate and hence total variable costs. Of course, control of fixed costs is always financially prudent, regardless of the type of reimbursement.

Conversely, there is one positive feature of the variable cost structure under capitation. With two elements to control, the clinic has more opportunity to lower the variable cost rate under capitation than under fee-for-service reimbursement. The key is the ability of Atlanta's managers to control utilization. If **both** utilization and per visit costs can be reduced, the clinic can reap greater benefits (profits) than are possible under fee-for-service reimbursement.

Projected P&L Statement Analysis

Table 5.9 contains three projected P&L statements in this capitated environment. The three volume levels shown are the same as those contained in Table 5.6 for a fee-for-service environment. To begin, start with the middle column—the one that contains the expected 75,000 patient visits. The bottom line, $419,038, is the same as in the fee-for-service analysis, which reinforces the point that, at least superficially, the capitated contract is not inherently better or worse than the fee-for-service contract.

	Number of Visits		
	69,165	75,000	82,500
Total revenues	$7,500,000	$7,500,000	$7,500,000
Total variable costs ($28.18 × volume)	1,949,070	2,113,500	2,324,850
Total contribution margin	$5,550,930	$5,386,500	$5,175,150
Fixed costs	4,967,462	4,967,462	4,967,462
Profit	$ 583,468	$ 419,038	$ 207,688

Although the profit at 75,000 visits is the same, some of the values in the projected analyses and their economic meanings differ. For example, although total revenues are $7,500,000, it is a flat amount in Table 5.9, while it varies with volume in Table 5.6. The variable cost rate is the same in both tables—$28.18 per visit. However, because each visit does not result in additional revenue, the revenue per visit is zero in Table 5.9 and the contribution margin is −$28.18.

What would happen if the clinic experienced more visits than predicted? If the number of visits increases by 10 percent, or by 7,500, to 82,500, the right column in Table 5.9 shows that profit would decrease by $419,038 − $207,688 = $211,350. This occurs because total revenues stay constant while costs increase at a rate of $28.18 for each additional visit. With 7,500 additional visits, the clinic's costs increase by 7,500 × $28.18 = $211,350. Obviously this is quite in contrast to the significant increase in profit at this volume level that occurs in a fee-for-service environment (see Table 5.6).

Under capitation, a decrease in visits will improve the profitability of the clinic. When the number of visits decreases to 69,165, which is the breakeven point in a fee-for-service environment, profit in a capitated environment increases by $164,430 to $583,468. This increase is explained by the decrease in visits (5,835) multiplied by the contribution margin (−$28.18), which results in a $164,430 decrease in costs while revenues remain constant.

The Importance of Utilization

Table 5.9 provides information on the impact of utilization changes on profitability. The center column, the base case, is once again our starting point. With an assumed utilization of four visits for each of Peachtree's 18,750 members, 75,000 visits result in a projected profit of $419,038.

However, if Atlanta's managers are not able to limit utilization to the level forecasted (or less), the clinic's profit would fall. Assume that realized utilization is actually 4.4 visits per member, rather than the 4.0 forecasted. This higher utilization would result in 4.4 × 18,750 = 82,500 visits, which produces the profit of $207,688 shown in the right column in Table 5.9. Because revenues are fixed and total costs are tied to volume, higher utilization leads to higher costs and lower profit. With the same 82,500 visits, but total variable costs of $2,324,850 at the higher utilization rate, the variable cost per member increases to $2,324,850 / 18,750 = $124.99, which could also be found by multiplying 4.4 visits per member by the variable cost rate of $28.18.

The left column of Table 5.9 shows that the clinic's profitability would increase to $583,468 if utilization was reduced to 3.69 visits per member, producing about 69,165 total visits. With lower utilization, total variable costs are reduced and profit increases. The key point is that the ability of a provider to control utilization is the primary key to profitability in a capitated environment. Less utilization means lower total costs, and lower total costs mean greater profit.

In our initial discussion of profit analysis, we introduced the concept of operating leverage, which is related to the cost structure of the organization— the higher the proportion of fixed costs, the greater the operating leverage. In a fee-for-service environment, high operating leverage means a low variable cost rate and a high per visit contribution margin, and hence high risk in that small volume decreases lead to large reductions in profitability. On the other hand, small volume increases can have a significant positive impact on the bottom line.

Under capitation, the situation is reversed because the per visit contribution margin is negative. Whereas a higher proportion of fixed costs drives the positive per visit contribution margin even higher under fee-for-service reimbursement, it drives the negative per visit contribution margin toward zero under capitation. In fact, if all of Atlanta Clinic's costs were fixed, its contribution margin would be zero, and the clinic's profit would be assured regardless of the number of visits, assuming that they fall within the relevant range. (We will have more to say about this in the next major section.)

The Importance of the Number of Members

Table 5.10 contains the projected P&L statements under capitation, recast to focus on the number of members. Assuming a per member utilization of four visits per year, a 10 percent membership increase to 20,625 members increases the projected profit by about 128 percent. However, if membership declines to 17,291, the clinic just breaks even.

We can use the breakeven equation to verify the breakeven point:

$$\text{Total revenues} \quad - \quad \text{Total variable costs} \quad - \text{Fixed costs} = \text{Profit}$$

$$(\$400 \times \text{Members}) - (\$112.72 \times \text{Members}) - \$4,967,462 = \$0$$

$$\$287.28 \times \text{Members} = \$4,967,462$$

$$\text{Members} = 17,291.$$

Thus, breakeven analysis reaffirms that the clinic needs 17,291 members in its contract with the Alliance to break even, given the assumed cost structure,

TABLE 5.10
Atlanta Clinic:
2008 Projected
P&L Statements
(based on
17,291; 18,750;
and 20,625
members)

	Number of Members		
	17,291	18,750	20,625
Total revenues ($400 × number of members)	$6,916,400	$7,500,000	$8,250,000
Total variable costs ($112.72 × members)	1,949,042	2,113,500	2,324,850
Total contribution margin	$4,967,358	$5,386,500	$5,925,150
Fixed costs	4,967,462	4,967,462	4,967,462
Profit	($ 104)	$ 419,038	$ 957,688

which in turn assumes utilization of four visits per member and a variable cost rate of $28.18 per visit.

Assuming constant per member utilization, more members increases profitability because additional members create additional revenues that presumably exceed their incremental (variable) costs. Indeed, the DOL concept can be applied here. As shown in Table 5.10, a 10 percent increase to 20,625 members from a base case membership of 18,750 results in a (roughly) 128.5 percent increase in profit (from $419,038 to $957,688, or by $538,650). Thus, each 1 percent increase in membership increases profitability by 12.85 percent. Similarly, if membership decreases to the breakeven point of 17,291, a decrease of 7.8 percent, profitability falls by 7.8% × 12.85 ≈ 100%, which leads to a profit of zero.

Self-Test Questions

1. Under capitation, what is the difference between a CVP graph with the number of visits on the X axis versus one with the number of members on the X axis?
2. What is unique about the contribution margin under capitation?
3. Why is utilization management so important in a capitated environment?
4. Why is the number of members so important in a capitated environment?

The Impact of Cost Structure on Financial Risk

The financial risk of a healthcare provider, at least in theory, is minimized by having a cost structure that "matches" its revenue structure. To illustrate, consider a clinic with all payers using fee-for-service reimbursement and hence revenues directly related to volume. If the clinic's cost structure consisted of all variable costs (no fixed costs), then each visit would incur costs but at the same time create revenues. Assuming that the per visit revenue amount exceeds the variable cost rate (per visit costs), the clinic would "lock in" a profit on each visit. The total profitability of the clinic would be uncertain, as it is tied to volume, but the ability of the clinic to generate a profit would be guaranteed.

At the other extreme, consider a clinic that is totally capitated. In this situation, assuming a fixed number of covered lives, the clinic's revenue stream is fixed regardless of volume. Now, to match the revenue and cost structures, the clinic must have all fixed (no variable) costs. Assuming that annual fixed revenue exceeds annual fixed costs, the clinic has a guaranteed profit at the end of the year.

Note that in both illustrations, the key to minimizing risk (ensuring a profit) is to create a cost structure that matches the revenue structure: variable costs for fee-for-service revenues and fixed costs for capitated revenues. Of course, "real world" problems occur when a provider tries to implement a cost structure that matches its revenue structure. First, very few providers are reimbursed solely on a fee-for-service or a capitated basis. Most providers face a mix of reimbursement methods. Still, most providers are either predominantly fee-for-service or predominantly capitated.

Second, providers do not have complete control over their cost structures. It is impossible for providers to create cost structures with all variable or all fixed costs. Nevertheless, managers can take actions to change their existing cost structure to one that is more compatible with the revenue structure (has less risk). For example, assume a medical group practice is reimbursed almost exclusively on a per procedure basis. To minimize financial risk, the practice can take such actions as pay physicians on a per procedure basis and use per procedure leases for diagnostic equipment. The greater the proportion of variable costs in the practice's cost structure, the lower its financial risk.

Self-Test Questions

1. Explain this statement: To minimize financial risk, match the cost structure to the revenue structure.
2. What cost structure would minimize risk if a provider had all fee-for-service reimbursement?
3. What cost structure would minimize risk if a provider were entirely capitated?
4. What are the real world constraints on creating matching cost structures?

Key Concepts

Managers rely on managerial accounting information to plan for and control a business's operations. A critical part of managerial accounting information is the measurement of costs and the use of this information in profit analysis. The key concepts of this chapter are:

- Costs can be classified by their relationship to the *amount of services provided*.
- *Variable costs* are those costs that are expected to increase and decrease

with volume (patient days, number of visits, and so on), while *fixed costs* are the costs that are expected to remain constant regardless of volume within some *relevant range*. *Semi-fixed costs* are those that are fixed within ranges that are less than the relevant range.

- The relationship between cost and activity (volume) is called *cost behavior* or *underlying cost structure*.
- *Profit analysis*, often called *cost-volume-profit (CVP) analysis*, is an analytical technique that typically is used to analyze the effects of volume changes on revenues, costs, and profit.
- A *projected profit and loss (P&L) statement* is a profit projection that, in a profit analysis context, uses assumed values for volume, price, and costs.
- *Breakeven analysis* is used to estimate the volume needed (or the value of some other variable) for the organization to break even in profitability.
- *Accounting breakeven* occurs when revenues equal accounting costs, while *economic breakeven* occurs when revenues equal accounting costs **plus** some profit target.
- *Contribution margin* is the difference between unit price and the *variable cost rate*, or per unit revenue minus per unit variable cost. Hence, contribution margin is the per unit dollar amount available to first cover an organization's fixed costs and then to contribute to profits.
- *Operating leverage* reflects the extent to which an organization's costs are fixed. It is measured by the *degree of operating leverage (DOL)*. Assuming fee-for-service reimbursement, a business with a high DOL has more risk than a business with a low DOL because DOL measures the impact of utilization changes on profits. Thus, in a fee-for-service environment, high-DOL businesses benefit most from increases in utilization. Conversely, high-DOL businesses are hurt the most when utilization falls.
- In *marginal analysis*, the focus is on the incremental (marginal) profitability associated with increasing or decreasing volume.
- A *capitated environment* dramatically changes the situation for providers vis-à-vis a fee-for-service environment. In essence, a capitated provider takes on the insurance function.
- Under capitation, the revenue per unit of volume, when measured traditionally, is zero. Thus, provider risk is minimized with a high DOL (high fixed costs), which results in a low variable cost rate and a small but negative contribution margin.
- The keys to success in a capitated environment are to manage (reduce) utilization and increase the number of members covered.
- To minimize financial risk, a provider should strive to attain a cost structure that matches its revenue structure.

In Chapter 6, the discussion of managerial accounting continues with an examination of the second major classification of costs, which is based on the relationship of costs to the subunit being analyzed.

Questions

5.1 Explain the differences between fixed costs, semi-fixed costs, and variable costs?

5.2 Total costs are made up of what components?

5.3 a. What is cost-volume-profit (CVP) analysis?
   b. Why is it so useful to health services managers?

5.4 a. Define contribution margin.
   b. What is its economic meaning?

5.5 a. Write out and explain the equation for volume breakeven.
   b. What role does contribution margin play in this equation?

5.6 a. What is operating leverage?
   b. How is it measured?

5.7 What elements of profit analysis change when a provider moves from a fee-for-service to a discounted fee-for-service environment?

5.8 What are the critical differences in profit analysis when conducted in a capitated environment versus a fee-for-service environment?

5.9 How do provider incentives differ when the provider moves from a fee-for-service to a capitated environment?

5.10 a. What cost structure is best when a provider is capitated? Explain.
   b. What cost structure is best when a provider is reimbursed mostly by fee for service? Explain.

Problems

5.1 Consider the CVP graphs below for two providers operating in a fee-for-service environment:
   a. Assuming the graphs are drawn to the same scale, which provider has the greater fixed costs? The greater variable cost rate? The greater per unit revenue?
   b. Which provider has the greater contribution margin?
   c. Which provider needs the higher volume to break even?
   d. How would the graphs above change if the providers were operating in a discounted fee-for-service environment? In a capitated environment?

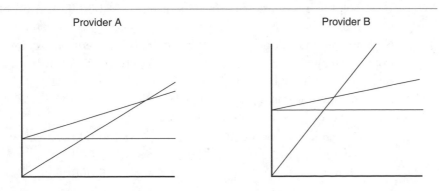

Provider A   Provider B

5.2 Consider the data in the table below for three independent health services organizations:

	Revenues	Total Variable Costs	Fixed Costs	Total Costs	Profit
a.	$2,000	$1,400	?	$2,000	?
b.	?	1,000	?	1,600	$2,400
c.	4,000	?	$600	?	400

Fill in the missing data indicated by question marks.

5.3 Assume that a radiologist group practice has the following cost structure:

Fixed costs	$500,000
Variable cost per procedure	$25
Charge (revenue) per procedure	$100

Furthermore, assume that the group expects to perform 7,500 procedures in the coming year.

a. Construct the group's base case projected profit and loss statement.
b. What is the group's contribution margin? What is its breakeven point?
c. What volume is required to provide a pretax profit of $100,000? A pretax profit of $200,000?
d. Sketch out a CVP analysis graph depicting the base case situation.
e. Now assume that the practice contracts with one HMO, and the plan proposes a 20 percent discount from charges. Redo questions a, b, c, and d under these conditions.

5.4 General Hospital, a not-for-profit acute care facility, has the following cost structure for its inpatient services:

Fixed costs	$10,000,000
Variable cost per inpatient day	$200
Charge (revenue) per inpatient day	$1,000

The hospital expects to have a patient load of 15,000 inpatient days next year.

a. Construct the hospital's base case projected P&L statement.
b. What is the hospital's breakeven point?
c. What volume is required to provide a profit of $1,000,000? A profit of $500,000?
d. Now assume that 20 percent of the hospital's inpatient days come from a managed care plan that wants a 25 percent discount from charges. Should the hospital agree to the discount proposal?

5.5 You are considering starting a walk-in clinic. Your financial projections for the first year of operations are as follows:

Revenues (10,000 visits)	$400,000
Wages and benefits	220,000
Rent	5,000

Depreciation	30,000
Utilities	2,500
Medical supplies	50,000
Administrative supplies	10,000

Assume that all costs are fixed, except supply costs, which are variable. Furthermore, assume that the clinic must pay taxes at a 30 percent rate.

a. Construct the clinic's projected P&L statement.

b. What number of visits is required to break even?

c. What number of visits is required to provide you with an after-tax profit of $100,000?

5.6 Review the walk-in clinic data presented in Problem 5.5. Construct projected profit and loss statements at volume levels of 8,000, 9,000, 10,000, 11,000, and 12,000 visits.

a. Assume that the base case forecast is 10,000 visits. What is the clinic's degree of operating leverage (DOL) at this volume level? Confirm the net incomes at the other volume levels using the DOL combined with the percent changes in volume.

b. Now assume that the base case volume is 9,000 visits. What is the DOL at this volume?

5.7 Grandview Clinic has fixed costs of $2 million and an average variable cost rate of $15 per visit. Its sole payer, an HMO, has proposed an annual capitation payment of $150 for each of its 20,000 members. Past experience indicates the population served will average two visits per year.

a. Construct the base case projected profit and loss statement on the contract.

b. Sketch two CVP analysis graphs for the clinic—one with number of visits on the X axis and one with number of members on the X axis. Compare and contrast these graphs with the one in Problem 5.3.d.

c. What is the clinic's contribution margin on the contract? How does this value compare with the value in Problem 5.3.b?

d. What profit gain can be realized if the clinic can lower per member utilization to 1.8 visits?

Notes

1. The term *management accounting* is sometimes used in place of managerial accounting. Although some accountants differentiate between managerial and management accounting, the differences are small and beyond the scope of this book. Thus, for purposes here, managerial accounting and management accounting are the same.

2. Semi-fixed costs are sometimes called *semi-variable costs*.

References

For a more in-depth treatment of cost measurement in health services organizations, see

Finkler, S. A., and D. M. Ward. 2006. *Accounting Fundamentals for Health Care Management.* Sudbury, MA: Jones and Bartlett.

Finkler, S. A., D. M. Ward, and J. J. Baker. 2007. *Essentials of Cost Accounting for Health Care Organizations.* Sudbury, MA: Jones and Bartlett.

Nowicki, M. 2006. *HFMA's Introduction to Hospital Accounting.* Chicago: Health Administration Press/Healthcare Financial Management Association.

Young, D. W. 2003. *Management Accounting in Health Care Organizations.* New York: Jossey-Bass.

In addition, see

Barnett, P., and A. Hendricks (eds). 1999. "Developments in Cost Methodology: Lessons from VA Research." *Medical Care* (April).

Berger, S. H. 2004. "Ten Ways to Improve Healthcare Cost Management." *Healthcare Financial Management* (August): 76–80.

Boles, K. E., and S. T. Fleming. 1996. "Breakeven Under Capitation." *Health Care Management Review* (Winter): 38–47.

Davis, K., R. Otwell, and J. Barber. 2004. "Managing Costs Through Clinical Quality Improvement." *Healthcare Financial Management* (July): 52–58.

Eastaugh, S. R. 2001. "Hospital Costs and Specialization: Benefits of Trimming Product Lines." *Journal of Health Care Finance* (Fall): 61–71.

Glandon, G. L., and M. A. Counte. 1995. "An Analysis of the Adoption of Managerial Innovation: Cost Accounting Systems in Hospitals." *Health Services Management Research* (November): 243–251.

Kazahay, G. 2005. "Harnessing Technology to Redesign Labor Cost Management Reports." *Healthcare Financial Management* (April): 94–100.

Kilgore, M. L., S. J. Steindel, and J. A. Smith. 1999. "Cost Analysis for Decision Support: The Case of Comparing Centralized Versus Distributed Methods for Blood Gas Testing." *Journal of Healthcare Management* (May/June): 207–215.

Shackelford, L. 1999. "Measuring Productivity Using RBRVS Cost Accounting." *Healthcare Financial Management* (January): 67–69.

Smith, B., and R. B. Hardaway. 2004. "Making the Tough Choices for Cost Control." *Healthcare Financial Management* (July): 76–84.

COST ALLOCATION

Learning Objectives

After studying this chapter, readers will be able to:

- Explain why proper cost allocation is important to health services organizations.
- Define a cost driver and explain the characteristics of a good driver as opposed to a poor one.
- Describe the three primary methods used to allocate overhead costs among revenue producing departments.
- Apply cost-allocation principles across a wide range of situations within health services organizations.

Introduction

In Chapter 5 we discussed the classification of costs according to their relationship to volume. In this chapter we introduce the second primary classification of costs—the relationship between costs and the subunit being analyzed (e.g., a department, service, or third-party payer contract). In essence, we will see that some costs are unique to the subunit being analyzed, while some costs stem from resources that belong to the organization as a whole. Once it is recognized that some costs are organizational in nature rather than specific to a subunit, it becomes necessary to create a system that allocates organizational costs to subunits. Although some of this chapter's material is conceptual in nature, much of it involves the application of various allocation techniques. Thus, a considerable portion of the chapter is devoted to examples of cost allocation in different settings.

Direct Versus Indirect (Overhead) Costs

Some costs—about 50 percent of a health services organization's cost structure—are unique to the reporting subunit and hence usually can be identified with relative certainty. To illustrate, consider a hospital's clinical laboratory. Certain costs are unique to the laboratory: for example, the salaries and benefits for the technicians who work there and the costs of the equipment and supplies used to conduct the tests. These costs, which would not occur if the laboratory were closed, are classified as the *direct costs* of the department.

Unfortunately, direct costs constitute only a portion of the laboratory's entire cost structure. The remaining resources used by the laboratory are **not** unique to the laboratory; the laboratory uses many shared resources of the hospital as a whole. For example, the laboratory shares the organization's physical space as well as its infrastructure, which includes information systems, utilities, housekeeping, maintenance, medical records, and general administration. The costs that are not borne solely by the laboratory are called *indirect*, or *overhead, costs*.

Indirect costs, in contrast to direct costs, are much more difficult to measure at the subunit level for the precise reason that they arise from shared resources—that is, if the laboratory were closed, the indirect costs would not disappear. Perhaps some indirect costs could be reduced, but the hospital still requires a basic infrastructure to operate its remaining departments. The direct/indirect classification has relevance only at the subunit level; if the unit of analysis is the entire organization, all costs are direct by definition.

Note that the cost classifications (fixed/variable and direct/indirect) overlay one another. That is, fixed costs typically include both direct and indirect costs, while variable costs can include both direct and indirect costs (although in most cases variable costs contain only direct costs). Conversely, direct costs usually include fixed and variable costs, while indirect costs typically include only fixed costs.

Introduction to Cost Allocation

A critical part of cost measurement at the subunit level is the assignment, or allocation, of indirect costs. *Cost allocation* is essentially a pricing process within the organization whereby managers allocate the costs of one department to other departments. Because this pricing process does not occur in a market setting, no objective standard exists that establishes the price for the transferred services. Thus, cost allocation within a business must, to the extent possible, establish prices that proxy those that would be set under market conditions.

What costs within a health services organization must be allocated? Typically, the overhead costs of the business, such as those incurred by administrators, facilities management personnel, financial staffs, and housekeeping and maintenance personnel, must be allocated to those departments that generate revenues for the organization (generally patient services departments). The allocation of support costs to patient services departments is necessary because there would be no need for support costs if there were no patient services departments. Thus, decisions regarding pricing and service offerings by the patient services departments must be based on the *full costs* associated with each service, including both direct and overhead (indirect) costs. Clearly, the proper allocation of overhead costs is essential to good decision making within health services organizations.

The *goal* of cost allocation is to assign all of the costs of an organization to the activities that cause them to be incurred. Ideally, health services managers would like to track and assign costs by individual patient, physician, diagnosis, reimbursement contract, and so on. With complete cost data accessible in the organization's managerial accounting system, managers can make better decisions regarding cost control, what services should be offered, and how these services should be priced. Of course, the more complex the managerial accounting system, the higher the costs of developing, implementing, and operating the system. As in all situations, the benefits associated with more accurate cost data must be weighed against the costs required to develop such data.

Interestingly, much of the motivation for more accurate cost allocation systems comes from the recipients of overhead services. Managers at all levels within health services organizations are coming under increased pressure to optimize economic performance, which translates into reducing costs. Indeed, many department heads are being evaluated, and hence compensated and promoted, primarily on the basis of economic results, assuming that performance along other dimensions is satisfactory. For such a performance evaluation system to work, all parties must perceive the cost allocation process to be accurate and fair because managers are being held accountable for both the direct and the indirect costs of their departments. In other words, department heads are being held accountable for the full costs associated with services performed by their departments.

1. What is meant by the term *cost allocation*?
2. What is the goal of cost allocation?
3. Why is cost allocation important to health services managers?

Self-Test Questions

Cost Allocation Basics

To assign costs from one activity to another, two important elements must be identified: a cost pool and a cost driver. A *cost pool* is a grouping of costs that must be allocated, while a *cost driver* is the criterion upon which the allocation is made. To illustrate, a hospital may allocate housekeeping costs to its other departments on the basis of the size of each department's physical space. The logic here is that the amount of housekeeping resources expended in each department is directly related to the physical size of that department. In this situation, total housekeeping costs would be the cost pool, and the number of square feet of occupied space would be the cost driver.

When the cost pool is divided by the cost driver, the result is the overhead *allocation rate*. Thus, in the housekeeping illustration, the allocation rate is total housekeeping costs of the organization divided by the total space (square footage) occupied by the departments receiving the allocation. This procedure results in an allocation rate measured in dollar cost per square foot of space utilized. In the patient services departments, total costs would include not only the direct costs of each department but also an allocation for the cost of providing housekeeping services made on the basis of the amount of occupied space. Clearly, the development of meaningful allocation rates enhances the ability of managers to make judgments concerning price negotiations, service profitability, and cost reduction.

Cost Pools

Typically, a cost pool consists of the all of the direct costs of one support department. However, if the services of a single support department differ substantially and the patient services departments use different relative amounts, it may be beneficial to separate the costs of that support department into multiple pools.

For example, suppose a hospital's Financial Services department provides two significantly different services: patient billing and budgeting. Furthermore, assume that the Routine Care department uses proportionally more patient billing services than does the Laboratory department, but the Laboratory uses proportionally more budgeting services than does Routine Care. In this situation, it would be best to create two cost pools for one support department. To do this, the total costs of Financial Services must be divided into a billing pool and a budgeting pool. Then, cost drivers must be chosen for each pool and the costs allocated to the patient services departments as described in the following sections.

Cost Drivers

Perhaps the most important step in the cost allocation process is the identification of proper cost drivers. Traditionally, overhead costs were aggregated across all support departments and then divided by a rough measure of organizational output, resulting in an allocation rate of some dollar amount of generic overhead per unit of output. For example, the total inpatient overhead costs of a hospital might be divided by total inpatient days, giving an allocation rate of so many dollars per patient day, which was called the *per diem overhead rate*. If a hospital had 72,000 patient days in 2007, and total inpatient overhead costs were $36 million, the overhead allocation rate would be $36,000,000 / 72,000 = $500 per patient day (per diem). Regardless of the type of patients treated within an inpatient services department (adult versus child, trauma versus illness, acute versus critical care, and so on), the $500 per diem allocation rate would be applied to determine the total indirect cost allocation for that department.

However, it is clear that not all overhead costs are tied to the number of patient days. For example, overhead costs associated with admission, discharge, and billing are typically not related to the number of patient days but to the number of admissions. Thus, tying all overhead costs to a single cost driver improperly allocates such costs, which distorts reported costs for patient services, and hence raises concerns about the effectiveness of decisions based on such costs. In state-of-the-art cost management systems, the various types of overhead costs are separated into different cost pools and the most appropriate cost driver for each pool is identified.

The theoretical basis for identifying cost drivers is the extent to which costs from a pool actually vary as the value of the driver changes. For example, does a department with 10,000 square feet of space use twice the amount of housekeeping services as a department with only 5,000 square feet of space? The better the relationship (correlation) between actual resource expenditures at each subunit and the cost driver, the better the cost driver and hence the better the resulting cost allocations.

Good cost drivers possess two characteristics. First, and perhaps the less important of the two, is *fairness*—that is, do the cost drivers chosen result in an allocation that is fair to the patient services departments? The second, and perhaps more important, characteristic is *cost control*—that is, do the cost drivers chosen create incentives for departments to use less overhead services? For example, there is little that patient services department managers can do to influence overhead cost allocations if the cost driver is patient days. In fact, the action needed to reduce the overhead allocation, reduction in patient days, would likely lead to negative financial consequences for the organization. A good cost driver will encourage patient services department managers to take overhead cost reduction actions that do not have negative implications for the organization. The remainder of this chapter emphasizes the importance of good cost drivers, including several illustrations that distinguish good drivers from poor ones.

The Allocation Process

The steps involved in allocating overhead costs are summarized in Table 6.1, which illustrates how Prairie View Clinic allocated its housekeeping costs for 2008.[1] First, the cost pool must be established. In this case, the clinic is allocating housekeeping costs, so the cost pool is the projected total costs of the Housekeeping department, $100,000.

Next, the best cost driver must be identified. After considerable investigation, Prairie View's managers concluded that the best cost driver for housekeeping costs is labor hours—that is, the number of hours of housekeeping services required by the clinic's departments is the variable most closely related to the actual cost of providing these services. The intent here, of course, is to pick the cost driver that provides the most accurate cause-and-effect relationship between the use of housekeeping services and the costs of the Housekeeping

Step One: Determine the Cost Pool
   The departmental costs to be allocated are for the Housekeeping department, which has total budgeted costs for 2008 of $100,000.

Step Two: Determine the Cost Driver
   The best cost driver was judged to be the number of hours of housekeeping services provided. An expected total of 10,000 hours of such services will be provided in 2008 to those departments that will receive the allocation.

Step Three: Calculate the Allocation Rate
   $100,000 / 10,000 hours = $10 per hour of housekeeping services provided.

Step Four: Determine the Allocation Amount
   Physical Therapy utilizes 3,000 hours of housekeeping services, so its allocation of Housekeeping department overhead is $10 × 3,000 = $30,000.

department. For 2008, Prairie View's managers estimate that Housekeeping will provide 10,000 hours of service to the departments that will receive the allocation.

Now that the cost pool and cost driver have been defined and measured, the allocation rate is established by dividing the expected total overhead cost (the cost pool) by the expected total volume of the cost driver: $100,000 / 10,000 hours = $10 per hour of services provided.

The final step in the process is to make the allocation to each department. To illustrate the allocation, consider Physical Therapy (PT)—one of Prairie View's patient services departments. For 2008, PT is expected to use 3,000 hours of housekeeping services, so the dollar amount of housekeeping overhead allocated to PT is $10 × 3,000 = $30,000. Other departments within the clinic will also use housekeeping services, and their allocations would be made in a similar manner. The $10 allocation rate per hour of services used is multiplied by the amount of each department's utilization of housekeeping services to obtain the dollar allocation. When all departments are considered, the entire clinic is projected to use 10,000 hours of housekeeping services, so the total amount allocated across the entire clinic must be $10 × 10,000 = $100,000, which is the amount in the cost pool. For any department, the amount allocated depends on both the allocation rate and the amount of overhead services used.

Self-Test Questions

1. What are the definitions of a cost pool, a cost driver, and an allocation rate?
2. Under what conditions should a single overhead department be divided into multiple cost pools?
3. On what theoretical basis are cost drivers chosen?
4. What two characteristics make a good cost driver?
5. What are the four steps in the cost allocation process?

Cost Allocation Methods

Mathematically, cost allocation can be accomplished in a variety of ways, and the method used is somewhat discretionary. No matter what method is chosen, all support department costs eventually must be allocated to the departments (primarily, patient services departments) that create the need for those costs.

The key differences among the methods are how support services provided by one department are allocated to **other support departments**. The direct method totally ignores services provided by one support department to another; the reciprocal method recognizes all of the intrasupport department services; and the step-down method represents a compromise that recognizes some, but not all, of the intrasupport department services. Regardless of the method, all of the support costs within an organization ultimately are allocated from support departments to the departments that generate revenues for the organization and hence create the need for the support services.

Figure 6.1 summarizes the three allocation methods. Prairie View Clinic, which is used in the illustration, has three support departments (Human Resources, Housekeeping, and Administration) and two patient services departments (Physical Therapy and Internal Medicine).

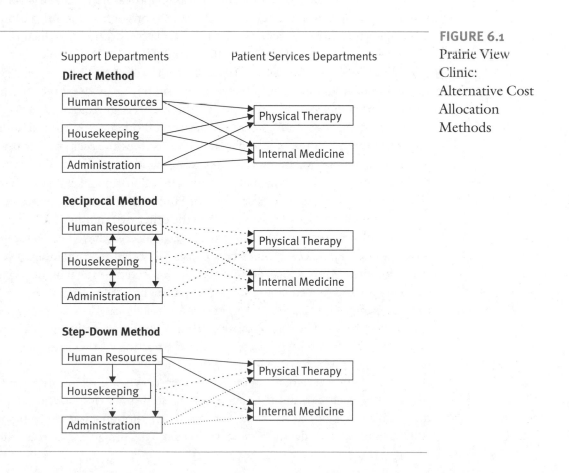

FIGURE 6.1
Prairie View
Clinic:
Alternative Cost
Allocation
Methods

Under the *direct method*, shown in the top section of Figure 6.1, each support department's costs are allocated directly to the patient services departments that use the services. In the illustration, both Physical Therapy and Internal Medicine use the services of all three support departments, so the costs of each support department are allocated to both patient services departments. The key feature of the direct method—and the feature that makes it relatively simple to apply—is that none of the costs of providing support services is allocated to other support departments. In effect, under the direct method, only the direct costs of the support departments are allocated to the patient services departments because no indirect costs have been created by intrasupport department allocations.

As shown in the center section of Figure 6.1, the *reciprocal method* recognizes the support department interdependencies between Human Resources, Housekeeping, and Administration, and hence it generally is considered to be more accurate and objective than the direct method. The reciprocal method derives its name from the fact that it recognizes all of the services that departments provide to and receive from other departments. The good news is that this method captures all of the intrasupport department relationships, so no information is ignored and no biases are introduced into the cost allocation process. The bad news is that the reciprocal method relies on the simultaneous solution of a series of equations representing the utilization of intrasupport department services. Thus, it is relatively complex, which makes it difficult to explain to department heads and more costly to implement.

The *step-down method*, which is shown in the lower section of Figure 6.1, represents a compromise between the simplicity of the direct method and the complexity of the reciprocal method. It recognizes some of the intrasupport department effects that the direct method ignores, but it does **not** recognize the full range of interdependencies as does the reciprocal method. The step-down method derives its name from the sequential, stair-step pattern of the allocation process, which requires that the allocation takes place in a specific sequence. First, all the direct costs of Human Resources are allocated to both the patient services departments and the other two support departments. Human Resources is then *closed out* because all its costs have been allocated. Next, Housekeeping costs, which now consist of both direct and indirect costs (the allocation from Human Resources), are allocated to the patient services departments and the remaining support department—Administration. Finally, the direct and indirect costs of Administration are allocated to the patient services departments. The final allocation from Administration includes Human Resources and Housekeeping costs because a portion of these support costs have been "stepped down" to Administration.

The critical difference between the step-down and reciprocal methods is that after each allocation is made in the step-down method, a support department is removed from the process. Even though Housekeeping and Administration provide support services back to Human Resources, these indirect costs are not recognized because Human Resources is removed from the allocation process after the initial allocation. Such costs are recognized in the reciprocal method.

1. What are the three primary methods of cost allocation?
2. Explain how they differ?

Self-Test Questions

Direct Method Illustration

The best way to gain a more in-depth understanding of cost allocation is to work through several allocation illustrations. We will begin with the direct method. As shown in Table 6.2, Kensington Hospital has three revenue-producing patient services departments, or *profit centers*: Routine Care, Laboratory, and Radiology. Hospital costs are divided into those costs attributable to the profit centers (direct costs) and those costs attributable to the support departments (overhead costs). Of course, the overhead costs are direct costs to the support departments (*cost centers*), but when they are allocated these direct costs become indirect (overhead) costs to the profit centers (patient services departments).

The data show that the revenues for each of the patient services departments are much greater than their direct costs. Furthermore, Kensington's projected total revenues of $27,000,000 exceed the hospital's projected total costs of $25,450,000. However, the aggregate revenue and cost amounts provide no information to Kensington's managers concerning the profitability of each patient services department. To determine true profitability by profit center, the **full costs** of providing patient services, including both direct and indirect costs, must be measured. Only then can the hospital's managers develop rational pricing and cost control strategies.

As previously discussed, three decisions are required when allocating costs: defining the cost pools, choosing the cost drivers, and choosing the method of allocation. We will begin by illustrating the direct method of cost allocation. The step-down method is discussed in a later section.

The cost pools (total costs) for the support departments are given in the lower section of Table 6.2. Financial Services costs are $1,500,000; Facilities costs equal $3,800,000; Housekeeping costs are $1,600,000; Administration costs total $4,400,000; and Personnel costs equal $2,550,000. Thus, overhead costs at the hospital total $13,850,000, which ultimately must be allocated to the hospital's three patient services departments. Kensington's managers believe that little is to be gained by dividing any of the support departments into multiple cost pools, so each support department constitutes one cost pool.

The next step in the allocation process is to identify the best cost drivers for each cost pool. Table 6.3 provides a summary of the support departments

TABLE 6.2

Kensington
Hospital:
2008 Revenue
and Cost
Projections

Projected Revenues by Patient Services Department	
Routine Care	$ 16,000,000
Laboratory	5,000,000
Radiology	6,000,000
Total revenues	$27,000,000

Projected Costs for All Departments	
Patient Services Departments (Direct Costs):	
Routine Care	$ 5,500,000
Laboratory	3,300,000
Radiology	2,800,000
Total costs	$ 11,600,000
Support Services Departments (Overhead Costs):	
Financial Services	$ 1,500,000
Facilities	3,800,000
Housekeeping	1,600,000
Administration	4,400,000
Personnel	2,550,000
Total costs	$13,850,000
Total costs of both patient and support services	$25,450,000
Projected profit	$ 1,550,000

and their assigned cost drivers. Unfortunately, the selection of cost drivers is not an easy process, and to a large extent the usefulness of the entire cost allocation process depends on choosing the most appropriate drivers. As discussed later, Kensington's selection of cost drivers, like many selections made in real-world situations, is somewhat of a compromise between accuracy and simplicity.

The cost driver chosen for Financial Services is patient services revenue. Financial Services provides a full range of financial support to the hospital. The bulk of its efforts are devoted to patient accounts, but it is also involved in financial and managerial accounting, budgeting and report preparation, and a host of other financial tasks. Tying the allocation of this support department to the amount of patient services revenues assumes a strong positive relationship between the amount of financial services provided to each patient services department and revenues generated by that department. Clearly, patient services revenue is a relatively rough cost driver, and hence the resulting cost allocation has limitations. In the next section, we discuss the benefits of moving from a poor cost driver to a better one.

The amount of space used (square footage) is the basis for allocating the costs of Facilities. This cost driver is often used by health services organizations to allocate the initial costs of land, buildings, and equipment as well as

Support Services Department	Cost Driver	TABLE 6.3
		Kensington
		Hospital:
Financial Services	Patient services revenue	Assigned Cost
Facilities	Space utilization (square footage)	Drivers
Housekeeping	Labor hours	
Administration	Salary dollars	
Personnel	Salary dollars	

the costs of maintenance and other facilities services. The logic applied here is that the patient services departments with the most space require the most facilities and hence the most facilities support. Of course, this assumption does not always hold. For example, in any year, Facilities may be required to support a special large project for one of the patient services departments that results in costs that far exceed that department's proportional space utilization. Nevertheless, over the long run at Kensington Hospital, the relative costs of Facilities utilization by the patient services departments track closely with the space occupied by those departments.

Two of the remaining support departments, Administration and Personnel, also use a relatively poor cost driver, salary dollars. Thus, if Radiology has payroll costs that are five times larger than those of Laboratory, Radiology will be charged (allocated) five times as much of the costs incurred by Administration and Personnel. This cost driver is often used, but in reality it is not very precise. Thus, the allocated costs from Administration and Personnel probably do not accurately represent the relative amounts of utilization of these overhead services.

Housekeeping has chosen perhaps the best cost driver—namely, the number of labor hours of housekeeping services consumed. In many organizations, housekeeping costs are allocated on the basis of square footage, using the logic that the amount of space occupied by a department accurately reflects housekeeping efforts and hence costs. This assumption may or may not be valid, however. In effect, large space departments may be subsidizing small space departments, such as emergency services, where space may be limited but the intensity of work requires a significant amount of housekeeping services. To account for such situations at Kensington Hospital, Housekeeping is using a better cost driver—one that is more closely aligned to the actual resources expended in providing support to the patient services departments.

The development and use of the best cost driver is a cost-benefit issue. Housekeeping must now devote resources to tracking where their workers spend their time, an effort that would not be required if the cost driver were square footage. The benefit, of course, is a cost driver that makes it easier for Kensington's senior managers to hold department heads responsible for both direct and indirect costs. If the head of Radiology does not like the amount of housekeeping costs that are being charged to the department, he or she can do something about it: use less Housekeeping services. With an inferior cost driver, such as square footage, there is little that patient services department heads can do if they do not like the Housekeeping allocation. In most cases, reduction of square footage is not a very practical way to deal with excessive housekeeping costs.

However, with labor hours consumed as the cost driver, the cost control solution for patient services department heads is to reduce the amount of Housekeeping services used. If all patient services department heads are made to think this way by having the right incentive system in place, ultimately the hospital will discover it is as efficient as possible in using housekeeping services. In the long run, the direct costs of the Housekeeping department, currently $1,600,000, will fall as these services are more efficiently used. In reality, the secondary benefit of choosing a better cost driver is a more equitable allocation. The primary benefit is that a good cost driver creates an incentive to use less of the support service, which ultimately leads to lower overhead costs for the organization.

Table 6.4 contains the initial data necessary for the allocation. The first column of Table 6.4 lists the patient services departments. The amounts of the chosen cost drivers consumed by each patient services department are listed after that: patient services revenue used for allocating Financial Services costs, square footage used for Facilities allocations, housekeeping labor hours used for Housekeeping allocations, and departmental salary dollars used for both Administration and Personnel allocations.

If Kensington were using the step-down or reciprocal allocation methods, the information shown in Table 6.4 would have included the support departments because the data would be needed for intrasupport department allocations. By using the direct method, the hospital ignores intrasupport department dependencies, so the totals indicated at the bottom of each column reflect only the use of support services by the patient services departments, which are allocated all of the support costs.

Table 6.5 combines the dollar amount of each cost pool with the total amount of each cost driver to derive the allocation rates. For example, the cost pool (direct costs) for Financial Services totals $1,500,000, which will be

TABLE 6.4
Kensington
Hospital:
Patient Services
Departmental
Summary Data

Department	Patient Services Revenues	Square Feet	Housekeeping Labor Hours	Salary Dollars
Routine Care	$16,000,000	199,800	76,000	$ 5,709,000
Laboratory	5,000,000	39,600	6,000	2,035,000
Radiology	6,000,000	61,200	9,000	2,439,000
Total	$27,000,000	300,600	91,000	$10,183,000

Department	Cost Pool (Total Costs)	Cost Driver	Total Utilization	Allocation Rate
Financial Services	$1,500,000	Patient revenue	$27,000,000	$0.05556
Facilities	3,800,000	Square feet	300,600	12.64
Housekeeping	1,600,000	Labor hours	91,000	17.58
Administration	4,400,000	Salary dollars	$10,183,000	0.432
Personnel	2,550,000	Salary dollars	$10,183,000	0.250

TABLE 6.5
Kensington Hospital: Overhead Allocation Rates

allocated as indirect (overhead) costs to the patient services departments that have a total of $27,000,000 in patient services revenues. The allocation rate for Financial Services, therefore, is $1,500,000 / $27,000,000 = $0.05556 per dollar of patient services revenue.

As previously mentioned, the allocation of indirect costs can be viewed as an internal pricing mechanism. Thus, the heads of the revenue-producing departments can look at Table 6.5 and see the rate that they are being charged for support services, which amounts to:

- $0.05556 for each dollar of patient services revenue generated for Financial Services support.
- $12.64 per square foot of space used for Facilities support.
- $17.58 per labor hour consumed for Housekeeping support.
- $0.432 per salary dollar paid to department employees for Administrative overhead.
- $0.250 per salary dollar for Personnel support.

If Radiology pays a technician $10 an hour in direct labor costs for each hour the technician works, the department will also be charged 0.432 × $10.00 = $4.32 for Administrative overhead and 0.250 × $10.00 = $2.50 for Personnel overhead, plus additional allocations for Financial Services, Facilities, and Housekeeping support.

Having two support services, in this case Administration and Personnel, that use the same cost driver, salary dollars, is not unusual. However, the allocation rate is different for the two support departments because they have different cost pool amounts.

The final step in the allocation process is to calculate the actual dollar allocation to each of the patient services departments, which is shown in Table 6.6. The support departments are listed in the first column, along with the applicable allocation rate, while the patient services departments are listed across the top. To illustrate the calculations, consider Routine Care. It produces $16,000,000 in patient services revenue, and the overhead allocation rate for Financial Services is $0.05556 per dollar of patient services revenue, so the allocation for such support is 0.05556 × $16,000,000 = $888,960.

TABLE 6.6
Kensington Hospital: Final Allocations

Support Department	Routine Care		Patient Services Department Laboratory		Radiology	
Financial Services ($0.0556)	× $16,000,000 =	$ 888,960	× $5,000,000 =	$ 277,800	× $6,000,000 =	$ 333,360
Facilities ($12.64)	× 199,800 =	2,525,472	× 39,600 =	500,544	× 61,200 =	773,568
Housekeeping ($17.58)	× 76,000 =	1,336,080	× 6,000 =	105,480	× 9,000 =	158,220
Administration ($0.432)	× 5,709,000 =	2,466,288	× 2,035,000 =	879,120	× 2,439,000 =	1,053,648
Personnel ($0.250)	× 5,709,000 =	1,427,250	× 2,035,000 =	508,750	× 2,439,000 =	609,750
Total indirect costs		$ 8,644,050		$ 2,271,694		$ 2,928,546
Direct costs		$ 5,500,000		$ 3,300,000		$ 2,800,000
Total costs		$ 14,144,050		$ 5,571,694		$ 5,728,546

Total indirect costs = $8,644,050 + $2,271,694 + $2,928,546 = $13,844,290.

Total costs = $14,144,050 + $5,571,694 + $5,728,546 = $25,444,290.

Note: Because of rounding in the allocation process, the totals here differ slightly from the values contained in Table 6.2.

Furthermore, Routine Care has 199,800 square feet of space; with a Facilities rate of $12.64 per square foot, its allocation for Facilities support is $12.64 × 199,800 = $2,525,472.

The allocations to Routine Care for Housekeeping, Administration, and Personnel services support shown in Table 6.6 were calculated similarly. The end result is that $8,644,050 out of a total of $13,850,000 of the indirect (overhead) costs of Kensington Hospital are allocated to Routine Care. Routine Care also has direct costs of $5,500,000, so the full (total) costs of the department, including both direct and indirect, are $8,644,050 + $5,500,000 = $14,144,050. The cost allocations and total cost calculations for Laboratory and Radiology shown in Table 6.6 were done in a similar manner.

For general management purposes, understanding the mechanics of the allocation is less important than recognizing the value of choosing good cost drivers. The cost driver for Housekeeping (i.e., the number of service hours provided) is good in the sense that it reflects the true level of effort expended by this department in support of the patient services departments. The patient services department heads are being fairly charged for Housekeeping services, and more importantly, patient services managers can take actions to lower the allocated amounts by reducing the amount of these services used.

In closing this illustration, note how Table 6.6, after the allocation process, reconciles with Table 6.2, before the allocation process. First, as shown in Table 6.2, total support services (overhead) costs are $13,850,000. This is the same amount (except for a rounding difference) shown in Table 6.6 as the total overhead allocated to the patient services departments: $8,644,050 (to Routine Care) + $2,271,694 (to Laboratory) + $2,928,546 (to Radiology) = $13,844,290. The total after-allocation costs of $25,444,290 shown in Table 6.6 also equals the original forecast for total costs in Table 6.2 of $25,450,00 (again, except for a rounding difference).

---

1. Briefly outline the allocation procedures used by Kensington Hospital.
2. What underlying characteristic creates a good cost driver?
3. What is the most important organizational benefit derived from the selection of a good cost driver?

Self-Test Questions

Changing to a Better Cost Driver

The Kensington Hospital example in the previous section illustrated the direct method of cost allocation. Now we build upon the previous illustration, but the focus here is on the benefits of moving from a poor cost driver to a better one.

Kensington historically has allocated the $1,500,000 in Financial Services costs on the basis of the dollar volume of patient services provided.

However, it was widely recognized by the managers involved that this driver is not highly correlated with the actual amount of overhead services provided to each patient services department, and hence it was not perceived as being fair. More importantly, it did not create an incentive for overhead cost reduction because patient services department heads would not reduce the amount of services provided (and hence reduce revenues) just to lower their overhead allocations.

A through analysis of the work done by Financial Services indicated that its primary task in support of the patient services departments is generating third-party payer billings and collecting on those bills. Thus, the conclusion was drawn that the cost of providing financial services is more highly correlated with the number of bills generated than with patient services revenues, so number of bills was chosen as the new cost driver.

Table 6.7 contains the new cost allocations for Financial Services as well as a comparison with the allocations under the old (patient services revenue) driver. Note that the allocations have changed substantially. Because the average amount of a Routine Care bill is much higher than the average amounts of Laboratory or Radiology bills, Routine Care has significantly fewer bills than the other patient services departments in spite of its significantly higher revenues. Thus, the new Financial Services allocation is very much lower than the amount under the old driver for Routine Care, but it is much higher for Laboratory and Radiology.

The move to a different cost driver represents more than just change for the sake of change. It represents an attempt by Kensington's managers to base the allocation on the actual amount of support provided by Financial Services to each patient services department. By doing so, the overhead allocation will have economic meaning and hence will be perceived by patient services department heads as being fair. Furthermore, the new cost driver will encourage patient services department heads to reduce their utilization of Financial Services support and hence lower Kensington's overhead costs.

In spite of the improvement that results from the change, the new cost driver is not perfect. Other changes could be made to improve the allocation even more. For example, the Financial Services department performs tasks other than billing, such as generating numerous reports for the organization, including both financial statements and budget reports. Indeed, the department has one analyst whose full-time job is creating and interpreting budget reports. (Budgeting is discussed in detail in Chapter 8.) A better allocation of Financial Services costs, therefore, may require that Financial Services be separated into two (or more) cost pools, each with its own cost driver. If this were done, some proportion of the department's total costs of $1,500,000 would be assigned to report preparation, and a separate cost driver would be identified to allocate these costs to the other departments.

Even though an even better cost driver may be developed, the change that has taken place is still meaningful. Cost accounting studies generally

TABLE 6.7
Kensington
Hospital: New
Financial
Services
Allocations

Utilization of Financial Services

Patient Services Department	Number of Bills required
Routine Care	3,200
Laboratory	60,300
Radiology	36,500
Total	100,000

Allocation Rate

$1,500,000 / 100,000 = $15.00 per bill.

Allocations

	New	Old	Difference
Routine Care	$15.00 × 3,200 = $ 48,000	$ 888,960	−$840,960
Laboratory	15.00 × 60,300 = 904,500	277,800	+626,700
Radiology	15.00 × 36,500 = 547,500	333,360	+214,140
Total	$1,500,000	≈$1,500,000	$ 0

have shown that the relationship between overhead cost usage and volume, measured either by revenues or units of service, is not very strong. Indeed, use of volume as the cost driver often results in systematic, as opposed to random, errors in cost allocation. Volume-based allocation schemes create a bias against larger revenue-producing departments by overallocating their costs, while the overhead costs of smaller revenue-producing departments are underallocated. This bias occurs largely because a volume-based cost driver fails to recognize the economies of scale inherent in larger departments in the utilization of overhead services. For example, it probably costs no more to bill a third-party payer for $5,000 than it does to bill for $500 in terms of the resources required to produce and transmit the bill and to monitor and collect the payment. Yet a revenue-based allocation scheme would tend to allocate more financial services costs to a patient services department with relatively high charges than to a department with relatively low charges that had exactly the same patient load and hence the same number of bills.

Although the cost driver (allocation) change made above appears to be a zero-sum game (i.e., one patient services department benefits while the other two lose), the decision to make the change was not really difficult for Kensington's senior managers. With a better cost driver, the hospital has moved to a more equitable allocation of Financial Services costs, even though it may not seem that way to the department heads who saw their allocated amounts increase. However, those departments with allocation increases for Financial Services (Laboratory and Radiology) are now being allocated their fair share of those overhead expenses. They were formerly being subsidized by the Routine Care department whose allocation was too high.

In additon, the heads of revenue-producing departments can now reap the benefits of their efforts to make the billing process more efficient. If the head of Laboratory does not like the new higher allocation, he or she can do something about it—generate fewer bills. The task must be done without lowering the total billing amount, which may not be easy. In fact, the effort will probably have to be done jointly with Financial Services, and perhaps with the cooperation of third-party payers.

The critical point is that patient services department heads are now motivated to participate in making the billing process more efficient. If Laboratory can cut the number of bills in half, it can cut its allocation in half. If other patient services departments can do this, Kensington will eventually discover that it can get along with fewer resources devoted to Financial Services and can thus reduce total overhead costs. A reduction in overhead costs is the ultimate benefit of moving to a better cost driver. A well-chosen cost driver makes department heads accountable for the use of support department resources, which is the starting point in gaining control of overhead costs within any organization.

Self-Test Questions

1. What are the advantages of changing from a poor cost driver to a better one?
2. What are the costs involved in the change?
3. Why is good cost allocation critical to good decision making?

Step-Down Method Illustration

We close our cost allocation illustrations with a simple example of the step-down method. Fargo Medical Associates, which has two support departments (Financial Services and Administration) and two patient services departments (Home Care and Diagnostic Services), will be used. In the previous illustration, support department costs were allocated directly to the patient services departments, with no recognition of intrasupport department services. Now we will recognize, at least partially, that support departments provide services to each other.

The allocation is summarized in Table 6.8. Under the step-down method, a new decision is needed; which of the two support departments is the most primary (i.e., which support department provides more services to the other). In this illustration, we assume that Administration provides more support to Financial Services than Financial Services provides to Administration. Thus, in the step-down process, the first support department to be allocated is Administration.[2]

In the step-down method, the $312,425 in Administration direct costs are allocated not only to the revenue-producing departments but also to

TABLE 6.8
Fargo Medical
Associates:
Step-Down
Allocation of
Administration
and Financial
Services Costs

Initial Allocation of Administration Department Costs:

Administration costs = $312,425.

Allocation rate = $312,425/$4,307,281 = $0.072534 per dollar of payroll.

	Financial Services	Home Care	Diagnostic Services	Total
Payroll costs	$ 505,321	$3,376,845	$ 425,115	$ 4,307,281
Percent of total	11.7%	78.4%	9.9%	100.0%
Allocation	$ 36,653	$ 244,937	$ 30,835	$ 312,425

Subsequent Allocation of Financial Services Department Costs:

Financial Services costs = $665,031 + $36,653 = $701,684.

Allocation rate = $701,684/14,456 = $48.539 per bill.

Number of bills		10,508	3,948	14,456
Percent of total		72.7%	27.3%	100.0%
Allocation	$ 0	$ 510,051	$ 191,633	$ 701,684

Financial Services, the other support department. Thus, the initial allocation in the top section of Table 6.8 shows that Administration costs are allocated to Financial Services in addition to the Home Care and Diagnostic Services patient services departments.

The allocation of Administration costs is made using payroll costs of the receiving departments as the cost driver. The total payroll for Fargo, less the Administration department, is $4,307,281, so the $312,425 in Administration costs are allocated at a rate of $312,425 / $4,307,281 = $0.072534 per dollar of payroll. For example, the allocation of Administration costs to Financial Services is 0.072534 × $505,321 = $36,653, while the allocation to Home Care is 0.072534 × $3,376,845 = $244,937. The key point is that under the step-down method, overhead costs are allocated both to other support departments and to patient services departments. Table 6.8 places Financial Services in the allocation scheme, while similar tables under the direct method listed only patient services departments.

Now that Administration costs have been allocated across both support and patient services departments, the role of Administration in the allocation process is finished. The next step is to allocate Financial Services costs, which now include both direct costs plus the indirect costs from the allocation for Administration overhead. This allocation is shown in the bottom section of Table 6.8. Although Financial Services has only $665,031 in direct costs, the total amount to be allocated is $701,684 because it includes $36,653 of allocated Administration overhead. Because some of the costs of Administration now flow through Financial Services, the allocation of Financial Services costs to the patient services departments is somewhat greater than it would be using the direct method. However, the allocation of Administration costs to the patient services departments is less under the step-down method than under the direct method because some costs that had been allocated directly to patient services departments are now allocated to another support department.

The step-down method of allocation is somewhat more complicated than the direct method. However, a good managerial accounting system can accomplish either allocation method quite easily. The real disadvantage of the step-down method is that it is more difficult for department heads to understand, especially in large, complex organizations. Still, for the reasons discussed previously (equity and cost control), managers want the best possible allocation system. In addition, CMS requires that the step-down method be used in reporting Medicare costs. Thus, in practice, the step-down method dominates the others in terms of usage.

Self-Test Questions	1. What is the primary difference between the direct and step-down methods of cost allocation? 2. Why might organizations adopt a more complicated allocation system?

Activity-Based Costing

Our discussion thus far has focused on *traditional* costing methods. In essence, the traditional methods begin with aggregate costs, typically at the department level. Overhead costs are then allocated downstream to the patient services departments. Thus, traditional methods can be thought of as top-down allocation. Although traditional costing works well for estimating costs at the department level, its usefulness for estimating the costs of activities within or across departments, such as individual tests, services, or diagnoses, is limited.

Activity-based costing (ABC) is a relatively new allocation system that is gaining popularity in the health services industry. ABC uses an upstream approach to cost allocation. Its premise is that all costs within an organization stem from *activities;* hence its name. In fact, the term *cost driver*, which has been used throughout this chapter, originated with ABC—a cost driver is the basic activity that causes costs to be incurred in the first place. In ABC, because activities are the focus of the cost accounting system, costs can be more easily assigned to individual patients, individual physicians, particular diagnoses, a reimbursement contract, a managed care population, and so on.

The key to cost allocation under ABC is to identify the activities that are performed to provide a particular service and then aggregate the costs of the activities. The steps required to implement ABC are as follows:

- Identify the relevant activities.
- Determine the cost of each activity, including both direct and indirect.
- Determine the cost drivers for the activity.
- Collect activity data for each service.
- Calculate the total cost of the service by aggregating activity costs.

To illustrate the ABC concept, suppose that the seven activities performed at a family practice clinic are (1) patient check-in, including insurance verification, (2) preliminary assessment, (3) diagnosis, (4) treatment, (5) prescription writing, (6) patient check-out, and (7) third-party payer billing. Furthermore, assume that the clinic has 10,000 visits annually, split evenly between two services: A and B. Before we go further, note that this example is highly simplified. Its purpose is merely to give you a flavor of how ABC works.

Table 6.9 contains the initial data and allocation rate calculations. For example, the annual costs of patient check-in, consisting of clerical labor and supplies (direct costs) plus space and other overhead (indirect costs), are $50,000 to support 10,000 total visits, giving an allocation rate of $5 per visit. Also, the total (direct labor by a nurse and overhead) costs required to conduct the initial assessment is $75,000, spread over (5,000 visits × 5 minutes for A) + (5,000 visits × 10 minutes for B) = 25,000 + 50,000 = 75,000 minutes annually, giving an allocation rate of $1 per minute.

As shown in Table 6.10, the final step is to aggregate the activity costs for each service. Note that this is done on a per visit basis. For example, for Service A, the cost of check-in is 1 visit × $5.00 = $5.00; the cost of assessment is 5 minutes per visit × $1.00 = $5.00; and the cost of diagnosis is 10 minutes per visit × $2.00 = $20.00. Other activity costs for Service A and Service B were calculated in a similar manner.

The end result of summing the individual activity costs associated with each service is a total cost of $75.10 for Service A and $130.40 for service B. The ability of the family practice to estimate the costs of its individual services allows the services to be priced properly (on the basis of costs). In addition, cost control is made easier because the activities, and hence resource expenditures, associated with each service have been clearly identified.

Note that the total annual costs of providing Service A are 5,000 visits × $75.10 = $375,500, while the total costs for B are 5,000 visits × $130.40 = $652,000. Because there are only two services in this simple example, the total costs of the practice are $375,500 + $652,000 = $1,027,500, which equals the total cost amount identified in Table 6.9.

TABLE 6.9
ABC Illustration: Initial Data and Allocation Rate Calculation

Activity	Annual Costs	Cost Driver	Service A	Service B	Total	Allocation Rate
				Activity Data		
Check-in	$ 50,000	Number of visits	5,000	5,000	10,000	$ 5.00
Assessment	75,000	Number of minutes per visit	5	10	75,000	1.00
Diagnosis	250,000	Number of minutes per visit	10	15	125,000	2.00
Treatment	450,000	Number of minutes per visit	10	20	150,000	3.00
Prescription	2,500	Drugs prescribed per visit	0.5	2.0	12,500	0.20
Check-out	50,000	Number of visits	5,000	5,000	10,000	5.00
Billing	150,000	Number of bills per visit	1.0	2.0	15,000	10.00
Total costs	$1,027,500					

TABLE 6.10

ABC Illustration: Final Aggregation of Activity Costs per Visit

Activity	Cost Driver	Rate	Service A		Service B	
			Consumption	Cost	Consumption	Cost
Check-in	Number of visits	$ 5.00	1	$ 5.00	1	$ 5.00
Assessment	Number of minutes	1.00	5	5.00	10	10.00
Diagnosis	Number of minutes	2.00	10	20.00	15	30.00
Treatment	Number of minutes	3.00	10	30.00	20	60.00
Prescription	Number of drugs	0.20	0.5	0.10	2.0	0.40
Check-out	Number of visits	5.00	1	5.00	1	5.00
Billing	Number of bills	10.00	1.0	10.00	2.0	20.00
Total cost per service				$75.10		$130.40

Clearly, ABC holds great promise for healthcare providers. The ability to assess the costs of individual services provides managers with much better information regarding the true costs of providing services. However, the information and resource requirements to establish an ABC system far exceed those required for a traditional cost allocation system. For this reason, traditional cost allocation still dominates the scene, but ABC is becoming more prevalent as the need for better cost data becomes more important and providers invest in newer and more powerful managerial accounting systems.

Self-Test Questions
1. What are the key differences between traditional and activity based costing?
2. Why does ABC hold so much promise for healthcare providers?

Final Thoughts on Cost Allocation

This chapter has been more mechanical than conceptual, but readers should not lose sight of the basic principles of cost allocation. The primary goal of cost allocation is to allocate as many costs as possible to those activities that create the need for the costs. In addition, to be an effective allocation system, the cost drivers used must meet two tests. First, a good cost allocation system must be fair; managers must believe that the overhead allocations to their departments truly reflect the amount of overhead services consumed. Second, the allocation process should foster cost reduction within the organization. To ensure fairness and cost control incentives, cost drivers must reflect those factors that truly influence the amount of overhead services consumed.

In any organization, the better the cost allocation process meets these two tests, the better the managerial decisions will be. After all, costs play a major role in provider decisions such as what prices to charge, what services to offer, and how much clinical managers should be paid. If the cost allocation system is faulty, those decisions may be flawed, and the financial condition of the business and employee morale will be degraded. Although the allocation process may seem rather mundane, the more confidence that all managers have in its validity, the better the organization will function.

Self-Test Questions
1. What is the goal of cost allocation?
2. What are the two primary tests that good cost allocation processes pass?
3. Why is the cost allocation process important to health services managers?

Key Concepts

This chapter focuses on cost allocation. The key concepts of this chapter are:
- *Direct costs* are the unique and exclusive resources used only by one unit

of an organization, such as a department, and therefore are fairly easy to measure.

- *Indirect costs,* in contrast, are inherently difficult to measure because these costs constitute a shared resource of the organization as a whole, such as administrative costs.

- The *goal* of cost allocation is to assign as many costs of an organization as possible directly to the activities that cause them to be incurred.

- *Cost allocation* is a critical part of the costing process because it addresses the issue of how to assign the costs of support activities to the revenue-producing (patient services) departments.

- The motivation to improve cost allocation systems comes largely from the increasing pressure to optimize economic performance within health services organizations and the resultant managerial incentive systems that focus on financial parameters.

- A *cost pool* is a dollar amount of overhead services to be allocated. In general, a cost pool consists of the total costs of one support department. However, under some circumstances, it may be better to divide the costs of a support department into multiple cost pools.

- A *cost driver* is the basis for making allocations from a cost pool. The identification of good *cost drivers* is essential to a sound cost allocation system.

- Cost drivers are chosen on the basis of their positive *correlation* with the amount of overhead services used.

- A good cost driver both will be perceived by department heads as being *fair* and will promote *cost reduction* within the organization.

- There are three primary *methods for cost allocation*: direct, reciprocal, and step-down.

- The *direct method* recognizes no intrasupport department services. Thus, support department costs are allocated exclusively to patient services departments.

- The *reciprocal method* recognizes all intrasupport department services. Unfortunately, the reciprocal method is difficult to implement because it requires the simultaneous solution of a series of equations.

- The *step-down method* represents a compromise that recognizes some of the intrasupport department services.

- Regardless of the allocation method, all costs eventually end up in the patient services departments.

- *Activity-based costing (ABC)* allocates costs on the basis of activities and hence aggregates costs from the basic components that create costs in the first place.

- ABC can provide a much more meaningful allocation of costs because costs can be assigned to individual patients, diagnoses, patient populations, and so on.

- ABC requires a very sophisticated and costly managerial accounting information system.

Although this chapter contains a great deal of detail, the most important point to remember is that a sound cost allocation system is required in making good pricing and service decisions, which is the topic of discussion in the next chapter.

Questions

6.1 What are the primary differences between direct and indirect costs?

6.2 What is the goal of cost allocation?

6.3 a. What are the three primary methods of cost allocation?
    b. What are the differences among them?

6.4 a. What is a cost pool?
    b. What is a cost driver?
    c. How is the cost allocation rate determined?

6.5 Under what circumstances should an overhead department be divided into multiple cost pools?

6.6 Effective cost drivers, and hence the resulting allocation system, must have what two important attributes?

6.7 Briefly describe (illustrate) the cost allocation process. (To keep things simple, use the direct method for your illustration.)

6.8 Which is the better cost driver for the costs of a hospital's Financial Services department: patient services department revenues or number of bills generated? Explain your rationale.

6.9 How does activity-based costing (ABC) differ from traditional costing approaches?

Problems

6.1 The Housekeeping Services department of Ruger Clinic, a multispecialty practice in Toledo, Ohio, had $100,000 in direct costs during 2007. These costs must be allocated to Ruger's three revenue-producing patient services departments using the direct method. Two cost drivers are under consideration: patient services revenue and hours of housekeeping services used. The patient services departments generated $5 million in total revenues during 2007, and to support these clinical activities, they used 5,000 hours of housekeeping services.
    a. What is the value of the cost pool?
    b. What is the allocation rate if:
        - patient services revenue is used as the cost driver?
        - hours of housekeeping services is used as the cost driver?

6.2 Refer to Problem 6.1. Assume that the three patient services departments are Adult Services, Pediatric Services, and Other Services. The patient services revenue and hours of housekeeping services for each department are:

Department	Revenue	Housekeeping Hours
Adult Services	$3,000,000	1,500
Pediatric Services	1,500,000	3,000
Other Services	500,000	500
Total	$5,000,000	5,000

a. What is the dollar allocation to each patient services department if patient services revenue is used as the cost driver?
b. What is the dollar allocation to each patient services department if hours of housekeeping support are used as the cost driver?
c. What is the difference in the allocation to each department between the two drivers?
d. Which of the two drivers is better? Why?

The following data pertain to the Problems 6.3 through 6.6:
St. Benedict's Hospital has three support departments and four patient services departments. The direct costs to each of the support departments are:

General Administration	$2,000,000
Facilities	5,000,000
Financial Services	3,000,000

Selected data for the three support and four patient services departments are:

Department	Patient Services Revenue	Space (Square Feet)	Housekeeping Labor Hours	Salary Dollars
Support:				
General Administration		10,000	2,000	$1,500,000
Facilities		20,000	5,000	3,000,000
Financial Services		15,000	3,000	2,000,000
Total		45,000	10,000	$6,500,000
Patient Services:				
Routine Care	$30,000,000	400,000	150,000	$12,000,000
Intensive Care	4,000,000	40,000	30,000	5,000,000
Diagnostic Services	6,000,000	60,000	15,000	6,000,000
Other Services	10,000,000	100,000	25,000	7,000,000
Total	$50,000,000	600,000	220,000	$30,000,000
Grand total	$50,000,000	645,000	230,000	$36,500,000

6.3 Assume that the hospital uses the direct method for cost allocation. Furthermore, the cost driver for General Administration and Financial Services is patient services revenue, while the cost driver for Facilities is space utilization.

a. What are the appropriate allocation rates?

b. Use an allocation table similar to Table 6.6 to allocate the hospital's overhead costs to the patient services departments.

6.4 Assume that the hospital uses salary dollars as the cost driver for General Administration, housekeeping labor hours as the cost driver for Facilities, and patient services revenue as the cost driver for Financial Services. (The majority of the costs of the Facilities department are devoted to housekeeping services.)

a. What are the appropriate allocation rates?

b. Use an allocation table similar to the one used for Problem 6.3 to allocate the hospital's overhead costs to the patient services departments.

c. Compare the dollar allocations with those obtained in Problem 6.3. Explain the differences.

d. Which of the two cost driver schemes is better? Explain your answer.

6.5 Now assume that the hospital uses the step-down method for cost allocation, with salary dollars as the cost driver for General Administration, housekeeping labor hours as the cost driver for Facilities, and patient services revenue as the cost driver for Financial Services. Assume also that General Administration provides the most services to other support departments, followed closely by Facilities. Financial Services provides the least services to the other support departments.

a. Use an allocation table to allocate the hospital's overhead costs to the patient services departments.

b. Compare the dollar allocations with those obtained in Problem 6.4. Explain the differences.

c. Is the direct method or the step-down method better for cost allocation within St. Benedict's? Explain your answer.

6.6 Return to the direct method of cost allocation and use the same cost drivers as specified in Problem 6.4 for General Administration and Facilities. However, assume that $2,000,000 of Financial Services costs are related to billing and managerial reporting and $1,000,000 are related to payroll and personnel management activities.

a. Devise and implement a cost allocation scheme that recognizes that Financial Services has two widely different functions.

b. Is there any additional information that would be useful in completing Part a?

c. What are the costs and benefits to St. Benedict's of creating two cost pools for Financial Services?

6.7 Consider the following data for a clinical laboratory:

Activity	Annual Costs	Cost Driver	Test A	Test B	Test C	Test D
				Activity Data		
Receive specimen	$ 10,000	Number of tests	2,000	1,500	1,000	500
Equipment set up	25,000	Number of minutes per test	5	5	10	10
Run test	100,000	Number of minutes per test	1	5	10	20
Record results	10,000	Number of minutes per test	2	2	2	4
Transmit results	5,000	Number of minutes per test	3	3	3	3
Total costs	$150,000					

a. Using ABC techniques, determine the allocation rate for each activity.

b. Now, using this allocation rate, estimate the total cost of performing each test.

c. Verify that the total annual costs aggregated from individual test costs equal the total annual costs of the laboratory given in the table above.

Notes

1. Cost allocation takes place both for historical purposes, in which realized costs over the past year are allocated, and for planning purposes, in which estimated future costs are allocated to aid in pricing and other decisions. The examples in this chapter generally assume that the purpose of the allocation is for pricing, and so the data presented are estimated for the coming year—2008.

2. If the two support departments were Human Resources and Housekeeping, the decision regarding which department to allocate first may be more difficult because each of these departments provides significant support to the other. In such a situation, the best allocation method may be the reciprocal method (see Figure 6.1).

References

Baker, J. J. 1995. "Activity-Based Costing for Integrated Delivery Systems." *Journal of Health Care Finance* (Winter): 57–61.

Baker, J. J., and G. F. Boyd. 1997. "Activity-Based Costing in the Operating Room at Valley View Hospital." *Journal of Health Care Finance* (Fall): 1–9.

Greene, J. K., and A. Metwalli. 2001. "The Impact of Activity Based Cost Accounting on Health Care Capital Investment Decisions." *Journal of Healthcare Finance* (Winter): 50–64.

Hill, N. T., and E. L. Johns. 1994. "Adoption of Costing Systems by U.S. Hospitals." *Hospital & Health Services Administration* (Winter): 521–537.

Hoyt, R. E., and C. M. Lay. 1995. "Linking Cost Control Measures to Health Care Services by Using Activity-Based Information." *Health Services Management Research* (November): 221–233.

Meeting, D. T., and R. O. Harvey. 1998. "Strategic Cost Accounting Helps Create a Competitive Edge." *Healthcare Financial Management* (December): 43–51.

Muise, M. L., and B. A. Amoia. 2006. "Step Up to the Step-Down Method." *Healthcare Financial Management* (May): 72–77.

Pedan, A., and J. J. Baker. 2002. "Allocating Physicians' Overhead Cost to Services: An Econometric Accounting-Activity Based-Approach." *Journal of Healthcare Finance* (Fall): 57–75.

Ramsey, R. H., IV. 1994. "Activity-Based Costing for Hospitals." *Hospital & Health Services Administration* (Fall): 385–396.

Ridderstolpe, L., et al. 2002. "Clinical Process Analysis and Activity-Based Costing at a Heart Center." *Journal of Medical Systems* (August): 309–322.

Ross, T. K. 2004. "Analyzing Health Care Operations Using ABC." *Journal of Health Care Finance* (Spring): 1–20.

Sides, R. W. 2000. "Cost Analysis Helps Evaluate Contract Profitability." *Healthcare Financial Management* (February): 63–66.

Stiles, R. A., and S. S. Mick. 1997. "What is the Cost of Controlling Quality." *Hospital & Health Services Administration* (Summer): 193–204.

Upda, S. 1996. "Activity-Based Costing for Hospitals." *Health Care Management Review* (Summer): 83–96.

———. 2001. "Activity Cost Analysis: A Tool to Cost Medical Services and Improve Quality of Care." *Managed Care Quarterly* (Summer): 34–41.

West, D. A., T. D. West, and P. J. Malone. 1998. "Managing Capital and Administrative (Indirect) Costs To Achieve Strategic Objectives: The Dialysis Clinic Versus the Outpatient Clinic." *Journal of Health Care Finance* (Winter): 20–34.

Zeller, T. L., G. Siegel, G. Kaciuba, and A. H. Lau. 1999. "Using Activity-Based Costing to Track Resource Use in Group Practices." *Healthcare Financial Management* (September): 46–50.

Young, D. W. 2007. "The folly of Using RCCs and RVUs for Intermediate Product Costing." *Healthcare Financial Management* (April): 100–106.

PRICING AND
SERVICE DECISIONS

Learning Objectives

After studying this chapter, readers will be able to:

- Describe the difference between providers as price setters and providers as price takers, and how this difference affects pricing and service decisions.
- Explain the difference between full cost and marginal cost pricing.
- Describe how target costing is used.
- Explain how accounting and actuarial information are used to make pricing and service decisions.
- Conduct basic analyses to set prices and determine service offerings under both fee-for-service and capitation.

Introduction

One of the most important uses of managerial accounting data involves either establishing a price for a particular service or, given a price, determining whether or not the service will be profitable. For example, in a charge-based environment, managers of healthcare providers must set prices on the services that their organizations offer. Managers also must determine whether or not to offer volume discounts to valued payer groups, such as managed care plans or business coalitions, and how large these discounts should be. Such decisions are called *pricing decisions*.

In many situations, insurers, especially governmental and managed care plans, dictate the reimbursement amount. Therefore, health services managers are not setting prices but must decide whether or not the payment is sufficient to assume the risks associated with providing services to the covered populations. These decisions are called *service decisions*. Because service decision analyses are similar to pricing decision analyses, the two types of analyses are discussed jointly.

Pricing and service decisions affect a business's revenues and costs and hence its financial condition, which ultimately determines the business's long-term viability. The importance of such decisions is easy to understand. In essence, pricing and service decisions determine both the strategic direction of the business and the ability of the organization to survive and prosper. In this chapter, the focus is on the analyses behind such decisions, including doing so in a capitated environment.

Healthcare Providers and the Power to Set Prices

Two extremes exist regarding the power of healthcare providers to set prices. At one extreme, providers have no power whatsoever and must accept the reimbursement levels set by the marketplace. At the other extreme, providers can set any prices (within reason) they desire, and payers must accept those prices. Clearly, few real-world markets for healthcare services support such extreme positions across all payers. Nevertheless, thinking in such terms can help health services managers better understand the pricing and service decisions they face.

Providers as Price Takers

As discussed throughout the book, healthcare services are provided in an increasingly competitive marketplace. As providers respond to market competition, managers must assess the ability of their organizations to influence the prices paid for the services offered. If the organization is one of a large number of providers in a service area with a large number of commercial fee-for-service purchasers (payers), and if little distinguishes the services offered by different providers, economic theory suggests that prices will be set by local supply-and-demand conditions. Thus, the actions of a single participant, whether the participant is a provider or a payer, cannot influence the prices set in the marketplace. In such a perfectly competitive market, healthcare providers are said to be *price takers* because they are constrained by the prices set in the marketplace.

Although very few markets for healthcare services are perfectly competitive, some payers, notably government payers and managed care plans with market power, can set reimbursement levels on a "take-it-or-leave-it" basis. In this situation, as in competitive markets, providers also are price takers in the sense that they have very little influence over reimbursement rates. Because many markets either are somewhat competitive or are dominated by large payer groups, and because governmental payers cover a significant proportion of the population, most providers probably qualify as price takers for a large percentage of their revenue.

As a general rule, providers that are price takers must take price as a given and concentrate managerial efforts on cost structure and utilization to ensure that their services are profitable. From a purely financial perspective, a price-taking provider should offer all services with costs that are less than the given price, even if that price has fallen because of discounting or other market actions.

Although the pure financial approach to service decisions is obviously simplistic, it does raise an important managerial accounting issue: What costs are relevant to the decision at hand? To ensure long-term sustainability, prices must cover full costs. However, prices that do not cover full costs may be acceptable for short periods, and it might be in the provider's long-run best interests to do so. This matter is discussed in the next major section.

Providers as Price Setters

In contrast to the previous discussion, healthcare providers with market dominance enjoy large market shares and hence exercise some pricing power. Within limits, such providers can decide what prices to set on the services offered. Furthermore, if a provider's services can be differentiated from others on the basis of quality, convenience, or some other characteristic, the provider also has the ability, again within limits, to set prices on the differentiated services. Healthcare providers that have such pricing power are called *price setters*.

The situation would be much easier for managers if a provider's status as a price taker or price setter were fixed for all payers for all services for long periods of time. Unfortunately, the market for healthcare services is ever changing, and hence providers can quickly move from one status to the other. For example, the merger of two healthcare providers may create sufficient market power to change two price takers, as separate entities, into one price setter, as a combined entity. Furthermore, providers can be price takers for some services and price setters for others or price takers for some payers and price setters for others. To make matters even more complicated, a large provider that serves separate market areas may be a price taker for a particular service in one geographical market yet be a price setter in another geographical market.

1. What is the difference between a price taker and a price setter?
2. Are healthcare providers generally either price takers or price setters exclusively? Explain your answer.

Self-Test Questions

Price Setting Strategies

When providers are **price setters**, alternative strategies can be used to price healthcare services. Unfortunately, no single strategy is most appropriate in all situations. In this section, we discuss two of the price setting strategies most frequently used by health services organizations.

Full Cost Pricing

Full cost pricing recognizes that to remain viable in the long run, health services organizations must set prices that recover all costs associated with operating the business. Thus, the full cost of a service, whether a patient day in a hospital, a visit to a clinic, a laboratory test, or the treatment of a particular diagnosis must include the following: (1) the direct variable costs of providing the service, (2) the direct fixed costs, and (3) the appropriate share of the overhead expenses of the organization.

Because of the difficulties inherent in allocating overhead costs (as discussed in Chapter 6), the full costs of an individual service are difficult to measure with precision and hence have to be viewed with some skepticism. Nevertheless, in the aggregate, revenues must cover both direct and overhead costs, and hence prices in total must cover all costs of an organization. Furthermore, all businesses need profits to survive in the long run. In not-for-profit businesses, prices must be set high enough to provide the profits needed to support asset replacement and to meet growth targets. In addition, for-profit providers must provide equity investors with an explicit financial return on their investment. The bottom line here is that, to cover all costs, including economic costs, full cost pricing must cover accounting costs plus a profit target.

Marginal Cost Pricing

In economics the *marginal cost* of an item is the cost of providing one additional unit of output, whether that output is a product or service. For example, suppose that a hospital currently provides 40,000 patient days of care. Its marginal cost, based on inpatient day as the unit of output, is the cost of providing the 40,000th day of care. In this situation, it is likely that fixed costs, both direct and overhead, have already been covered by reimbursements associated with the existing patient base (the 40,000 patient days), so the marginal cost that must be covered consists solely of the variable costs associated with an additional one-day stay. In most situations, no additional labor costs would be involved; additional personnel would not be hired nor overtime required. The marginal cost, therefore, consists of expenses such as laundry, food and expendable supplies, and any additional utility services consumed during that day. Obviously, the marginal cost associated with one additional patient day is far less than the full cost, which must include all direct fixed and overhead costs plus a profit component.

Many proponents of government programs such as Medicare and Medicaid argue that payments to providers should be made on the basis of marginal rather than full costs. The argument here is that some price above marginal cost is all that is required for the provider to "make money" on government-sponsored patients. By implication, nongovernmental payers would cover all base costs. However, what would happen if all payers for a particular provider set reimbursement rates based on marginal costs? If such a situation occurred, the organization would not recover its total costs, including both direct and overhead, and hence would ultimately fail.

Should any prices be set on the basis of marginal costs? In **theory**, the answer is no. For prices to be equitable, all payers should pay their fair share in covering providers' total costs. Furthermore, if *marginal cost pricing* should be adopted, which payer(s) should receive its benefits by being charged lower prices? Should it be the government because it is taxpayer funded, or should it be the last payer to contract with the provider? There are no good answers to these questions, so the easy way out, at least conceptually, is to require all payers to pay full costs and hence equitably share the burden of the organization's total costs.

However, as a practical matter, it may make sense for healthcare providers to occasionally use marginal cost pricing to attract a new patient clientele or to retain an existing clientele (i.e., gain or retain market share). To survive in the long run, however, businesses must earn revenues that cover their full costs. Thus, either marginal cost pricing must be a temporary measure or the organization must employ *cross-subsidization* (*price shifting*). In such situations, some patients or covered populations are overcharged for services, as compared to full costs, while others are undercharged.

Historically, price shifting was used by providers to support services, such as emergency care, teaching and research, and indigent care, which were not self-supporting. Without such price shifting strategies, many providers would not have been able to offer a full range of services. Payers were willing to accept price shifting because the additional burden was not excessive. Today, however, overall healthcare costs have risen to the point where the major purchasers of healthcare services are not willing to support the costs associated with providing services to others, and hence purchasers are demanding prices that cover only true costs, without cross-subsidies. Payers perhaps rightly believe that they do not have the moral responsibility to fund healthcare services for those outside of their covered populations.

1. Describe two common pricing strategies used by price setters and their implications for financial survivability. 2. What is cross-subsidization (price shifting)? 3. Is cross-subsidization used by providers as frequently today as it was in the past? If not, why?	**Self-Test Questions**

Target Costing

Target costing is a management strategy that helps providers deal with situations in which they are **price takers**. Target costing assumes the price for a service is a given, and then subtracts the desired profit on that service to obtain the target cost level. If possible, management then will reduce the full cost of the service to the target level, with a goal of continuous cost reduction that will eventually push costs below the target. Essentially, target costing backs into the cost at which a healthcare service must be provided in the long run to attain a given profitability target.

Perhaps the greatest value of target costing lies in the fact that it forces managers to take very seriously the prices set by external forces; that is, it recognizes that the purchasers of healthcare services do not really care whether or not prices are based on the underlying costs of the services provided. Thus, to ensure financial survival, providers must attain cost structures compatible with the revenue stream. Providers that cannot lower costs to the level required to make a profit will ultimately fail.

Setting Prices on Individual Services

The best way to understand the mechanics of pricing and service decisions is to work through several illustrations. The first example illustrates the basic approach to setting prices on individual services.

Assume that the managers of Windsor Community Hospital, a not-for-profit provider, are planning to offer a new outpatient service. The hospital's managerial accountants have estimated the following cost data for the service:

Variable cost per visit	$10
Annual direct fixed costs	$100,000
Annual overhead allocation	$25,000

Furthermore, the hospital's marketing staff believes that demand for the new service will be 5,000 visits during its first year of operation.

To begin, Windsor's managers want to know what price must be set on each visit for the service to break even during the first year. To answer this question, we will apply the profit (CVP) analysis method discussed in Chapter 5, but now our focus is on price breakeven rather than volume breakeven. For *accounting breakeven*, the expected profit of the service must be zero, so revenues less costs must equal zero. One way to calculate the breakeven price is to express the relationship between revenues, costs, and profit in equation form:

$$\text{Total revenues} - \text{Total costs} = \$0$$
$$\text{Total revenues} - \text{Total variable costs} - \text{Direct fixed costs} - \text{Overhead} = \$0$$
$$(5{,}000 \times \text{Price}) - (5{,}000 \times \$10) - \$100{,}000 - \$25{,}000 = \$0$$
$$(5{,}000 \times \text{Price}) - \$175{,}000 = \$0$$
$$5{,}000 \times \text{Price} = \$175{,}000$$
$$\text{Price} = \$175{,}000 \, / \, 5{,}000 = \$35.$$

Thus, under the utilization and cost assumptions developed by Windsor's managers, a price of $35 per visit must be set on the new service to break even in the accounting sense.

Of course, Windsor's managers want the service to earn a profit and hence to achieve *economic breakeven*. Suppose the goal is to make a profit of $100,000 on the new service. The calculations above show that costs at 5,000 visits are expected to total $175,000. Thus, to make a profit of $100,000, service revenues must total $175,000 + $100,000 = $275,000. With 5,000 visits, the price must be set at $275,000 / 5,000 = $55 per visit.

Up to this point, the analysis has focused on full cost pricing. Suppose that Windsor's managers wanted to price the service aggressively to quickly build market share. What price would be set under marginal cost pricing? Now the service must only cover the variable (marginal) cost of $10 per visit, so a price of $10 is all that is required. This price, which is well below the accounting breakeven of $35 and the economic breakeven of $55, would result in a loss of $125,000 ($100,000 in direct fixed costs and $25,000 in overhead) during the first year the service is offered, assuming that the aggressive pricing does not affect the 5,000-visit utilization estimate.

What price should Windsor's managers actually set on the new service? It should be obvious to readers that a great deal of judgment is required to make this decision. One important consideration is the relationship between price and utilization, which the analysis has ignored by assuming that the service would produce 5,000 visits regardless of price. A more complete analysis would examine the effect of different prices *and* utilization levels on profits. Another consideration is how easy it would be to increase the price that is initially set. If price increases are expected to be met with a great deal of resistance, then pricing low to gain market share today might not be a good long-run strategy.

1. Briefly explain the process for pricing individual services.
2. What do you think the price should be on Windsor's new service? Justify your answer.

Self-Test Questions

Setting Prices Under Capitation

The second illustration focuses on how one hospital priced a new capitated product.

Base Case Analysis

Table 7.1 contains relevant 2008 forcasted revenue and cost data for Montana Medical Center (MMC), a 350-bed, not-for-profit hospital. According to its managers' best estimates, MMC is expecting to earn a profit (net income) of $1,662,312 in 2008. The data consist first of a worksheet, which breaks down the cost data by payer. Here, the assumption is that all payers use fee-for-service reimbursement, including discounted fee-for-service. The Table 7.1 cost data also include the hospital's cost structure, broken down by variable

TABLE 7.1

Montana
Medical Center:
Projected Payer
Worksheet and
P&L Statement
for 2008

Payer	Number of Admissions	Average Revenue per Admission	Revenue by Payer	Variable Cost per Admission	Total Variable Costs	Contribution Margin
Payer Worksheet:						
Medicare	4,268	$7,327	$ 31,271,636	$2,529	$10,793,772	$20,477,864
Medicaid	5,895	5,448	32,115,960	1,575	9,284,625	22,831,335
Montana Care	828	4,305	3,564,540	1,907	1,578,996	1,985,544
Managed Care	1,885	3,842	7,242,170	1,638	3,087,630	4,154,540
Blue Cross	332	5,761	1,912,652	2,366	785,512	1,127,140
Commercial	1,408	11,770	16,572,160	2,969	4,180,352	12,391,808
Self-Pay	1,289	2,053	2,646,317	1,489	1,919,321	726,996
Other	1,149	11,539	13,258,311	3,085	3,544,665	9,713,646
Total	17,054		$108,583,746		$35,174,873	$73,408,873
Weighted average		$6,367		$2,063		

P&L Statement:

Total revenues	$108,583,746
Variable costs	35,174,873
Contribution margin	$ 73,408,873
Fixed costs	71,746,561
Profit	$ 1,662,312

costs; fixed costs, including both direct and overhead (the $71,746,561 given in the P&L statement); and contribution margin.

To illustrate the data, consider MMC's Medicare patients. Medicare is expected to provide the hospital with 4,268 admissions at an average revenue of $7,327 per admission, for total revenues of 4,268 × $7,327 = $31,271,636. Expected variable cost per admission for a Medicare patient is $2,529, which results in expected total variable costs of 4,268 × $2,529 = $10,793,772. The difference between expected total revenues and the expected total variable costs produces a forecasted total contribution margin of $31,271,636 − $10,793,772 = $20,477,864 for the Medicare patient group. This total contribution margin is combined with the total contribution margins of the other payer groups to produce an expected aggregate total contribution margin for the hospital of $73,408,873. As shown in the P&L statement portion of Table 7.1, the total contribution margin both covers MMC's forecasted fixed costs of $71,746,561 and produces an expected profit of $1,662,312.

MMC's managers are considering taking a bold strategic action—offering a capitated plan for inpatient services. One of the first tasks that must be performed is setting the price for the new plan. Table 7.2 contains the key assumptions inherent in the pricing decision. The hospital's managers believe that about 13 percent of the current patient base would be converted to the capitated plan. To be conservative, the assumption was made that no additional patients would be generated. Thus, at least initially, patients in the capitated plan would come from MMC's current patient base. In effect,

MMC would have to cannibalize from its own business with the expectation of protecting current market share and using the capitated plan as a marketing tool to expand market share in the future.

Assumptions also have been made regarding where the cannibalization would occur and the number of admissions under the capitated plan. These data are provided in Points 2 and 3 of Table 7.2. The patient mix assumptions will be important when costs are estimated for the new plan.

MMC's managers believe, at least initially, that hospital utilization will be unaffected by the conversion of some patients from fee-for-service contracts to capitation. Another expectation is that variable costs for the new plan would be the same as experienced in the past with each payer group. These are two **very important** assumptions. MMC's managers are assuming that the utilization and delivery of healthcare services for the capitated population will be exactly the same as for the fee-for-service population. This is probably a reasonable starting assumption given that the capitated population will represent only a small portion of MMC's overall business. However, if increased managed care penetration in MMC's service area leads to a greater proportion of capitated patients, both utilization patterns and the underlying cost structure are likely to change as the hospital responds to the incentives created.

Finally, and perhaps most importantly in terms of pricing strategy, the capitated price that MMC plans to offer to the market must result in the same profit ($1,662,312) as expected if the hospital were to remain totally fee-for-service. The underlying logic here is that MMC's managers want to experiment with capitation, but they are unwilling to do so at the expense of the bottom line. This pricing goal, and the expected cost structure of

---

1. The capitated plan will initially enroll the following percentages of the hospital's current patients:
    a. Medicaid: 20 percent
    b. Commercial: 40 percent
    c. Self-pay: 40 percent
2. Assuming that utilization rates are not affected by the change to a capitated plan, admissions from the capitated group are expected to total $(0.20 \times 5,895) + (0.40 \times 1,408) + (0.40 \times 1,289) = 2,258$.
3. Based on current coverage information, the patient population under capitation (number of enrollees) would be 25,000.
4. Variable costs for capitated patients will remain the same as currently estimated for each payer group.
5. Total fixed costs will remain the same.
6. All other assumptions inherent in the Table 7.1 forecast hold for the capitated plan.
7. The goal for the price set for capitated enrollees will be to generate, at a minimum, the profit forecasted in Table 7.1 under fee-for-service reimbursement.

TABLE 7.2
Montana
Medical Center:
Initial
Assumptions for
a Capitated Plan

serving the capitated population, therefore, will drive the monthly premium established for the capitated product. If the goal of preserving the bottom line while adding the new product proves to be unattainable, MMC's managers would have to reevaluate their initial pricing strategy.

Table 7.3 contains an analysis similar to the one shown in Table 7.1, except that Table 7.3 includes the proposed capitated plan. Changes from the Table 7.1 values are shown in **boldface**. For example, the entire first line of the worksheet, labeled "Capitated," is in boldface because this is MMC's new product line, which does not appear in Table 7.1. Also in boldface are selected values on the Medicaid, commercial, and self-pay lines, because these values will change because of the shift of some of these payer groups' patients to the capitated plan.

Notice that the Table 7.3 volume levels reflect the expected patient shifts from fee-for-service to capitation. For example, the Medicaid group reflects the 20 percent decrease resulting from patients shifting to the capitated plan: $0.80 \times 5,895 = 4,716$. The commercial and self-pay payer groups also reflect their 40 percent losses in admissions to the new plan. In total, the capitated plan is expected to siphon off $0.20 \times 5,895 = 1,179$ Medicaid admissions, $0.40 \times 1,408 = 563$ commercial admissions, and $0.40 \times 1,289 = 516$ self-pay admissions, for a total of 2,258 admissions.

For now, pass by the revenue columns in Table 7.3 and focus on the variable cost columns for the capitated patients. Because each capitated patient is expected to have the same variable cost as under the previous plans, variable costs for the capitated plan are expected to total $(1,179 \times \$1,575) + (563 \times \$2,969) + (516 \times \$1,489) = \$4,296,794$.[1] With an expected number of admissions of 2,258, the average variable cost per capitated admission is $\$4,296,794 / 2,258 = \$1,903$.

Now consider the revenue columns. To keep the projected profit the same as in Table 7.1, revenues must total $108,583,746. Furthermore, expected total revenues from all payer groups except the new plan amount to $94,473,163. Thus, the capitated plan must bring in revenue of $108,583, − $94,473,163 = $14,110,583 to achieve MMC's target profit. This calculation can be thought of as working backward on (or up) the projected P&L statement shown at the bottom of Table 7.3.

With expected admissions at 2,258, the average revenue per admission can be calculated as $\$14,110,583 / 2,258 = \$6,250$. However, this implied average revenue per admission has no real meaning in a capitated plan because MMC will not be charging these patients on a per admission basis. The calculated per admission revenue value of $6,250 is a *fee-for-service equivalent revenue*, and every worker at MMC must recognize that the hospital will not actually receive $6,250 per admission under the new plan. As MMC's patients move from fee-for-service to capitation, revenue will be based on enrollment rather than admissions.

With all this information at hand, MMC's managers now can price the new plan. Total revenues of $14,110,583 are required from 25,000 enrollees,

Payer	Number of Admissions	Average Revenue per Admission	Revenue by Payer	Variable Cost per Admission	Total Variable Costs	Contribution Margin
Payer Worksheet:						
Capitated	**2,258**	$ 6,250	$ 14,110,583	$1,903	$ 4,296,794	$ 9,813,789
Medicare	4,268	7,327	31,271,636	2,529	10,793,772	20,477,864
Medicaid	**4,716**	5,448	**25,692,768**	1,575	**7,427,700**	**18,265,068**
Montana Care	828	4,305	3,564,540	1,907	1,578,996	1,985,544
Managed Care	1,885	3,842	7,242,170	1,638	3,087,630	4,154,540
Blue Cross	332	5,761	1,912,652	2,366	785,512	1,127,140
Commercial	**845**	11,770	**9,943,296**	2,969	**2,508,211**	**7,435,085**
Self-Pay	**773**	2,053	**1,587,790**	1,489	**1,151,593**	**436,198**
Other	1,149	11,539	13,258,331	3,085	3,544,665	9,713,646
Total	17,054		$108,583,746		$35,174,873	$73,408,873
Weighted average		$ 6,367		$2,063		

TABLE 7.3
Montana Medical Center: Projected Analysis Assuming 25,000 Enrollees and Constant Net Income

Annual capitated revenue requirements = $14,110,583/25,000 = $564.42 per member.
Monthly capitated revenue requirements = $564.42/12 = $47.04 per member per month (PMPM).

P&L Statement:

Total revenues	$ 108,583,746
Variable costs	35,174,873
Contribution margin	$ 73,408,873
Fixed costs	71,746,561
Profit	$ 1,662,312

Note: Some rounding differences occur in the table.

so the annual revenue per enrollee is $14,110,583 / 25,000 = $564.42. Because premiums are normally expressed on a *per member per month (PMPM)* basis, the annual revenue requirement must be divided by 12 to obtain $47.04 PMPM. This PMPM charge is what MMC's managers would set as the initial price when marketing the new plan.

Scenario Analysis

The previous section illustrated how MMC's managers could establish a price for a new capitated plan. However, a good pricing analysis goes well beyond the base case analysis (or *base case scenario*), which uses the most likely estimates for all input variables—number of enrollees, variable costs, and so on. The second part of a complete pricing analysis involves *scenario analysis*, whereby MMC's managers assess the impact of assumption changes in key variable values from their base case values by creating alternative scenarios.[2]

Additional Enrollees

Table 7.4 repeats the analysis, but now the assumption is that 10,000 **new** enrollees are added to the capitated plan. Coupled with the base case estimate of 25,000 enrollees from MMC's other payer groups, total enrollment in the capitated plan is increased to 35,000. The assumptions are that the new

TABLE 7.4

Montana Medical Center: Projected Analysis Assuming 35,000 Enrollees at $47.04 PMPM

Payer	Number of Admissions	Average Revenue per Admission	Revenue by Payer	Variable Cost per Admission	Total Variable Costs	Contribution Margin
Payer Worksheet:						
Capitated	**3,161**	$6,250	$ **19,754,816**	$1,903	$ **6,015,512**	$**13,739,304**
Medicare	4,268	7,327	31,271,636	2,529	10,793,772	20,477,864
Medicaid	4,716	5,448	25,692,768	1,575	7,427,700	18,265,068
Montana Care	828	4,305	3,564,540	1,907	1,578,996	1,985,544
Managed Care	1,885	3,842	7,242,170	1,638	3,087,630	4,154,540
Blue Cross	332	5,761	1,912,652	2,366	785,512	1,127,140
Commercial	845	11,770	9,943,296	2,969	2,508,211	7,435,085
Self-Pay	773	2,053	1,587,790	1,489	1,151,593	436,198
Other	1,149	11,539	13,258,331	3,085	3,544,665	9,713,646
Total	**17,957**		$ 114,227,979		$**36,893,591**	$**77,334,388**
Weighted average		**$6,361**		**$2,055**		

P&L Statement:

Total revenues	$ **114,227,979**
Variable costs	36,893,591
Contribution margin	$ **77,334,388**
Fixed costs	71,746,561
Profit	$ **5,587,827**

Note: Some rounding differences occur in the table.

enrollees would use hospital services at the same rate as current plan members, and the variable cost per admission would be the same for the new enrollees as for the existing 25,000 enrollees. Furthermore, no additional fixed costs would be required to handle the increased volume.

Those entries that differ from Table 7.3 are boldfaced. The addition of new capitated enrollees does not affect any of the other payer groups, so the changes in Table 7.4 are limited to the first line of the payer worksheet, the totals and averages, and the P&L statement. Adding 10,000 enrollees increases MMC's total revenues by $114,227,979 − $108,583,746 = $5,644,233 but only increases total variable costs by $36,893,591 − $35,174,873 = $1,718,718, thus resulting in a total contribution margin gain of $5,644,233 − $1,718,718 = $3,925,515. Assuming that fixed costs remain at $71,746,561, the entire amount of the contribution margin increase will flow to the bottom line, so projected profit will increase by a like amount.

An alternative way to consider the effect of additional enrollees on the bottom line is to examine the contribution margin on capitated patients. Each additional enrollee brings in $47.04 × 12 = $564.48 per year, but what about the cost side? The 35,000 enrollees are expected to have 3,161 admissions, for an average rate of 3,161 / 35,000 = 0.0903 admissions per enrollee, so the expected variable cost per enrollee is 0.0903 × $1,903 = $171.84. Thus, the contribution margin per enrollee is $564.48 − $171.84 = $392.64, and 10,000 new enrollees would add $3,926,400 to the bottom line, which is the same as calculated previously (except for a rounding difference).

This analysis confirms the benefit that would accrue to MMC if the capitated plan does indeed result in increasing the hospital's market share. Note, however, that the increased market share analysis has several key assumptions—notably, that the premium remains at $47.04 PMPM, that utilization and costs associated with new enrollees are the same as for the initial cannibalized enrollees, and that no additional fixed costs are required.

Reduced Premium

What would happen if the initial premium of $47.04 PMPM has to be lowered to $40 to be attractive in the marketplace? To examine the effects of a lower premium, consider the analysis presented in Table 7.5. In this case, the assumption is that a premium of $40 results in the same 35,000 enrollees as analyzed in the last scenario. The only changes from Table 7.4 stem from the reduced revenues associated with lowering the premium from $47.04 PMPM to $40 PMPM, or by $7.04 PMPM. The loss of annual revenue of 35,000 × $7.04 × 12 = $2,956,800, with no offsetting reduction in costs, flows directly to the bottom line. The end result is a corresponding reduction in projected profit (except for a rounding difference).

TABLE 7.5 Montana Medical Center: Projected Analysis Assuming 35,000 Enrollees at $40 PMPM

Payer	Number of Admissions	Average Revenue per Admission	Revenue by Payer	Variable Cost per Admission	Total Variable Costs	Contribution Margin
Payer Worksheet:						
Capitated	3,161	**$5,315**	$ 16,800,000	$1,903	$ 6,015,512	**$10,784,488**
Medicare	4,268	7,327	31,271,636	2,529	10,793,772	20,477,864
Medicaid	4,716	5,448	25,692,768	1,575	7,427,700	18,265,068
Montana Care	828	4,305	3,564,540	1,907	1,578,996	1,985,544
Managed Care	1,885	3,842	7,242,170	1,638	3,087,630	4,154,540
Blue Cross	332	5,761	1,912,652	2,366	785,512	1,127,140
Commercial	845	11,770	9,943,296	2,969	2,508,211	7,435,085
Self-Pay	773	2,053	1,587,790	1,489	1,151,593	436,198
Other	1,149	11,539	13,258,331	3,085	3,544,665	9,713,646
Total	17,957		$ 111,273,163		$ 36,893,591	$ 74,379,573
Weighted average		**$6,197**		$2,055		

P&L Statement:

Total revenues	$ 111,273,163
Variable costs	36,893,591
Contribution margin	$ 74,379,573
Fixed costs	71,746,561
Profit	$ 2,633,012

Note: Some rounding differences occur in the table.

Premium Breakeven

It would be useful for MMC's managers to know what premium would be required to obtain the original forecasted profit of $1,662,312 (see Tables 7.1 and 7.3), assuming a capitated plan enrollment of 35,000. By using a spreadsheet model, MMC's managers found that a PMPM premium of about $37.69 would produce a projected profit of $1,662,312. Therefore, MMC could lower the premium to that amount, if necessary, to obtain 35,000 enrollees, without reducing its profit below the initial forecast. Furthermore, MMC could set the premium as low as $33.73 and still reach accounting breakeven (i.e., zero profit), assuming 35,000 enrollees.

The Value of Utilization and Cost Reduction

Finally, consider the value inherent in utilization and cost reduction efforts. Suppose that MMC actually obtained 25,000 enrollees at a premium of $47.04. The expected net income in this scenario is $1,662,312 (see Table 7.3). However, assume that MMC instituted a utilization review program that lowered the annual utilization rate for capitated enrollees from the current 0.0903 admissions per enrollee to 0.08 admissions per enrollee, for a reduction of about 11 percent. Furthermore, assume that MMC conducted a review of its clinical guidelines for capitated patients, resulting in a variable cost per admission reduction from $1,903 per admission to $1,800 per admission, or by about 5 percent. The results of such utilization and cost control efforts are shown in Table 7.6.

TABLE 7.6
Montana
Medical Center:
Projected
Analysis
Assuming
25,000
Enrollees at
$47.04 PMPM
Plus Utilization
and Cost-
Containment
Measures

Payer	Number of Admissions	Average Revenue per Admission	Revenue by Payer	Variable Cost per Admission	Total Variable Costs	Contribution Margin
Payer Worksheet:						
Capitated	**2,000**	**$7,055**	**$ 14,110,583**	**$1,800**	**$ 3,600,000**	**$10,510,583**
Medicare	4,268	7,327	31,271,636	2,529	10,793,772	20,477,864
Medicaid	4,716	5,448	25,692,768	1,575	7,427,700	18,265,068
Montana Care	828	4,305	3,564,540	1,907	1,578,996	1,985,544
Managed Care	1,885	3,842	7,242,170	1,638	3,087,630	4,154,540
Blue Cross	332	5,761	1,912,652	2,366	785,512	1,127,140
Commercial	845	11,770	9,943,296	2,969	2,508,211	7,435,085
Self-Pay	773	2,053	1,587,790	1,489	1,151,593	436,198
Other	1,149	11,539	13,258,331	3,085	3,544,665	9,713,646
Total	16,796		$108,583,746		$34,478,079	$ 74,105,667
Weighted average		**$6,465**		**$2,053**		

P&L Statement:	
Total revenues	$ 108,583,746
Variable costs	**34,478,079**
Contribution margin	$ **74,105,667**
Fixed costs	71,746,561
Profit	$ **2,359,106**

Note: Some rounding differences occur in the table.

Again, the changes from Table 7.3 occur on the first line of the payer worksheet, along with aggregate and average values. The overall result is that variable costs, both for capitated patients and in total, are lowered by $35,174,873 − $34,478,079 = $696,794, so projected profit increases to $1,662,312 + $696,794 = $2,359,106. A reduction in utilization alone produces a cost savings of $490,616, and a reduction in variable cost per admission alone produces a cost savings of $232,754. Each effort, therefore, contributes to the projected increase in MMC's profitability.[3] The benefits of cost containment would be even greater if the program could be applied to all payer groups rather than only to the capitated patients.

Note, though, that MMC would have to incur costs to establish and run the utilization and cost containment programs, so the real question is not what is the benefit of such programs, but what is the **net** benefit. The programs should be undertaken only if the estimated annual costs are less than the projected $696,794 annual benefit. Of course, the greater the number of patients that are brought under these programs, the greater the gross annual benefit and the greater the costs could be and still make the programs financially worthwhile.

Self-Test Questions

1. Briefly explain why the base case analysis required the calculation to move up the profit and loss statement rather than down (the normal direction).
2. How are capitated revenue requirements typically expressed?
3. What is scenario analysis, and why is it so critical to good pricing decisions?
4. What is the most uncertain variable in MMC's capitated plan pricing analysis?

Setting Managed Care Plan Premium Rates

A primary finance task within healthcare insurers is the development of premium rates. In this section, we illustrate several methods that an insurer (or managed care plan or integrated delivery system) can use to estimate the payments it must make to its providers to provide health services to a defined population. These payments are then aggregated and combined with the insurer's own costs to set the premium rate. **Rates typically are developed as if all providers in the system were capitated because the final premium rate will be quoted on a PMPM basis. However, actual reimbursement to the providers in the plan (or system) could be by capitation, discounted fee-for-service, or any other method.** Typically, different classes of providers would be reimbursed using different methods.

To illustrate premium development, assume that BetterCare, Inc., a large HMO, must develop a bid to submit to Big Business, a major employer in BetterCare's service area. To keep the illustration manageable, assume that most of the medically necessary in-area services can be provided by a single hospital that offers both inpatient and outpatient services (including emergency room services), a single nursing home, a panel of primary care physicians, and a panel of specialist physicians. In addition, BetterCare must budget for covered care to be delivered out of area when its members are traveling and for a small amount of specialty services that will be provided outside of the physician panel. Thus, to develop its bid, BetterCare has to estimate the amount of payments to this set of providers for the covered population, plus allow for administrative expenses and profits.

Institutional Rates

The *fee-for-service approach* is often used to set the within-system hospital in-patient capitation rate. This method is based on expected utilization and fee-for-service charges rather than underlying costs, although there clearly should be a link between charges and costs. To illustrate, assume that BetterCare targets 400 inpatient days (in area) for each 1,000 members, or 0.400 inpatient days per member. Furthermore, BetterCare believes that a fair fee-for-service charge in a competitive environment would be $1,200 per inpatient day. The number of inpatient days reflects a highly managed working-age population, and the fee-for-service charge is designed to cover all hospital costs, including profits, in an efficiently run hospital that operates in a highly competitive environment. The inpatient cost PMPM is found this way:

$$\text{Inpatient cost PMPM} = \frac{\text{Per member utilization rate} \times \text{Fee-for-service rate}}{12}$$

$$= \frac{0.400 \times \$1,200}{12} = \$40.00 \text{ PMPM.}$$

Thus, using the fee-for-service method, BetterCare estimates that inpatient costs for Big Business's HMO enrollees is $40 PMPM. Note, however, that even though the cost for inpatient services is estimated on a PMPM basis, actual payment to the hospital for services to the covered population would likely be on a per diem basis.

The rates for out-of-area hospital usage, hospital outpatient visits, and skilled nursing home stays were developed using the fee-for-service method also. Here is a summary of BetterCare's estimates for these services:

Service	Annual Usage per Member	Fee-for-Service Rate	Capitation Rate PMPM
Out-of-area inpatient days	0.045	$1,495	$5.61
Outpatient surgeries	0.050	2,082	8.68
Emergency room visits	0.125	238	2.48
Skilled nursing home days	0.005	350	0.15
			$16.92

Here, each PMPM rate was calculated by multiplying annual utilization by the fee-for-service rate and then dividing the product by 12 to get the PMPM rate. The end result is a capitation estimate of $16.92 PMPM for the services listed. Note, however, that actual payments to these providers typically would be made on a fee-for-service basis (usually discounted). With a PMPM rate of $40 for area inpatient services and a rate of $16.92 for other institutional services, the total PMPM for institutional services is $40.00 + $16.92 = $56.92.

Physician Rates

The *cost approach* will be used to estimate physicians' costs for Big Business's enrollees. This method, which is the most common for setting physicians' payments, is based on utilization and underlying costs as opposed to charges. Again, the starting point is expected patient utilization, but now it is for primary care and specialty physicians' services rather than for institutional services. The expected utilization of physicians' services is then translated into the number of full-time equivalent (FTE) physicians required to treat the covered population, which depends on physician productivity. Next, the cost for physician services is estimated by multiplying the number of physicians required by the average cost per physician, including base compensation, fringe benefits, and malpractice premiums. Finally, an amount is added for clinical and administrative support for physicians, to recognize that physicians must incur heavy overhead costs to support their practices.

In developing its rate for primary care physicians, BetterCare made the following assumptions:

- On average, each enrollee makes 3 visits to a primary care physician per year.
- Each primary care physician can handle 4,000 patient visits per year.
- Total compensation per primary care physician is $175,000 per year.

Given these assumptions, one way to calculate primary physicians' costs is to recognize that each enrollee will require $3 / 4{,}000 = 0.00075$ physicians, for an annual cost of $0.00075 \times \$175{,}000 = \$131.25$ per enrollee. Thus, the cost PMPM $= \$131.25 / 12 = \$10.94$, and the rate that BetterCare will propose to Big Business will include a payment of $10.94 PMPM for primary care physician compensation.

The rate for specialists' care is developed in a similar way. The end result is an annual cost per member of $170.40, giving a PMPM of $\$170.40 / 12 = \$14.20$. The rate that BetterCare will propose to Big Business will therefore include a payment of $14.20 PMPM for specialist physician compensation.

Thus far, the PMPM rate for physicians' compensation has been estimated, but BetterCare's analysis has not accounted for the other costs associated with physicians' practices. First, on average, physicians require 5.7

FTEs for clinical and administrative support, and each supporting staff member receives an average of $45,000 per year in total compensation. Because the physician requirement to support one member is 0.00075 primary care plus 0.00060 specialists, for a total of 0.00135 physicians, each covered life will require 0.00135 × 5.7 × $45,000 = $346.28 to cover physicians' staff costs, or $346.28 / 12 = $28.86 PMPM.

Next, expenditures on supplies, including administrative, medical, and diagnostic, at physicians' practices average $10 per visit, and members are expected to make 4.2 visits per year to both primary and specialty care physicians. Thus, the annual cost per member is $42, and the cost PMPM is estimated to be $42 / 12 = $3.50 PMPM. Finally, facilities expenses, including depreciation, rent, utilities, and so on, are estimated at $6 PMPM.

BetterCare has estimated numerous categories of costs attributable solely to physicians. For ease, assume that BetterCare plans to contract with a single medical group practice to provide all physicians' services and to pay the group a capitated rate. The total capitation rate for the medical group would be as follows:

Primary care	$10.94	PMPM
Specialist care	14.20	
Support staff	28.86	
Supplies	3.50	
Facilities	6.00	
Subtotal	$63.50	PMPM
Profit (10%)	6.35	
In-area total	$69.85	PMPM
Outside referrals	5.40	
Total	$75.25	PMPM

The $75.25 PMPM rate for the medical group is the aggregate of the rates previously developed for physicians' services, plus two additional elements. First, BetterCare believes that a fair profit markup on medical services is 10 percent, so $6.35 PMPM is allowed for profit on the in-area physician subtotal of $69.85 PMPM. Second, $5.40 PMPM is allocated to cover referrals outside the group practice when needed either because a particular specialty is not available within the group or because the covered member is outside the service area. Finally, note that the medical group may not capitate all of its physicians even though it receives a capitated rate from BetterCare.

In general, capitation rates paid to individual physicians include adjustments for the types of patients assigned. Thus, an alternative method for calculating provider costs uses utilization data broken down by age and gender. This *demographic approach* focuses on the characteristics of the population being served, which is then coupled with cost or fee-for-service data to estimate the capitation rate. Table 7.7 illustrates the demographic approach by applying it to the population that would be served if BetterCare wins the

| | Demographics | | Cost per Member per Month | | | | | |
| | | | Primary Care | | Specialist/Referral | | Hospital/Other | |
Age Band	Male	Female	Male	Female	Male	Female	Male	Female
0–1	1.9%	1.9%	$72.25	$72.25	$48.30	$48.30	$46.71	$46.71
2–4	2.8	2.8	31.13	31.13	17.05	17.05	25.42	25.42
5–19	12.4	12.4	16.97	16.97	17.20	17.20	23.96	23.96
20–29	11.4	15.4	16.19	24.47	28.35	75.78	18.07	86.85
30–39	9.6	10.0	20.04	26.99	35.76	68.42	38.94	92.04
40–49	5.3	5.7	25.21	30.07	50.17	63.10	83.87	81.64
50–59	3.6	3.6	31.88	34.96	72.45	73.39	125.80	104.43
60+	0.7	0.5	38.32	39.35	112.88	90.56	189.69	136.672
Total	47.7%	52.3%						
Male/female cost			$10.87	$13.99	$16.26	$28.73	$20.66	$36.26
Total service cost			$24.86		$44.99		$56.92	

TABLE 7.7
Demographic-Based Rates

contract to provide an HMO plan for Big Business. The male/female costs were calculated by multiplying the population percentages for each sex by the applicable costs PMPM. The total cost for each service is the sum of the male and female costs.

The total cost for physicians, $24.86 + $44.99 = $69.85 PMPM, is the same as BetterCare estimated using the cost approach. If the data are consistent, both methods should lead to the same capitation rate. However, with the demographic approach, the PMPM rates paid to individual physicians can be tailored to reflect the age and gender characteristics of each physician's assigned patients. Also, the hospital/other institutional capitation rate of $56.92 PMPM is the same as the rate obtained using the fee-for-service approach. Clearly, the data were fudged so the results would be consistent. In most cases, PMPM rates that are developed using different methodologies will be different, and hence a great deal of judgment must be applied in the rate setting process.

Setting the Final Rate

The goal in this illustration is to set a premium rate that BetterCare can use to make a bid to cover Big Business's employees. Thus far, the PMPM rates required to pay all the providers needed to serve the population have been estimated for both in-area and out-of-area services. The assumption is that pharmacy and durable medical equipment (DME) benefits will be handled separately, or *carved out*, and that the cost of these benefits would be $107 PMPM. After all costs have been considered, BetterCare's managers conclude that they should submit a bid of $275.05 PMPM. Included in the overall bid amount is $23.92 PMPM for contract administration and $11.96 to build reserves and earn a profit. Thus, of the $275.05 PMPM premium that BetterCare would receive from Big Business, $35.88 (13%) would be retained by the HMO and $239.17 (87%) would be paid out to providers, if expectations are met.

Hospital inpatient	$ 40.00	PMPM
Other institutional	16.92	
Pharmacy and DME benefits	107.00	
Physician care	75.25	
Total medical care costs	$239.17	PMPM
HMO costs:		
Administration	$ 23.92	PMPM
Contribution to reserves/profits	11.96	
Total HMO costs	$ 35.88	PMPM
Total premium	$275.05	PMPM

Note that the monthly revenue to providers would be about 10 percent higher than the estimated PMPM rates because enrollees will be required to make copayments for selected services.

BetterCare's bid most likely will be subject to market forces—that is, there will be multiple bidders for Big Business's health contract. If Better-Care's bid is to be accepted, it must offer the right combination of price and quality. If BetterCare's costs and therefore bid is too high, or its quality is too low, it will not get the contract. In that case, it must reassess its cost and quality structure to ensure that it is competitive on future bids.

Self-Test Questions

1. Briefly describe the following three methods for developing premium rates:
   • Fee-for-service approach
   • Cost approach
   • Demographic approach
2. Of the three approaches, which one would be the most accurate? Which approach is the easiest to apply in practice?
3. It is common to express premium rates as PMPM. Does this mean that all providers will be capitated?

Using Relative Value Units (RVUs) to Set Prices

A *relative value unit (RVU)* measures the amount of resources consumed to provide a particular service. Its use in healthcare pricing and reimbursement was influenced primarily by the RBRVS (Resource Based Relative Value System), which uses RVUs to set Medicare payments for physician services. Here, we use the RVU concept to price services for a hospital's clinical laboratory.

Note that using RVUs to estimate costs and ultimately to set prices is simply an application of activity-based costing (ABC), which was discussed in Chapter 6.

To keep the illustration manageable, assume that the clinical laboratory performs only four tests. Furthermore, an in-depth study by the department head and financial staff identified the number of RVUs required to perform each test. To begin, they defined one RVU as equal to five minutes of technicians' time, $10 worth of laboratory equipment use, and $5 worth of laboratory supplies. Then, each of the four tests conducted in the laboratory was examined in detail to determine the time, test equipment, and supplies required to perform one test. The result was the RVU estimates given in the second column of Table 7.8. The RVUs for each test were then multiplied by the number of tests performed annually, and the products were summed to obtain the total RVUs for the laboratory—165,000.

Now assume that the annual costs of the laboratory, including overhead, total $250,000. The laboratory volume and cost estimates could be historical, or they could be budgeted values for the coming year. With these estimates, it is now possible to estimate the cost per RVU by dividing total costs by total RVUs:

$$\$250,000/165,000 = \$1.52 \text{ per RVU.}$$

Finally, the cost associated with each test is merely the number of RVUs assigned to the test multiplied by the $1.52 per RVU cost.

To obtain a price list for the laboratory, assume that the hospital wants to make a 20 percent profit margin on its laboratory services, so each test's price must be 25 percent higher than its cost. The profit-adjusted charge (price) per RVU then becomes $1.52 × 1.25 = $1.90.[4] Table 7.9 lists the price for each test. For example, a very simple urinalysis would be priced at $9.50, while a very complex tissue analysis would be priced at $380.

The goal of RVU pricing is to create prices that reflect the cost of the resources used to provide the service. Of course, the key to the fairness of RVU pricing is how well the number of RVUs assigned to each service actually matches the cost of the resources consumed. Because of the difficulties involved in initially assigning RVU values to services, this method is used most

Test	Number of RVUs	Number of Tests Performed Annually	Total RVUs	
Urinalysis	5	5,000	25,000	
Blood typing	10	4,000	40,000	
Blood cell count	50	1,000	50,000	
Tissue analysis	200	250	50,000	
			165,000	

TABLE 7.8
Clinical Laboratory RVU Analysis

TABLE 7.9
Clinical
Laboratory Price
List

Test	Number of RVUs	Price per RVU	Test Price
Urinalysis	5	$1.90	$ 9.50
Blood typing	10	1.90	19.00
Blood cell count	50	1.90	95.00
Tissue analysis	200	1.90	380.00

often when RVU values have already been estimated, such as for procedures performed by physicians.

Self-Test Questions

1. What is a relative value unit (RVU)?
2. Explain how RVUs can be used to estimate costs and set prices on individual services?

Making Service Decisions (Contract Analysis)

The primary focus of the previous illustrations was price setting. This illustration moves to a related decision—the service decision.

Base Case Analysis

County Health Plan (CHP), an HMO with 40,000 members, has proposed a new contract that would capitate Baptist Memorial Hospital for all inpatient services provided to CHP's commercial enrollees whose primary care physicians are affiliated with the hospital. The proposal calls for a capitation payment of $35 PMPM for the first year of the contract. Baptist's managers must decide whether or not to accept the proposal.

To begin the analysis, Baptist's managed care analysts developed the inpatient actuarial data contained in Table 7.10. The data are presented under two levels of utilization management. The data in the top section are based on a loosely managed population in Baptist's service area. These data represent a bare minimum of utilization management effort and hence reflect relatively poor utilization management practices. The bottom section contains data that represent the best-observed practices throughout the United States. These data are based on hospitals located in service areas that have extremely high managed care penetration. The differences between the two data sets illustrate the potential for improved financial performance that comes with more sophisticated utilization management systems. Both sets of data reflect populations with characteristics similar to CHP's commercial enrollees.

To illustrate the calculations, consider the top line in the top section (General). Under loosely managed utilization, the covered population is expected to use 157 days of general medical services for each 1,000 enrollees. Furthermore, the costs associated with one day of such services total $1,500.

Loosely Managed (Sub-optimal) Utilization:

Service Category	Inpatient Days per 1,000 Enrollees	Average Cost per Day	Average Cost per Member per Month*
General	157	$1,500	$19.62
Surgical	132	1,800	19.80
Psychiatric	71	700	4.14
Alcohol/Drug abuse	38	500	1.58
Maternity	42	1,500	5.25
Total medical costs	440	$1,374	$50.39
Administrative costs			2.80
Risk (profit) margin			2.80
Total PMPM			$55.99

Tightly Managed (Optimal) Utilization:

Service Category	Inpatient Days per 1,000 Enrollees	Average Cost per Day	Average Cost per Member per Month*
General	79	$1,600	$10.53
Surgical	58	1,900	9.18
Psychiatric	13	800	0.87
Alcohol/Drug abuse	4	600	0.20
Maternity	26	1,600	3.47
Total medical costs	180	$1,617	$24.25
Administrative costs			1.35
Risk (profit) margin			1.35
Total PMPM			$26.95

*Based on 40,000 members (enrollees).
Note: Some rounding differences occur in the table.

TABLE 7.10
CHP/Baptist Memorial Hospital: Contract Analysis Under Two Utilization Management Scenarios

Thus, the general services costs for each 1,000 enrollees are expected to be 157 × $1,500 = $235,500, or $19.62 PMPM. Calculations for other inpatient services were performed similarly and added to obtain total medical costs of $50.39 PMPM.

There are two additional categories of costs beside medical costs. Each section of the table has lines for administrative costs and risk (profit) margin. *Administrative costs* include costs incurred in managing the contract, such as costs associated with patient verification, utilization management, quality assurance, and member services. The second category of nonmedical costs is the *risk (profit) margin*. Because Baptist would be bearing inpatient utilization risk for the covered population, it builds in a margin both to provide a profit on the contract commensurate with the risk assumed and to create a reserve that could be tapped if utilization, and hence costs, exceeds the amount estimated. It is Baptist's practice to allow 10 percent of the total premium for these two nonmedical costs, so medical costs represent 90 percent of the total premium. For example, in the upper section of Table 7.10, $0.9 \times$ Total Premium = $50.39, so Total Premium = $50.39 / 0.9 = $55.99. Furthermore, it is Baptist's policy to split the $55.99 − $50.39 = $5.60 in nonmedical costs evenly between the two categories, so administrative costs and risk (profit) margin are allocated $2.80 each.[5]

Table 7.10 sends a strong message to Baptist's managers regarding the acceptability of CHP's $35 PMPM contract offer. If Baptist were to accept the offer, and then loosely manage the enrollee population, it would lose $55.99 − $35 = $20.99 PMPM on the contract. The costs in Table 7.10 represent full costs as opposed to only variable (marginal) costs. Therefore, Baptist may be able to carry the contract in the short-run, but it would not be able to sustain the contract over time. On the other hand, if Baptist could manage the enrollee population in accordance with "best observed practices," it would make a profit of $35 − $26.95 = $8.05 PMPM on the contract.

The contract also can be analyzed in accounting, rather than actuarial, terms. This format, along with the required worksheets, is shown in Table 7.11. Again, focus on the loosely managed section. In Table 7.11, instead of showing inpatient days per 1,000 enrollees as in Table 7.10, inpatient days are expressed in terms of the total number of enrollees, which is expected to be 40,000 for this contract. Thus, using utilization data from Table 7.10, the total number of patient days of general medical services is $157 \times 40,000 = 6,280$. With an estimated cost of $1,500 per day, total costs for general medical services amount to $6,280 \times \$1,500 = \$9,420,000$. The costs for all service categories were calculated in the same way and, for all service categories, total $24,192,000. Each nonmedical service cost was calculated as $40,000 \times \$2.80 \times 12 = \$1,344,000$, resulting in total costs under loosely managed utilization of $26,880,000.

Regardless of the level of utilization management, revenues from the contract are expected to total $40,000 \times \$35 \times 12 = \$16,800,000$. Thus, the projected P&L statements in simplified form consist of this revenue amount minus total costs under each utilization scenario. The end result is an expected net loss of $10,080,000 under loosely managed utilization and a profit of $3,864,000 under tightly managed utilization.

What should Baptist's managers do regarding the contract? For now, the decision appears simple: accept the contract if the hospital can tightly manage utilization or reject the contract if it can not. Unfortunately, the base case contract analysis, like many financial analyses, raises more questions than it answers. This demonstrates that analyses conducted to help with pricing and service decisions tend more often to raise managers' awareness of potential consequences than offer simple solutions.

COST WORKSHEETS:
Loosely Managed (Sub-optimal) Utilization:

Service Category	Inpatient Days per 40,000 Enrollees	Average Cost per Day	Total Annual Costs
General	6,280	$1,500	$ 9,420,000
Surgical	5,280	1,800	9,504,000
Psychiatric	2,840	700	1,988,000
Alcohol/Drug abuse	1,520	500	760,000
Maternity	1,680	1,500	2,520,000
Total medical costs	17,600	$1,374	$ 24,192,000
Administrative costs			1,344,000
Risk (profit) margin			1,344,000
Total annual costs			$ 26,880,000

Tightly Managed (Optimal) Utilization:

Service Category	Inpatient Days per 40,000 Enrollees	Average Cost per Day	Total Annual Costs
General	3,160	$1,600	$ 5,056,000
Surgical	2,320	1,900	4,408,000
Psychiatric	520	800	416,000
Alcohol/Drug abuse	160	600	96,000
Maternity	1,040	1,600	1,664,000
Total medical costs	7,200	$1,617	$ 11,640,000
Administrative costs			648,000
Risk (profit) margin			648,000
Total annual costs			$ 12,936,000

P&L STATEMENTS:
Loosely Managed (Sub-optimal) Utilization:

Total revenues	$16,800,000
Total costs	26,880,000
Profit (Loss)	($10,080,000)

Tightly Managed (Optimal) Utilization:

Total revenues	$16,800,000
Total costs	12,936,000
Profit (Loss)	$ 3,864,000

TABLE 7.11
CHP/Baptist Memorial Hospital: Projected Cost Worksheets and P&L Statements

Note: Some rounding differences occur in the table.

What else would Baptist's managers want to know prior to making the decision? One key element of information is the cost structure (fixed versus variable) associated with the contract. Even though the analyses indicate that the contract is unprofitable under loosely managed utilization, the analysis has been on a full cost basis. If the costs associated with the contract consist of

50 percent fixed costs and 50 percent variable costs, the variable cost PMPM in the worst case (loosely managed utilization) would be $0.50 \times \$55.99 = \$28.00$. At a premium of \$35, the marginal PMPM contribution margin is $\$35 - \$28 = \$7$. Thus, even under loose management, the premium would at least cover the contract's variable costs. If Baptist cannot afford to lose the market share associated with CHP's members, its managers may deem the contract acceptable in the short run. Assuming that the hospital can improve its utilization management over time, eventually it will be able to cover the total costs associated with the contract.

Cost structure is not the only variable that can change over time. Perhaps Baptist can demonstrate superior quality and negotiate a higher premium over time. On the down side, perhaps CHP will gain additional market power over time and attempt to push the premium even lower. These are just a few of the imponderables that Baptist's managers must consider when making the service decision.

Self-Test Questions

1. Why does utilization management play such an important role in pricing and service decisions under capitation?
2. Why are nonmedical costs included in the analysis?
3. What would you do regarding the contract if you were the CEO of Baptist Memorial Hospital?
4. What other factors should Baptist's managers consider when making the capitation contract decision?

Key Concepts

Managers rely on managerial accounting and actuarial information to help make pricing and service decisions. Pricing decisions involve setting prices on services for which the provider is a price setter, while service decisions involve whether or not to offer a service when the price is set by the payer (the provider is a price taker). The key concepts of this chapter are:

- *Pricing* and *service strategies* are linked to an organization's financial statements and the need for revenues to (1) cover the full cost of doing business and (2) provide the profits necessary to acquire new technologies and offer new services.
- *Price takers* are healthcare providers that have to accept, more or less, the prices set in the marketplace for their services, including the prices set by governmental insurers.
- *Price setters* are healthcare providers whose services can be differentiated from others, either by market share or by quality or other differences, such that they have the ability to set the prices on some or all of their services.
- *Full cost pricing* permits businesses to recover all costs, including both

fixed and variable costs and direct and indirect costs, while *marginal cost pricing* recovers only variable costs.

- Purchasers of healthcare services are now exercising considerable market power, thereby restricting the ability of providers to *cross-subsidize (price shift)*.
- *Target costing* is a concept that takes the prices paid for healthcare services as a given and then determines the cost structure necessary for financial survival given the prices set.
- Three primary techniques are used to develop capitation rates: the *fee-for-service approach*, the *cost approach*, and the *demographic approach*.
- Pricing and service decisions are supported by a variety of analyses that use both actuarial and accounting data. Typically, such analyses include a *base case*, which uses the most likely estimates for all input values, plus a *scenario analysis* that considers the effects of alternative assumptions.
- One common method for setting prices, especially for medical practices, is to use *relative value units (RVUs)* to measure the amount of resources consumed by individual services.

In the next chapter, our coverage of managerial accounting continues with a discussion of planning and budgeting.

Questions

7.1 a. Using a healthcare provider (e.g., a hospital) to illustrate your answer, explain the difference between a price setter and a price taker.
    b. Can most providers be classified strictly as either a price setter or a price taker?
7.2 Explain the essential differences between full cost and marginal cost pricing strategies.
7.3 What would happen financially to a health services organization over time if its prices were set at:
    a. Full costs
    b. Marginal costs
7.4 a. What is cross-subsidization (price shifting)?
    b. Is it as prevalent today as it has been in the past?
7.5 a. What is target costing?
    b. Suppose a hospital was offered a capitation rate for a covered population of $40 per member per month (PMPM). Briefly explain how target costing would be applied in this situation.
7.6 What is the role of information systems in pricing decisions?
7.7 Compare and contrast the following three methods for developing capitation rates: fee-for-service approach, cost approach, and demographic approach.

7.8 a. What is scenario analysis as applied to pricing and service decisions?
   b. Why is it such an important part of the process?
7.9 a. Define a relative value unit (RVU).
   b. Explain how RVUs can be used to set prices on individual services.

Problems

7.1 Assume that the managers of Fort Winston Hospital are setting the price on a new outpatient service. Here are relevant data estimates:

Variable cost per visit	$5.00
Annual direct fixed costs	$500,000
Annual overhead allocation	$50,000
Expected annual utilization	10,000 visits

   a. What per visit price must be set for the service to break even? To earn an annual profit of $100,000?
   b. Repeat Part a, but assume that the variable cost per visit is $10.
   c. Return to the data given in the problem. Again repeat Part a, but assume that direct fixed costs are $1,000,000.
   d. Repeat Part a assuming both a $10 variable cost and $1,000,000 in direct fixed costs.

7.2 The Audiology department at Randall Clinic offers many services to the clinic's patients. The three most common, along with cost and utilization data, are:

Service	Variable Cost per Service	Annual Direct Fixed Costs	Annual Number of Visits
Basic examination	$ 5	$50,000	3,000
Advanced examination	7	30,000	1,500
Therapy session	10	40,000	500

   a. What is the fee schedule for these services, assuming that the goal is to cover only variable and direct fixed costs?
   b. Assume that the Audiology department is allocated $100,000 in total overhead by the clinic, and the department director has allocated $50,000 of this amount to the three services listed above. What is the fee schedule assuming that these overhead costs must be covered? (To answer this question, assume that the allocation of overhead costs to each service is made on the basis of number of visits.)
   c. Assume that these services must make a combined profit of $25,000. Now what is the fee schedule? (To answer this question, assume that the profit requirement is allocated in the same way as overhead costs.)

7.3 Allied Laboratories is combining some of its most common tests into one-price packages. One such package will contain three tests that have the following variable costs:

	Test A	Test B	Test C
Disposable syringe	$3.00	$3.00	$3.00
Blood vial	0.50	0.50	0.50
Forms	0.15	0.15	0.15
Reagents	0.80	0.60	1.20
Sterile bandage	0.10	0.10	0.10
Breakage/losses	0.05	0.05	0.05

When the tests are combined, only one syringe, form, and sterile bandage will be used. Furthermore, only one charge for breakage/losses will apply. Two blood vials are required and reagent costs will remain the same (reagents from all three tests are required).

a. As a starting point, what is the price of the combined test assuming marginal cost pricing?

b. Assume that Allied wants a contribution margin of $10 per test. What price must be set to achieve this goal?

c. Allied estimates that 2,000 of the combined tests will be conducted during the first year. The annual allocation of direct fixed and overhead costs total $40,000. What price must be set to cover full costs? What price must be set to produce a profit of $20,000 on the combined test?

7.4 Assume that Valley Forge Hospital has only the following three payer groups:

Payer	Number of Admissions	Average Revenue per Admission	Variable Cost per Admission
PennCare	1,000	$5,000	$3,000
Medicare	4,000	4,500	4,000
Commercial	8,000	7,000	2,500

The hospital's fixed costs are $38 million.

a. What is the hospital's net income?

b. Assume that half of the 100,000 covered lives in the commercial payer group will be moved into a capitated plan. All utilization and cost data remain the same. What PMPM rate will the hospital have to charge to retain their Part a net income?

c. What overall net income would be produced if the admission rate of the capitated group were reduced from the commercial level by 10 percent?

d. Assuming that the utilization reduction also occurs, what overall net income would be produced if the variable cost per admission for the capitated group were lowered to $2,200?

7.5 Bay Pines Medical Center estimates that a capitated population of 50,000 would have the following base case utilization and total cost characteristics:

Service Category	Inpatient Days per 1,000 Enrollees	Average Cost per Day
General	150	$1,500
Surgical	125	1,800
Psychiatric	70	700
Alcohol/Drug abuse	38	500
Maternity	42	1,500
Total	440	$1,374

In addition to medical costs, Bay Pines allocates 10 percent of the total premium for administration/reserves.

   a. What is the PMPM rate that Bay Pines must set to cover medical costs plus administrative expenses?

   b. What would be the rate if a utilization management program would reduce utilization within each patient service category by 10 percent? By 20 percent?

   c. Return to the initial base case utilization assumption. What rate would be set if the average cost on each service were reduced by 10 percent?

   d. Assume that both utilization and cost reductions were made. What would the premium be?

7.6 Assume that a primary care physician practice performs only physical examinations. However, there are three levels of examination—I, II, and III—that vary in depth and complexity. An RVU analysis indicates that a Level I examination requires 10 RVUs, a Level II exam 20 RVUs, and a Level III exam 30 RVUs. The total costs to run the practice, including a diagnostic laboratory, amount to $500,000 annually, and the numbers of examinations administered annually are 2,400 Level I, 800 Level II, and 400 Level III.

   a. Using RVU methodology, what is the estimated cost per type of examination?

   b. If the goal of the practice is to earn a 20 percent profit margin on each examination, how should the examinations be priced?

Notes

1. The values in Tables 7.1 and 7.3 were obtained from a spreadsheet analysis, which does not round to the nearest dollar. Thus, there are some minor rounding differences when the calculations are made by hand.

2. This type of analysis is also called a *sensitivity analysis* because its purpose is to determine how sensitive the results are to changes in the underlying assumptions. However, in Chapter 16, we will use the term "sensitivity analysis" to describe a very particular type of analysis, so we will call the analysis here "scenario analysis."

3. The two cost savings amounts total $490,616 + $232,754 = $723,370, which is $26,576 greater than the $696,794 savings actually realized if both efforts are undertaken. This apparent anomaly occurs because a reduction in admissions lowers the value of the reduction in variable costs by $258 \times \$103 = \$26,574$, which, except for a rounding difference, equals $723,370 − $696,794 = $26,576.

4. To make a 20 percent profit margin, Profit / Price = (Price − Cost) / Price = 0.20. Solving for price as a function of cost gives Price = Cost / 0.80 = 1.25 × Cost. In the example, each RVU has a profit component of $1.90 − $1.52 = $0.38, which gives a profit margin of $0.38 / $1.90 = 0.20 = 20%.

5. Baptist's managers use the same 10 percent nonmedical cost allocation for both the loosely and tightly managed utilization scenarios. One could argue that the greater the utilization management effort, the higher the administrative costs. Thus, it might be better to allocate a greater percentage for administrative costs in the tightly managed scenario than in the loosely managed scenario. In fact, administrative costs could require a higher dollar allocation under tightly managed utilization, even though the overall premium amount is lower.

References

Anderson, G. F., et al. 1990. "Setting Payment Rates for Capitated Systems: A Comparison of Various Alternatives." *Inquiry* (Fall): 225–233.

Baker, J. J., P. Chiverton, and V. Hines. 1998. "Identifying Costs for Capitation in Psychiatric Case Management." *Journal of Health Care Finance* (Spring). 41–44.

Benz, P. D., and R. V. Nagelhout. 1986. "Evaluating Pricing for Health Care Service Contracts." *Journal of Health Care Finance* (Winter): 59–78.

Berlin, M. F., et al. 1997. "RVU Costing Applications." *Healthcare Financial Management* (Nov): 73–74.

Cleverley, W. O. 2003. "What Price is Right." *Healthcare Financial Management* (April): 64–70.

Cleverley, W. O., and J. Cleverley. 2007. "Setting Defensible and Appropriate Prices in Healthcare." *Healthcare Executive* (January/February): 9–12.

Heshmat, S. 1997. "Managed Care and the Relevant Costs for Pricing." *Health Care Management Review* (Winter): 82–85.

Healthcare Financial Management Association (HFMA). 2004. "Strategic Price Setting: Ensuring Your Financial Viability Through Price Modeling." *Healthcare Financial Management* (July): 97–98.

Horowitz, J. L., and M. A. Kleinman. 1994. "Advanced Pricing Strategies for Hospitals in Contracting with Managed Care Organizations." *Journal of Health Care Finance* (Fall): 90–100.

Jacobs, P., and C. R. Franz. 1985. "Developing Pricing Policies by Diagnostic Group." *Healthcare Financial Management* (January): 50–52.

Keough, C. L., and A. Ruskin. 2004. "Medicare Implications of Discounts to the Uninsured." *Healthcare Financial Management* (July): 40–43.

Nugent, M. 2004. "The Price Is Right?" *Healthcare Financial Management* (December): 56–62.

————. 2006. "Picking Up the Pace: Accelerating Your Pricing Competency." *Healthcare Financial Management* (October): 62–70.

Pederson, C. D. 2005. "Cost-Based Pricing and the Underperforming Physician Group." *Healthcare Financial Management* (October): 62–68.

Pickard, J. G., R. A. Friedman, and T. J. Johnson. 1991. "Repricing Plan Yields Realistic Revenue Enhancement." *Healthcare Financial Management* (May): 45–52.

Rosko, M. D., and C. E. Carpenter. 1994. "Hospital Markups: Responses to Environmental Pressures in Pennsylvania." *Hospital & Health Services Administration* (Spring): 3–16.

Smith, B. F., and R. B. Hardaway. 2005. "Time for a Price Check?" *Healthcare Financial Management* (October): 55–60.

West, T. D., E. A. Balas, and D. A. West. 1996. "Contrasting RCC, RVU, and ABC for Managed Care Decisions." *Healthcare Financial Management* (Aug): 54–61.

Wichmann, R., and R. Clark. 2006. "Developing a Defensible Pricing Strategy." *Healthcare Financial Management* (October): 72–80.

PLANNING AND BUDGETING

Learning Objectives

After studying this chapter, readers will be able to:

- Describe the overall planning process and the key components of the financial plan.
- Discuss briefly the format and use of several types of budgets.
- Explain the difference between a static budget and a flexible budget.
- Create a simple operating budget.
- Use variance analysis to assess financial performance and identify operational areas of concern.
- Explain the construction and use of a cash budget.

Introduction

Planning and budgeting play a critical role in the finance function of all health services organizations. In fact, one could argue (and usually win the argument) that planning and budgeting are the most important of all finance-related tasks.

Planning encompasses the overall process of preparing for the future. Because of its importance to organizational success, most health services managers, especially at large organizations, spend a great deal of time on activities related to planning. *Budgeting* is an offshoot of the planning process. A set of *budgets* is the basic managerial accounting tool used to tie together planning and control functions. In general, organizational plans focus on the long-term big picture, whereas budgets address the details of both planning for the immediate future and, through the control mechanism, ensuring that current performance is consistent with organizational plans and goals.

This chapter first introduces the planning process and then discusses how budgets are used within health services organizations. In particular, the chapter focuses on how managers can use flexible budgets and variance analysis to help exercise control over current operations. Unfortunately, in an introductory book, only the surface of these very important topics can be scratched.[1]

The Planning Process

Financial plans and budgets are developed within the framework of the business's overall *strategic plan*. Thus, we begin our discussion with an overview of strategic planning.

Values Statement

The "guiding light" for the strategic plan is an organization's values statement, because values represent the core priorities that define the culture of an organization. In general, the values statement contains a list of four to six values that provide the basic beliefs that underlie the strategic plan. To illustrate, consider the following values statement of Bayside Memorial Hospital, a not-for-profit acute care hospital:

- To treat everyone with respect and dignity
- To trust in all relationships
- To be compassionate in comfort and care
- To do the right thing at the right time for the right reason
- To be patient and tolerant
- To achieve excellence and ensure quality

Mission and Vision Statements

The *mission statement*, which must conform to the values of the organization, defines its overall purpose and reason for existence. The mission may be defined either very specifically or in more general terms, but, at a minimum, it must describe what the organization does and for whom. For example, an investor-owned medical equipment manufacturer might state that its mission is "to provide our customers with state-of-the-art diagnostic systems at the lowest attainable cost, which will also maximize benefits to our employees and stockholders."

Mission statements for not-for-profit businesses normally are stated in different terms; but the reality of competition in the health services industry forces all businesses, regardless of ownership, to operate in a manner consistent with financial viability. Bayside's mission statement is as follows:

The mission of Bayside Memorial Hospital is to

- provide comprehensive, state-of-the-art patient services.
- emphasize caring and other human values in the treatment of patients and in relations among employees, medical staff, and community.
- provide employees and medical staff with maximum opportunities to achieve their personal and professional goals.

Vision statements usually are developed concurrently with the mission statement. The most effective vision statements are brief, single-sentence statements that describe the desired position of the organization at a future point in time—say, ten years. The intent is to provide a single goal that motivates managers, employees, and the medical staff. Bayside's vision statement is "to be the regional leader in providing state-of-the-art compassionate care in a humanistic environment."

In addition to providing limited guidance regarding management and employee behavior at Bayside, the mission and vision statements provide managers with a framework for establishing specific goals and objectives.

Corporate Goals

The mission and vision statements contain the general philosophy and approach of the organization, as well as its long-term aspiration, but they do not provide managers with specific operational goals. *Corporate goals* set forth specific goals that management strives to attain. Corporate goals generally are qualitative in nature, such as "keeping the firm's research and development efforts at the cutting edge of the industry." Multiple goals are established, and they should be changed over time as conditions change. Furthermore, a firm's corporate goals should be challenging yet realistically attainable.

Bayside Memorial Hospital divides its corporate goals into the following five major areas:

1. *Quality and Customer Satisfaction*
   - To make quality performance the goal of each employee
   - To be recognized by our patients as the provider of choice in our market area
   - To identify and resolve as rapidly as possible areas of patient dissatisfaction

2. *Medical Staff Relations*
   - To identify and develop timely channels of communication among all members of the medical staff, management, and board of directors
   - To respond in a timely manner to all medical staff concerns brought to the attention of management
   - To make Bayside Memorial Hospital a more desirable location to practice medicine
   - To develop strategies to enhance the mutual commitment of the medical staff, administration, and board of directors for the benefit of the hospital's stakeholders
   - To provide the highest quality, most cost-effective medical care through a collaborative effort of the medical staff, administration, and board of directors

3. *Human Resources Management*
   - To be recognized as the customer service leader in our market area
   - To develop and manage human resources to make Bayside Memorial Hospital the most attractive location to work in our market area

4. *Financial Performance*
   - To maintain a financial condition that permits us to be highly competitive in our market area
   - To develop the systems necessary to identify inpatient and outpatient costs by unit of service

5. *Health Systems Management*
   - To be a leader in applied technology based on patient needs
   - To establish new services and programs in response to patient needs
   - To be in the forefront of electronic medical records (EMR) technology

Of course, these goals occasionally conflict, and when they do Bayside's senior managers have to make judgments regarding which one takes precedence.

Corporate Objectives

Once an organization has defined its mission, vision, and goals, it must develop objectives designed to help it achieve its stated goals. *Corporate objectives* are generally quantitative in nature, such as specifying a target market share, a target return on equity (ROE), a target earnings per share growth rate, or a target EVA (economic value added). Furthermore, the extent to which corporate objectives are met is commonly used as a basis for managers' compensation. To illustrate, consider Bayside's financial performance goal of maintaining a financial condition that permits the hospital to be highly competitive in its market area. These objectives are tied to that goal:

- To maintain or exceed the hospital's current 4.3 percent operating margin
- To maintain or exceed the hospital's current 7.3 percent total margin
- To increase the hospital's debt ratio to the range of 35–40 percent; however, this objective will not be attained by accepting new projects that will lower the hospital's profit margin
- To maintain the hospital's liquidity as measured by the current ratio in the range of 2.0 to 2.5
- To increase fixed asset utilization as measured by the fixed asset turnover ratio to 1.5

Corporate objectives give managers precise targets to shoot for. But the objectives must support the business's mission, vision, and goals, and must be chosen carefully so that they are challenging yet attainable in a few years' time.

1. Briefly, describe the nature and use of the following corporate planning tools:
   a. Values statement
   b. Mission statement
   c. Vision statement
   d. Corporate goals
   e. Corporate objectives
2. Why do financial planners need to be familiar with the business's strategic plan?

Operational Planning

Whereas strategic planning provides general guidance, along with specific goals and objectives, operational planning provides a roadmap for executing a business's strategic plan. The key document in operational planning is the business's *operating plan*, which contains the detailed guidance necessary to meet corporate objectives. In other words, the operating plan provides the "how to" or perhaps "how we expect to" portion of an organization's overall plan for the future. Operating plans can be developed for any time horizon, but most firms use a five-year horizon, and thus the term *five-year plan* has become common. In a five-year plan, the plans are most detailed for the first year, with each succeeding year's plan becoming less specific.

Table 8.1 outlines the key elements of Bayside Memorial Hospital's five-year plan, with an expanded section for the financial plan. A full outline would require several pages, but Table 8.1 provides some insights into the format and contents of a five-year plan. Note that the first two chapters of the operating plan are drawn from the organization's strategic plan.

Table 8.2 contains the hospital's annual financial planning schedule. This schedule illustrates the fact that for most organizations the financial planning process is essentially continuous. For Bayside, much of the financial planning function takes place at the department level, with technical assistance from the marketing, planning, and financial staffs. Larger businesses, with divisions, would focus the planning process at the divisional level. Each division would have its own mission and goals, as well as objectives and budgets designed to support its goals; and these plans, when consolidated, would constitute the overall corporate plan.

The first part of the *financial plan* (Chapter 7.C of the five-year plan) focuses on financial condition, investments, and financing at the organizational level. Its first component is a review of the business's current financial condition, which provides the basis, or starting point, for the remainder of the financial plan. (Insights into how this is accomplished are presented in Chapter 17.) Next, the capital budget, which outlines future capital investment (i.e., long-term asset purchases), is presented. (Capital budgeting procedures are discussed in Chapters 14 and 15.) This information feeds into the forecasted financial statements, which are projected for the next five years.[2] Finally, the organization's external financing requirements are listed, along with a plan for obtaining these funds. (Financing decisions will be covered in Chapters 11, 12, and 13.) As can be seen from its content, Section 1 of the financial plan provides an overview of the financial future of the organization.

Section 2 of the financial plan concerns current asset and current liability management, which often is called *working capital management*. Here, the plan provides overall guidance regarding day-to-day, short-term financial operations. (The cash budget is discussed later in the chapter. The remainder of working capital management is covered in Chapter 16.) In essence, Section 2 of the financial plan provides short-term operating benchmarks for all levels of management.

The managerial accounting portion (Section 3) provides financial goals at the micro level—for example, by division, contract, or diagnosis—and is

Months	Action
April–May	Marketing department analyzes national and local economic factors likely to influence Bayside's patient volume and reimbursement rates. At this time, a preliminary volume forecast is prepared for each service line.
June–July	Operating departments prepare new project (long-term asset) requirements as well as operating cost estimates based on the preliminary volume forecast.
August–September	Financial analysts evaluate proposed capital expenditures and department operating plans. Preliminary forecasted financial statements are prepared with emphasis on Bayside's overall sources and uses of funds and forecasted financial condition.
October–November	All previous input is reviewed and the hospital's five-year plan is drafted by the planning, financial, and departmental staffs. At this stage, the operating and cash budgets are finalized. Any changes that have occurred since the beginning of the planning process are incorporated into the plan.
December	The five-year plan, including all budgets for the coming year, is approved by the hospital's executive committee and then submitted to the board of directors for final approval.

TABLE 8.2
Bayside Memorial Hospital: Annual Financial Planning Schedule

used to control operations through frequent comparisons with actual results. In essence, this portion contains the budgets that provide the benchmarks that managers should be striving to attain throughout the year.

If financial planning were compared to planning a cross-country road trip, Section 1 of the financial plan could be thought of as a roadmap of the United States, which provides the overview, while Sections 2 and 3 could be thought of as the state maps, which provide the details.

1. What is the primary difference between strategic and operating plans?
2. What is the most common time horizon for operating plans?
3. Briefly describe the contents of a typical financial plan.
4. What is the primary difference between Sections 1 and 3 of the financial plan?

Self-Test Questions

Introduction to Budgeting

Budgeting involves detailed plans, expressed in dollar terms, which specify how resources will be obtained and used during a specified period of time. In general, budgets rely heavily on revenue and cost estimates, so the budgeting process applies many of the managerial accounting concepts presented in Chapters 5, 6, and 7.

To be of most use, managers must think of budgets not as accounting tools but as managerial tools. Budgets are more important to managers than to accountants because budgets provide the means to plan and communicate operational expectations within an organization. Every manager within an organization must be aware of the plans made by other managers and by the organization as a whole, and budgets provide the means of communication. In addition, the budgeting process and the resultant final budget provide the means for senior managers to allocate financial resources among competing demands within an organization.

Although planning, communication, and allocation are important purposes of the budgeting process, perhaps the greatest value of budgeting is that it establishes financial benchmarks for control. When compared to actual results, budgets provide managers with feedback about the relative financial performance of the entity—whether it is a department, diagnosis, contract, or the organization as a whole. Such comparisons help managers evaluate the performance of individuals, departments, product lines, reimbursement contracts, and so on.

Finally, budgets provide managers with information about what needs to be done to improve performance. When actual results fall short of those specified in the budget, managers use *variance analysis* to identify the areas that caused the subpar performance. In this way, managerial resources can be brought to bear on those areas of operations that offer the most promise for financial improvement. In addition, the information developed by comparing actual results with expected (planned) results (i.e., the control process) is useful in improving the overall accuracy of the planning process. Managers want to meet budget targets, and hence most managers will think long and hard when those targets are being developed.

Self-Test Questions	1. What is budgeting?
	2. What are its primary purposes and benefits?

Budget Types

Although an organization's immediate financial expectations are expressed in a document called *the budget* (or *master budget*), in most organizations "the budget" is actually composed of several different budgets. Unlike a business's financial statements, budget formats are not specified by external parties, so the contents and format of the budget are dictated by the business's mission and structure and by managerial preferences. That said, several types of budgets are used either formally or informally at virtually all health services organizations.

Statistics Budget

The *statistics budget* is the cornerstone of the budgeting process in that it specifies the patient volume and resource assumptions used in other budgets. Because the statistics budget feeds into all other budgets, accuracy is particularly important. Note that the statistics budget does not provide detailed information on required resources such as staffing or short-term operating asset requirements, but it provides general guidance.

Some organizations, especially smaller ones, may not have a separate statistics budget but instead may incorporate data directly into the revenue and expense budgets or perhaps into a single operating budget. The advantage of having a separate statistics budget is that it forces all other budgets within the organization to use the same set of volume and resource assumptions. Unfortunately, volume estimates, which are the heart of the statistics budget and which drive all other forecasts, are among the most difficult to make.

To illustrate the complexities of volume forecasting, consider the volume forecast procedures followed by Bayside Memorial Hospital. To begin, the demand for services is divided into four major groups: inpatient, outpatient, ancillary, and other services. Volume trends in each of these areas over the past five years are plotted, and a first approximation forecast is made, assuming a continuation of past trends. Next, the level of population growth and disease trends are forecasted. For example, what will be the growth in the over-65 population in the hospital's service area? These forecasts are used to develop volume by major diagnoses and to differentiate between normal services and critical care services.

Bayside's managers then analyze the competitive environment. Consideration is given to such factors as the hospital's inpatient and outpatient capacities, its competitors' capacities, and new services or service improvements that either Bayside or its competitors might institute. Next, Bayside's managers consider the effect of the hospital's planned pricing actions on volume. For example, does the hospital have plans to raise outpatient charges to boost profit margins or to lower charges to gain market share and utilize excess capacity? If such actions are expected to affect volume forecasts, these forecasts must be revised to reflect the expected impact. Marketing campaigns and changes in managed care plan contracts also affect volume, so probable developments in these areas must be considered.

If the hospital's volume forecast is off the mark, the consequences can be serious. First, if the market for any particular service expands more than Bayside has expected and planned for, the hospital will not be able to meet its patients' needs. Potential patients will end up going to competitors, and Bayside will lose market share and perhaps miss a major opportunity. However, if its projections are overly optimistic, Bayside could end up with too much capacity, which means higher than necessary costs because of excess facilities and staff.

Revenue Budget

Detailed information from the statistics budget feeds into the *revenue budget*, which combines volume and reimbursement data to develop revenue forecasts. Bayside's planners consider the hospital's pricing strategy for managed care plans, conventional fee-for-service contracts, and private pay patients as well as trends in inflation and third-party payer reimbursement, all of which affect operating revenues.

The end result is a compilation of operating revenue forecasts by service, both in the aggregate—for example, inpatient revenue—and on an individual diagnosis basis. The individual diagnosis forecasts are summed and then compared with the aggregate service group forecasts. Differences are reconciled, and the result is an operating revenue forecast for the hospital as a whole but with breakdowns by service categories and by individual diagnoses.

In addition to operating revenues, other revenues, such as interest income on investments and lease payments on medical office buildings, must be forecasted. Note that in all revenue forecasts both the amount and the *timing* are important. Thus, the revenue budget must forecast not only the amount of revenue but also when the revenue is expected to occur, typically by month. (As we discuss later, budgets generally follow accrual accounting concepts, so the revenue focus is on reported revenue as opposed to cash flow.)

Expense Budget

Like the revenue budget, the *expense budget* is derived from data in the statistics budget. The focus here is on the costs of providing services rather than the resulting revenues. The expense budget typically is divided into labor (salaries, wages, and fringe benefits, including travel and education) and nonlabor components. The nonlabor components include expenses associated with such items as depreciation, leases, utilities, and administrative and medical supplies. Expenses normally will be broken down into fixed and variable components. (As discussed later in this chapter, cost structure information is required if an organization uses flexible budgeting techniques.)

Operating Budget

For larger organizations, the *operating budget* is a combination of the revenue and expense budgets. For smaller businesses, the statistics, revenue, and expense budgets often are combined into a single operating budget. Because the operating budget (and, by definition, the revenue and expense budgets) is prepared using accrual accounting methods, it can be roughly thought of as a forecasted income statement. However, unlike the income statement, which is typically prepared at the organizational level, operating budgets are prepared at the subunit level—say, a department or product line. Because of its overall importance to the budgeting process, most of this chapter focuses on the operating budget.

Cash Budget

Finally, the *cash budget* focuses on the organization's cash position. Because the operating budget and its component budgets use accrual accounting, they do not provide cash flow information. Like the statement of cash flows, which recasts the income statement to focus on cash, the cash budget recasts the operating budget to focus on the actual flow of cash into and out of a business. Thus, the cash budget tells managers whether the business is projected to generate excess cash, which will have to be invested, or to experience a cash shortfall, which will have to be covered in some way.

The primary difference between a cash budget and a forecasted statement of cash flows is time period. The projected statement of cash flows generally is prepared on an annual (and perhaps quarterly) basis and is used for long-term planning. Conversely, the cash budget is prepared on a monthly, weekly, or daily basis and is used for short-term cash management. Cash budgeting will be discussed later in this chapter, while its implications for cash management will be discussed in Chapter 16.

1. What are some of the budget types used within health services organizations?
2. Briefly describe the purpose and use of each.
3. How are the statistics budget, revenue and expense budgets, and operating budget related?
4. How does the cash budget differ from the operating budget? From the statement of cash flows?

Self-Test Questions

Budget Decisions

In addition to deciding on the types of budgets to be used within an organization, managers must make several other decisions regarding the budget process.

Timing

Virtually all health services organizations have annual budgets, which set the standards for the coming year. However, it would take too long for managers to detect adverse trends if budget feedback were provided solely on an annual basis, so most organizations also have quarterly budgets, while some have monthly, weekly, or even daily budgets. Not all budget types or subunits within an organization have to use the same timing pattern. Additionally, many organizations prepare budgets for one or more *out years*, or years beyond the next budget year, which are more closely aligned with financial planning than with operational control.

Conventional Versus Zero-Based Budgets

Traditionally, health services organizations have used the *incremental/decremental*, or *conventional, approach* to budgeting. In this approach, the previous budget is used as the starting point for creating the new budget. Each line on the old budget is examined, and then adjustments are made to reflect changes in circumstances. In this approach, it is common for many budget changes to be applied more or less equally across departments and programs. For example, labor costs might be assumed to increase at the same inflation rate for all departments and programs within an organization. In essence, the traditional approach to budgeting assumes that prior budgets are based on operational rationality, so the main issue is determining what changes (typically minor) must be made to the previous budget to account for changes in the operating environment.

As its name implies, *zero-based budgeting* starts with a clean slate.[3] For example, departments begin with a budget of zero. Department heads then must fully justify every line item in their budgets. In effect, departments and programs must justify their contribution (positive or negative) to the organization's financial condition each budget period. In some situations, department and program heads must create budgets that show the impact of alternative funding levels. Senior management then can use this information to make rational decisions about where cuts could be made in the event of financial constraints.

Conceptually, zero-based budgeting is superior to conventional budgeting. Indeed, when zero-based budgeting was first introduced in the 1970s, it was widely embraced. However, the managerial resources required for zero-based budgeting far exceed those required for conventional budgeting. Therefore, many organizations that initially adopted zero-based budgeting soon concluded that its benefits were not as great as its costs. There is evidence, however, that zero-based budgeting is making a comeback among health services organizations, primarily because market forces are requiring providers to implement cost-control efforts on a more or less continuous basis.

As a compromise, some health services organizations use conventional budgeting annually but then use a zero-based budget on a less frequent basis—say, every five years. An alternative is to use the conventional approach on 80 percent of the budget each year and the zero-based approach on 20 percent. Then, over every five-year period, the entire budget will be subjected to zero-based budgeting. This approach takes advantage of the benefits of zero-based budgeting without creating a budgeting process in any year that is too time-consuming for managers.

Top-Down Versus Bottom-Up Budgets

The budget affects virtually everyone in the organization, and individuals' reactions to the budgeting process can have considerable influence on an organization's overall effectiveness. Thus, one of the most important decisions regarding budget preparation is whether the budget should be created top-down or bottom-up.

In the *bottom-up*, or *participatory, approach*, budgets are developed first by department or program managers. Presumably, such individuals are most knowledgeable regarding their departments' or programs' financial needs. The department budgets are submitted to the finance department for review and compilation into the organizational budget, which then must be approved by senior management. Unfortunately, the aggregation of department or program budgets often results in an organizational budget that is not financially feasible. In such cases, the component budgets must be sent back to the original preparers for revision, which starts a negotiation process aimed at creating a budget acceptable to all parties, or at least to as many parties as possible.

A more authoritarian approach to budgeting is the *top-down approach*, in which little negotiation takes place between junior and senior managers. This approach has the advantages of being relatively expeditious and reflecting top management's perspective from the start. However, by limiting involvement and communication, the top-down approach often results in less commitment among junior managers and employees than does the bottom-up approach. Most people will perform better and make greater attempts to achieve budgetary goals if they have played a prominent role in setting those goals. The idea of participatory budgeting is to involve as many managers, and even employees, as possible in the budgetary process.

1. What time periods are used in budgeting? 2. What are the primary differences between conventional and zero-based budgets? 3. What are the primary differences between top-down and bottom-up budgets?	**Self-Test Questions**

Constructing a Simple Operating Budget

Table 8.3 contains the 2007 operating budget for Carroll Clinic, a large, inner city, primary care facility. Most operating budgets are more complex than this illustration, which has purposely been kept simple for ease of discussion.

As with most financial forecasts, the starting point for the operating budget, which was developed in October of 2006, is patient volume. *A volume projection* gives managers a starting point for making revenue and cost estimates. As shown in Part I of Table 8.3, Carroll Clinic's expected patient volume for 2007 comes from two sources: a fee-for-service (FFS) population expected to total 36,000 visits and a capitated population expected to average 30,000 members. Historically, annual utilization by the capitated population

TABLE 8.3

Carroll Clinic: 2007 Operating Budget

I.	*Volume Assumptions:*			
	A.	FFS	36,000	visits
	B.	Capitated lives	30,000	members
		Number of member months	360,000	
		Expected utilization per member-month	0.15	
		Number of visits	54,000	visits
	C.	Total expected visits	90,000	visits
II.	*Revenue Assumptions:*			
	A.	FFS	$ 25	per visit
			× 36,000	expected visits
			$ 900,000	
	B.	Capitated lives	$ 3	PMPM
			× 360,000	actual member months
			$ 1,080,000	
	C.	Total expected revenues	$ 1,980,000	
III.	*Cost Assumptions:*			
	A.	Variable Costs:		
		Labor	$ 1,200,000	(48,000 hours at $25/hour)
		Supplies	150,000	(100,000 units at $1.50/unit)
		Total variable costs	$ 1,350,000	
		Variable cost per visit	$ 15	($1,350,000/90,000)
	B.	Fixed Costs:		
		Overhead, plant, and equipment	$ 500,000	
	C.	Total expected costs	$ 1,850,000	
IV.	*Pro Forma Profit and Loss (P&L) Statement:*			
		Revenues:		
		FFS	$ 900,000	
		Capitated	1,080,000	
		Total	$ 1,980,000	
		Costs:		
		Variable:		
		FFS	$ 540,000	
		Capitated	810,000	
		Total	$ 1,350,000	
		Contribution margin	$ 630,000	
		Fixed costs	500,000	
		Projected profit	$ 130,000	

has averaged 0.15 visits per member-month, so in 2007 this population, which is expected to total $30,000 \times 12 = 360,000$ member-months, will provide $360,000 \times 0.15 = 54,000$ visits. In total, therefore, Carroll's patient base is expected to produce $36,000 + 54,000 = 90,000$ visits. Armed with this Part I volume projection, Carroll's managers can proceed with revenue and cost projections.

Part II contains revenue data. The clinic's net collection for each FFS visit averages $25. Some visits will generate greater revenues, and some will generate less. On average, though, expected revenue is $25 per visit. Thus, 36,000 visits would produce $25 × 36,000 = $900,000 in FFS revenues. In addition, the premium for the capitated population is $3 PMPM, which would generate a revenue of $3 × 360,000 member-months = $1,080,000. Considering both patient sources, total revenues for the clinic are forecasted to be $900,000 + $1,080,000 = $1,980,000 in 2007.

Because of the uncertainty inherent in the clinic's volume estimates, it is useful to recognize that total revenues will be $1,980,000 only if the volume forecast holds. In reality, Total revenues = ($25 × Number of FFS visits) + ($3 × Number of capitated member-months). If the actual number of FFS visits is more or less than 90,000 in 2007, or the number of capitated lives (and hence member-months) is something other than 30,000, the resulting revenues will be different from the $1,980,000 forecast.

Part III of Table 8.3 focuses on expenses. To support the forecasted 90,000 visits, the clinic is expected to use 48,000 hours of medical labor at an average cost of $25 per hour, for a total labor expense of 48,000 × $25 = $1,200,000. Thus, labor costs are expected to average $1,200,000 / 90,000 = $13.33 per visit in 2007. In reality, all labor costs are not variable, but there are a sufficient number of workers who either work part-time or are paid on the basis of productivity to closely tie labor hours to the number of visits.

Supplies expense, the bulk of which is inherently variable in nature, historically has averaged about $1.50 per bundle (unit) of supplies, with 100,000 units expected to be used to support 90,000 visits. (A unit of supplies is a more or less standard package that contains both administrative and clinical supplies.) Thus, supplies expense is expected to total $150,000, or $150,000 / 90,000 = $1.67 on a per visit basis. Taken together, Carroll's labor and supplies variable costs are forecasted to be $13.33 + $1.67 = $15 per visit in 2007. The same amount can be calculated by dividing total variable costs by the number of visits: $1,350,000 / 90,000 = $15.

Finally, the clinic is expected to incur $500,000 of fixed costs in 2007, primarily administrative overhead, labor costs, depreciation, and lease expense. Therefore, to serve the anticipated 90,000 visits, costs are expected to consist of $1,350,000 in variable costs plus $500,000 in fixed costs, for a total of $1,850,000. Again, it is important to recognize that some costs (in Carroll's case, a majority of costs) are tied to volume. Thus, total costs can be expressed as ($15 × Number of visits) + $500,000. If the actual number of visits in 2007 is more or less than 90,000, then total costs will differ from the $1,850,000 budget estimate.

The final section (Part IV) of Table 8.3 contains Carroll Clinic's budgeted 2007 profit and loss (P&L) statement, the heart of the operating budget. The difference between the projected revenues of $1,980,000 and the projected variable costs of $1,350,000 produces a total contribution margin of $630,000. Deducting the forecasted fixed costs of $500,000 results in a budgeted profit of $130,000. The true purpose of the operating budget is to set financial goals for the clinic. In effect, the operating budget can be thought of as a contract between the organization and its managers. Thus, the $130,000 profit forecast becomes the overall profit benchmark for the clinic in 2007, and individual managers will be held accountable for the revenues and expenses needed to meet the budget.

Self-Test Questions

1. What are some of the key assumptions required to prepare an operating budget?
2. Do the required assumptions depend on the type of organization and the nature of its reimbursement contracts?
3. Why is the budgeted profit and loss (P&L) statement so important?

Variance Analysis

Variance analysis, which focuses on differences (variances) between realized values and forecasts, is an important technique for controlling financial performance. This section includes a discussion of the basics of variance analysis, including flexible budgeting, as well as an illustration of the process.

Variance Analysis Basics

In accounting, a *variance* is the difference between an actual (realized) value and the budgeted value, often called a *standard*. Note that the accounting definition of variance is different from the statistical definition, although both meanings connote a difference from some base value. In effect, *variance analysis* is an examination and interpretation of differences between what has actually happened and what was planned. If the budget is based on realistic expectations, variance analysis can provide managers with very useful information. Variance analysis does not provide all the answers, but it does help managers ask the right questions.

Variance analysis is essential to the managerial control process. Actions taken in response to variance analysis often have the potential to dramatically improve the operations and financial performance of the organization. For example, many variances are controllable, so managers can take actions to avoid unfavorable variances in the future. The primary focus of variance analysis should not be to assign blame for unfavorable results. Rather, the goal of variance analysis is to uncover the cause of operational problems so that these problems can be avoided, or at least minimized, in the future. Unfortunately, not all variances are controllable by management. Nevertheless, knowledge of such variances is essential to the overall management and well-being of the organization. It may be necessary to revise plans, for example, to tighten controllable costs in an attempt to offset unfavorable cost variances in areas that are beyond managerial control.

Static Versus Flexible Budgets

To be of maximum use to managers, variance analysis must be approached systematically. The starting point for such analyses is the *static budget*, which is the original approved budget unadjusted for differences between planned and actual (realized) volumes. However, at the end of a budget period, it is unlikely that realized volume will equal budgeted volume, and it would be very useful to know which variances are due to volume forecast errors and which variances are caused by other factors.

To illustrate this concept, consider Carroll Clinic's 2007 operating budget contained in Table 8.3. The profit projection, $130,000, is predicated on specific volume assumptions: 36,000 visits for the FFS population and 360,000 member-months, resulting in 54,000 visits, for the capitated population. At the end of the year, the clinic's managers will compare actual profits with budgeted profits. The problem, of course, is that it is highly unlikely that actual profits will be based on 36,000 fee-for-service visits and 360,000 member months (with 54,000 visits) for the capitated population. Thus, if Carroll's managers were to merely compare the realized profit with the $130,000 profit in the static budget, they would not know whether any profit difference is caused by volume differences or underlying operational differences.

To provide an explanation of what is driving the profit variance, managers must create a flexible budget. A *flexible budget* is one in which the static budget has been adjusted to reflect the actual volume achieved in the budget period. Essentially, flexible budgets are an after-the-fact device to tell managers what the results would have been under the volume level actually attained, **assuming all other budgeting assumptions are held constant**. The flexible budget permits a more detailed analysis than is possible with a static budget. However, a flexible budget requires the identification of variable and fixed costs and hence places a larger burden on the organization's managerial accounting system.

Variance Analysis Illustration

To illustrate variance analysis, consider Carroll's static budget for 2007 (Table 8.3), which projects a profit of $130,000. Data used for variance analysis is tracked in various parts of Carroll's managerial accounting information system throughout the year, and variance analyses are performed monthly. This allows managers to take necessary actions during the year to positively influence annual results. For purposes of this illustration, however, the monthly feedback is not shown. Rather, the focus is on the year-end results, which are contained in Table 8.4.

TABLE 8.4
Carroll Clinic:
2007 Results

I.	*Volume:*		
	A. FFS	40,000	visits
	B. Capitated lives	30,000	members
	Number of member months	360,000	
	Actual utilization per member-month	0.20	
	Number of visits	72,000	visits
	C. Total actual visits	112,000	visits

II.	*Revenues:*		
	A. FFS	$ 24	per visit
		× 40,000	actual visits
		$ 960,000	
	B. Capitated lives	$ 3	PMPM
		× 360,000	actual member months
		$ 1,080,000	
	C. Total actual revenues	$ 2,040,000	

III.	*Costs:*		
	A. Variable Costs:		
	Labor	$ 1,557,400	(59,900 hours at $26/hour)
	Supplies	234,600	(124,800 units at $1.88/unit)
	Total variable costs	$ 1,792,000	
	Variable cost per visit	$ 16	($1,792,000/112,000)
	B. Fixed Costs:		
	Overhead, plant, and equipment	$ 500,000	
	C. Total actual costs	$ 2,292,000	

IV. Profit and Loss Statement:		
Revenues:		
FFS	$ 960,000	
Capitated	1,080,000	
Total	$ 2,040,000	
Costs:		
Variable:		
FFS	$ 640,000	
Capitated	1,152,000	
Total	$ 1,792,000	
Contribution margin	$ 248,000	
Fixed costs	500,000	
Actual profit	($ 252,000)	

Creating the Flexible Budget

Table 8.5 contains three sets of data for 2007. The static budget, which is taken from Table 8.3, is the forecast made at the beginning of 2007; the actual results, taken from Table 8.4, reflect what actually happened. The flexible budget in the center column of Table 8.5 reflects projected revenues and costs

	Static Budget	Flexible Budget	Actual Results
Assumptions:			
FFS visits	36,000	40,000	40,000
Capitated visits	54,000	72,000	72,000
Total	90,000	112,000	112,000
Revenues:			
FFS	$ 900,000	$1,000,000	$ 960,000
Capitated	1,080,000	1,080,000	1,080,000
Total	$1,980,000	$2,080,000	$2,040,000
Costs:			
Variable:			
FFS	$ 540,000	$ 600,000	$ 640,000
Capitated	810,000	1,080,000	1,152,000
Total	$1,350,000	$1,680,000	$1,792,000
Contribution margin	$ 630,000	$ 400,000	$ 248,000
Fixed costs	500,000	500,000	500,000
Profit	$ 130,000	($ 100,000)	($ 252,000)

TABLE 8.5
Carroll Clinic:
Static and
Flexible
Budgets and
Actual Results
for 2007

at the **realized (actual) volume**, as opposed to the projected volume, **but incorporates all other assumptions that went into the static (original) budget**. By analyzing differences in these three data sets, Carroll's managers can gain insights into why the clinic ended the year with a loss.

Note that the flexible budget maintains the original budget assumptions of Revenues = ($25 × Number of FFS visits) + ($3 × Number of capitated member-months) and Expenses = ($15 × Number of FFS visits) + ($15 × Number of capitated visits) + $500,000. However, the flexible budget *flexes* (adjusts) revenues and costs to reflect actual volume levels. Thus, in the flexible budget column, Revenues = ($25 × 40,000) + ($3 × 360,000) = $1,000,000 + $1,080,000 = $2,080,000, and Expenses = ($15 × 40,000) + ($15 × 72,000) + $500,000 = $600,000 + $1,080,000 + $500,000 = $1,680,000 + $500,000 = $2,180,000.

The flexible budget can be described as follows. The $2,080,000 in total revenues is what the clinic **would have expected** at the start of the year if the volume estimates had been 40,000 FFS visits and a capitated membership of 30,000. In addition, the total variable costs of $1,680,000 in the flexible budget are the costs that Carroll **would have expected** for 40,000 FFS visits and 72,000 capitated visits (based on a membership of 30,000). By definition, the fixed costs should be the same, within a reasonable range, no matter what the volume level. On net, the $100,000 loss shown on the flexible budget represents the profit expected given the initial assumed revenue, cost, and volume relationships, coupled with a forecasted volume that equals the realized volume.

Conducting the Variance Analysis

As explained earlier, *variance analysis* involves comparing two amounts, with the variance being the difference between the values. For example, if at the beginning of the year, a hospital expected to make a profit of $2 million, but actual results were a profit of $3 million, the variance would be $1 million. The expected value, in this case $2 million of profits, is often called the *standard* because it is the profit goal of the hospital (the standard to be reached) as expressed in the budget. As you will see from the following paragraphs, most variances are calculated in more-or-less the same way.

To begin Carroll Clinic's variance analysis, consider the data contained in Table 8.5. The *total*, or *profit*, *variance* is the difference between the realized profit and the static profit. Thus, Profit variance = Actual profit − Static profit, or (−$252,000) − $130,000 = −$382,000. In words, Carroll's 2007 profitability was $382,000 below *standard*, or $382,000 less than expected. Although this large negative variance should generate considerable concern among Carroll's managers, a more detailed analysis is required to determine the underlying causes.

Perhaps the first question that Carroll's management would want answered is this: Is the large negative loss (as compared to expectations) due to a revenue shortfall, cost overruns, or both? Figure 8.1 shows the −$382,000 profit variance at the top, and then breaks it down into its revenue and cost components. In calculating all variances, we are using definitions (given in the bottom of each variance table) that show "bad" results as a negative number.[4]

The *revenue variance* shown in Figure 8.1 is Actual revenues − Static revenues = $2,040,000 − $1,980,000 = $60,000, which, because it is a positive variance, tells Carroll's managers that realized revenues were actually $60,000 **higher** than expected. However, the *cost variance* of Static costs − Actual costs = $1,350,000 − $1,792,000 = −$442,000 indicates that realized costs were **much greater** than expected. (Remember that our convention is that positive variances are "good" and negative variances are "bad.") The net effect of the revenue and cost variances is the $60,000 + (−$442,000) = −$382,000 profit variance. By breaking down the profit variance into revenue and cost components, it is readily apparent that the major cause of Carroll's poor financial performance in 2007 was that costs were too high. However, the analysis thus far does not discriminate between cost overruns caused by volume forecast errors and those caused by other factors.

Regarding the revenue variance, it would be nice to know if the greater-than-expected revenues were due to greater-than-expected volume or greater-than-expected prices (reimbursement). Figure 8.2 examines the revenue variance in more detail. Here, the $60,000 positive revenue variance is de-

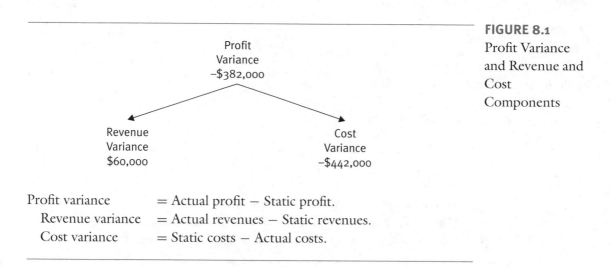

FIGURE 8.1

Profit Variance
and Revenue and
Cost
Components

composed into volume and price variances. The *volume variance* is Flexible revenues − Static revenues = $2,080,000 − $1,980,000 = $100,000 and the *price variance* is Actual revenues − Flexible revenues = $2,040,000 − $2,080,000 = −$40,000. These variances tell Carroll's managers that a higher-than-expected volume should have resulted in revenues being $100,000 greater than expected in 2007. However, this potential revenue increase was partially offset by the fact that realized prices (reimbursement) were less than expected. The end result of higher volume at lower prices is realized revenue that was $60,000 higher than forecasted. Note that to keep this illustration manageable, the number of covered lives (enrollment) was the same in both the static and actual budgets. If this had not been the case, two flexible budgets would be required and the volume variance would have two components. (Refer to the note at the bottom of Figure 8.2.)

Now let's change our focus to the cost side of the variance analysis. Figure 8.3 breaks the −$442,000 cost variance into volume and management components. The *volume variance* of Static costs − Flexible costs = $1,350,000 − $1,680,000 = −$330,000 indicates that a large portion of the $442,000 cost overrun was caused by the incorrect volume forecast: Higher-than-expected volume resulted in higher-than-expected costs. This higher-than-expected volume would not be a financial problem if it were the result of fee-for-service patients, in which case higher costs as a result of higher volume would likely be more than offset by higher revenues. However, the fact that a majority of the higher volume (18,000 of 22,000 visits) came from capitated patients means that there was no matching revenue increase.

In addition to the problem of higher-than-expected volume, $112,000 of the $442,000 cost overrun was caused by other factors. This amount is the so-called *management variance*, which is calculated as Flexible costs − Actual costs = $1,680,000 − $1,792,000 = −$112,000. The management variance gets its name from the assumption that any cost variances not caused

FIGURE 8.2

Revenue
Variance and
Volume and
Cost
Components

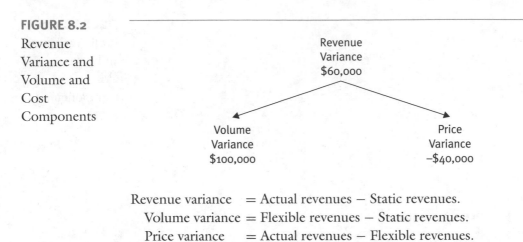

Revenue variance   = Actual revenues − Static revenues.
  Volume variance = Flexible revenues − Static revenues.
  Price variance   = Actual revenues − Flexible revenues.

Note: In our example, there are no enrollment differences. However, if some patients are capitated, and there are enrollment differences between expected and realized budgets, the situation becomes more complex. Then, it is necessary to create two flexible budgets: (1) one flexed for both enrollment and utilization and (2) one flexed only for enrollment. With two flexible budgets, volume variances can be calculated for both changes in the number of covered lives and changes in utilization.

Volume variance   = Flexible (enrollment and utilization) revenues − Static revenues.
  Enrollment variance   = Flexible (enrollment) revenues − Static revenues.
  Utilization variance   = Flexible (enrollment and utilization) revenues − Flexible (enrollment) revenues.

by volume forecast inaccuracies are a result of either good or bad management performance. The theory here is that most managers have very limited (if any) control over the volume of services supplied, but they do have control over factors such as the amount of labor used, wage rates, supplies utilization and costs, and so forth. Thus, the $112,000 cost overrun classified as a management variance can be influenced by managerial actions. If all standards in the static budget except the volume estimate were met, the cost overrun would have been only $330,000, and not the $442,000 realized.

To attempt to eliminate the managerial variance in future years, Carroll's managers must determine precisely where the cost overruns lie. The primary resources involved in operating costs are labor and supplies, so it would be valuable to learn which of the two areas contributed most to the management variance. Perhaps a more probing investigation can be made within labor and supplies: Is too much of each resource being used or is too much money being paid for what is being used? The variance calculations necessary to answer these questions are not overly complex, but they are lengthy, so we will only discuss the results here.

A further variance analysis indicates that only a very small portion of the labor cost overrun was caused by productivity problems; the vast majority of the overrun was caused by higher-than-expected wage rates. This suggests that Carroll's managers have to take a close look to ensure that they are not paying more than the local market for labor dictates. Of course, Carroll managers

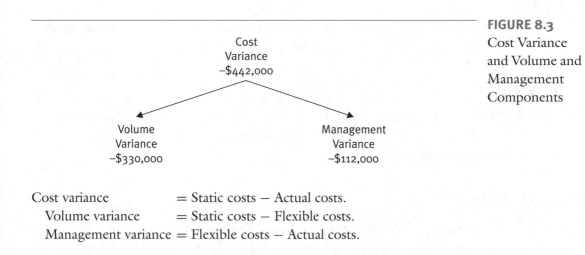

FIGURE 8.3

Cost Variance
and Volume and
Management
Components

want to have quality employees, but at the same time, they must be concerned about labor costs.

Finally, the variance analysis shows that the supplies cost overrun was a result, almost totally, of price increases; supplies usage was almost on target when volume differences were accounted for. Thus, it would be prudent for management to investigate the clinic's purchasing policy to see if prices can be lowered through such actions as changing vendors, making larger purchases at a single time, joining a purchasing alliance, or just negotiating better.

Final Comments on Variance Analysis

It is important to recognize that the Carroll Clinic example presented here was meant to illustrate variance analysis techniques as opposed to illustrate a complete analysis. A complete analysis would encompass many more variances. Furthermore, at most organizations, variance analysis would be conducted at the department level as well as at other sublevels, such as service or contract lines, in addition to the organization as a whole. Nevertheless, the Carroll Clinic example is sufficient to give readers a good feel for how variance analysis is conducted as well as its benefits to the organization.

Variance analysis helps managers identify the factors that cause realized profits to be different from those expected. If profits are higher than expected, managers can see why and then try to further exploit those factors in the future. If profits are lower than expected, managers can identify the causes and then embark on a plan to correct the deficiencies. Larger health services organizations have made significant improvements in their use of variance analysis. The benefit of expanding the level of information detail is that it is easier for managers to isolate and presumably rectify problem areas. Fortunately, the marginal cost of obtaining such detailed information is lower now than ever before because large amounts of managerial accounting information are being generated at many health services organizations, both to support cost-control efforts and to aid in pricing and service decisions.

The Cash Budget

Thus far, our discussion of budgeting has focused on the operating budget. As shown in the Carroll Clinic illustration, the operating budget, along with the budgetary control process, provides managers with numerous insights into the efficiency of an organization's operations. However, the operating budget is based on accrual accounting principles and hence does not provide managers with much information about a business's cash position. This situation is corrected by the *cash budget*.

To create a cash budget, managers begin by forecasting volume, revenue, and collections data. Then they forecast both fixed asset acquisition and inventory requirements, along with the times when such payments must be made. Finally, this information is combined with cash outlay projections for operating and financial expenses such as wages and benefits, interest payments, tax payments, and so on. All this collection and payment information is then combined to show the organization's projected cash inflows and outflows over some specified period. Generally, "the cash budget" consists of individual monthly cash budgets forecasted for one year, plus a more detailed daily or weekly cash budget for the coming month. The monthly cash budget is used for liquidity planning purposes, and the daily or weekly budget is used for actual cash control.

Creating a cash budget does not require the application of a complex set of accounting rules. Rather, all the entries in a cash budget represent the actual movement of cash into or out of the organization. To illustrate, Table 8.6 contains a monthly cash budget that covers six months of 2008 for Madison Homecare, a small, for-profit home health care company. Madison's cash budget, which is broken down into three sections, is typical, although there is a great deal of variation in formats used by different organizations. Also, for ease of illustration, the cash budget has been constrained to relatively few lines.

The first section of Madison's cash budget contains the *collections worksheet*, which translates the billing for services provided into cash revenues. Because of its location in a summer resort area, Madison's patient volume, and hence billings, peak in July. However, like most health services organizations, Madison rarely collects when services are provided. What is relevant from a

	Mar	Apr	May	June	July	Aug	Sept	Oct	
Collections Worksheet:									**TABLE 8.6**
1. Billed charges	$50,000	$50,000	$100,000	$150,000	$200,000	$100,000	$100,000	$50,000	Madison
2. Collections:									Homecare:
a. Within 30 days			19,600	29,400	39,200	19,600	19,600	9,800	May Through
b. 30–60 days			35,000	70,000	105,000	140,000	70,000	70,000	October Cash
c. 60–90 days			5,000	5,000	10,000	15,000	20,000	10,000	Budget
3. Total collections			$ 59,600	$104,400	$154,200	$174,600	$109,600	$89,800	
Supplies Worksheet:									
4. Amount of supplies ordered	$10,000	$15,000	$20,000	$10,000	$10,000	$5,000			
5. Payments made for supplies		$10,000	$15,000	$20,000	$10,000	$10,000	$5,000		
Net Cash Gain (Loss):									
6. Total collections (from Line 3)			$ 59,600	$104,400	$154,200	$174,600	$109,600	$89,800	
7. Total purchases (from Line 5)			$ 10,000	$ 15,000	$ 20,000	$ 10,000	$ 10,000	$ 5,000	
8. Wages and salaries			60,000	70,000	80,000	60,000	60,000	60,000	
9. Rent			2,500	2,500	2,500	2,500	2,500	2,500	
10. Other expenses			1,000	1,500	2,000	1,000	1,000	500	
11. Taxes			20,000				20,000		
12. Payment for capital assets						50,000			
13. Total payments			$ 73,500	$109,000	$104,500	$123,500	$ 93,500	$ 68,000	
14. Net cash gain (loss)			($ 13,900)	($ 4,600)	$ 49,700	$ 51,100	$ 16,100	$ 21,800	
Surplus/Deficit Summary:									
15. Cash at beginning with no borrowing			$ 15,000	$ 1,100	($ 3,500)	$ 46,200	$ 97,300	$113,400	
16. Cash at end with no borrowing			$ 1,100	($ 3,500)	$ 46,200	$ 97,300	$113,400	$135,200	
17 Target cash balance			10,000	10,000	10,000	10,000	10,000	10,000	
18. Cumulative surplus (deficit)			($ 8,900)	($ 13,500)	$ 36,200	$ 87,300	$103,400	$125,200	

cash budget perspective is not when services are provided or when billings occur but when cash is collected. Based on previous experience, Madison's managers know that most collections occur 30 to 60 days after billing. In fact, Madison's managers have created a collections table that allows them to forecast, with some precision, the timing of collections. This table was used to convert the billings shown on Line 1 of Table 8.6 into the collection amounts shown on Lines 2 and 3.

To illustrate the relationship between billings and collections, consider the $100,000 of billed charges forecasted for May. Of this amount, $19,600 is expected to be collected in May (within 30 days), $70,000 is expected to be collected in June (30–60 days after billing), and $10,000 is expected to be collected in July (60–90 days after billing). Thus, of the $100,000 in May billings, $19,600 + $70,000 + $10,000 = $99,600 is expected to be collected, so a very small amount ($400) is forecasted to be a bad debt loss.

The next section of Madison's cash budget is the *supplies worksheet*, which accounts for both the amount of supplies purchased and timing differences between when supplies are ordered and when the resulting bills are paid. Madison's patient volume forecasts, which are used to predict the billing amounts shown on Line 1, are also used to forecast the supplies (primarily medical) needed to support patient services. These supplies are ordered and received one month prior to expected usage, as shown on Line 4. However, Madison's suppliers do not demand immediate payment. Rather, Madison has, on average, 30 days to pay for supplies after they are received. Thus, the actual payment occurs one month after purchase, as shown on Line 5.

The next section combines data from the collections and supplies worksheets with other projected cash outflows to show the *net cash gain (loss)* for each month. Cash from collections is shown on Line 6. Lines 7 through 12 list cash payments that are expected to be made during each month, including payments for supplies. Then all payments are summed, with the total shown on Line 13. The difference between expected cash receipts and cash payments, Line 6 minus Line 13, is the net cash gain or loss during the month, which is shown on Line 14. For May, there is a forecasted net cash outflow of $13,900, with the parentheses indicating a negative cash flow.

Although Line 14 contains the "meat" of the cash budget, Lines 15 through 18 (the *surplus/deficit summary*) extend the basic budget data to show Madison's monthly forecasted cumulative cash position. Line 15 shows the forecasted cash on hand at the beginning of each month, assuming that no borrowing takes place. Madison is expected to enter the budget period, the beginning of May, with $15,000 of cash on hand. For each succeeding month, Line 15 is merely the value shown on Line 16 for the previous month. The values on Line 16, which are obtained by adding Lines 14 and 15, show the cash on hand at the end of each month, assuming no borrowing takes place. For May, Madison expects a cash loss of $13,900 on top of a starting balance of $15,000, for an ending cash balance of $1,100, in the absence of any borrowing. This amount is the cash at beginning with no borrowing amount for June shown on Line 15.

To continue, Madison's target cash balance (i.e., the amount that it wants on hand at the beginning of each month), which is shown on Line 17, is $10,000. The target cash balance is subtracted from the forecasted ending cash with no borrowing amount to determine the firm's monthly deficit (shown in parentheses) or surplus (shown without parentheses). Because Madison expects to have ending cash, as shown on Line 16, of only $1,100 in May, it will have to obtain $1,100 − $10,000 = −$8,900 to bring the cash account up to the target balance of $10,000. If this amount is borrowed, as opposed to obtained from other sources such as liquidating marketable securities, the total loan outstanding will be $8,900 at the end of May. (The assumption here is that Madison will not have any loans outstanding on May 1 because the beginning cash balance exceeds the firm's target balance.)

The cumulative cash surplus or deficit is shown on Line 18; a positive value indicates a cash surplus, while a negative value indicates a deficit. The surplus cash or deficit shown on Line 18 is a **cumulative amount**. Thus,

Madison is projected to require $8,900 in May; it has a cash shortfall during June of $4,600, as reported on Line 14, so its total deficit projected for the end of June is $8,900 + $4,600 = $13,500, as shown on Line 18.

The same procedures are followed in subsequent months. Patient volume and billings are projected to peak in July, accompanied by increased payments for supplies, wages, and other items. However, collections are projected to increase by a greater amount than costs, and Madison expects a $49,700 net cash inflow during July. This amount is sufficient to pay off the cumulative loan (if one is used) of $13,500 and have a $36,200 cash surplus on hand at the end of the month.

Patient volume, and the resulting operating costs, is expected to fall sharply in August, but collections will be the highest of any month because they will reflect the high June and July billings. As a result, Madison would normally be forecasting a healthy $101,100 net cash gain during the month. However, the company expects to make a cash payment of $50,000 to purchase a new computer system during August, so the forecasted net cash gain is reduced to $51,100. This net gain adds to the surplus, so August is projected to end with $87,300 in surplus cash. If all goes according to the forecast, later cash surpluses will enable Madison to end this budget period with a surplus of $125,200.

The cash budget is used by Madison's managers for liquidity planning purposes. For example, the Table 8.6 cash budget indicates that Madison will need to obtain $13,500 in total to get through May and June. Thus, if the firm does not have any marketable securities to convert to cash, it will have to arrange a loan, typically a line of credit, to cover this period. Furthermore, the budget indicates a $125,200 cash surplus at the end of October. Madison's managers will have to consider how these funds can best be used. Perhaps the money should be returned to owners as dividends or bonuses, or perhaps it should be used for fixed asset acquisitions or be temporarily invested in marketable securities for later use within the business. This decision will be made on the basis of Madison's overall financial plan.

This brief illustration shows the mechanics and managerial value of the cash budget. However, before concluding the discussion, several additional points need to be made. First, if cash inflows and outflows are not uniform during the month, a monthly cash budget could seriously understate a business's peak financing requirements. The data in Table 8.6 show the situation expected on the last day of each month, but on any given day during the month it could be quite different. For example, if all payments had to be made on the fifth of each month, but collections came in uniformly throughout the month, Madison would need to borrow cash to cover within-month shortages. Looking at August, the $123,500 of cash payments would occur before the full amount of the $174,600 in collections has been made. In this situation, some amount of cash would be needed to cover shortfalls in August, even though the end of month cash flow after all collections had been made is positive. Because Madison's cash flows do occur unevenly during each month, it also prepares weekly cash budgets to forecast within-month shortages.

Also, because the cash budget represents a forecast, all the values in the table are **expected** values. If actual patient volume, collection times, supplies purchases, wage rates, and so on differ from forecasted levels, the projected cash deficits and surpluses will be incorrect. Thus, there is a reasonable chance that Madison may end up needing to obtain a larger amount of funds than is indicated on Line 18. Because of the uncertainty of the forecasts, spreadsheets are particularly well suited for constructing and analyzing cash budgets. For example, Madison's managers could change any assumption—say, projected monthly volume or the time third-party payers take to pay—and the cash budget would automatically and instantly be recalculated. This would show Madison's managers exactly how the firm's cash position changes under alternative operating assumptions. Typically, such an analysis is used to determine the size of the credit line needed to cover temporary cash shortages.[5] In Madison's case, such an analysis indicated that a $20,000 line is sufficient.

Self-Test Questions	1. Considering all the information in the operating budget, why do organizations need a cash budget?
	2. Does the cash budget require an extensive knowledge of accounting principles?
	3. In your view, what is the most important line of the cash budget?

Key Concepts

Planning and budgeting are important managerial activities. In particular, budgets allow health services managers to plan for and set expectations for the future, assess financial performance on a timely basis, and ensure that operations are carried out in a manner consistent with expectations. The key concepts of this chapter are:

- *Planning* encompasses the overall process of preparing for the future, while *budgeting* is the accounting process that ties together planning and control functions.
- The *strategic plan*, which provides broad guidance for the future, is the foundation of any organization's planning process. More detailed managerial guidance is contained in the *operating plan*, often called the *five-year plan*.
- The *financial plan*, which is the financial portion of the operating plan, contains a *long-term plan*, *working capital management plan*, and *managerial accounting plan*.

- *Budgeting* provides a means for communication and coordination of organizational expectations as well as allocation of financial resources. In addition, budgeting establishes benchmarks for control.
- There are several types of budgets, including the *statistics budget*, *revenue budget*, *expense budget*, *operating budget*, and *cash budget*.
- The *conventional approach* to budgeting uses the previous budget as the basis for constructing the new budget. *Zero-based budgeting* begins each budget as a clean slate, and hence all entries have to be justified each budget period.
- *Bottom-up budgeting*, which begins at the unit level, encourages maximum involvement by junior managers. Conversely, *top-down budgeting*, which is less participatory in nature, is a more efficient way to communicate senior management's views.
- The *operating budget* is the basic budget of an organization in that it sets the profit target for the budget period.
- A *variance* is the difference between a budgeted (planned) value, or *standard*, and the actual (realized) value. *Variance analysis* examines differences between budgeted and realized amounts with the goal of finding out why things went either badly or well.
- A budget that fully reflects realized results is called the *actual budget*. When the original, or *static budget*, is recast to reflect the actual volume of patients treated, leaving all other assumptions unchanged, the result is called a *flexible budget*. To be most useful, variance analysis examines differences between the actual, flexible, and static budgets.
- A *cash budget*, which is the primary cash management tool, forecasts the cash inflows and outflows of an organization with the goal of identifying expected surpluses and shortfalls.
- In general, *monthly* cash budgets are used for planning purposes while *weekly* or *daily* budgets are used for cash management purposes.

This chapter concludes the discussion of managerial accounting. Chapter 9 begins the examination of basic financial management concepts.

Questions

8.1 Why are planning and budgeting so important to an organization's success?

8.2 Briefly describe the planning process. Be sure to include summaries of the strategic, operating, and financial plans.

8.3 Describe the components of a financial plan.

8.4 How are the statistics, revenue, expense, and operating budgets related?

8.5 a. What are the advantages and disadvantages of conventional budgeting versus zero-based budgeting?

    b. What organizational characteristics create likely candidates for zero-based budgeting?

8.6 If you were the CEO of Bayside Memorial Hospital, would you advocate a top-down or bottom-up approach to budgeting? Explain your rationale.

8.7 What is variance analysis?

8.8 a. Explain the relationships among the static budget, flexible budget, and actual results.

    b. Assume that a group practice has both capitated and fee-for-service (FFS) patients. Furthermore, the number of capitated enrollees has changed over the budget period. In order to calculate the volume variance and break it down into enrollment and utilization components, how many flexible budgets must be constructed?

8.9 a. What is a cash budget and how is it used?

    b. Should depreciation expense appear on a cash budget? Explain your answer.

Problems

8.1 Consider the following 2007 data for Newark General Hospital (in millions of dollars):

	Static Budget	Flexible Budget	Actual Results
Revenues	$4.7	$4.8	$4.5
Costs	4.1	4.1	4.2
Profits	0.6	0.7	0.3

    a. Calculate and interpret the profit variance.

    b. Calculate and interpret the revenue variance.

    c. Calculate and interpret the cost variance.

    d. Calculate and interpret the volume and price variances on the revenue side.

    e. Calculate and interpret the volume and management variances on the cost side.

    f. How are the variances calculated above related?

8.2 Here are the 2007 **revenues** for the Wendover Group Practice Association for four different budgets, in thousands of dollars:

Static Budget	Flexible (Enrollment/Utilization) Budget	Flexible (Enrollment) Budget	Actual Results
$425	$200	$180	$300

    a. What does the budget data tell you about the nature of Wendover's patients: Are they capitated or fee-for-service? (Hint: See the note to Figure 8.2.)

    b. Calculate and interpret the following variances:
- Revenue variance
- Volume variance
- Price variance
- Enrollment variance
- Utilization variance

8.3 Here are the budgets of Brandon Surgery Center for the most recent historical quarter, in thousands of dollars:

	Static	Flexible	Actual
Number of surgeries	1,200	1,300	1,300
Patient revenue	$2,400	$2,600	$2,535
Salary expense	1,200	1,300	1,365
Non-salary expense	600	650	585
Profit	$ 600	$ 650	$ 585

The center assumes that all revenues and costs are variable and hence tied directly to patient volume.

    a. Explain how each amount in the flexible budget was calculated. (Hint: Examine the static budget to determine the relationship of each budget line to volume.)

    b. Determine the variances for each line of the profit and loss statement, both in dollar terms and in percentage terms. (Hint: Each line has a total variance, a volume variance, and a management variance.)

    c. What do the Part b results tell Brandon's managers about the surgery center's operations for the quarter?

8.4 Refer to Carroll Clinic's 2007 operating budget contained in Table 8.3. Instead of the actual results reported in Table 8.4, assume the results reported below:

Carroll Clinic: New 2007 Results		
I. *Volume:*		
A. FFS	34,000	visits
B. Capitated lives	30,000	members
Number of member months	360,000	
Actual utilization per		
member-month	0.12	
Number of visits	43,200	visits
C. Total actual visits	77,200	visits

II. *Revenues:*

A.	FFS	$ 28	per visit
		× 34,000	actual visits
		$ 952,000	
B.	Capitated lives	$ 2.75	PMPM
		× 360,000	actual member months
		$ 990,000	
C.	Total actual revenues	$1,942,000	

III. *Costs:*

A.	Variable Costs:		
	Labor	$1,242,000	(46,000 hours at $27/hour)
	Supplies	126,000	(90,000 units at $1.40/unit)
	Total variable costs	$1,368,000	
	Variable cost per visit	$ 17.72	($1,368,000/77,200)
B.	Fixed Costs:		
	Overhead, plant, and equipment	$ 525,000	
C.	Total actual costs	$1,893,000	

IV. *Profit and Loss Statement:*

Revenues:		
FFS	$ 952,000	
Capitated	990,000	
Total	$1,942,000	
Costs:		
Variable:		
FFS	$ 602,487	
Capitated	765,513	
Total	$1,368,000	
Contribution margin	$ 574,000	
Fixed costs	525,000	
Actual profit	$ 49,000	

a. Construct Carroll's flexible budget for 2007.

b. What are the profit variance, revenue variance, and cost variance?

c. Consider the revenue variance. What is the component volume variance? The price variance?

d. Break down the cost variance into volume and management components.

e. Break down the management variance into labor, supplies, and fixed costs variances.

f. Interpret your results. In particular, focus on the differences between the variance analysis here and the Carroll Clinic illustration presented in the chapter.

8.5 Refer to Problem 8.4. Assume the results reported in that problem hold, except that a difference existed among budgeted, static enrollment and realized enrollment. The corrected results are:

Carroll Clinic: Corrected 2007 Results

I.   *Volume:*

   A.   FFS   34,000   visits

   B.   Capitated lives   31,000   members

       Number of member months   372,000

       Actual utilization per

          member-month   0.11613

          Number of visits   43,200   visits

   C.   Total actual visits   77,200   visits

II. *Revenues:*

   A.   FFS $ 28   per visit

                   × 34,000   actual visits

               $ 952,000

   B.   Capitated lives $ 2.75   PMPM

                  × 372,000   actual member months

              $1,023,000

   C.   Total actual revenues $1,975,000

III. *Costs:*

   A.   Variable Costs:

       Labor $1,242,000   (46,000 hours at $27/hour)

       Supplies   126,000   (90,000 units at $1.40/unit)

          Total variable costs $1,368,000

       Variable cost per visit $ 17.72   ($1,368,000/77,200)

   B.   Fixed Costs:

       Overhead, plant,

          and equipment $ 525,000

   C.   Total actual costs $1,893,000

IV. *Profit and Loss Statement:*

       Revenues:

          FFS $ 952,000

          Capitated   1,023,000

          Total $1,975,000

       Costs:

         Variable:

          FFS $ 602,487

          Capitated   765,513

          Total $1,368,000

       Contribution margin $ 607,000

       Fixed costs   525,000

       Actual profit $ 82,000

---

a. Construct Carroll's flexible budgets for 2007. (Hint: Because of a change in enrollment, creating three flexible budgets is necessary. See the note to Figure 8.2.)

b. What are the profit variance, revenue variance, and cost variance?

   c. Focus on the revenue side. What is the volume variance? The price variance? Break the volume variance into enrollment and utilization components. How does your answer here differ from your corresponding answer to Problem 8.4?

   d. Now consider the cost side. What are the volume and management variances? Break down the management variance into labor, supplies, and fixed costs variances.

   e. Interpret your results. In particular, focus on the differences between the variance analysis here and the one in Problem 8.4.

Notes

1. For more information on planning, see Alan M. Zuckerman, *Healthcare Strategic Planning* (Health Administration Press, 2005). For more information on budgeting processes in general, see William R. Lalli (editor), *Handbook of Budgeting* (Wiley, 2003). For more information on budgeting within healthcare organizations, see William J. Ward, Jr., *Health Care Budgeting and Financial Management for Non-Financial Managers* (Album House, 1994).

2. Financial statement forecasting is an important function of any business's financial staff. However, this discussion will be left to other texts. For more information, see Louis C. Gapenski, *Understanding Health Care Financial Management, 5th ed.* (AUPHA Press/Health Administration Press, 2007), Chapter 14.

3. For an extensive discussion of zero-based budgeting within hospitals, see Matthew M. Person, III, *The Zero-Base Hospital* (Health Administration Press, 1997).

4. Variances can be defined so the resulting value is either a positive or a negative number. For example, when cost variances are calculated, they can be defined so that a negative variance means costs less than standard, which is good, or costs greater than standard, which is bad, depending on which value is subtracted from the other. In this example, all variances have been defined so that a negative number indicates an undesirable variance and not necessarily that the realized value is less than the standard. For example, a higher-than-standard wage rate would be a negative variance, indicating that the variance is harmful to the clinic, even though realized wages were higher than that expected.

5. A *credit line* is an agreement between a borrower and a financial institution that obligates the institution to furnish credit over a time period, typically a year, up to the agreed-upon amount. The borrower may use some, all, or none of the credit line. Usually, credit lines require borrowers to pay an upfront fee for the credit guarantee, called a *commitment fee*, as well as interest charges on the amount of credit actually used.

References

Barr, P. 2005. "Flexing Your Budget." *Modern Healthcare* (September 12): 24–26.

Berlin, M. F., and M. R. Budzyuski. 1998. "Budget Variance Analysis Using RVUs." *Medical Group Management Journal* (November—December): 50–52.

Cardamone, M. A., M. Shaver, and R. Worthman. 2004. "Business Planning: Reasons, Definitions, and Elements." *Healthcare Financial Management* (April): 40–46.

Clark, J. J. 2005. "Improving Hospital Budgeting and Accountability: A Best Practice Approach." *Healthcare Financial Management* (July): 78–83.

Ginter, P. M., L. M. Swayne, and W. Jack Duncan. 1998. *Strategic Management of Health Care Organizations.* Malden, MA: Blackwell.

Herkimer, A. G., Jr. 1988. *Understanding Health Care Budgeting.* Rockville, MD: Aspen.

Healthcare Financial Management Association (HFMA). 2004. "How Are Hospitals Financing the Future—Core Competencies in Capital Planning." *Healthcare Financial Management* (July): 44–49.

Maitland, D. 1993. "Flexible Budgeting and Variance Analysis: Why Leave Staff Nurses in the Dark?" *Hospital Cost Accounting* (December): 1–8.

Person, M. M., III. 1997. *The Zero-Base Hospital.* Chicago: Health Administration Press.

Sorensen, D., and D. Sullivan. 2005. "Managing Trade-Offs Makes Budgeting Processes Pay Off." *Healthcare Financial Management* (November): 54–60.

Basic Financial Management Concepts

Before we discuss the details of the financial management of healthcare organizations, it is essential that you gain some fundamental knowledge of two very important basic topics.

The first topic is time value analysis. Most financial management decisions involve future dollar amounts. For example, when a physician group practice uses debt financing, it is obligated to make a series of future (principal and interest) payments to the lender. Or, when a hospital builds an outpatient surgery center, it expects the investment to provide a series of future cash flows when the center is up and running. In order to estimate the financial impact of these transactions, future dollar amounts must be valued. The process of doing this is called time value analysis, and Chapter 9 provides the concepts necessary to perform this analysis.

The second major topic in Part IV is financial risk and required return. Virtually all financial decisions involve risk. To illustrate, there is the risk that the physician group practice that obtained debt financing will not be able to make the required payments. Or, there is the risk that the cash flows expected from the hospital's new outpatient surgery center will be less than those forecasted when the center was built. Situations like this involve financial risk, and to make good financial decisions, managers must be able to define and measure such risk. Furthermore, risk must be incorporated into the decision process by setting a required rate of return that is tied to the risk of the transaction. Chapter 10 provides the tools required to understand financial risk and how it is translated into required return.

TIME VALUE ANALYSIS

Learning Objectives

After studying this chapter, readers will be able to:

- Explain why time value analysis is so important to healthcare financial management.
- Find the present and future values for lump sums, annuities, and uneven cash flow streams.
- Solve for interest rate and number of periods.
- Explain and apply the opportunity cost principle.
- Measure the financial return on an investment in both dollar and percentage terms.
- Create an amortization table.
- Describe and apply stated, periodic, and effective annual interest rates.

Introduction

The monetary (economic) value of any asset, whether a *financial asset*, such as a stock or a bond, or a *real asset*, such as a piece of diagnostic equipment or an ambulatory surgery center, is based on future cash flows. However, a dollar to be received in the future is worth less than a current dollar because a dollar in hand today can be invested in an interest-bearing account and hence can be worth more than one dollar in the future.[1] Because current dollars are worth more than future dollars, financial management decisions must account for cash flow timing differences.

The process of assigning appropriate values to cash flows that occur at different points in time is called *time value analysis* or *discounted cash flow analysis*. It is an important part of healthcare financial management because most financial analyses involve the valuation of future cash flows. In fact, of all the financial analysis techniques that are discussed in this book, none is more important than time value analysis. The concepts presented here are the cornerstones of most financial analyses, so a thorough understanding of time value concepts is essential to good financial decision making.

Time Lines

The creation of a *time line* is the first step in time value analysis, especially when first learning time value concepts. Time lines make it easier to visualize when the cash flows in a particular analysis occur. To illustrate the time line concept, consider the following five-period time line:

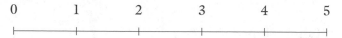

Time 0 is any starting point (typically the time of the first cash flow in an analysis); Time 1 is one period from the starting point, or the end of Period 1; Time 2 is two periods from the starting point, or the end of Period 2; and so on. Thus, the numbers on top of the tick marks represent end-of-period values. Often, the periods are years, but other time intervals such as quarters, months, or days are also used when needed to fit the timing of the cash flows being evaluated. If the time periods are years, the interval from 0 to 1 would be Year 1, and the tick mark labeled 1 would represent both the end of Year 1 and the beginning of Year 2.

Cash flows are shown on a time line directly below the tick marks that indicate the point in time that they are expected to occur. The interest rate that is relevant to the analysis is sometimes shown directly above the time line in the first period. Additionally, unknown cash flows—the ones to be determined in the analysis—are sometimes indicated by question marks. To illustrate, consider the following time line:

$$
\begin{array}{ccccc}
0 & \quad 5\% \quad & 1 & 2 & 3 \\
\hline
-\$100 & & & & ?
\end{array}
$$

In this situation, the interest rate for each of the three periods is 5 percent, an investment of $100 is made at Time 0, and the Time 3 value is the unknown. The $100 is an *outflow* because it is shown as a negative cash flow. (Outflows are sometimes designated by parentheses rather than by minus signs.) In more complicated analyses, it is essential to use the proper signs to get the correct answer. Furthermore, many financial calculators and some spreadsheet functions require that signs be attached to cash flows in time value analyses, even simple ones, before the calculation can be completed. Thus, to ensure that readers are familiar with the sign convention used in time value analyses, we will use them on most illustrations.

Time lines are essential when learning time value concepts, but even experienced analysts use time lines when dealing with complex problems. The time line may be an actual line, as illustrated above, or it may be a series of columns (or rows) on a spreadsheet. Time lines will be used extensively in the remainder of this book, so get into the habit of creating time lines when conducting analyses that involve future cash flows.

Self-Test Questions

1. Draw a three-year time line that illustrates the following situation: An investment of $10,000 at Time 0; inflows of $5,000 at the end of Years 1, 2, and 3; and an interest rate of 10 percent during the entire three years.
2. Why is sign convention important in time value analyses?

Future Value of a Lump Sum (Compounding)

The process of going from today's values, or *present values*, to future values is called *compounding*. Although compounding is not used extensively in health-care finance, it is the best starting point for learning time value analysis. To illustrate *lump sum* compounding, which deals with a single starting amount, suppose that the manager of Meridian Clinics deposits $100 in a bank account that pays 5 percent annual interest (interest is credited to the account at the end of each year). How much would be in the account at the end of one year? To begin, here are the terms that are used in this time value analysis:

- $PV = \$100 =$ present value, or beginning amount, of the account.
- $I = 5\% =$ interest rate the bank pays on the account per year. The interest amount, which is paid at the end of the year, is based on the balance at the beginning of each year. Note that in "by hand" time value calculations, I must be expressed as a decimal, so $I = 0.05$.
- $INT =$ dollars of interest earned during each year, which equals the beginning amount multiplied by the interest rate. Thus, $INT = PV \times I$.
- $FV_N =$ future value, or ending amount, of the account at the end of N years. Whereas PV is the value now, or *present value*, FV_N is the value N years into the *future* after the interest earned has been added to the account.
- $N =$ number of years involved in the analysis.

In this example, $N = 1$, so FV_N can be calculated as follows:

$$FV_N = FV_1 = PV + INT$$
$$= PV + (PV \times I)$$
$$= PV \times (1 + I).$$

The future value at the end of one year, FV_1, equals the present value multiplied by (1.0 plus the interest rate). This future value relationship can be used to find how much $100 will be worth at the end of one year, if it is invested in an account that pays 5 percent interest:

$$FV_1 = PV \times (1 + I) = \$100 \times (1 + 0.05) = \$100 \times 1.05 = \$105.$$

What would be the value of the $100 if Meridian Clinics left the money in the account for five years? Here is a time line that shows the amount at the end of each year:

	0	1	2	3	4	5
	5%					
Beginning amount	−$100					
Interest earned		$ 5	$ 5.25	$ 5.51	$ 5.79	$ 6.08
End-of-year amount		105	110.25	115.76	121.55	127.63.

Note the following points:

- The account is opened with a deposit of $100. This is shown as an outflow at Year 0.
- Meridian earns $100 × 0.05 = $5 of interest during the first year, so the amount in the account at the end of Year 1 is $100 + $5 = $105.
- At the start of the second year, the account balance is $105. Interest of $105 × 0.05 = $5.25 is earned on the now larger amount, so the account balance at the end of the second year is $105 + $5.25 = $110.25. The Year 2 interest, $5.25, is higher than the first year's interest, $5, because $5 × 0.05 = $0.25 in interest was earned on the first year's interest.
- This process continues, and because the beginning balance is higher in each succeeding year, the interest earned increases in each year.
- The total interest earned, $27.63, is reflected in the final balance, $127.63, at the end of Year 5.

To better understand the mathematics of compounding, note that the Year 2 value, $110.25, is equal to:

$$FV_2 = FV_1 \times (1 + I)$$
$$= PV \times (1 + I) \times (1 + I)$$
$$= PV \times (1 + I)^2$$
$$= \$100 \times (1.05)^2 = \$110.25.$$

Furthermore, the balance at the end of Year 3 is:

$$FV_3 = FV_2 \times (1 + I)$$
$$= PV \times (1 + I)^3$$
$$= \$100 \times (1.05)^3 = \$115.76,$$

Continuing the calculation to the end of Year 5 gives:

$$FV_5 = \$100 \times (1.05)^5 = \$127.63.$$

These calculations show that a pattern clearly exists in future value calculations. In general, the future value of a lump sum at the end of N years can be found by applying this equation:

$$FV_N = PV \times (1 + I)^N.$$

Future values, as well as most other time value problems, can be solved three ways: regular calculator, financial calculator, or spreadsheet.

To use a regular calculator, multiply the PV by $(1 + I)$ for N times or use the *Regular* exponential function to raise $(1 + I)$ to the Nth power and then multiply the *Calculator* result by the PV. Perhaps the easiest way to find the future value of $100 after *Solution* five years when compounded at 5 percent is to enter $100, then multiply this amount by 1.05 for five times. If the calculator is set to display two decimal places, the answer would be $127.63:

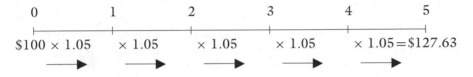

As denoted by the arrows, compounding involves moving to the **right** along the time line. In fact, the term *compounding* is used for finding future values because future values increase, or compound, over time.

Financial calculators have been programmed to solve many types of time *Financial* value analyses, including future value of a lump sum. In effect, the future *Calculator* value equation is programmed directly into the calculator. With a financial *Solution* calculator, the future value is found using three of the following five time value input keys[2]:

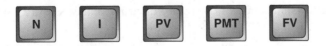

Note that these keys correspond to the five time value variables that are commonly used:

- N = number of periods.
- I = interest rate per period.
- PV = present value.
- PMT = payment. (This key is used only if the cash flows involve an annuity, which is a series of equal payments. Annuities are discussed in a later section.)
- FV = future value.

Also, note that this chapter deals with time value analyses that involve only four of the variables at any one time. Three of the variables will be known, and the calculator will solve for the fourth, unknown variable. In Chapter 11, when bond valuation is discussed, all five variables will be included in the analysis.

To find the future value of $100 after five years at 5 percent interest using a financial calculator, just enter PV = 100, I = 5, and N = 5, and then press the FV key. The answer, 127.63 (rounded to two decimal places), will appear. As stated previously, many financial calculators require that cash flows be designated as either inflows or outflows (entered as either positive or negative values). Applying this logic to the illustration, Meridian deposits the initial amount, which is an outflow to the firm, and takes out, or receives, the ending amount, which is an inflow to the firm. If the calculator requires this sign convention, the PV would be entered as −100. (If the PV was entered as 100, a positive value, the calculator would display −127.63 as the answer.) The calculator solution can be shown pictorially as follows:

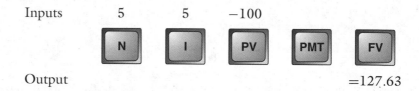

Inputs   5   5   −100

Output   =127.63

Also, some calculators require the user to press a *Compute* key before pressing the FV key. Finally, financial calculators permit specifying the number of decimal places that are displayed, even though 12 (or more) significant digits are actually used in the calculations. Two places are generally used for answers in dollars or percentages, and four places for decimal answers. The final answer, however, should be rounded to reflect the accuracy of the input values; it makes no sense to say that the return on a particular investment is 14.63827 percent when the cash flows are highly uncertain. **The nature of the analysis dictates how many decimal places should be displayed.**

Spreadsheet Solution

	A	B	C	D
1				
2	5	Nper	Number of periods	
3	$ 100.00	Pv	Present value	
4	5.0%	Rate	Interest rate	
5				
6	$ 127.63	=100*(1.05)^5 (entered into Cell A6)		
7				
8	$ 127.63	=A3*(1+A4)^A2 (entered into Cell A8)		
9				
10	$ 127.63	=FV(A4,A2,,−A3) (entered into Cell A10)		

Spreadsheet programs, such as Excel, are ideally suited for time value analyses. For simple time value calculations, it is easy to enter the appropriate formula directly into the spreadsheet. For example, you could enter the spreadsheet version of the future value equation into Cell A6: =100*(1.05)^5. Here, = tells the spreadsheet that a formula is being entered into the cell; * is the spreadsheet multiplication sign; and ^ is the spreadsheet exponential, or power, sign. When this formula is entered into Cell A6, the value $127.63 appears in the cell (when formatted with a dollar sign to two decimal places). Note that different spreadsheet programs use slightly different syntax in their time value analyses. The examples presented in this text use Excel syntax.

In most situations, it is more useful to enter a formula that can accommodate changing input values than to embed these values directly in the formula, so it would be better to solve this future value problem with this formula: =A3*(1+A4)^A2, as done in Cell A8. Here, the present value ($100) is contained in Cell A3, the interest rate (0.05, which is displayed as 5%) in Cell A4, and the number of periods (5) in Cell A2. With this formula, future values can be easily calculated with different starting amounts, interest rates, or number of years by changing the values in the input cells.

In addition to entering the appropriate time value formulas, most time value solutions are preprogrammed in the spreadsheet software. The preprogrammed time value formulas are called *functions*. Like any formula, a time value function consists of a number of arithmetic calculations combined into one statement. By using functions, spreadsheet users can save the time and tedium of building formulas from scratch.

Each function begins with a unique name that identifies the calculation to be performed, along with one or more *arguments* (the input values for the calculation) enclosed in parentheses. The best way to access the time value functions is to use the spreadsheet's *function wizard* (also called the *paste function*). For this future value problem, first move the cursor to Cell A10 (the cell where you want the answer to appear). Then click on the function wizard, select Financial for the function category and FV (future value) for the function name, and enter A4 for Rate, A2 for Nper (number of periods), and −A3 for Pv. (Note that the Pmt and Type entries are left blank for this problem. Also, note that the cell address entered for Pv has a minus sign. This is necessary for the answer to be displayed as a positive number.) Finally, press OK and the result, $127.63, appears in Cell A10.

Note that most of the spreadsheet solutions shown in this book follow a similar format. The input values and the output are contained in Column A. If a spreadsheet function is used in the solution, the input value (argument) names are shown in Column B to the right of the input values. In addition, the formula or function used to calculate the output is shown in Column B to the right of the output value. Finally, Column C contains the descriptive input names.

The most efficient way to solve most problems that involve time value is to use a financial calculator or spreadsheet.[3] However, the basic mathematics behind the calculations must be understood to set up complex problems before solving them. In addition, the underlying logic must be understood to comprehend stock and bond valuation, lease analysis, capital budgeting analysis, and other important healthcare financial management topics.

The Power of Compounding

The "power of compounding" is a phrase that emphasizes the fact that a relatively small starting value can grow to a large amount, even when the rate of growth (interest rate) is modest, when invested over a long period. For example, assume that a new parent places $1,000 in a stock mutual fund to help pay the child's college expenses, which are expected to begin in 18 years. The investment is assumed to earn a return of 10 percent per year, which is a reasonable estimate by historical standards. After 18 years, the value of the mutual fund account would be $5,560, which is not an inconsequential sum.

Now, assume that the money was meant to help fund the child's retirement, which is assumed to occur 65 years into the future. The value of the mutual fund account at that time would be $490,371, or nearly a **half-million dollars**. Imagine that: $1,000 grows to nearly half a million all because of the power of compounding. The moral of this story is clear: When saving for retirement, or for any other purpose, start early.

Self-Test Questions	1. What is a lump sum?
	2. What is compounding? What is interest on interest?
	3. What are three solution techniques for solving lump sum compounding problems?
	4. How does the future value of a lump sum change as the time is extended and as the interest rate increases?
	5. What is meant by the power of compounding?

Present Value of a Lump Sum (Discounting)

Suppose that GroupWest Health Plans, which has premium income reserves to invest, has been offered the chance to purchase a low-risk security from a local broker that will pay $127.63 at the end of five years. A local bank is currently offering 5 percent interest on a five-year certificate of deposit (CD), and GroupWest's managers regard the security offered by the broker as having the same risk as the bank CD. The 5 percent interest rate available on the bank CD is GroupWest's *opportunity cost rate*. (Opportunity costs are discussed in detail in the next section.) How much would GroupWest be willing to pay for the security that promises to pay $127.63 in five years?

The future value example presented in the previous section showed that an initial amount of $100 invested at 5 percent per year would be worth $127.63 at the end of five years. Thus, GroupWest should be indifferent to the choice between $100 today and $127.63 at the end of five years. Today's

$100 is defined as the *present value*, or *PV*, of $127.63 due in five years when the opportunity cost rate is 5 percent. If the price of the security being offered is exactly $100, GroupWest could buy it or turn it down because that is the security's "fair value." If the price is less than $100, GroupWest should buy it, while if the price is greater than $100, GroupWest should decline the offer.

Conceptually, the present value of a cash flow due N years in the future is the amount which, if it were on hand today, would grow to equal the future amount when compounded at the opportunity cost rate. Because $100 would grow to $127.63 in five years at a 5 percent interest rate, $100 is the present value of $127.63 due five years in the future when the opportunity cost rate is 5 percent. In effect, the present value tells us what amount would have to be invested to earn the opportunity cost rate. If the investment can be obtained for a lesser amount, a higher rate will be earned. If the investment costs more than the present value, the rate earned will be less than the opportunity cost rate.

Finding present values is called *discounting*, and it is simply the reverse of compounding: if the PV is known, compound to find the FV; if the FV is known, discount to find the PV. Here are the solution techniques used to solve this discounting problem.

```
0       1       2       3       4       5
   5%
 |---+---|---+---|---+---|---+---|---+---|

 ?                               $127.63
```

To develop the discounting equation, solve the compounding equation for PV:

Compounding: $FV_N = PV \times (1 + I)^N$

Discounting: $PV = \dfrac{FV_N}{(1 + I)^N}$

The equations show us that compounding problems are solved by multiplication, while discounting problems are solved by division.

Enter $127.63 and divide it five times by 1.05:

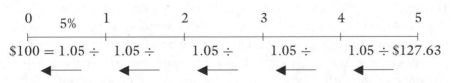

```
0       1         2         3         4         5
   5%
 |---+---|----+----|----+----|----+----|----+----|
$100 = 1.05 ÷  1.05 ÷    1.05 ÷    1.05 ÷    1.05 ÷ $127.63
   ◄───     ◄───      ◄───      ◄───      ◄───
```

Regular Calculator Solution

As shown by the arrows, discounting is moving left along a time line. As with compounding, the term *discounting* is descriptive. As we move left along a time line, values get smaller, or *discount*, over time.

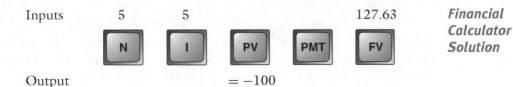

Inputs	5	5			127.63
	N	I	PV	PMT	FV
Output			= −100		

Financial Calculator Solution

Spreadsheet
Solution

	A	B	C	D
1				
2	5	Nper	Number of periods	
3	$ 127.63	Fv	Future value	
4	5.0%	Rate	Interest rate	
5				
6	$ 100.00	=A3/(1+A4)^A2 (entered into Cell A6)		
7				
8	$ 100.00	=PV(A4,A2,,–A3) (entered into Cell A8)		
9				
10				

One solution would be to enter the applicable formula, as shown to the right of Cell A6: =A3/(1+A4)^A2. Here, the future value ($127.63) is contained in Cell A3, the interest rate (0.05, which is displayed as 5%) in Cell A4, and the number of periods (5) in Cell A2. With this formula, present values easily can be calculated with different starting future amounts, interest rates, or number of years.

The function approach is illustrated in Cell A8. First, move the cursor to that cell (the cell where you want the answer to appear). Then, click on the function wizard, select Financial for the function category and Pv (present value) for the function name, and enter A4 for Rate, A2 for Nper (number of periods), and −A3 for Fv. (Note that the Pmt and Type entries are left blank for this problem. Also, note that the cell address entered for Fv has a minus sign. This is necessary for the answer to be displayed as a positive number.) Finally, press OK and the result, $100.00, appears in Cell A8.

Discounting at Work

At relatively high interest rates, funds due in the future are worth very little today, and even at moderate discount rates, the present value of a sum due in the distant future is quite small. To illustrate discounting at work, consider 100-year bonds. A bond is a type of debt security in which an investor loans some amount of principal—say, $1,000—to a company (borrower), which in turn promises to pay interest over the life of the bond and to return the principal amount at maturity. Typically, the longest maturities for bonds are 30–40 years, but in the early 1990s, several companies, including Columbia/HCA Healthcare (now HCA), issued 100-year bonds.

At first blush, it might appear that anyone who would buy a 100-year bond must be irrational because there is little assurance that the borrower will even be around in 100 years to repay the amount borrowed. However, consider the present value of $1,000 to be received in 100 years. If the discount rate is 7.5 percent, which is roughly the interest rate that was set on the bond, the present value is a mere $0.72. Thus, the time value of money eroded the value of the bond's principal repayment to the point that it was worth less than $1 at the time the bond was issued. This tells us that the value of the bond when it was sold was based primarily on the interest stream received in the early years of ownership, and that the payments expected during the later years contributed little to the bond's initial $1,000 value. Thus, the risk of not recovering the initial $1,000 principal amount did not have a large impact on investors' willingness to buy the bond.

Opportunity Costs

In the last section, the *opportunity cost* concept was used to set the discount rate on the time value analysis of GroupWest's investment offer. The opportunity cost concept plays a critical role in time value analysis. To illustrate, suppose an individual found the winning ticket for the Florida lottery and now has $1 million to invest. Should the individual assign a cost to these funds? At first blush it might appear that this money has zero cost because its acquisition was purely a matter of luck. However, as soon as the lucky individual thinks about what to do with the $1 million, he or she has to think in terms of the opportunity costs involved. By using the funds to invest in one alternative—for example, in the stock of Health Management Associates (HMA)—the individual forgoes the opportunity to make some other investment—for example, buying U.S. Treasury bonds. Thus, there is an opportunity cost associated with any investment planned for the $1 million, even though the lottery winnings were "free."

Because one investment decision automatically negates all other possible investments with the same funds, the cash flows expected to be earned from any investment must be discounted at a rate that reflects the return that could be earned on forgone investment opportunities. The problem is that the number of forgone investment opportunities is virtually infinite, so which one should be chosen to establish the opportunity cost rate? The opportunity cost rate to be applied in time value analysis is the rate that could be earned on alternative investments **of similar risk**. It would not be logical to assign a very low opportunity cost rate to a series of very risky cash flows, or vice versa. This concept is one of the cornerstones of healthcare finance, so it is worth repeating. **The opportunity cost rate (i.e., the discount rate) applied to investment cash flows is the rate that could be earned on alternative investments of similar risk.**

It is very important to recognize that the discounting process itself accounts for the opportunity cost of capital (i.e., the loss of use of the funds for other purposes). In effect, discounting a potential investment at, say, 10 percent, produces a present value that provides a 10 percent return. Thus, if the investment can be obtained for less than its present value, it will earn more than its opportunity cost of capital and hence is a good investment. Alternatively, if the cost of the investment is greater than its present value, it will earn less than its opportunity cost of capital and hence is a bad investment. It is also important to note that the opportunity cost rate does not depend on the source of the funds to be invested. Rather, **the primary determinant of this rate is the riskiness of the cash flows being discounted.** Thus, the same 10 percent opportunity cost rate would be applied to this potential investment regardless of whether the funds to be used for the investment were won in a lottery, taken out of petty cash, or obtained by selling some securities.

Generally, opportunity cost rates are obtained by looking at rates that could be earned, or more precisely, rates that are expected to be earned, on securities such as stocks or bonds. Securities are usually chosen to set opportunity cost rates because their expected returns are more easily estimated than rates of return on real assets such as hospital beds, MRI machines, and the like. Furthermore, as discussed in Chapter 12, securities generally provide the minimum return appropriate for the amount of risk assumed, so securities returns provide a good benchmark for other investments.

To illustrate the opportunity cost concept, assume that Oakdale Community Hospital is considering building a nursing home. The first step in the financial analysis is to forecast the cash flows that the nursing home is expected to produce. These cash flows, then, must be discounted at some opportunity cost rate to determine their present value. Would the hospital's opportunity cost rate be (1) the expected rate of return on a bank CD; (2) the expected rate of return on the stock of Manor Care, which operates a large number of nursing homes and assisted living centers; or (3) the expected rate of return on pork belly futures? (Pork belly futures are investments that involve commodity contracts for delivery at some future time.) The answer is the expected rate of return on Manor Care's stock because that is the rate of return available to the hospital on **alternative investments of similar risk**. Bank CDs are very low-risk investments, so they would understate the opportunity cost rate in owning a nursing home. Conversely, pork belly futures are very high-risk investments, so that rate of return is probably too high to apply to Oakdale's nursing home investment.[4]

The source of the funds used for the nursing home investment is **not relevant** to the analysis. Oakdale may obtain the needed funds by borrowing, by soliciting contributions, or by using excess cash accumulated from profit retention. The discount rate applied to the nursing home cash flows depends only on the riskiness of those cash flows and the returns available on alternative investments of similar risk, not on the source of the investment funds.

At this point, you may question the ability of real-world analysts to assess the riskiness of a cash flow stream or to choose an opportunity cost rate with any confidence. Fortunately, the process is not as difficult as it may appear here because businesses have benchmarks that can be used as starting points. (Chapter 13 contains a discussion of how benchmark opportunity cost rates are established for capital investments, while Chapter 15 presents a detailed discussion on how the riskiness of a cash flow stream can be assessed.)

1. Why does an investment have an opportunity cost rate even when the funds employed have no explicit cost?
2. How are opportunity cost rates established?
3. Does the opportunity cost rate depend on the source of the investment funds?

Self-Test Questions

Solving for Interest Rate and Time

At this point, it should be obvious that compounding and discounting are reciprocal processes. Furthermore, four time value analysis variables have been presented: PV, FV, I, and N. If the values of three of the variables are known, the value of the fourth can be found with the help of a financial calculator or spreadsheet. Thus far, the interest rate, I, and the number of years, N, plus either PV or FV have been given in the illustrations. In some situations, however, the analysis may require solving for either I or N.[5]

Solving for Interest Rate (I)

Suppose that Family Practice Associates (FPA), a primary care group practice, can buy a bank CD for $78.35 that will return $100 after five years. In this case, PV, FV, and N are known, but I, the interest rate that the bank is paying, is not known.

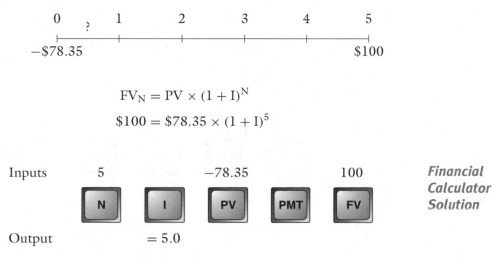

$$FV_N = PV \times (1 + I)^N$$

$$\$100 = \$78.35 \times (1 + I)^5$$

Financial Calculator Solution

Spreadsheet Solution

	A	B	C	D
1				
2	5	Nper	Number of periods	
3	$ (78.35)	Pv	Present value	
4	$ 100.00	Fv	Future value	
5				
6				
7				
8	5.00%	=RATE(A2,,A3,A4) (entered into Cell A8)		
9				
10				

Here, the spreadsheet function named RATE is used to solve for I, as illustrated to the right of Cell A8. First, click on the function wizard, select Financial for the function category and RATE for the function name, and enter A2 for Nper (number of periods), A3 for Pv (present value), and A4 for Fv (future value). (Note that the Pmt and Type entries are left blank for this problem. Also note that the Pv was entered as a negative number, as shown on the time line.) Finally, press OK and the result, 5%, appears in Cell A8. (Note that some spreadsheet programs display the answer in decimal form unless the cell is formatted to display in percent.)

Solving for Time (N)

Suppose that the bank told FPA that a certificate of deposit pays 5 percent interest each year, that it costs $78.35, and that at maturity the group would receive $100. How long must the funds be invested in the CD? In this case, Pv, Fv, and I are known, but N, the number of periods, is not known.

$$
\begin{array}{ccccccc}
0 & & 1 & 2 & & N-1 & N \\
\vdash & 5\% & \!\!\!\!\dashv & \!\!\!\!\dashv & \cdots & \!\!\!\!\dashv & \\
-\$78.35 & & & & & & \$100
\end{array}
$$

$$FV_N = PV \times (1 + I)^N$$

$$\$100 = \$78.35 \times (1.05)^N$$

Financial Calculator Solution

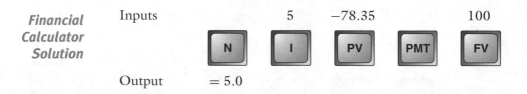

Inputs   5   −78.35   100

| N | I | PV | PMT | FV |

Output   = 5.0

	A	B	C	D
1				
2	5.00%	Rate	Interest rate	
3	$ (78.35)	Pv	Present value	
4	$ 100.00	Fv	Future value	
5				
6				
7				
8	5.00	=NPER(A2,,A3,A4) (entered into Cell A8)		
9				
10				

Spreadsheet Solution

To solve for time, the spreadsheet function named NPER (number of periods) is used. To begin, place the cursor in Cell A8 and click on the function wizard. Then, select Financial for the function category and NPER for the function name, and enter A2 for Rate, A3 for Pv, and A4 for Fv. (Note that the Pmt and Type entries are left blank for this problem. Also, note that the Pv was entered as a negative number, as shown on the time line.) Finally, press OK and the result, 5.0, appears in Cell A8.

Self-Test Questions

1. What are a few real-world situations that may require you to solve for interest rate or time?
2. Can financial calculators and spreadsheets easily solve for interest rate or time?

Annuities

Whereas lump sums are single values, an *annuity* is a series of **equal payments at fixed intervals** for a specified number of periods. Annuity *payments*, which are given the symbol PMT or Pmt, can occur at the beginning or end of each period. If the payments occur at the end of each period, as they typically do, the annuity is an *ordinary*, or *deferred*, *annuity*. If payments are made at the beginning of each period, the annuity is an *annuity due*. Because ordinary annuities are far more common in time value problems, when the term *annuity* is used in this book (or in general), payments are assumed to occur at the end of each period. Furthermore, we begin our discussion of annuities by focusing on ordinary annuities.

Ordinary Annuities

If Meridian Clinics were to deposit $100 at the end of each year for three years in an account that paid 5 percent interest per year, how much would Meridian accumulate at the end of three years? The answer to this question is the *future value of the annuity*, which for ordinary annuities coincides with the final payment.

Regular Calculator Solution

One approach to the problem is to compound each individual cash flow to Year 3.

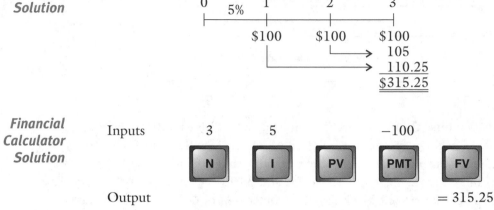

Financial Calculator Solution

Inputs	3	5		−100	
	N	I	PV	PMT	FV

Output   = 315.25

In annuity problems, the PMT key is used in conjunction with either the PV or FV key.

Spreadsheet Solution

	A	B	C	D
1				
2	3	Nper	Number of periods	
3	$ (100.00)	Pmt	Payment	
4	5.0%	Rate	Interest rate	
5				
6				
7				
8	$ 315.25	=FV(A4,A2,A3) (entered into Cell A8)		
9				
10				

Here, we again use the future value function, but now we will use the payment (Pmt) entry in the function wizard to recognize that the problem involves annuities. Place the cursor in Cell A8. Then, click on the function wizard, select Financial for the function category and FV (future value) for the function name, and enter A4 for Rate, A2 for Nper (number of periods), and A3 for Pmt. (Note that the Pv and Type entries are left blank for this problem.) Finally, press OK and the result, $315.25, appears in Cell A8.

Suppose that Meridian Clinics was offered the following alternatives: a three-year annuity with payments of $100 at the end of each year or a lump sum payment today. Meridian has no need for the money during the next three years. If it accepts the annuity, it would deposit the payments in an account that pays 5 percent interest per year. Similarly, the lump sum payment would be deposited into the same account. How large must the lump sum payment be today to make it equivalent to the annuity? The answer to this question is the *present value of the annuity*, which for ordinary annuities occurs one period prior to the first payment.

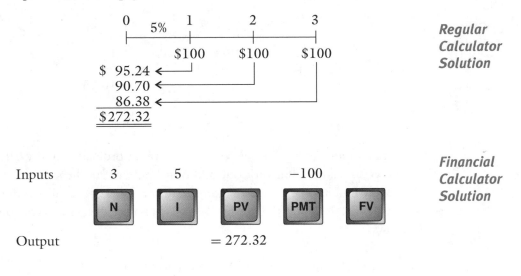

Regular Calculator Solution

Financial Calculator Solution

	A	B	C	D
1				
2	3	Nper	Number of periods	
3	$ (100.00)	Pmt	Payment	
4	5.0%	Rate	Interest rate	
5				
6				
7				
8	$ 272.32	=PV(A4,A2,A3) (entered into Cell A8)		
9				
10				

Spreadsheet Solution

Here we use the present value function, but again with a payment entry to recognize that the problem involves annuities. Place the cursor in Cell A8. Then click on the function wizard, select Financial for the function category and PV for the function name, and enter A4 for Rate, A2 for Nper (number of periods), and A3 for Pmt. (Note that the Fv and Type entries are left blank for this problem.) Finally, press OK and the result, $272.32, appears in Cell A8.

One especially important application of the annuity concept relates to loans with constant payments, such as mortgages, auto loans, and many bank loans to businesses. Such loans are examined in more depth in a later section on amortization.

Annuities Due

If the three $100 payments in the previous example had been made at the beginning of each year, the annuity would have been an *annuity due*. The future value of an annuity due occurs one period after the final payment, while the future value of a regular annuity coincides with the final payment. Here are the solution techniques for the **future value of an annuity due**.

*Regular
Calculator
Solution*

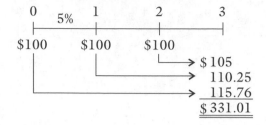

In the case of an annuity due, as compared with an ordinary annuity, all the cash flows are compounded for one additional period, and hence the future value of an annuity due is greater than the future value of a similar ordinary annuity by $(1 + I)$. Thus, the future value of an annuity due also can be found as follows:

$$FV \text{ (Annuity due)} = FV \text{ of a regular annuity } \times (1 + I)$$

$$= \$315.25 \times 1.05 = \$331.01.$$

*Financial
Calculator
Solution*

Most financial calculators have a switch or key marked DUE or BEGIN that permits the switching of the mode from end-of-period payments (ordinary annuity) to beginning-of-period payments (annuity due). When the beginning-of-period mode is activated, the calculator will normally indicate the changed mode by displaying the word BEGIN or some other symbol. To deal with annuities due, change the mode to the beginning of period and proceed as before. Because most problems will deal with end-of-period cash flows, do not forget to switch the calculator back to the END mode.

*Spreadsheet
Solution*

	A	B	C	D
1				
2	3	Nper	Number of periods	
3	$ (100.00)	Pmt	Payment	
4	5.0%	Rate	Interest rate	
5				
6	$ 331.01	=FV(A4,A2,A3,,1) (entered into Cell A6)		
7				
8	$ 331.01	=FV(A4,A2,A3)*(1+A4) (entered into Cell A8)		
9				
10				

One approach (as shown in Cell A6) is to use the spreadsheet future value (FV) function but with a "1" entered for Type (as opposed to a blank). Now the spreadsheet treats the entries as an annuity due, and $331.01 is displayed as the answer.

As an alternative, note that the solution is the same as for an ordinary annuity, except the result must be multiplied by (1 + Rate), which is (1 +

A4) in this example. This solution approach is given in Cell A8. The result, $331.01, is the future value of the annuity due.

Here are the solution techniques for the **present value of an annuity due**.

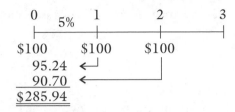

Regular Calculator Solution

Because the payments are shifted to the left, each one is discounted for one less year. Thus, the present value of an annuity due is larger than that of a similar regular annuity.

Note that the present value of an annuity due can be thought of as the present value of an ordinary annuity that is compounded for one additional period, so it also can be found as follows:

$$\text{PV(Annuity due)} = \text{PV of a regular annuity} \times (1 + \text{I})$$

$$= \$272.32 \times 1.05 = \$285.94$$

Activate the beginning of period mode (i.e., the BEGIN mode), and then proceed as before. Again, because most problems will deal with end-of-period cash flows, do not forget to switch the calculator back to the END mode.

Financial Calculator Solution

Spreadsheet Solution

	A	B	C	D
1				
2	3	Nper	Number of periods	
3	$ (100.00)	Pmt	Payment	
4	5.0%	Rate	Interest rate	
5				
6	$ 285.94	=PV(A4,A2,A3,,1) (entered into Cell A6)		
7				
8	$ 285.94	=PV(A4,A2,A3)*(1+A4) (entered into Cell A8)		
9				
10				

As with future value, one approach (as shown in Cell A6) is to use the spreadsheet present value (PV) function but with a "1" entered for Type (as opposed to a blank). Now the spreadsheet treats the entries as an annuity due, and $285.94 is displayed as the answer.

Note that the alternative solution is the same as for an ordinary annuity, except the function in Cell A8 is multiplied by (1 + A4). The result, $285.94, is the present value of the annuity due.

1. What is an annuity?
2. What is the difference between an ordinary annuity and an annuity due?
3. Which annuity has the greater future value: an ordinary annuity or an annuity due? Why?
4. Which annuity has the greater present value: an ordinary annuity or an annuity due? Why?

Perpetuities

Most annuities call for payments to be made over some finite period of time—for example, $100 per year for three years. However, some annuities go on indefinitely, or perpetually, and hence are called *perpetuities*. The present value of a perpetuity is found as follows:

$$\text{PV (Perpetuity)} = \frac{\text{Payment}}{\text{Interest rate}} = \frac{\text{PMT}}{\text{I}}.$$

Perpetuities can be illustrated by some securities issued by the Canadian Healthcare Board. Each security promises to pay $100 annually in perpetuity (forever). What would each security be worth if the opportunity cost rate, or discount rate, is 10 percent? The answer is $1,000:

$$\text{PV (Perpetuity)} = \frac{\$100}{0.10} = \$1,000.$$

	A	B	C	D
1				
2				
3	$ 100.00	Pmt	Payment	
4	10.0%	Rate	Interest rate	
5				
6				
7				
8	$ 1,000.00	=A3/A4 (entered into Cell A8)		
9				
10				

Or, using a spreadsheet, merely enter the perpetuity formula into a cell, as shown here in Cell A8.

Suppose interest rates, and hence the opportunity cost rate, rose to 15 percent. What would happen to the security's value? The interest rate increase would lower its value to $666.67:

$$\text{PV (Perpetuity)} = \frac{\$100}{0.15} = \$666.67.$$

Assume that interest rates fell to 5 percent. The rate decrease would increase the perpetuity's value to $2,000:

$$PV \text{ (Perpetuity)} = \frac{\$100}{0.05} = \$2,000.$$

The value of a perpetuity changes dramatically when opportunity costs (interest rates) change. All securities' values are affected by interest rate changes, but some, like perpetuities, are more sensitive to interest rate changes than others, such as short-term government bonds. The risks associated with interest rate changes are discussed in more detail in Chapter 11.

---

1. What is a perpetuity?
2. What happens to the value of a perpetuity when interest rates increase or decrease?

Self-Test Questions

Uneven Cash Flow Streams

The definition of an annuity (or perpetuity) includes the words "constant amount," so annuities involve payments that are the same in every period. Although some financial decisions, such as bond valuation, do involve constant payments, most important healthcare time value analyses involve uneven, or nonconstant, cash flows. For example, the financial evaluation of a proposed outpatient clinic or MRI facility rarely involves constant cash flows.

In general, the term *lump sum* is used with a single cash flow; the term *payment (PMT)* is reserved for annuity situations in which there are multiple constant lump sums; and the term *cash flow (CF)* is used when there is a series of uneven lump sums. Financial calculators are set up to follow this convention. When dealing with uneven cash flows, the CF function, rather than the PMT key, is used.

Present Value

The present value of an uneven cash flow stream is found as the sum of the present values of the individual cash flows of the stream. For example, suppose that Wilson Memorial Hospital is considering the purchase of a new x-ray machine. The hospital's managers forecast that the operation of the new machine would produce the following stream of cash inflows (in thousands of dollars):

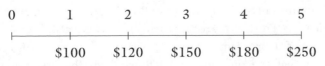

What is the present value of the new x-ray machine investment if the appropriate discount rate (i.e., the opportunity cost rate) is 10 percent?

Regular Calculator Solution The PV of each lump sum cash flow can be found using a regular calculator, and then these values are summed to find the present value of the stream, $580,950:

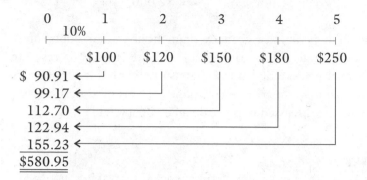

Financial Calculator Solution The present value of an uneven cash flow stream can be solved with most financial calculators by using the following steps:

- Input the individual cash flows, in chronological order, into the *cash flow register*, where they usually are designated as CF_0 and CF_j (CF_1, CF_2, CF_3, and so on) or just CF_j (CF_0, CF_1, CF_2, CF_3, and so on).
- Enter the discount rate.
- Push the *NPV* key.

For this problem, enter 0, 100, 120, 150, 180, and 250 in that order into the calculator's cash flow register; enter $I = 10$; then push NPV to obtain the answer, 580.95. Note that an implied cash flow of zero is entered for CF_0.

Three points should be noted about the calculator solution. First, when dealing with the cash flow register, the term NPV, rather than PV, is used to represent present value. The letter N in NPV stands for the word *net*, so NPV is the abbreviation for net present value. Net present value means the sum or net of the present values of a cash flow stream. Often, the stream will consist of both inflows and outflows, but the stream here contains all inflows.

Second, annuity cash flows within any uneven cash flow stream can be entered into the cash flow register most efficiently on most calculators by using the N_j key. This key allows the user to specify the number of times a constant payment occurs within the stream. (Some calculators prompt the user to enter the number of times each cash flow occurs.)

Finally, amounts entered into the cash flow register remain there until the register is cleared. Thus, if a problem had been previously worked with eight cash flows, and a problem is worked with only four cash flows, the calculator assumes that the final four cash flows from the first calculation belong to the second calculation. Be sure to clear the register before starting a new time value analysis.

	A	B	C	D
1				
2	10.0%	Rate	Interest rate	
3				
4	$ 100	Value 1	Year 1 CF	
5	$ 120	Value 1	Year 2 CF	
6	$ 150	Value 1	Year 3 CF	
7	$ 180	Value 1	Year 4 CF	
8	$ 250	Value 1	Year 5 CF	
9				
10	$ 580.95	=NPV(A2,A4:A8) (entered into Cell A10)		

Spreadsheet Solution

The NPV function calculates the present value of a stream, called a spreadsheet *range*, of cash flows. First, the cash flow values must be entered into consecutive cells in the spreadsheet, as shown above in Cells A4 through A8. Next, the discount (opportunity cost) rate must be placed into a cell (as in Cell A2 above). Then, place the cursor in Cell A10, use the function wizard to select Financial and NPV, and then enter A2 as Rate and A4:A8 as Value 1. Press OK and the value $580.95 is displayed in the cell. (Note that the Value 1 entry is the range of cash flows contained in Cells A4 through A8. Also, note that NPV stands for *net present value*, which indicates that the resulting present value is the net of the present values of two or more cash flows.)

The NPV function assumes that cash flows occur at the **end** of each period, so NPV is calculated as of the **beginning** of the period of the first cash flow specified in the range, which is one period before that cash flow occurs. Because the cash flow specified as the first flow in the range is a Year 1 value, the calculated NPV occurs at the beginning of Year 1, or the end of Year 0, which is correct for this illustration. However, if a Year 0 cash flow is included in the range, the NPV would be calculated at the beginning of Year 0, or the end of Year −1, which typically is incorrect. This problem will be addressed in the next major section.

Future Value

The future value of an uneven cash flow stream is found by compounding each payment to the end of the stream and then summing the future values.

The future value of each lump sum cash flow can be found, using a regular calculator, by summing these values to find the future value of the stream, $935,630:

Regular Calculator Solution

$$
\begin{array}{cccccc}
0 & 1 & 2 & 3 & 4 & 5 \\
\end{array}
$$

0	1	2	3	4	5
10%					
	$100	$120	$150	$180	$ 250.00
					198.00
					181.50
					159.72
					146.41
					$ 935.63

Financial Calculator Solution   Some financial calculators have a net future value key (NFV) that, after the cash flows have been entered into the cash flow register, can be used to obtain the future value of an uneven cash flow stream. However, analysts generally are more concerned with the present value of a cash flow stream than with its future value. The reason, of course, is that the present value represents the value of the investment today, which then can be compared to the cost of the investment—whether a stock, bond, x-ray machine, or new clinic—to make the investment decision.

Spreadsheet Solution   Most spreadsheet programs do not have a function that computes the future value of an uneven cash flow stream. However, future values can be found by building a formula in a cell that replicates the regular calculator solution.

Self-Test Questions

1. Give two examples of financial decisions that typically involve uneven cash flows.
2. Describe how present values of uneven cash flow streams are calculated using a regular calculator, using a financial calculator, and using a spreadsheet.
3. What is meant by *net present value*?

Using Time Value Analysis to Measure Return on Investment (ROI)

In most investments, an individual or a business spends cash today with the expectation of receiving cash in the future. The financial attractiveness of such investments is measured by *return on investment (ROI)*, or just *return*. There are two basic ways of expressing ROI: in dollar terms and in percentage terms.

To illustrate the concept, let's reexamine the cash flows expected to be received if Wilson Memorial Hospital buys its new x-ray machine (shown on the time line in thousands of dollars). In the last section, we determined that the present value of these flows, when discounted at a 10 percent rate, is $580,950:

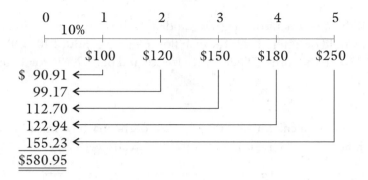

Dollar Return

The $580,950 calculated above represents the present value of the cash flows that the x-ray machine is **expected** to provide to Wilson Memorial Hospital, assuming a 10 percent discount rate (opportunity cost of capital). This result tells us that a 10 percent return on a $580,950 investment would produce a cash flow stream that is identical to one being discounted.

To measure the *dollar return* on the investment, the cost of the x-ray machine must be compared to the present value of the expected benefits (the cash inflows). If the machine will cost $500,000 and the present value of the inflows is $580,950, then the expected dollar return on the machine is $580,950 − $500,000 = $80,950. Note that this measure of dollar return incorporates time value, and hence opportunity costs, through the discounting process. The opportunity cost inherent in the use of the $500,000 is accounted for because the 10 percent discount rate reflects the return that could be earned on alternative investments of similar risk. By virtue of the $80,950 excess, the x-ray machine has an expected present value that is $80,950 more than would occur if it had only a 10 percent return, which is the opportunity cost rate. Thus, the x-ray machine makes sense financially because it creates an excess dollar return for the hospital.

The dollar return process can be combined into a single calculation by adding the cost of the x-ray machine to the time line:

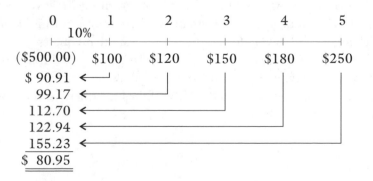

Financial Now, with the investment outlay (cost) added to the time line, the following
Calculator cash flows would be entered into the cash flow register: −500, 100, 120, 150,
Solution 180, and 250, in that order. Then, enter I = 10 and push *NPV* to obtain the
answer, 80.95.

Spreadsheet As in the financial calculator solution, the cost of the machine must be added
Solution to the cash flow data. Here, it is added to the spreadsheet range:

	A	B	C	D
1				
2	10.0%	Rate	Interest rate	
3	$ (500)		Year 0 CF	
4	$ 100	Value 1	Year 1 CF	
5	$ 120	Value 1	Year 2 CF	
6	$ 150	Value 1	Year 3 CF	
7	$ 180	Value 1	Year 4 CF	
8	$ 250	Value 1	Year 5 CF	
9				
10	$ 80.95	=NPV(A2,A4:A8)+A3 (entered into Cell A10)		

Note that the situation here is the same as in the previous cash flow stream,
except that there is an initial investment outlay of $500 added in Cell A3.
Because the NPV of the cash inflows in Cells A4 through A8 represents the
value one period before the first (A4) cash flow, all that must be done is to
add the investment outlay to the calculated NPV. This is done in Cell A10
above by adding A3 to the NPV function, and the result, $80.95, appears in
that cell.

Rate of Return

The second way to measure the ROI of an investment is by *rate of return*, or
percentage return. This measures the interest rate that must be earned on the
investment outlay to generate the expected cash inflows. In other words, this
measure provides the expected periodic rate of return on the investment. If
the cash flows are annual, as in this example, the rate of return is an annual
rate. In effect, we are solving for I—the interest rate that equates the sum of
the present values of the cash inflows to the dollar amount of the cash outlay.

Mathematically, if the sum of the present values of the cash inflows
equals the investment outlay, then the NPV of the investment is forced to $0.
This relationship is shown here:

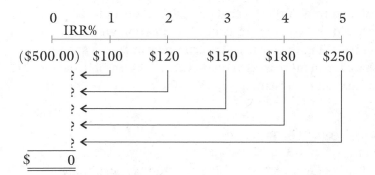

Note that the rate of return on an investment, particularly an investment in plant or equipment, typically is called the *internal rate of return* (*IRR*), a somewhat archaic term that often is used instead of ROI, or just rate of return. Although a trial-and-error procedure could be used on a regular calculator to determine the rate of return, it is better to use a financial calculator or spreadsheet.

Use the same cash flows that were entered to solve for NPV: −500, 100, 120, 150, 180, and 250. However, now push the IRR button to obtain the answer—15.3 percent.

Financial Calculator Solution

Spreadsheet Solution

	A	B	C	D
1				
2	10.0%	Guess	Interest rate	
3	$ (500)	Values	Year 0 CF	
4	$ 100	Values	Year 1 CF	
5	$ 120	Values	Year 2 CF	
6	$ 150	Values	Year 3 CF	
7	$ 180	Values	Year 4 CF	
8	$ 250	Values	Year 5 CF	
9				
10	15.3%	=IRR(A3:A8,A2) (entered into Cell A10)		

The IRR function is used to calculate rate of return. Choose Financial and IRR on the function wizard, then enter A3:A8 as Values and A2 as Guess. The result, 15.3%, appears in Cell A10, the cell that has the IRR function in it. (Note that IRR stands for internal rate of return. Also, note that a starting guess is required to calculate the IRR because the methodology used by the spreadsheet IRR function is actually a trial-and-error process that requires a starting point.)

The IRR of 15.3 percent tells the hospital's managers that the expected rate of return on the x-ray machine exceeds the opportunity cost rate by 15.3 − 10.0 = 5.3 percentage points. Thus, the expected rate of return is higher than that available on alternative investments of similar risk (the required rate of return), and hence the x-ray machine makes financial sense. Note that both the dollar (NPV) return and the percentage (IRR) return indicate that the x-ray machine should be acquired. In general, the two methods lead to the same conclusion regarding the financial attractiveness of an investment.

We will have much more to say about financial returns in Chapters 11, 12, and 14. For now, an understanding of the basic concept is sufficient.

Self-Test Questions

1. What does the term *ROI* mean?
2. Differentiate between dollar return and rate of return.
3. Is the calculation of financial return an application of time value analysis? Explain your answer.
4. What role does the opportunity cost rate play in calculating financial returns?

Semiannual and Other Compounding Periods

In all the examples thus far, we assumed that interest is earned (compounded) once a year, or annually. This is called *annual compounding*. Suppose, however, that Meridian Clinics puts $100 into a bank account that pays 6 percent annual interest, but it is compounded *semiannually*. How much would the clinic accumulate at the end of one year, two years, or some other period? Semiannual compounding means that interest is paid each six months, so interest is earned more often than under annual compounding.

The Effect of Semiannual Compounding

To illustrate semiannual compounding, assume that the $100 is placed into the account for three years. The following situation occurs under **annual** compounding:

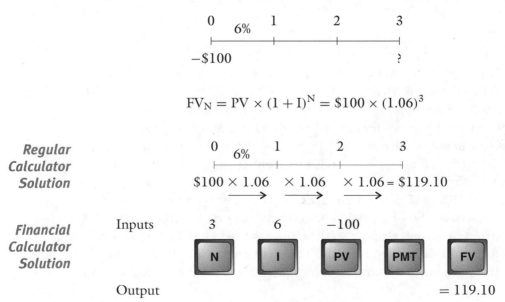

$$FV_N = PV \times (1 + I)^N = \$100 \times (1.06)^3$$

	A	B	C	D
1				
2		3	Nper	Number of periods	
3	$	100.00	Pv	Present value	
4		6.0%	Rate	Interest rate	
5				
6	$	119.10	=100*(1.06)^3 (entered into Cell A6)	
7				
8	$	119.10	=A3*(1+A4)^A2 (entered into Cell A8)	
9				
10	$	119.10	=FV(A4,A2,,-A3) (entered into Cell A10)	

Now, consider what happens under **semiannual** compounding. Because interest rates usually are stated as annual rates, this situation would be described as 6 percent interest, compounded semiannually. With semiannual compounding, N = 2 × 3 = 6 semiannual periods, and I = 6 / 2 = 3% per semiannual period. Here is the solution.

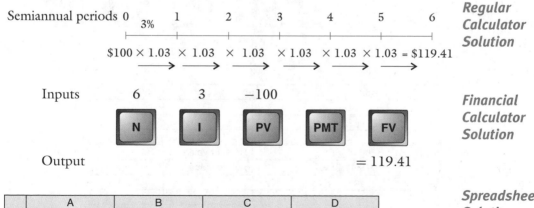

$$FV_N = PV \times (1 + I)^N = \$100 \times (1.03)^6$$

	A	B	C	D
1				
2		6	Nper	Number of periods	
3	$	100.00	Pv	Present value	
4		3.0%	Rate	Interest rate	
5				
6	$	119.41	=100*(1.03)^6 (entered into Cell A6)	
7				
8	$	119.41	=A3*(1+A4)^A2 (entered into Cell A8)	
9				
10	$	119.41	=FV(A4,A2,,-A3) (entered into Cell A10)	

The $100 deposit grows to $119.41 under semiannual compounding, but it grows only to $119.10 under annual compounding. This result occurs because interest on interest is being earned more frequently under semiannual compounding.

Stated Versus Effective Interest Rates

Throughout the economy, different compounding periods are used for different types of investments. For example, bank accounts often compound interest monthly or daily, most bonds pay interest semiannually, and stocks generally pay quarterly dividends.[6] Furthermore, the cash flows that stem from capital investments such as hospital wings or diagnostic equipment can be analyzed in monthly, quarterly, or annual periods or even some other interval. To properly compare time value analyses with different compounding periods, they need to be put on a common basis, which leads to a discussion of *stated interest rates* versus *effective annual rates.*

The stated interest rate in the Meridian Clinics's semiannual compounding example is 6 percent. The effective annual rate is the rate that produces the same ending (i.e., future) value under annual compounding. In the example, the effective annual rate is the rate that would produce a future value of $119.41 at the end of Year 3 under **annual compounding**. The solution is 6.09 percent, as found here using a financial calculator and a spreadsheet:

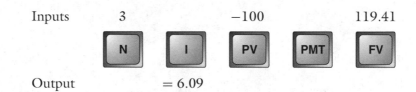

Inputs	3		−100		119.41
	N	I	PV	PMT	FV

Output   = 6.09

	A	B	C	D
1				
2				
3	3	Nper	Number of periods	
4	$ (100.00)	Pv	Present value	
5	$ 119.41	Fv	Future value	
6				
7				
8	6.09%	=RATE(A3,A4,A5) (entered into Cell A8)		
9				
10				

Thus, if one bank offered to pay 6 percent interest with semiannual compounding on a savings account, while another offered 6.09 percent with annual compounding, they both would be paying the same effective annual rate because the ending value is the same under both sets of terms:

Semiannual periods 0   3%   1   2   3   4   5   6

$100 × 1.03 × 1.03 × 1.03 × 1.03 × 1.03 × 1.03 = $119.41

Years   0   6.09%   1   2   3

$100 ×1.0609 ×1.0609 ×1.0609 = $119.41

In general, the effective annual rate (EAR) can be determined, given the stated rate and number of compounding periods per year, by using this equation:[7]

$$\text{Effective annual rate (EAR)} = (1 + I_{Stated}/M)^M - 1.0,$$

where I_{Stated} is the stated (i.e., the annual) interest rate and M is the number of compounding periods per year. The term I_{Stated} / M is the *periodic* interest rate, so the EAR equation can be recast as:

$$\text{Effective annual rate (EAR)} = (1 + \text{Periodic rate})^M - 1.0.$$

To illustrate the use of the EAR equation, the effective annual rate when the stated rate is 6 percent and semiannual compounding occurs is 6.09 percent:

$$EAR = (1 + 0.06/2)^2 - 1.0$$
$$= (1.03)^2 - 1.0$$
$$= 1.0609 - 1.0 = 0.0609 = 6.09\%,$$

which confirms the answer that we obtained previously.

As shown in the preceding calculations, semiannual compounding, or for that matter any compounding that occurs more than once a year, can be handled in two ways. First, the input variables can be expressed as periodic variables rather than annual variables. In the Meridian Clinics example, use N = 6 periods rather than N = 3 years, and I = 3% per period rather than I = 6% per year. Second, find the effective annual rate and then use this rate as an annual rate over the number of years. In the example, use I = 6.09% and N = 3 years.

For another illustration, consider the interest rate charged on credit cards. Many banks charge 1.5 percent per month and, in their advertising, state that the annual percentage rate (APR) is 18 percent.[8] However, the true cost rate to credit card users is the effective annual rate of 19.6 percent:

$$EAR = (1 + \text{Periodic rate})^M - 1.0$$
$$= (1.015)^{12} - 1.0 = 0.196 = 19.6\%.$$

Self-Test Questions

1. What changes must be made in the calculations to determine the future value of an amount being compounded at 8 percent semiannually versus one being compounded annually at 8 percent?
2. Why is semiannual compounding better than annual compounding from an investor's standpoint?
3. How does the effective annual rate differ from the stated rate?
4. How does the periodic rate differ from the stated rate?

Amortized Loans

One important application of time value analysis involves loans that are to be paid off in equal installments over time, including automobile loans, home mortgage loans, and most business debt other than very short-term loans and bonds. If a loan is to be repaid in equal periodic amounts—monthly, quarterly, or annually—it is said to be an *amortized loan*. The word *amortize* comes from the Latin *mors*, meaning *death*, so an amortized loan is one that is killed off over time.

To illustrate, suppose Santa Fe Healthcare System borrows $1 million from the Bank of New Mexico, to be repaid in three equal installments at the end of each of the next three years. The bank is to receive 6 percent interest on the loan balance that is outstanding at the beginning of each year. The first task in analyzing the loan is to determine the amount that Santa Fe must repay each year, or the annual payment. To find this value, recognize that the loan amount represents the present value of an annuity of PMT dollars per year for three years, discounted at 6 percent.

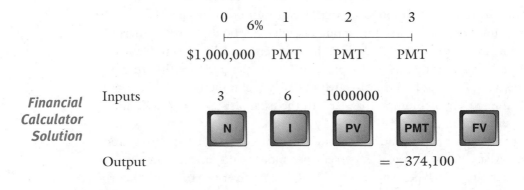

Financial Calculator Solution

	A	B	C	D
1				
2	6.0%	Rate	Interest rate	
3	3	Nper	Number of periods	
4	$ 1,000,000	Pv	Present value	
5				
6				
7				
8	$ 374,110	=PMT(A2,A3,-A4) (entered into Cell A8)		
9				
10				

Spreadsheet Solution

Therefore, if Santa Fe pays the bank $374,110 at the end of each of the next three years, the percentage cost to the borrower, and the rate of return to the lender, will be 6 percent.

Each payment made by Santa Fe consists partly of interest and partly of repayment of principal. This breakdown is given in the *amortization schedule* shown in Table 9.1. The interest component is largest in the first year, and it declines as the outstanding balance of the loan is reduced over time. For tax purposes, a taxable business borrower reports the interest payments in Column 3 as a deductible cost each year, while the lender reports these same amounts as taxable income.

Financial calculators are often programmed to calculate amortization schedules; simply key in the inputs and then press one button to get each entry in Table 9.1.

Year	Beginning Amount (1)	Payment (2)	Interest[a] (3)	Repayment of Principal[b] (4)	Remaining Balance (5)
1	$1,000,000	$ 374,110	$ 60,000	$ 314,110	$685,890
2	685,890	374,110	41,153	332,957	352,933
3	352,933	374,110	21,177	352,933	0
		$1,122,330	$122,330	$1,000,000	

TABLE 9.1 Loan Amortization Schedule

[a]Interest is calculated by multiplying the loan balance at the beginning of each year by the interest rate. Therefore, interest in Year 1 is $1,000,000 × 0.06 = $60,000; in Year 2 it is $685,890 × 0.06 = $41,153; and in Year 3 it is $352,933 × 0.06 = $21,177.
[b]Repayment of principal is equal to the payment of $374,110 minus the interest charge for each year.

1. When constructing an amortization schedule, how is the periodic payment amount calculated?
2. Does the periodic payment remain constant over time?
3. Do the principal and interest components remain constant over time? Explain your answer.

Self-Test Questions

Key Concepts

Financial decisions often involve situations in which future cash flows must be valued. The process of valuing future cash flows is called *time value analysis*. The key concepts of this chapter are:

- *Compounding* is the process of determining the *future value (FV)* of a lump sum or a series of payments.
- *Discounting* is the process of finding the *present value (PV)* of a future lump sum or series of payments.
- An *annuity* is a series of equal, periodic *payments (PMT)* for a specified number of periods.
- An annuity that has payments that occur at the end of each period is called an *ordinary* annuity.
- If each annuity payment occurs at the beginning of the period rather than at the end, the annuity is an *annuity due*.
- A *perpetuity* is an annuity that lasts forever.
- If an analysis that involves more than one lump sum does not meet the definition of an annuity, it is called an *uneven cash flow stream*.
- The financial consequence of an investment is measured by *return on investment (ROI)*, or just *return*, which can be expressed either in *dollar terms* or in *percentage (rate of return) terms*.
- An *amortized* loan is one that is paid off in equal amounts over some specified number of periods. An *amortization schedule* shows how much of each payment represents interest, how much is used to reduce the principal, and how much of the principal balance remains on each payment date.
- The *stated rate* is the annual rate normally quoted in financial contracts.
- The *periodic rate* equals the stated rate divided by the number of compounding periods per year.
- If compounding occurs more frequently than once a year, it is often necessary to calculate the *effective annual rate*, which is the rate that produces the same results under annual compounding as obtained with more frequent compounding.

Time value analysis will be applied in subsequent chapters, so the contents of this chapter are very important. Readers should feel comfortable with this material before moving ahead.

Questions

9.1 a. What is an opportunity cost rate?
    b. How is this rate used in time value analysis?
    c. Is this rate a single number that is used in all situations?

9.2 What is the difference between a lump sum, an annuity, and an unequal cash flow stream?

9.3 Great Lakes Health Network's net income increased from $3.2 million in 1997 to $6.4 million in 2007. The total growth rate over the ten years is 100 percent, while the annual growth rate is only about 7.2 percent, which is much less than 100 percent divided by ten years.
   a. Why does this relationship hold?
   b. Which growth rate has more meaning—the total rate over ten years or the annualized rate?

9.4 Would you rather have a savings account that pays 5 percent compounded semiannually or one that pays 5 percent compounded daily? Explain your answer.

9.5 The present value of a perpetuity is equal to the payment divided by the opportunity cost (interest) rate: $PV = PMT/I$. What is the future value of a perpetuity?

9.6 When a loan is amortized, what happens over time to the size of the total payment, interest payment, and principal payment?

9.7 Explain the difference between the stated rate, periodic rate, and effective annual rate.

9.8 What are three techniques for solving time value problems?

9.9 Explain the concept of return on investment (ROI) and the two different approaches to measuring ROI.

Problems

9.1 Find the following values for a lump sum assuming annual compounding:
   a. The future value of $500 invested at 8 percent for one year
   b. The future value of $500 invested at 8 percent for five years
   c. The present value of $500 to be received in one year when the opportunity cost rate is 8 percent
   d. The present value of $500 to be received in five years when the opportunity cost rate is 8 percent

9.2 Repeat Problem 9.1 above, but assume the following compounding conditions:
   a. Semiannual
   b. Quarterly

9.3 What is the effective annual rate (EAR) if the stated rate is 8 percent and compounding occurs semiannually? Quarterly?

9.4 Find the following values assuming a regular, or ordinary, annuity:
   a. The present value of $400 per year for ten years at 10 percent
   b. The future value of $400 per year for ten years at 10 percent
   c. The present value of $200 per year for five years at 5 percent
   d. The future value of $200 per year for five years at 5 percent

9.5 Repeat Problem 9.4, but assume the annuities are annuities due.

9.6 Consider the following uneven cash flow stream:

Year	Cash Flow
0	$ 0
1	250
2	400
3	500
4	600
5	600

a. What is the present (Year 0) value if the opportunity cost (discount) rate is 10 percent?

b. Add an outflow (or cost) of $1,000 at Year 0. What is the present value (or net present value) of the stream?

9.7 Consider another uneven cash flow stream:

Year	Cash Flow
0	$2,000
1	2,000
2	0
3	1,500
4	2,500
5	4,000

a. What is the present (Year 0) value of the cash flow stream if the opportunity cost rate is 10 percent?

b. What is the value of the cash flow stream at the end of Year 5 if the cash flows are invested in an account that pays 10 percent annually?

c. What cash flow today (Year 0), in lieu of the $2,000 cash flow, would be needed to accumulate $20,000 at the end of Year 5? (Assume that the cash flows for Years 1 through 5 remain the same.)

d. Time value analysis involves either discounting or compounding cash flows. Many healthcare financial management decisions, such as bond refunding, capital investment, and lease versus buy, involve discounting projected future cash flows. What factors must executives consider when choosing a discount rate to apply to forecasted cash flows?

9.8 What is the present value of a perpetuity of $100 per year if the appropriate discount rate is 7 percent? Suppose that interest rates doubled in the economy and the appropriate discount rate is now 14 percent. What would happen to the present value of the perpetuity?

9.9 Assume that you just won $35 million in the Florida lottery, and hence the state will pay you 20 annual payments of $1.75 million each beginning immediately. If the rate of return on securities of similar risk to the lottery earnings (e.g., the rate on 20-year U.S. Treasury bonds) is 6 percent, what is the present value of your winnings?

9.10 An investment that you are considering promises to pay $2,000 semiannually for the next two years, beginning six months from now. You have determined that the appropriate opportunity cost (discount) rate is 8 percent, compounded quarterly. What is the value of this investment?

9.11 Consider the following investment cash flows:

Year	Cash Flow
0	($1,000)
1	250
2	400
3	500
4	600
5	600

a. What is the return expected on this investment measured in dollar terms if the opportunity cost rate is 10 percent?

b. Provide an explanation, in economic terms, of your answer.

c. What is the return on this investment measured in percentage terms?

d. Should this investment be made? Explain your answer.

9.12 Epitome Healthcare has just borrowed $1,000,000 on a five-year, annual payment term loan at a 15 percent rate. The first payment is due one year from now. Construct the amortization schedule for this loan.

9.13 Assume that $10,000 was invested in the stock of General Medical Corporation with the intention of selling after one year. The stock pays no dividends, so the entire return will be based on the price of the stock when sold. The opportunity cost of capital on the stock is 10 percent.

a. To begin, assume that the stock sale nets $11,500. What is the dollar return on the stock investment? What is the rate of return?

b. Assume that the stock price falls and the net is only $9,500 when the stock is sold. What is the dollar return and rate of return?

c. Assume that the stock is held for two years. Now, what is the dollar return and rate of return?

Notes

1. Even if no investment opportunities existed, a dollar in hand would still be worth more than a dollar to be received in the future because a dollar today can be used for immediate consumption, whereas a future dollar cannot.

2. On some financial calculators, the keys are buttons on the face of the calculator; on others, the time value variables are shown on the display after accessing the time value menu. Also, some calculators use different symbols to represent the number of periods and interest rate. Finally, financial calculators today are quite powerful in that they can easily solve relatively complex time value of money problems. To focus on concepts rather than mechanics, all the illustrations in this chapter and the remainder of the book assume that cash flows occur at the end or beginning of a period and that there is only one cash flow per period. Thus, to follow the illustrations, financial calculators must be set to one period per year, and it is not necessary to use the calendar function.

3. Time value problems also can be solved using mathematical multipliers obtained from tables. At one time, tables were the most efficient way to solve time value problems, but calculators and spreadsheets have made tables obsolete.

4. Actually, owning a single nursing home is riskier than owning the stock of a firm that has a large number of nursing homes with geographical diversification. Also, an owner of Manor Care's stock can easily sell the stock if things go sour, whereas it would be much more difficult for Oakdale to sell its nursing home. These differences in risk and liquidity suggest that the true opportunity cost rate is probably higher than the return that is expected from owning Manor Care's stock. However, direct ownership of a nursing home implies control, while ownership of the stock of a large firm usually does not. Such control rights would tend to reduce the opportunity cost rate. The main point here is that in practice it may not be possible to obtain a "perfect" opportunity cost rate. Nevertheless, an imprecise one is better than none at all.

5. The *Rule of 72* gives a simple and quick method for judging the effect of different interest rates on the growth of a lump sum deposit. To find the number of years required to double the value of a lump sum, merely divide the number 72 by the interest rate paid. For example, if the interest rate is 10 percent, it would take $72 / 10 = 7.2$ years for the money in an account to double in value. The calculator solution is 7.27 years, so the Rule of 72 is relatively accurate, at least when reasonable interest rates are applied. In a similar manner, the Rule of 72 can be used to determine the interest rate required to double the money in an account in a given number of years. To illustrate, an interest rate of $72 / 5 = 14.4$ percent is required to double the value of an account in five years. The calculator solution in this case is 14.9 percent, so the Rule of 72 again gives a reasonable approximation of the precise answer.

6. Some financial institutions even pay interest on accounts that is compounded *continuously*. However, continuous compounding is not relevant to healthcare finance, so it will not be discussed here.

7. Most financial calculators are programmed to calculate the EAR or, given the EAR, to find the stated rate. This is called *interest rate conversion*. Enter the stated rate and the number of compounding periods per year, and then press the EFF percent key to find the EAR.

8. The *annual percentage rate (APR)* and *annual percentage yield (APY)* are terms defined in Truth in Lending and Truth in Savings laws. APR is defined as Periodic rate × Number of compounding periods per year, so it ignores the consequences of compounding. Although the APR on a credit card with interest charges of 1.5 percent per month is $1.5\% \times 12 = 18\%$, the true effective annual rate is 19.6 percent.

References

The owner's manual for your calculator.

The reference manual for your spreadsheet software, or any of the after-market spreadsheet manuals.

CHAPTER 10

FINANCIAL RISK AND
REQUIRED RETURN

Learning Objectives

After studying this chapter, readers will be able to:

- Explain in general terms the concept of financial risk.
- Define and differentiate between stand-alone risk and portfolio risk.
- Define and differentiate between corporate risk and market risk.
- Explain the Capital Asset Pricing Model (CAPM) relationship between risk and required rate of return.
- Use the CAPM to determine required returns.

Introduction

Two of the most important concepts in healthcare financial management are financial risk and required return. What is financial risk, how is it measured, and what effect, if any, does it have on required return (opportunity cost rates) and hence on managerial decisions? Because so much of financial decision making involves risk and return, it is impossible to gain a good understanding of healthcare financial management without having a solid appreciation of risk and return concepts.

If investors—both individuals and businesses—viewed risk as a benign fact of life, it would have little impact on decision making. However, decision makers for the most part believe that if a risk must be taken, there must be a reward for doing so. Thus, an investment of higher risk, whether it is an individual investor's security investment or a radiology group's investment in diagnostic equipment, must offer a higher return to make it financially attractive.

In this chapter, basic risk concepts are presented from the perspective of both individual investors and businesses. Health services managers must be familiar with both contexts because investors supply the capital that businesses need to function. In addition, the chapter discusses the relationship between risk and required rate of return. To be truly useful in financial decision making, it is necessary to know the impact of risk on investors' views of investment acceptability.

The Many Faces of Financial Risk

Unfortunately, a full discussion of financial risk would take many chapters, perhaps even an entire book, because financial risk is a very complicated subject. First of all, the nature of financial risk depends on whether the investor is an individual or a business. Then, if the investor is an individual, it depends on the *investment horizon*, or the amount of time until the investment proceeds are needed. To make the situation even more complex, it may be difficult to define, measure, or translate financial risk into something usable for decision making. For example, the risk that individual investors face when saving for retirement is the risk that the amount of funds accumulated will not be sufficient to fund the lifestyle expected during the full term of retirement. Needless to say, translating such a definition of risk into investment goals is not easy. The good news is that our primary interest in this book is the financial risk inherent in businesses. Thus, our discussion can focus on the fundamental factors that influence the riskiness of real-asset investments, such as land, buildings, and equipment, and the securities that businesses sell to raise the capital needed to make those investments.

In spite of our focused approach to risk, two factors still come into play that complicate our discussion. The first complicating factor is that financial risk is seen both by businesses and the investors in businesses. There is some risk inherent in the business itself that depends on the type of business. For example, pharmaceutical firms are generally acknowledged to face a great deal of risk, while hospitals typically have less risk. Then, investors, primarily stockholders and debtholders (creditors), bear the riskiness inherent in the business, but as **modified by the nature of the securities they hold**. For example, the stock of Manor Care is more risky than its debt, although the risk of both securities depends on the inherent risk of a business that operates in the long-term care industry. The risk differential arises because of contractual differences between equity and debt: Debtholders have a fixed claim against the cash flows and assets of the business, while stockholders have a residual claim, or a claim to what is left after all other claimants have been paid.

The second complicating factor results from the fact that the riskiness of an investment depends on the context in which it is held. For example, a stock held alone (in isolation) is riskier than the same stock held as part of a large portfolio of stocks. Similarly, a magnetic resonance imaging (MRI) system operated independently is riskier than the same system operated as part of a large, geographically diversified business that owns and operates numerous types of diagnostic equipment.

Self-Test Question	1. What are the two complications that arise when dealing with financial risk in a business setting?

Introduction to Financial Risk

Generically, *risk* is defined as "a hazard; a peril; exposure to loss or injury." Thus, risk refers to the chance that an unfavorable event will occur. If a person engages in skydiving, he or she is taking a chance with injury or death; skydiving is risky. If a person gambles at roulette, he or she is not risking injury or death but is taking a *financial risk*. Even when a person invests in stocks or bonds, he or she is taking a risk in the hope of earning a positive rate of return. Similarly, when a healthcare business invests in new assets such as diagnostic equipment or new hospital beds or a new managed care plan, it is taking a financial risk.

To illustrate financial risk, consider two potential personal investments. The first investment consists of a one-year, $1,000 face value U.S. Treasury bill (or T-bill) that is bought for $950. Treasury bills are short-term federal debt that are sold at a *discount* (i.e., less than face value) and return *face*, or *par*, *value* at maturity. The investor expects to receive $1,000 at maturity in one year, so the anticipated rate of return on the T-bill investment is ($1,000 − $950) / $950 = $50 / $950 = 0.0526, or 5.26%. Using a financial calculator:

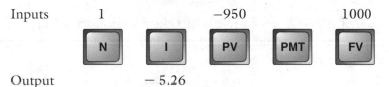

Inputs   1   −950   1000

N   I   PV   PMT   FV

Output   − 5.26

Or a spreadsheet:

	A	B	C	D
1				
2	1	Nper	Number of periods	
3	$ (950.00)	Pv	Present value	
4	$ 1,000	Fv	Future value	
5				
6				
7				
8	5.26%	=RATE(A3,,A4,A5) (entered into Cell A8)		
9				
10				

The $1,000 payment is fixed by contract (the T-bill promises to pay this amount), and the U.S. government is certain to make the payment, except for national disaster—a very unlikely event. Thus, there is virtually a 100 percent probability that the investment will actually earn the 5.26 percent rate of return that is expected. In this situation, the investment is defined as being *riskless*, or *risk free*.

Now, assume that the $950 is invested in a biotechnology partnership that will be terminated in one year. If the partnership develops a new commercially valuable product, its rights will be sold and $2,000 will be received from the partnership for a rate of return of ($2,000 − $950) / $950 = $1,050 / $950 = 1.1053 = 110.53%:

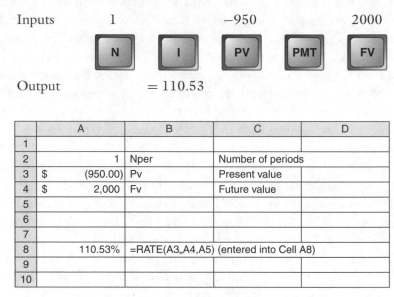

	A	B	C	D
1				
2	1	Nper	Number of periods	
3	$ (950.00)	Pv	Present value	
4	$ 2,000	Fv	Future value	
5				
6				
7				
8	110.53%	=RATE(A3,,A4,A5) (entered into Cell A8)		
9				
10				

But if nothing worthwhile is developed, the partnership would be worthless, no money would be received, and the rate of return would be ($0 − $950) / $950 = −1.00 = −100%:

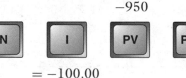

	A	B	C	D
1				
2	1	Nper	Number of periods	
3	$ (950.00)	Pv	Present value	
4	$ 0.01	Fv	Future value	
5				
6				
7				
8	−100.00%	=RATE(A3,,A4,A5) (entered into Cell A8)		
9				
10				

(Most financial calculators and spreadsheets give no solution when the future value is zero, but if a very small number, for example, 0.01, is entered for the future value, the solution for interest rate is −100.00.)

Now, assume that there is a 50 percent chance that a valuable product will be developed. In this admittedly unrealistic situation, the expected rate of return, a statistical concept that will be discussed shortly, is the same 5.26 percent as on the T-bill investment: $(0.50 \times 110.53\%) + (0.50 \times [-100\%])$

= 5.26%. However, the biotechnology partnership is a far cry from being riskless. If things go poorly, the realized rate of return will be −100 percent, which means that the entire $950 investment will be lost. Because there is a significant chance of actually earning a return that is far less than expected, the partnership investment is described as being very risky.

Thus, financial risk is related to the probability of earning a return less than expected. The greater the chance of earning a return **far below** that expected, the greater the amount of financial risk.[1]

1. What is a generic definition of risk?
2. Explain the general concept of financial risk.

Self-Test Questions

Risk Aversion

Why is it so important to define and measure financial risk? The reason is that, for the most part, both individual and business investors dislike risk. Suppose that a person was given the choice between a sure $1 million and the flip of a coin for either zero or $2 million. In the statistical sense, the expected dollar return on the coin flip is $1 million, the same amount as the sure thing. Thus, from a statistical standpoint, the return on both choices is the same. However, just about everyone confronted with this choice would take the sure $1 million. A person who takes the sure thing is said to be *risk averse*; a person who is indifferent between the two alternatives is *risk neutral*; and an individual who prefers the gamble to the sure thing is a *risk seeker*.

Of course, people and businesses do gamble and take other financial chances, so all of us at some time typically exhibit risk-seeking behavior. However, most individuals would never put a sizable portion of their wealth at risk, and most health services managers would never "bet the business." Most people are risk averse when it really matters.

What are the implications of risk aversion for financial decision making? First, given two investments with similar returns but different risk, investors will favor the lower-risk alternative. Second, investors will require higher returns on higher-risk investments. These behavioral outcomes of risk aversion have a significant impact on many facets of financial decision making and hence will appear over and over in this book.

1. What does the term *risk aversion* mean?
2. What are the implications of risk aversion for financial decision making?

Self-Test Questions

Probability Distributions

The chance that an event will occur is called *probability of occurrence*, or just *probability;* for example, when rolling a single die, the probability of rolling a two is one out of six, or $1 / 6 = 0.1667 = 16.67\%$. If all possible outcomes related to a particular event are listed, and a probability is assigned to each outcome, the result is a *probability distribution*. In the example of the roll of a die, the probability distribution looks like this:

Outcome	Probability
1	0.1667 = 16.67%
2	0.1667 = 16.67%
3	0.1667 = 16.67%
4	0.1667 = 16.67%
5	0.1667 = 16.67%
6	0.1667 = 16.67%
	1.0000 = 100%

The possible outcomes (i.e., the number of dots showing after the die roll) are listed in the left column, while the probability of each outcome is listed as both decimals and percentages in the right column. For a complete probability distribution, which must include all possible outcomes for an event, the probabilities must sum to 1.0, or 100 percent.

Probabilities can also be assigned to possible outcomes—in this case, returns—on both personal and business investments. If a person buys stock, the return will usually come in the form of *dividends* and *capital gains* (selling the stock for more than the person paid for it) or *losses* (selling the stock for less the person paid for it). Because all stock returns are uncertain, there is some chance that the dividends will not be as high as expected and that the stock price will not increase as much as expected or that it will even decrease. The higher the probabilities of dividends and stock price well below those expected, the higher the probability that the return will be significantly less than expected and hence the greater the risk.

To illustrate the concept using a business investment, consider a hospital evaluating the purchase of a new MRI system. The cost of the system is an investment, and the net cash inflows that stem from patient utilization provide the return. The net cash inflows, in turn, depend on the number of procedures, charge per procedure, payer discounts, operating costs, and so on. These values typically are not known with certainty but depend on factors such as patient demographics, physician acceptance, local market conditions, labor costs, and so on. Thus, the hospital actually faces a probability distribution of returns rather than a single return known with certainty. The greater the probability of returns well below the return anticipated, the greater the risk of the MRI investment.

Self-Test Questions   1. What is a probability distribution?
2. How are probability distributions used in financial decision making?

Expected and Realized Rates of Return

To be most useful, the concept of financial risk must be defined more precisely than just the chances of a return well below that anticipated. Table 10.1 contains the estimated return distributions developed by the financial staff of Norwalk Community Hospital for two proposed projects: an MRI system and a walk-in clinic. Here, each economic state reflects a combination of factors that dictate each project's profitability. For example, for the MRI project, the very poor economic state signifies a very competitive market and hence very low utilization, very high discounts on reimbursements, very high operating costs, and so on. Conversely, the very good economic state assumes very high utilization and reimbursement, very low operating costs, and so on. The economic states are defined in a similar fashion for the walk-in clinic.

The *expected rate of return*, defined in the statistical sense, is the weighted average of the return distribution, where the weights are the probabilities of occurrence. For example, the expected rate of return on the MRI system, $E(R_{MRI})$, is 10 percent:

$$
\begin{aligned}
E(R_{MRI}) = \ & \text{Probability of Return 1} \times \text{Return 1} \\
& + \text{Probability of Return 2} \times \text{Return 2} \\
& + \text{Probability of Return 3} \times \text{Return 3 and so on} \\
= \ & (0.10 \times [-10\%]) + (0.20 \times 0\%) + (0.40 \times 10\%) \\
& + (0.20 \times 20\%) + (0.10 \times 30\%) \\
= \ & 10\%.
\end{aligned}
$$

Calculated in a similar manner, the expected rate of return on the walk-in clinic is 15 percent.

The expected rate of return is the average return that would result, given the return distribution, if the investment were randomly repeated many times. In this illustration, if 1,000 clinics were built in different areas, each of which faced the return distribution given in Table 10.1, the average return on the 1,000 investments would be 15 percent, assuming the returns in each area

Economic State	Probability of Occurrence	Rate of Return if State Occurs	
		MRI	Clinic
Very poor	0.10	−10%	−20%
Poor	0.20	0	0
Average	0.40	10	15
Good	0.20	20	30
Very good	0.10	30	50
	1.00		

TABLE 10.1
Norwalk
Community
Hospital:
Estimated
Returns for Two
Proposed
Projects

are independent of one another (random). However, only one clinic would actually be built, and the realized rate of return may be less than the expected 15 percent. Therefore, the clinic investment (as well as the MRI investment) is risky.

Expected rate of return expresses expectations for the future. When the managers at Norwalk Community Hospital analyzed the MRI investment, they expected it to earn 10 percent. However, assume that economic conditions take a turn for the worse and the very poor economic scenario actually occurs. In this case, the *realized rate of return*, which is the rate of return that the investment actually produced as measured at termination, would be a negative 10 percent. It is the potential of realizing a minus 10 percent return on an investment that has an expected return of plus 10 percent that produces risk.

Note that in many situations, especially those arising in classroom illustrations, the expected rate of return is not even achievable. For example, an investment that has a 50 percent chance of a 5 percent return and a 50 percent chance of a 15 percent return has an expected rate of return of 10 percent. Yet, assuming the given distribution truly reflects the complete return potential of the investment, there is zero probability of actually realizing the 10 percent expected rate of return.

Self-Test Questions
1. How is the expected rate of return calculated?
2. What is the economic interpretation of the expected rate of return?
3. What is the difference between the expected rate of return and the realized rate of return?

Stand-Alone Risk

We can look at the two distributions in Table 10.1 and intuitively conclude that the clinic is more risky than the MRI system because the clinic has a chance of a 20 percent loss, while the worst possible loss on the MRI system is 10 percent. This intuitive risk assessment is based on the *stand-alone risk* of the two investments; that is, we are focusing on the riskiness of each investment under the assumption that it would be the business's only asset (operated in isolation). In the next section, portfolio effects will be introduced, but for now, let us continue our discussion of stand-alone risk.

Stand-alone risk depends on the "tightness" of an investment's return distribution. If an investment has a "tight" return distribution, with returns falling close to the expected return, it has relatively low stand-alone risk. Conversely, an investment with a return distribution that is "loose," and hence has values well below the expected return, is relatively risky in the stand-alone sense.

It is important to recognize that risk and return are **separate** attributes of an investment. An investment may have a very "tight" distribution of returns, and hence very low stand-alone risk, but its expected rate of return might be only 2 percent. In this situation, the investment probably would not be financially attractive, in spite of its low risk. Similarly, a high-risk investment with a sufficiently high expected rate of return would be attractive.

It is also important to recognize that the size of an investment does **not** affect its risk. For example, a $1,000 investment in Manor Care's bonds has the same risk as a $1,000,000 investment. The amount of capital (money) at risk does not change the riskiness of the investment—the bonds have a certain amount of risk regardless of the amount bought. What may differ, however, is the investor's ability to *bear* that risk. An individual with modest income may be able to bear the risk of the $1,000 investment but not the $1,000,000 investment. On the other hand, a large fixed-income mutual fund would easily be able bear the risk of the $1,000,000 investment. Remember, though, that the size of an investment does not change its inherent risk.

To be truly useful, any definition of risk must have some measure, or numerical value, so we need some way to specify the "degree of tightness" of an investment's return distribution. One such measure is *standard deviation*, which is often given the symbol "σ" (Greek lowercase sigma). Standard deviation is a common statistical measure of the dispersion of a distribution about its mean—the smaller the standard deviation, the "tighter" the distribution and hence the lower the riskiness of the investment. To illustrate the calculation of standard deviation, consider the estimated returns of the MRI investment, as listed in Table 10.1. Here are the steps:

1. The expected rate of return on the MRI, $E(R_{MRI})$, is 10 percent.
2. The *variance* of the return distribution is determined as follows:

$$\text{Variance} = (\text{Probability of Return 1} \times [\text{Rate of Return 1} - E(R_{MRI})]^2)$$
$$+ (\text{Probability of Return 2} \times [\text{Rate of Return 2} - E(R_{MRI})]^2)$$
$$\text{and so on}$$
$$= (0.10 \times [-10\% - 10\%]^2) + (0.20 \times [0\% - 10\%]^2)$$
$$+ (0.40 \times [10\% - 10\%]^2) + (0.20 \times [20\% - 10\%]^2)$$
$$+ (0.10 \times [30\% - 10\%]^2)$$
$$= 120.00.$$

Variance, like standard deviation, is a measure of the dispersion of a distribution about its expected value, but it is less useful than standard deviation because its measurement unit is percent (or dollars) squared, which has no economic meaning.

3. The standard deviation is defined as the square root of the variance:

$$\text{Standard deviation } (\sigma) = \sqrt{\text{Variance}}$$
$$= \sqrt{120.00} = 10.95\% \approx 11\%.$$

Note that most financial calculators and spreadsheet programs have built-in functions that calculate standard deviation. However, these functions assume that the distribution values entered have **equal probabilities** of occurrence and hence are **not** usable with the types of distributions contained in Table 10.1. Such functions are designed to handle *historical* data, such as annual returns over the past five years, as opposed to *forecasted* distributions with unequal probabilities of occurrence.

Using the same procedure, the clinic investment listed in Table 10.1 was found to have a standard deviation of returns of about 18 percent. Because the standard deviation of returns of the clinic investment is larger than that of the MRI investment, the clinic investment has more stand-alone risk than the MRI investment.

As a general rule, investments with higher expected rates of return have larger standard deviations than investments with smaller expected returns. This situation occurs in our MRI and clinic example. In situations where expected rates of return on investments differ substantially, standard deviation may not give a good picture of the stand-alone risk of one investment **relative** to another. The *coefficient of variation (CV)*, which is defined as the standard deviation of returns divided by the expected return, measures the **risk per unit of return** and hence standardizes the measurement of stand-alone risk. To illustrate, here are the CVs for the MRI and clinic investments:

$$\text{Coefficient of variation} = \frac{\sigma}{E(R)}.$$

$$CV_{MRI} = 11\%/10\% = 1.10.$$

$$CV_{Clinic} = 18\%/15\% = 1.20.$$

In this situation, the clinic investment has slightly more risk per unit of return, so it is riskier than the MRI as measured by both standard deviation and coefficient of variation. However, note that the clinic's stand-alone risk as measured by the coefficient of variation is not as great relative to the MRI as it is when measured by standard deviation. This difference in relative risk occurs because the clinic has a higher expected rate of return. Finally, note that the coefficient of variation has no units; it is just a raw number.

Self-Test Questions

1. What is stand-alone risk?
2. Are risk and return separate attributes of an investment? Explain.
3. Does the amount of money at risk affect the riskiness of an investment? Explain.
4. Define and explain two measures of stand-alone risk?
5. Is one measure better than another?

Portfolio Risk and Return

The preceding section introduced a risk measure—standard deviation—that applies to investments held in isolation. (We also introduced the coefficient of variation, but in most situations the standard deviation will suffice.) However, most investments are held not in isolation but as part of a collection, or *portfolio*, of investments. Individual investors typically hold portfolios of **securities** (i.e., stocks and bonds), while businesses generally hold portfolios of **projects** (i.e., product or service lines). When investments are held in portfolios, the primary concern of investors is not the realized rate of return on an individual investment but rather the realized rate of return on the entire portfolio. Similarly, the stand-alone risk of each individual investment in the portfolio is not important to the investor; what matters is the aggregate riskiness of the portfolio. Thus, the whole nature of risk and how it is defined and measured changes when one recognizes that investments are held not in isolation but as parts of portfolios.

Portfolio Returns

Consider the returns estimated for the seven investment alternatives listed in Table 10.2. The individual investment alternatives—Investments A, B, C, and D—could be projects under consideration by South West Clinics, Inc., or they could be stocks that are being evaluated as personal investments by Bruce Duncan. The remaining three alternatives in Table 10.2 are portfolios. Portfolio AB consists of 50 percent invested in Investment A and 50 percent in Investment B (e.g., $10,000 invested in A and $10,000 invested in B); Portfolio AC is an equal-weighted portfolio of Investments A and C; and Portfolio AD is an equal-weighted portfolio of Investments A and D. As shown in the bottom of the table, Investments A and B have 10 percent expected rates of return, while the expected rates of return for Investments C and D are 15 percent and 12 percent, respectively. Investments A and B have identical stand-alone risk as measured by standard deviation (11 percent), while Investments C and D have greater stand-alone risk than A and B.

Economic State	Probability of Occurrence	Rate of Return if State Occurs						
		A	B	C	D	AB	AC	AD
Very poor	0.10	−10%	30%	−25%	15%	10%	−17.5%	2.5%
Poor	0.20	0	20	−5	10	10	−2.5	5.0
Average	0.40	10	10	15	0	10	12.5	5.0
Good	0.20	20	0	35	25	10	27.5	22.5
Very good	0.10	30	−10	55	35	10	42.5	32.5
	1.00							
Expected rate of return		10.0%	10.0%	15.0%	12.0%	10.0%	12.5%	11.0%
Standard deviation		11.0%	11.0%	21.9%	12.1%	0.0%	16.4%	10.1%

TABLE 10.2
Estimated Returns for Four Individual Investments and Three Portfolios

The *expected rate of return on a portfolio, $E(R_p)$,* is the weighted average of the expected returns on the assets that make up the portfolio, with the weights being the proportion of the total portfolio invested in each asset:

$$E(R_p) = (w_1 \times E[R_1]) + (w_2 \times E[R_2]) + (w_3 \times E[R_3]) \text{ and so on.}$$

In this case, w_1 is the proportion of Investment 1 in the overall portfolio and $E(R_1)$ is the expected rate of return on Investment 1, and so on. Thus, the expected rate of return on Portfolio AB is 10 percent:

$$E(R_{AB}) = (0.5 \times 10\%) + (0.5 \times 10\%) = 5\% + 5\% = 10\%,$$

while the expected rate of return on Portfolio AC is 12.5 percent and on AD is 11 percent.

Alternatively, the expected rate of return on a portfolio can be calculated by looking at the portfolio's return distribution. To illustrate, consider the return distribution for Portfolio AC contained in Table 10.2. The portfolio return in each economic state is the weighted average of the returns on Investments A and C in that state. For example, the return on Portfolio AC in the very poor state is $(0.5 \times [-10\%]) + (0.5 \times [-25\%]) = -17.5\%$. Portfolio AC's return in each other state is calculated similarly. Portfolio AC's return distribution now can be used to calculate its expected rate of return:

$$E(R_{AC}) = (0.10 \times [-17.5\%]) + (0.20 \times [-2.5\%]) + (0.40 \times 12.5\%)$$
$$+ (0.20 \times 27.5\%) + (0.10 \times 42.5\%)$$
$$= 12.5\%.$$

This is the same value as that calculated from the expected rates of return of the two portfolio components:

$$(0.5 \times 10\%) + (0.5 \times 15\%) = 12.5\%.$$

After the fact, the actual, or realized, returns on Investments A and C will probably be different from their expected values, and hence the realized rate of return on Portfolio AC will likely be different from its 12.5 percent expected return.

Portfolio Risk: Two Investments

When an investor holds a portfolio of investments, the portfolio is in effect a stand-alone investment, so the **riskiness of the portfolio is measured by the standard deviation of portfolio returns**, the previously discussed measure of stand-alone risk. How does the riskiness of the individual investments in a portfolio combine to create the overall riskiness of the portfolio? Although the rate of return on a portfolio is the weighted average of the returns on the component investments, a portfolio's standard deviation (i.e., riskiness) is generally **not** the weighted average of the standard deviations of the individual components. The portfolio's riskiness may be smaller than the weighted average of each component's riskiness. Indeed, the riskiness of a portfolio may be less than the least risky portfolio component and, under certain conditions, a portfolio of risky investments may be even riskless.

A simple example can be used to illustrate this concept. Suppose that an individual is given the following opportunity: Flip a coin once; if it comes up heads, he or she wins $10,000, but if it comes up tails, the individual loses $8,000. This is a reasonable gamble in that the expected dollar return is (0.5 × $10,000) + (0.5 × [−$8,000]) = $1,000. However, it is highly risky because the individual has a 50 percent chance of losing $8,000. Thus, risk aversion would cause most individuals to refuse the gamble, especially if the $8,000 potential loss would result in financial hardship.

Alternatively, suppose that the individual is given the opportunity to flip the coin 100 times, and he or she would win $100 for each head but lose $80 for each tail. It is possible, although extremely unlikely, that the individual would flip all heads and win $10,000. It is also possible, and also extremely unlikely, that he or she would flip all tails and lose $8,000. But the chances are very high that the individual would actually flip close to 50 heads and 50 tails and net about $1,000. Even if he or she flipped a few more tails than heads, the individual would still make money on the gamble.

Although each flip is very risky in the stand-alone sense, taken collectively the flips are not very risky at all. In effect, the multiple flipping has created a portfolio of investments; each flip of the coin can be thought of as one investment, so the individual now has a 100-investment portfolio. Furthermore, the return on each investment is independent of the returns on the other investments: The individual has a 50 percent chance of winning on each flip of the coin regardless of the results of the previous flips. By combining the flips into a single gamble (i.e., into an investment portfolio), the risk associated with each flip of the coin is reduced. In fact, if the gamble consisted of a very large number of flips, almost all risk would be eliminated: The probability of a near-equal number of heads and tails would be extremely high, and the result would be a sure profit. The key to the risk reduction inherent in the portfolio is that the negative consequences of tossing a tail can be offset by the positive consequences of tossing a head.

To examine portfolio effects in more depth, consider Portfolio AB in Table 10.2. Each investment (A or B) has a standard deviation of returns of 10 percent and hence is quite risky when held in isolation. However, a portfolio of the two investments has a rate of return of 10 percent in every possible state of the economy, so it offers a riskless 10 percent return. This result is verified by the value of zero for Portfolio AB's standard deviation of return. The reason Investments A and B can be combined to form a riskless portfolio is that their returns move exactly opposite to one another. Thus, in economic states when A's returns are relatively low, those of B are relatively high, and vice versa, so the gains on one investment in the portfolio more than offset losses on the other.

The movement relationship of two variables (i.e., their tendency to move either together or in opposition) is called *correlation*. The *correlation coefficient, r*, measures this relationship. Investments A and B can be combined to form a riskless portfolio because the returns on A and B are *perfectly negatively correlated*, which is designated by $r = -1.0$. In every state where Investment A has a return higher than its expected return, Investment B has a return lower than its expected return, and vice versa.

The opposite of perfect negative correlation is *perfect positive correlation*, with $r = +1.0$. Returns on two perfectly positively correlated investments move up and down together as the economic state changes. When the returns on two investments are perfectly positively correlated, combining the investments into a portfolio will not lower risk because the standard deviation of the portfolio is merely the weighted average of the standard deviations of the two components.

To illustrate the impact of perfect positive correlation, consider Portfolio AC in Table 10.2. Its expected rate of return, $E(R_{AC})$, is 12.5 percent, while its standard deviation is 16.4 percent. Because of perfect positive correlation between the returns on A and C, Portfolio AC's standard deviation is the weighted average standard deviation of its components:

$$\sigma_{AC} = (0.5 \times 11.0\%) + (0.50 \times 21.95\%)$$

$$= 16.4\%.$$

There is no risk reduction in this situation. The risk of the portfolio is less than the risk of Investment C, but it is more than the risk of Investment A. Forming a portfolio does not reduce risk when the returns on the two components are perfectly positively correlated; the portfolio merely **averages** the risk of the two investments.

What happens when a portfolio is created with two investments that have positive, but not perfectly positive, correlation? Combining the two investments can eliminate some, but not all, risk. To illustrate, consider Portfolio AD in Table 10.2. This portfolio has a standard deviation of returns of 10.1 percent, so it is risky. However, Portfolio AD's standard deviation is not only less than the weighted average of its components' standard deviations, $(0.5 \times 11\%) + (0.5 \times 12.1\%) = 11.6\%$, it also is less than the standard deviation of each component. The correlation coefficient between the return distributions for A and D is 0.53, which indicates that the two investments are positively correlated, but they are not perfectly correlated because the coefficient is less than $+1.0$. Thus, combining two investments that are positively correlated, but not perfectly so, lowers risk but does not eliminate it.

Because correlation is the factor that drives risk reduction, a logical question arises: What is the correlation among the returns on "real-world" investments? Generalizing about the correlations among real-world investment alternatives is difficult. However, it is safe to say that the return distributions of two randomly selected investments—whether they are real assets in a hospital's portfolio of service lines or financial assets in an individual's investment portfolio—are virtually never perfectly correlated, and hence correlation coefficients are never −1.0 or +1.0. In fact, it is almost impossible to find actual investment opportunities with returns that are negatively correlated with one another, or even to find investments with returns that are uncorrelated ($r = 0$). Because all investment returns are affected to a greater or lesser degree by general economic conditions, investment returns tend to be positively correlated with one another. However, because investment returns are not affected identically by general economic conditions, returns on most real-world investments are not perfectly positively correlated.

The correlation coefficient between the returns of two randomly chosen investments will usually fall in the range of +0.4 to +0.8. Returns on investments that are similar in nature, such as two inpatient projects in a hospital or two stocks in the same industry, will typically have correlations at the upper end of this range. Conversely, returns on dissimilar projects or securities will tend to have correlations at the lower end of the range.

Portfolio Risk: Many Investments

Businesses are not restricted to two projects, and individual investors are not restricted to holding two-security portfolios. Most companies have tens, or even hundreds, of individual projects (i.e., product or service lines), and most individual investors hold many different securities or mutual funds that may be composed of hundreds of individual securities. Thus, what is most relevant to investment decision making is not what happens when two investments are combined into portfolios, but what happens when many investments are combined.

To illustrate the risk impact of creating large portfolios, consider Figure 10.1. The figure illustrates the riskiness inherent in holding **randomly selected** portfolios of one investment, two investments, three investments, four investments, and so on, considering the correlations that occur among real-world investments. The plot is based on **historical** annual returns on common stocks traded on the New York Stock Exchange (NYSE), but the conclusions reached are applicable to portfolios made up of any type of investment, including healthcare providers that offer many different types of services. The plot shows the average standard deviation of all one-investment (one-stock) portfolios, the average standard deviation of all possible two-investment portfolios, the average standard deviation of all possible three-investment portfolios, and so on.

The riskiness inherent in holding an average one-investment portfolio is relatively high, as measured by its standard deviation of annual returns. The average two-investment portfolio has a lower standard deviation, so holding

FIGURE 10.1
Portfolio Size
and Risk

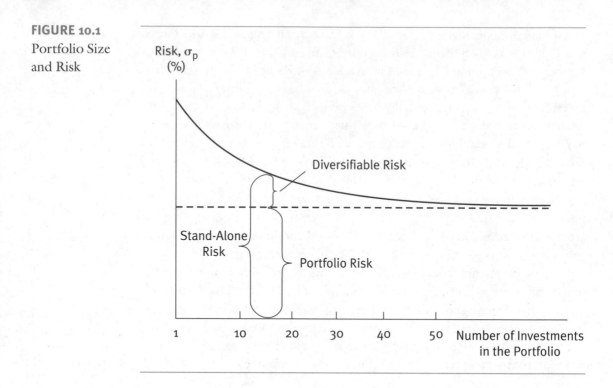

an average two-investment portfolio is less risky than holding a single in-vestment of average risk. The average three-investment portfolio has an even lower standard deviation of returns, so an average three-investment portfolio is even less risky than an average two-investment portfolio. As more invest-ments are randomly added to create larger and larger portfolios, the average riskiness of the portfolio decreases. However, as more and more investments are added, the incremental risk reduction of adding even more investments decreases, and regardless of how many are added, some risk always remains in the portfolio—even with a portfolio of thousands of investments, substantial risk remains.

The reason that all risk cannot be eliminated by creating a very large portfolio is that the returns on the component investments, although not perfectly so, are still positively correlated with one another. In other words, all investments, both real and financial, are affected to a lesser or greater degree by general economic conditions. If the economy booms, all investments tend to do well, while in a recession all investments tend to do poorly. It is the positive correlation among real-world investment returns that prevents investors from creating riskless portfolios.

Diversifiable Risk Versus Portfolio Risk

Figure 10.1 shows what happens as investors create ever larger portfolios. As the size of a randomly created portfolio increases, the riskiness of the portfolio decreases, so a large proportion of the stand-alone risk inherent in an individual investment can be eliminated if it is held as part of a large portfolio. For example, recent studies have found that a large stock portfolio has only about one-half the annual standard deviation of an average stock.

Thus, if a stock investor wanted to eliminate the maximum amount of stand-alone risk inherent in owning NYSE stocks, he or she would have to, at least in theory, own more than 3,000 stocks. Such a portfolio is called the *market portfolio* because it consists of the entire stock market (or at least one entire segment of the stock market). However, it is not necessary for individual investors to own a very large number of stocks to gain the risk-reducing benefit inherent in holding large portfolios. As illustrated in Figure 10.1, most of the benefit of diversification can be obtained by holding a *well-diversified portfolio* of about 50 **randomly selected** stocks. (A portfolio of 50 healthcare stocks, for example, is not well diversified because the stocks are in the same sector of the economy and hence are not randomly chosen.)

That part of the stand-alone riskiness of an individual investment that can be eliminated by diversification (i.e., by holding it as part of a well-diversified portfolio) is called *diversifiable risk*. That part of the stand-alone riskiness of an individual investment that cannot be eliminated by diversification is called *portfolio risk*. Thus, every investment, whether it is the stock of Manor Care held by an individual investor or an MRI system operated by a hospital, has some diversifiable risk that can be eliminated and some portfolio risk that cannot be diversified away. Not all investments benefit to the same degree from portfolio risk-reducing effects, and some portfolios are not truly well diversified. In general, however, any investment will have some of its stand-alone risk eliminated when it is held as part of a portfolio.

Diversifiable risk, as seen by individuals who invest in stocks, is caused by events that are unique to a single business, such as new product or service introductions, strikes, and lawsuits. Because these events are essentially random, their effects can be eliminated by diversification. When one stock in a large, well-diversified portfolio does worse than expected because of a negative event unique to that firm, another stock in the portfolio will do better than expected because of a firm-unique positive event. On average, bad events in some companies will be offset by good events in others, so lower-than-expected returns on one stock will be offset by higher-than-expected returns on another, leaving the investor with an overall portfolio return closer to that expected than would be the case if only a single stock were held.

The same logic can be applied to a firm with a portfolio of projects. Perhaps hospital returns generated from inpatient surgery are less than expected because of the trend toward outpatient procedures, but this may be offset by returns that are greater than expected on state-of-the-art diagnostic services. (If the hospital offered both inpatient and outpatient surgery, it would be *hedging* itself against the trend toward more outpatient procedures because reduced demand for inpatient surgery would be offset by increased demand for outpatient surgery.)

The point to be made here is that the negative impact of random events that are unique to a particular business, or to a particular product or service within a firm, can be offset by positive events in other businesses or in other products or services. Thus, the risk caused by random, unique events can be eliminated by portfolio diversification. Individual investors can diversify by holding many different securities, and businesses can diversify by offering many different products or services.

Note that not all investments benefit to the same degree from portfolio risk-reducing effects. Some have a large amount of diversifiable risk and hence have a great deal of risk reduction when they are added to a portfolio. Others do not benefit nearly as much from portfolio risk reduction—it depends on the investment and the portfolio. For example, consider adding the stock of Tenet Healthcare, a hospital management company, to two portfolios. The first portfolio consists of the stocks of 50 healthcare providers. The second portfolio consists of the stocks of 50 randomly selected firms from many different industries. Much less risk reduction will occur when the Tenet stock is added to the healthcare portfolio than when it is added to the randomly selected portfolio. The reason should be obvious. Tenet's returns are more highly correlated with healthcare providers than with firms in other industries. The lower the correlation, the greater the risk reduction.

This logic tells us that, potentially, there is more risk reduction inherent in adding a nursing home to a hospital business than there is in adding it to a long-term care business that already owns a large number of such investments. However, recognize that it is probably more difficult for managers of a hospital to manage a nursing home than it is for managers of a firm that specializes in such businesses.

Unfortunately, regardless of the situation, not all risk can be diversified away. Portfolio risk—the risk that remains even when well-diversified portfolios are created—stems from factors that systematically affect all stocks in a portfolio, such as wars, inflation, recessions, and high interest rates or all products or services offered by a business. For example, the increasing power of managed care organizations could lower reimbursement levels for all services offered by a hospital. No amount of diversification by the hospital (except, perhaps, moving into managed care) could eliminate this risk. Because portfolio risk cannot be eliminated, even well-diversified investors, whether they are individuals with large securities portfolios or diversified healthcare companies with many different service lines, face this type of risk.

Implications for Investors

The ability to eliminate a portion of the stand-alone riskiness inherent in individual investments has two significant implications for investors, whether the investor is an individual who holds securities or a business that offers products or services.

- Holding a single investment is *not* rational. Holding a large, well-diversified portfolio can eliminate much of the stand-alone riskiness inherent in individual investments. Investors who are risk averse should seek to eliminate all diversifiable risk. Individual investors can easily diversify their personal investment portfolios by buying many individual securities or mutual funds that hold diversified portfolios. Businesses cannot diversify their investments as easily as individuals, but businesses that offer a diverse line of products or services are less risky than businesses that rely on a single product or service.

- Because an investment held in a portfolio has less risk than one held in isolation, the traditional stand-alone risk measure of standard deviation is not appropriate for individual investments held in portfolios. Thus, it is necessary to rethink the definition and measurement of financial risk for such investments. (Note, though, that standard deviation remains the correct measure for the riskiness of an investor's entire **portfolio** because the portfolio is, in effect, a single investment held in isolation.)

1. What is a portfolio of assets?
2. What is a well-diversified portfolio?
3. What happens to the risk of a single asset when it is held as part of a portfolio of assets?
4. Explain the differences between stand-alone risk, diversifiable risk, and portfolio risk.
5. Why should all investors hold well-diversified portfolios rather than individual assets?
6. Is standard deviation the appropriate risk measure for an individual asset?
7. Is standard deviation the appropriate risk measure for an investor's portfolio of assets?

Self-Test Questions

Measuring the Risk of Investments Held in Portfolios

The stand-alone risk of individual investments is reduced when they are held as part of a portfolio, so standard deviation is **not** the relevant risk measure for such investments. Because investors are concerned with the overall riskiness of the portfolio, which **is** measured by standard deviation, the appropriate measure of risk for individual investments in the portfolio is the contribution of each one to the overall riskiness (standard deviation) of the portfolio. In this section, we describe how the portfolio risk of individual investments can be measured.

The Beta Coefficient

The most widely used measure of risk for investments held in portfolios is called the *beta coefficient*, or just *beta*. It measures the volatility of an investment's returns **relative to the volatility of the portfolio**. To illustrate the concept of beta, consider Table 10.3, which contains **historical** annual returns for three individual investments, H, M, and L, and for a large well-diversified portfolio, P. Five years of annual returns are displayed in the table, but three years of monthly returns, or some other combination, could have been chosen. Because the returns are historical (i.e., realized) rather than projected, the probability of occurrence of each return is the same: for five years of returns, each return has a probability of 100% / 5 = 20%. For now, the context does not matter; H, M, and L could be stocks that an individual investor is considering as an addition to Portfolio P, a stock portfolio, or they could be projects that are being evaluated by a hospital and hence would be added to the hospital's portfolio of services.

Figure 10.2 plots the historical annual returns on the three individual investments on the Y-axis versus returns on the portfolio on the X-axis. Investment M has the same volatility as the portfolio. (In fact, Investment M has the same historical returns as does the portfolio.) However, Investment H is more volatile than the portfolio: its returns ranged from −18 to 50 percent. Conversely, Investment L is less volatile than the portfolio: its returns ranged only from 2 to 19 percent.

Investments that are more volatile than the portfolio increase the riskiness of the portfolio when they are added, while investments that are less volatile decrease the riskiness of the portfolio. Thus, the amount of volatility of an investment, relative to the portfolio, measures the contribution of the investment to the overall riskiness of the portfolio, and hence relative volatility measures an individual investment's portfolio risk. Remember that an individual investment's **stand-alone risk** is defined as volatility about its mean (expected) return, so a completely different concept is being used to assess the **portfolio risk** of an individual investment.

How should the risks of Investments H, M, and L be measured, considering that they would be held as part of Portfolio P? In fact, the lines that are plotted on Figure 10.2 are regression lines in the statistical sense, and the

TABLE 10.3		Rate of Return			
Beta Coefficient Illustration	Year	H	M	L	Portfolio (P)
	1	35%	15%	8%	15%
	2	5	5	5	5
	3	−18	−5	2	−5
	4	40	25	18	25
	5	50	35	19	35

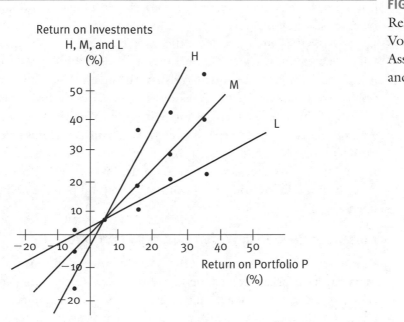

FIGURE 10.2

Relative Volatility of Assets H, M, and L

slope of each line measures the volatility of that investment **relative to** the volatility of the portfolio. (The slope of a regression line is a measure of its steepness and is defined as rise over run.) The regression line for Investment M has a slope, or *beta coefficient*, of 1.0, which shows that M has the same volatility as the portfolio and hence has average risk, where average is defined as the riskiness of the portfolio.[2] Investment H has a beta of 1.5, and hence it is 1.5 times as risky as the portfolio, while L, with a beta of 0.5, is only half as risky as Portfolio P.

A U.S. Treasury security that had a 5 percent realized return in each year over the same five-year period, if plotted on Table 10.3, would have a horizontal regression line and hence a slope of zero. Such an investment would have a beta of zero, which signifies no portfolio risk. In fact, such a Treasury security would have no stand-alone risk because a 5 percent rate of return in each year would result in both a standard deviation of zero and a beta of zero.

Theoretically, an investment could have a negative beta; the regression line for such an investment would slope downward. In this case, the investment's return would move opposite to the portfolio's return: in years when the portfolio's return was high, the investment's return would be low, and vice versa. Such an investment with returns that are negatively correlated with the portfolio's returns, has negative portfolio risk, which means that it would have a significant risk-reducing impact on the portfolio. Although it is possible to find investments in the real world that have negative betas based on **historical returns**, it is next to impossible to find an investment that is expected to have a negative beta on the basis of **future returns**. The reason is that the returns on all assets in a portfolio typically are affected in a more or less similar manner by external economic forces.

Note that, in Figure 10.2, the investment returns (the dots) do not all fall on the regression line. As previously discussed, the slope of the regression line (beta) measures the portfolio risk of the investment. The distance of the points, on average, from the regression line measures the investment's amount of diversifiable risk. The farther the points plot from the line, the greater the amount of risk that is diversified away when the investment is held as part of a portfolio. In effect, adding the investment to a portfolio forces the points to the regression line, because returns on other investments in the portfolio will drag the points above the line down to the line and pull the points below the line up to it.

Corporate Risk: Risk Within Business Portfolios

Businesses typically offer many products or services and thus can be thought of as having a large number (perhaps hundreds or even more) of individual activities, or *projects*. For example, most managed care organizations offer numerous healthcare plans to diverse groups of enrollees in numerous service areas. And many hospitals and hospital systems offer a large number of inpatient, outpatient, and even home health services that cover a wide geographical area and treat a wide range of illnesses and injuries. Thus, healthcare businesses, except for the very smallest, actually consist of a portfolio of projects.

What is the riskiness of an individual project to a business with many projects? Because the project is part of the business's portfolio of assets, its stand-alone risk is not relevant—the project is not held in isolation. The relevant risk of any project to a business with many projects is **its contribution to the business's overall risk**, or the impact of the project on the variability of the firm's overall rate of return. Some of the stand-alone riskiness of the project will be diversified away by combining the project with the firm's other projects. The remaining risk, which is the portfolio risk **in a business context**, is called *corporate risk*.

The quantitative measure of corporate risk is a project's *corporate beta*, or *corporate b*, which is the slope of the regression line that results when the project's returns are plotted on the Y-axis and the overall returns on the firm are plotted on the X-axis. If Table 10.3 and Figure 10.2 represented returns on three projects and the overall returns for AtlantiCare, a not-for-profit HMO, the betas for H, M, and L would be corporate betas. They would measure the contribution of each project to AtlantiCare's overall risk.

A project's corporate beta measures the volatility of returns on the project relative to the business as a whole, which has a corporate beta of 1.0. If a project's corporate beta is 1.5, such as for Project H, its returns are 1.5 times as volatile as the firm's returns. Such a project increases the volatility of AtlantiCare's overall returns and hence increases the riskiness of the business. A corporate beta of 1.0, such as for Project M, indicates that the project's returns have the same volatility as the firm's returns. Hence, the project has the same risk as AtlantiCare's *average project*, which is a hypothetical project with risk identical to the aggregate business (the portfolio). A corporate beta of 0.5, such as for Project L, indicates that the project's returns are less volatile than the firm's returns, so the project reduces AtlantiCare's overall risk.

In closing the discussion of corporate risk (the risk of individual projects within a business with many projects), it must be noted that we have glossed over the difficulties inherent in implementing the concept in practice. That discussion will take place in Chapter 15. However, the concept of corporate risk remains important to health services managers in spite of its implementation problems.

Market Risk: Risk Within Stock Portfolios

The previous section discussed the riskiness of business projects to an organization. This section discusses the riskiness of business projects to owners, which for investor-owned corporations are common stockholders. Why should health services managers be concerned about how stock investors view risk? The answer is simple: Stock investors are the suppliers of equity capital to investor-owned businesses, so they set the rates of return that such businesses must pay to raise that capital. In turn, these rates set the minimum profitability that investor-owned businesses must earn on the equity portion of their real-asset investments. Even managers of not-for-profit firms should have an understanding of how stock investors view risk because market-set required rates of return can influence the opportunity cost rates used in making real-asset investments within not-for-profit businesses. Chapter 13 discusses this topic in detail.

Because stock investors hold well-diversified portfolios of stocks, the relevant riskiness of an individual project undertaken by a company whose stock is held in the portfolio is the project's **contribution to the overall riskiness of that stock portfolio.** Some of the stand-alone riskiness of the project will be diversified away by combining the project with all the other projects in the stock portfolio. The remaining risk is called *market risk*, which is defined as the contribution of the project to the riskiness of a **well-diversified stock portfolio**.

How should a project's market risk be measured? A project's *market beta*, or *market b*, measures the volatility of the project's returns relative to the returns on a well-diversified portfolio of stocks, which represents a very large portfolio of individual projects. If Table 10.3 and Figure 10.2 represented returns on three projects and the overall returns on a well-diversified stock portfolio, the betas for H, M, and L would be *market betas*, and they would measure the market risk of the projects. The only difference between the discussion of market risk and the previous discussion of corporate risk is what defines the relevant portfolio. When focusing on **corporate risk**, the relevant portfolio is the business's overall portfolio of projects. When discussing

market risk, the relevant portfolio is a well-diversified stock portfolio (the market portfolio).

A project with a market beta of 1.5, such as for Project H, has returns that are 1.5 times as volatile as the returns on the market and hence increases the riskiness of a well-diversified stock portfolio. A market beta of 1.0 indicates that the project's returns have the same volatility as the market—such a project has the same market risk as the market portfolio. A market beta of 0.5 indicates that the project's returns are half as volatile as the returns on the market—such a project reduces the riskiness of a well-diversified stock portfolio.[3]

The two types of portfolio risk—corporate and market—are identical in concept. Both types of risk are defined as the contribution of the investment—in this case, a business project—to the overall riskiness of the portfolio. Also, both types of risk are measured by the volatility of the investment's returns relative to the volatility of the portfolio. The only difference between corporate and market risk is **what defines the portfolio**. In corporate risk, the portfolio is defined as the collection of projects held within a business; in market risk, the portfolio is defined as the collection of projects held within a well-diversified stock portfolio.

Finally, even though an individual investor's stock portfolio can be thought of as a portfolio of many separate projects, the portfolio actually consists of the stocks of individual firms. Individual investors, therefore, are most concerned with the aggregate risk and return characteristics of the companies they own rather than the risk and return characteristics of each company's projects. This logic leads investors to be more concerned with the company's (stock's) market beta than they are with the market betas of individual projects.

A stock's market beta is the slope of the line formed by regressing the individual firm's stock returns against the aggregate returns on the market. For example, the market beta of General Healthcare (GH) was recently reported to be 0.80. This means that an equity investment in GH is somewhat less risky to well-diversified stock investors than an average stock, which has a beta of 1.0. GH's corporate beta, like all other company's corporate betas, is 1.0 by definition. What is relevant to stock investors, because they hold portfolios of common stocks, is the firm's market beta, not its corporate beta.

Self-Test Questions

1. What is the definition of portfolio risk?
2. How is portfolio risk measured?
3. What is a corporate beta, and how is it estimated?
4. What is a market beta, and how is it estimated?
5. Briefly, what is the difference between corporate risk and market risk?
6. What is the difference between a project's market beta and the firm's market beta?

Portfolio Betas

Individual investors hold portfolios of stocks, each with its own market risk as measured by the stock's market beta, while businesses hold portfolios of projects, each with its own corporate beta and market beta. What impact does the beta of a portfolio component have on the overall portfolio's beta? The beta of any portfolio of investments, b_p, is simply the weighted average of the individual component betas:

$$b_p = (w_1 \times b_1) + (w_2 \times b_2) \text{ and so on.}$$

Here, b_p is the beta of the portfolio, which measures the volatility of the entire portfolio; w_1 is the fraction of the portfolio in Investment 1; b_1 is the beta coefficient of Investment 1; and so on.

   To illustrate, the stock of GH has a market beta of 0.8, indicating that its returns to stockholders are somewhat less volatile than the returns on a well-diversified stock portfolio (or average stock with a beta of 1.0). Each project within GH has its own market risk, however, as measured by its market beta. Some projects may have very high market betas (e.g., over 1.5), while other projects may have very low market betas (e.g., under 0.5). When all the projects are combined, the overall market beta of the company is 0.8.

   For ease of discussion, assume that GH has only the following three projects:

Project	Market Beta	Dollar Investment	Proportion
A	1.3	$ 15,000	15.0%
B	1.1	30,000	30.0
C	0.5	55,000	55.0
		$100,000	100.0%

The weighted average of the project market betas, which is the firm's market beta, is 0.8:

$$\text{Market } b_{GH} = (w_1 \times b_1) + (w_2 \times b_2) + (w_3 \times b_3)$$

$$= (0.15 \times 1.3) + (0.30 \times 1.1) + (0.55 \times 0.5)$$

$$= 0.8.$$

   Each project's market beta reflects its volatility relative to the market portfolio. Note that each of GH's fictitious projects also has a corporate beta that measures the volatility of the project's returns relative to that of the corporation as a whole. The weighted average of these project corporate betas must equal 1.0, which is the corporate beta of any business.

Self-Test Questions

1. How is the beta of a portfolio related to the betas of the components?
2. What is the value of the weighted average of all project corporate betas within a business?

Relevance of the Risk Measures

Thus far, the chapter has discussed in some detail three measures of financial risk—stand-alone, corporate, and market—but it is still unclear which risk is the most relevant in financial decision making. It turns out that the risk that is relevant to any financial decision depends on the particular situation at hand. When the decision involves a single investment that will be held in isolation, stand-alone risk is the relevant risk. Here, the risk and return on the portfolio is the same as the risk and return on the single asset in the portfolio. In this situation, the riskiness faced by the investor, whether the investor is an individual considering a single stock purchase or a business considering a sole MRI system investment, is defined in terms of returns less than expected, and the appropriate measure is the standard deviation (or coefficient of variation) of the return distribution.

In most decisions, however, the investment under consideration will not be held in isolation but will be held as part of an investment portfolio. Individual investors normally hold portfolios of securities, while businesses normally hold portfolios of real-asset investments (projects). Thus, it is clear that portfolio risk is more relevant to real-world decisions than is stand-alone risk. However, there are three distinct ownership situations that affect the relevancy of portfolio risk.

Large Investor-Owned Businesses

For large investor-owned businesses, the primary financial goal is shareholder wealth maximization. This means that managerial decisions should focus on risk and return as seen by the business's stockholders. Because stockholders tend to hold large portfolios of securities and hence a very large portfolio of individual projects, the most relevant risk of a project under consideration by a large for-profit firm is the project's contribution to a well-diversified stock portfolio (the market portfolio). Of course, this is the project's market risk. Many would argue, and we agree, that corporate and stand-alone risk cannot be disregarded in all situations. For example, corporate risk, which best measures the impact of the project on the financial condition of the business, clearly is relevant to the business's nonowner stakeholders, such as managers, employees, creditors, and suppliers, who should not be totally ignored. Also, the failure of a project that is large, relative to the business, could bring down the entire firm. Under such circumstances, the project clearly has high risk to stockholders even if its market risk is low. The bottom line here is that market risk should be of primary importance in large investor-owned businesses, but corporate and stand-alone risk should not be totally ignored.

Small Investor-Owned Businesses

For small investor-owned businesses, the situation is more complicated. Take, for example, a three-physician group practice. Here, there is no separation between management and ownership, and the situation is complicated by the fact that the business is also the owners' employer. In this case, the primary goal of the business is more likely to be maximization of owners' overall well-being than strict shareholder wealth maximization. For example, owner/managers may value leisure time, as exemplified by three afternoons of golf, as being more important than additional wealth creation. To complicate the situation even more, shareholder wealth now consists of both the value of the ownership position and the professional fees (salaries) derived from the business.

Thus, in small for-profit businesses, corporate risk is probably more relevant than market risk. The owner/managers would not want to place the viability of the business in jeopardy just to increase their expected ownership value by a small amount. Put another way, the owner/managers are not well diversified in regards to the business because a large proportion of their wealth comes from expected future employment earnings. Because of this, market risk loses relevance and corporate risk becomes most important. However, the potential relevance of stand-alone risk as described in the previous section also applies.

Not-for-Profit Businesses

Not-for-profit businesses do not have owners, and their goals stem from a mission that generally involves service to society. In this situation, market risk clearly is not relevant; the concern to managers is the impact of the project on the riskiness of the business, which is measured by a project's corporate risk. Thus, the risk measure most relevant here is corporate risk. Again, however, the stand-alone risk of large projects that could sink the business is relevant.

---

1. Explain the situations in which each of the risk types—stand-alone, corporate, and market risk—are relevant.

**Self-Test
Question**

Interpretation of the Risk Measures

It is important to recognize that none of the risk measures discussed can be interpreted without some standard of reference. For example, suppose that Investors' Healthcare, a large for-profit company, is evaluating a project that has a 0.7 coefficient of variation of returns. Does the project have high, low, or moderate stand-alone risk? We don't know the answer without more information. However, knowing that the business's average project has a coefficient of variation of returns of 0.4 enables us to state that the project has above-average stand-alone risk.

Similarly, suppose the project under consideration has a corporate beta of 1.4. We know that it has above-average corporate risk because any business in the aggregate, including Investors' Healthcare, has a corporate beta of 1.0. This same project might have a market beta of 1.2. This indicates that the project is riskier than the average project held in a large stock portfolio, but how does the project's market risk compare to the market risk of Investors' Healthcare? If the business (i.e., its stock) has a market beta of 0.9, the project also has above-average market risk as compared to the business as a whole. The point here is that risk is always interpreted against some standard because without a standard it is impossible to make judgments.

Which risk judgment is most relevant to Investors' Healthcare? As discussed in the previous section, market risk is most relevant because the business taking on the project is both large and investor owned, and hence managers should be most concerned about the impact of a new project on stockholders' risk. However, as explained in the previous section, corporate and stand-alone risk might also have some relevance. The good news here is that the proposed project has above-average risk, when compared to the business's average project, regardless of which risk measure is used.

Self-Test Question   1. How are risk measures interpreted?

The Relationship Between Risk and Required Return

This chapter contains a great deal of discussion about defining and measuring financial risk. However, being able to define and measure financial risk is of no value in financial decision making unless risk can be related to return; that is, the answer to this question is needed: How much return is required to compensate investors for assuming a given level of risk? In this section, the focus is on setting required rates of return on stock investments, but in other chapters the focus is on setting required rates of return on individual projects within businesses.

The Capital Asset Pricing Model (CAPM)

The relationship between the market risk of a stock, as measured by its market beta, and its required rate of return is given by the *Capital Asset Pricing Model (CAPM)*.

To begin, some basic definitions are needed:

- $E(R_e)$ = Expected rate of return on a stock. Because an investment in stocks is called an equity investment, we use the subscript "e" (as opposed to "s") to designate the return.

- $R(R_e)$ = Required rate of return on a stock. If $E(R_e)$ is less than $R(R_e)$, the stock would not be purchased or it would be sold if it was owned. If $E(R_e)$ was greater than $R(R_e)$, the stock should be bought, and a person would be indifferent about the purchase if $E(R_e) = R(R_e)$.
- RF = Risk-free rate of return. In a CAPM context, RF is generally measured by the return on long-term U.S. Treasury bonds.
- b = Market beta coefficient of the stock. The market beta of an average-risk stock is 1.0.
- $R(R_M)$ = Required rate of return on a portfolio that consists of all stocks, which is called the *market portfolio*. $R(R_M)$ is also the required rate of return on an average-risk ($b = 1.0$) stock. Note that in practice the market portfolio is proxied by some stock index such as the NYSE Index or the S&P 500 Index.
- RP_M = Market risk premium = $R(R_M)$ − RF. This is the additional return over the risk-free rate required to compensate investors for assuming average ($b = 1.0$) risk.
- RP_e = Risk premium on the stock = $[R(R_M) − RF] \times b = RP_M \times$ b. A stock's risk premium is less than, equal to, or greater than the premium on an average stock, depending on whether its beta is less than, equal to, or greater than 1.0. If $b = 1.0$, then $RP_e = RP_M$.

Using these definitions, the CAPM relationship between risk and required rate of return is given by the following equation, which is called the *Security Market Line (SML)*:

$$R(R_e) = RF + (R[R_M] − RF) \times b$$
$$= RF + (RP_M \times b).$$

In words, the SML tells us that the required rate of return on a stock is equal to the risk-free rate plus a premium for bearing the risk inherent in that stock investment. Furthermore, the risk premium consists of the premium required for bearing average ($b = 1.0$) risk, $RP_M = (R[R_M] − RF)$, multiplied by the beta coefficient of the stock in question. In effect, the market risk premium is adjusted up or down on the basis of the riskiness of the individual stock relative to that of the market (or an average stock).

To illustrate use of the SML, assume that the risk-free rate, RF, is 6 percent; the required rate of return on the market, $R[R_M]$, is 12 percent; and the market beta, b, of General Healthcare (GH) stock is 0.8. According to the SML, a stock investment in GH has a required rate of return of 10.8 percent:

$$R(R_{GH}) = 6\% + (12\% − 6\%) \times 0.8$$
$$= 6\% + (6\% \times 0.8)$$
$$= 6\% + 4.8\% = 10.8\%.$$

If the expected rate of return, $E(R_{GH})$, were 15 percent, investors should buy the stock because $E(R_{GH})$ is greater than $R(R_{GH})$. Conversely, if $E(R_{GH}) = 8\%$, investors should sell the stock because $E(R_{GH})$ is less than $R(R_{GH})$.

A stock with a beta of 1.5, one that is riskier than GH, would have a required rate of return of 15 percent:

$$R(R_{b=1.5}) = 6\% + (6\% \times 1.5)$$

$$= 6\% + 9\% = 15\%.$$

An average stock, with $b = 1.0$, would have a required return of 12 percent, which is the same as the market return:

$$R(R_{b=1.0}) = 6\% + (6\% \times 1.0)$$

$$= 6\% + 6\% = 12\% = R(R_M).$$

Finally, a stock with below-average risk, with $b = 0.5$, would have a required rate of return of 9 percent.

$$R(R_{b=0.5}) = 6\% + (6\% \times 0.5)$$

$$= 6\% + 3\% = 9\%.$$

The market risk premium, RP_M, depends on the degree of aversion that investors in the aggregate have to risk. In this example, T-bonds yielded RF = 6% and an average risk stock had a required rate of return of $R(R_M) = 12\%$, so $RP_M = 6$ percentage points. If investors' degree of risk aversion increased, $R(R_M)$ might increase to 14 percent, which would cause RP_M to increase to 8 percentage points. Thus, the greater the overall degree of risk aversion in the economy, the higher the required rate on the market and hence the higher the required rates of return on all stocks.

Also, values for the risk-free rate, RF, and the required rate of return on the market, $R(R_M)$, are influenced by inflation expectations. The higher investor expectations regarding inflation, the greater these values and hence the greater the required rates of return on all stocks.

The SML is often expressed in graphical form, as in Figure 10.3, which shows the SML when RF = 6% and $R(R_M) = 12\%$. Here are the relevant points concerning Figure 10.3:

- Required rates of return are shown on the vertical axis, while risk as measured by market beta is shown on the horizontal axis.
- Riskless securities have $b = 0$; therefore, RF is the vertical axis intercept.
- The slope of the SML reflects the degree of risk aversion in the economy. The greater the average investor's aversion to risk the

FIGURE 10.3
The Security
Market Line

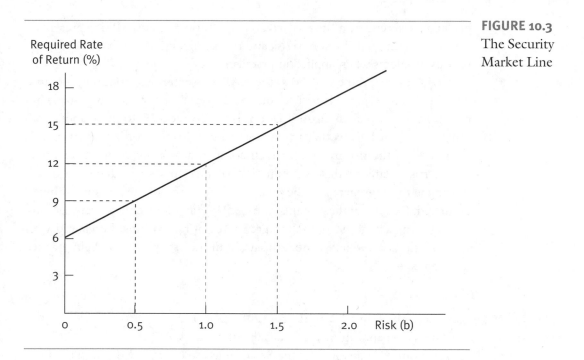

steeper the slope of the SML, the greater the risk premium for any
stock, and the higher the required rate of return on all stocks.
- The intercept on the Y (vertical) axis reflects the level of expected
  inflation. The higher inflation expectations, the greater both RF
  and $R(R_M)$. Thus, the higher the SML plots on the graph.
- The values previously calculated for the required rates of return on
  stocks with $b = 0.5$, 1.0, and 1.5 agree with the values shown on
  the graph.

Both the SML and a stock's position on it change over time because of
changes in interest rates, investors' risk aversion, and the individual company's
(stock's) beta. Thus, the SML, as well as a stock's risk, must be evaluated on
the basis of current information. The SML, its use, and how its input values
are estimated are covered in greater detail in Chapter 13.

Advantages and Disadvantages of the CAPM

A word of caution about beta coefficients and the CAPM is in order. To begin,
the CAPM is based on a very restrictive set of assumptions that does not conform well to real-world conditions. Second, although the concepts are logical,
the entire theory is based on expectations, while only historical data are available. Thus, the market betas that are calculated and reported in practice show
how volatile a stock has been in the **past**. However, conditions may change,
and a stock's **future volatility**—the item of real concern to investors—might

be quite different from its past volatility. Although the CAPM represents a very important contribution to risk and return theory, it does have potentially serious problems when applied in practice.

In spite of these concerns, the CAPM is extremely appealing because it is simple and logical. It focuses on the impact that a single investment has on a portfolio, which in most situations is the correct way to think about risk. Furthermore, it tells us that the required rate of return on an investment is composed of the risk-free rate, which compensates investors for time value, plus a risk premium that is a function of investors' attitudes toward risk bearing in the aggregate and the specific portfolio risk of the investment being evaluated. Because of these points, the CAPM is an important conceptual tool. However, its actual use to set required rates of return must be viewed with some caution. We will have more to say about the use of the CAPM in practice in Chapter 13.

Self-Test Questions

1. What is the Capital Asset Pricing Model (CAPM)?
2. What is the appropriate measure of risk in the CAPM?
3. Write out the equation for the Security Market Line (SML), and then graph it.
4. Describe the SML in words.
5. What are the advantages and disadvantages of the CAPM?

Key Concepts

This chapter has covered the very important topics of financial risk and required return. The key concepts of this chapter are:

- Risk definition and measurement is very important in financial management because decision makers, in general, are *risk averse* and hence require higher returns from investments that have higher risk.
- *Financial risk* is associated with the prospect of returns less than anticipated. The higher the probability of a return being far less than anticipated, the greater the risk.
- The riskiness of investments held in isolation, called *stand-alone risk*, can be measured by the dispersion of the rate of return distribution about its *expected value*. One commonly used measure of stand-alone risk is the *standard deviation* of the return distribution.
- Most investments are not held in isolation but as part of a *portfolio*. Individual investors hold portfolios of securities, and businesses hold portfolios of projects (i.e., products and services).
- When investments with returns that are less than perfectly positively correlated are combined in a portfolio, risk is reduced. The risk reduction occurs because less-than-expected returns on some investments are offset by greater-than-expected returns on other investments. However, among

real-world investments, it is impossible to eliminate all risk because the returns on all assets are influenced to a greater or lesser degree by overall economic conditions.

- That portion of the stand-alone risk of an investment that can be eliminated by holding the investment in a portfolio is called *diversifiable risk*, while the risk that remains is called *portfolio risk*.

- There are two different types of portfolio risk. *Corporate risk* is the riskiness of business projects when they are considered as part of a business's portfolio of projects. *Market risk* is the riskiness of business projects (or of the stocks of entire businesses) when they are considered as part of an individual investor's well-diversified portfolio of securities.

- Corporate risk is measured by a project's *corporate beta*, which reflects the volatility of the project's returns relative to the volatility of returns of the aggregate business.

- Market risk is measured by a project's or stock's *market beta*, which reflects the volatility of a project's (or stock's) returns relative to the volatility of returns on a well-diversified stock portfolio.

- *Stand-alone risk* is most relevant to investments held in isolation; *corporate risk* is most relevant to projects held by not-for-profit firms and by small owner-managed for-profit businesses; and *market risk* is most relevant to projects held by large investor-owned corporations.

- The *beta coefficient of a portfolio of investments* is the weighted average of the betas of the components of the portfolio, where the weights are the proportion of the overall investment in each component. Therefore, the weighted average of corporate betas of all projects in a business must equal 1.0, while the weighted average of all projects' market betas must equal the market beta of the firm's stock.

- The *Capital Asset Pricing Model (CAPM)* is an equilibrium model that describes the relationship between market risk and required rates of return.

- The *Security Market Line (SML)* provides the actual risk/required rate of return relationship. The required rate of return on any stock is equal to the risk-free rate plus the market risk premium times the stock's market beta coefficient: $R(R_e) = RF + [R(R_M) - RF] \times b = RF + (RP_M \times b)$.

This concludes the discussion of basic financial management concepts. The next chapter begins our coverage of long-term financing.

Questions

10.1 When considering stand-alone risk, the return distribution of a less risky investment is more peaked ("tighter") than that of a riskier investment. What shape would the return distribution have for an investment with (a) completely certain returns and (b) completely uncertain returns?

10.2 Stock A has an expected rate of return of 8 percent, a standard deviation of 20 percent, and a market beta of 0.5. Stock B has an expected rate of return of 12 percent, a standard deviation of 15 percent, and a market beta of 1.5. Which investment is the riskier? Why? (Hint: Remember that the risk of an investment depends on its context.)

10.3 a. What is risk aversion?
b. Why is risk aversion so important to financial decision making?

10.4 Explain why holding investments in portfolios has such a profound impact on the concept of financial risk.

10.5 Assume that two investments are combined in a portfolio.
a. In words, what is the expected rate of return on the portfolio?
b. What condition must be present for the portfolio to have lower risk than the weighted average of the two investments?
c. Is it possible for the portfolio to have lower risk than that of either investment?
d. Is it possible for the portfolio to be riskless? If so, what condition is necessary to create such a portfolio?

10.6 Explain the difference between portfolio risk and diversifiable risk.

10.7 What are the implications of portfolio theory for investors?

10.8 a. What are the two types of portfolio risk?
b. How is each type defined?
c. How is each type measured?

10.9 Under what circumstances is each type of risk—stand alone, corporate, and market—most relevant?

10.10 a. What is the Capital Asset Pricing Model (CAPM)? The security market line (SML)?
b. What are the weaknesses of the CAPM?
c. What is the value of the CAPM?

Problems

10.1 Consider the following probability distribution of returns estimated for a proposed project that involves a new ultrasound machine:

State of the Economy	Probability of Occurrence	Rate of Return
Very poor	0.10	−10.0%
Poor	0.20	0.0
Average	0.40	10.0
Good	0.20	20.0
Very good	0.10	30.0

a. What is the expected rate of return on the project?
b. What is the project's standard deviation of returns?

    c. What is the project's coefficient of variation (CV) of returns?

    d. What type of risk does the standard deviation and CV measure?

    e. In what situation is this risk relevant?

10.2 Suppose that a person won the Florida lottery and was offered a choice of two prizes: (1) $500,000 or (2) a coin-toss gamble in which he or she would get $1 million if a head were flipped and zero for a tail.

    a. What is the expected dollar return on the gamble?

    b. Would the person choose the sure $500,000 or the gamble?

    c. If he or she chooses the sure $500,000, is the person a risk averter or a risk seeker?

10.3 Refer to Table 10.2.

    a. Construct an equal-weighted (50/50) portfolio of Investments B and C. What is the expected rate of return and standard deviation of the portfolio? Explain your results.

    b. Construct an equal-weighted (50/50) portfolio of Investments B and D. What is the expected rate of return and standard deviation of the portfolio? Explain your results.

10.4 Suppose that the risk-free rate, RF, were 8 percent and the required rate of return on the market, $R(R_M)$, were 14 percent.

    a. Write out the Security Market Line (SML), and explain each term.

    b. Plot the SML on a sheet of paper.

    c. Suppose that inflation expectations increase such that the risk-free rate, RF, increases to 10 percent and the required rate of return on the market, $R(R_M)$, increases to 16 percent. Write out and plot the new SML.

    d. Return to the original assumptions in this problem. Now, suppose that investors' risk aversion increases and the required rate of return on the market, $R(R_M)$, increases to 16 percent. (There is no change in the risk-free rate because RF reflects the required rate of return on a riskless investment.) Write out and plot the new SML.

10.5 A few years ago, the *Value Line Investment Survey* reported the following market betas for the stocks of selected healthcare providers:

Company	Beta
Quorum Health Group	0.90
Beverly Enterprises	1.20
HEALTHSOUTH Corporation	1.45
United Healthcare	1.70

At the time these betas were developed, reasonable estimates for the risk-free rate, RF, and required rate of return on the market, $R(R_M)$, were 6.5 percent and 13.5 percent, respectively.

    a. What are the required rates of return on the four stocks?

    b. Why do their required rates of return differ?

    c. Suppose that a person is planning to invest in only one stock rather than a well-diversified stock portfolio. Are the required rates of return calculated above applicable to the investment? Explain your answer.

10.6 Suppose that Apex Health Services has four different projects. These projects are listed below, along with the amount of capital invested and estimated corporate and market betas:

Project	Amount Invested	Corporate Beta	Market Beta
Walk-in clinic	$ 500,000	1.5	1.1
MRI facility	2,000,000	1.2	1.5
Clinical laboratory	1,500,000	0.9	0.8
X-ray laboratory	1,000,000	0.5	1.0
	$5,000,000		

a. Why do the corporate and market betas differ for the same project?
b. What is the overall corporate beta of Apex Health Services? Is the calculated beta consistent with corporate risk theory?
c. What is the overall market beta of Apex Health Services?
d. How does the riskiness of Apex's stock compare with the riskiness of an average stock?
e. Would stock investors require a rate of return on Apex that is greater than, less than, or the same as the return on an average-risk stock?

10.7 Assume that HMA is evaluating the feasibility of building a new hospital in an area not currently served by the company. The company's analysts estimate a market beta for the hospital project of 1.1, which is somewhat higher than the 0.8 market beta of the company's average project. Financial forecasts for the new hospital indicate an expected rate of return on the equity portion of the investment of 20 percent. If the risk-free rate, RF, is 7 percent and the required rate of return on the market, $R(R_M)$, is 12 percent, is the new hospital in the best interest of HMA's shareholders? Explain your answer.

Notes

1. Defining financial risk as the probability of earning a return far below that expected is somewhat simplistic. As we discussed previously, there are many different ways of viewing financial risk. However, the simple definition presented here is a good starting point for discussing the types of risk that are most relevant to decisions made within health services organizations.

2. Consider what the slope of the line would be if the portfolio's returns were plotted on both the X and Y axes. The regression line would be a 45-degree line, which has a slope of 1.0. Thus, an average risk investment, as defined by the risk of the portfolio, has a slope of 1.0. In fact, Investment M has the same return distribution as Portfolio P, so the M regression line is identical to that for P.

3. In these illustrations, the same probability distributions are being used to illustrate both corporate risk and market risk. In reality, it is unlikely that returns on a particular firm and returns on the market portfolio would be the same. (The portfolio returns in the right column of Table 10.3 would not be identical for both a given firm and for the market portfolio.) This reality would cause the lines plotted in Figure 10.2 to have different slopes and hence different corporate and market betas—for example, Project H may have a corporate beta of 1.5 and a market beta of 1.2. In general, a project's corporate beta and market beta will differ.

References

Brigham, E. F., and M. C. Ehrhardt. 2005. *Financial Management: Theory and Practice*, chaps. 4 and 5. Fort Worth, TX: Thomson/South-Western.

Gapenski, L. C. 1992. "Project Risk Definition and Measurement in a Not-for-Profit Setting." *Health Services Management Research* (November): 216–24.

Long-Term Financing

Health services organizations need assets to provide services. For example, hospitals need facilities and equipment to provide inpatient and outpatient services, while clinics require similar (but somewhat different) assets to provide outpatient services. To obtain these assets, healthcare organizations need capital (money). A large hospital requires a very large amount of capital (some hospitals have more than $1 billion of capital), while a small home health business requires a relatively small amount of capital. Regardless of size, all health services organizations must have capital to acquire the facilities, equipment, inventories, and other assets needed to run the business.

There are many different types of capital available to health services organizations. Debt financing is supplied by lenders, while equity financing is obtained from owners in for-profit businesses and from the "community at large" in not-for-profit businesses. Because different types of financing have different characteristics, managers must understand how the types of capital differ and the impact of these differences on the risk and financial condition of the business. Furthermore, to better understand how capital suppliers decide how much to charge for capital, managers need to know how securities are valued.

Businesses have a choice regarding the amount of debt they use. Should a business use a small or large proportion of debt capital, as opposed to equity capital? This choice affects both the riskiness of the business and the cost of its financing, and hence its potential profitability.

The three chapters in this section introduce students to the types of capital available to health services organizations, how this capital is valued in the marketplace, and how the use of debt financing affects a business's risk and capital costs.

LONG-TERM DEBT FINANCING

Learning Objectives

After studying this chapter, readers will be able to:

- Describe how interest rates are set in the economy.
- Discuss the various types of long-term debt instruments and their features.
- Discuss the components that make up the interest rate on a debt security.
- Value debt securities.

Introduction

If a business is to operate, it must have assets. To acquire assets, it must raise *capital*. Capital comes in two basic forms: debt and equity. Historically, capital furnished by the owners of investor-owned businesses (i.e., stockholders of for-profit corporations) was called *equity* capital, while capital obtained by not-for-profit businesses from grants, contributions, and retained earnings was called *fund* capital. Both types of capital serve the same purpose in financing businesses—providing a permanent financing base without a contractually fixed cost—so today the term *equity* is often used to represent nonliability capital regardless of ownership type.

In addition to equity financing, most healthcare businesses use a considerable amount of *debt* financing, which is provided by *creditors*. For example, *Value Line* reports that, on average, healthcare providers finance their assets with 5 percent short-term debt (and liabilities), 30 percent long-term debt, and 65 percent equity as measured by balance sheet amounts. Thus, more than one-third of providers' financing comes from debt. In this chapter, many facets of debt financing are discussed, including important background material related to how interest rates are set in the economy. The discussion here focuses on long-term debt; short-term debt is discussed in Chapter 16.

The Cost of Money

Capital in a free economy is allocated through the price system. The *interest rate* is the price paid to obtain debt capital, whereas in the case of equity capital in for-profit firms, investors' returns come in the form of *dividends* and *capital gains* or *losses*. The four most fundamental factors that affect the supply of and demand for investment capital, and hence the cost of money, are investment opportunities, time preferences for consumption, risk, and inflation. To see how these factors operate, visualize the situation facing Lori Gibbs, an entrepreneur who is planning to found a new home health agency. Lori does not have sufficient personal funds to start the business, so she must supplement her equity capital with debt financing.

Investment Opportunities

If Lori estimates that the business will be highly profitable, she will be able to pay creditors a higher interest rate than if it is barely profitable. Thus, her ability to pay for borrowed capital depends on the business's *investment opportunities*. The higher the profitability of the business, the higher the interest rate that Lori can afford to pay lenders for use of their savings.

Time Preferences for Consumption

The interest rate lenders will charge depends in large part on their *time preferences for consumption*. For example, one potential lender, Jane Wright, may be saving for retirement, so she may be willing to loan funds at a relatively low rate because her preference is for future consumption. Another person, John Davis, may have a wife and several young children to clothe and feed, so he may be willing to lend funds out of current income, and hence forgo consumption, only if the interest rate is very high. John is said to have a high time preference for consumption and Jane a low time preference. If the entire population of an economy were living right at the subsistence level, time preferences for current consumption would necessarily be high, aggregate savings would be low, interest rates would be high, and capital formation would be difficult.

Risk

The *risk* inherent in the prospective home health care business, and thus in Lori's ability to repay the loan, would also affect the return lenders would require: the higher the risk, the higher the interest rate. Investors would be unwilling to lend to high-risk businesses unless the interest rate was higher than on loans to low-risk businesses.

Inflation

Finally, because the value of money in the future is affected by *inflation*, the higher the expected rate of inflation, the higher the interest rate demanded by savers. Debt suppliers must demand higher interest rates when inflation is high to offset the resulting loss of purchasing power.

Note that to simplify matters, the illustration implied that savers would lend directly to businesses that need capital, but in most cases the funds would actually pass through a *financial intermediary* such as a bank or a mutual fund.

Also, note that we used the interest rate on debt capital to illustrate the four factors, but the same logic applies to the cost of all investment capital.

Common Long-Term Debt Instruments

There are many different types of long-term debt, which in general is defined as debt that has a maturity greater than one year. Some types of long-term debt, such as home mortgages and auto loans, are used by individuals, while other types are use primarily by businesses. In this section, we discuss the long-term debt types most commonly used by healthcare businesses.

Term Loans

A *term loan* is a contract under which a borrower agrees to make a series of interest and principal payments, on specified dates, to a lender. Investment bankers are generally not involved; term loans are negotiated directly between the borrowing business and the lender. Typically, the lender is a financial institution such as a commercial bank, a mutual fund, an insurance company, or a pension fund, but it can also be a wealthy private investor. Most term loans have maturities of three to 15 years.

Like home mortgages, term loans are usually amortized in equal installments over the life of the loan, so part of the principal of the loan is retired with each payment. For example, Sacramento Cardiology Group has a $100,000 five-year term loan with Bank of America to fund the purchase of new diagnostic equipment. The interest rate on the fixed-rate loan is 10 percent, which obligates the group to five end-of-year payments of $26,379.75. Thus, loan payments total $131,898.75, of which $31,898.75 is interest and $100,000 is repayment of principal (i.e., the amount borrowed).

Term loans have three major advantages over bonds (the other major category of long-term debt, which we discuss in the next section): speed, flexibility, and low administrative costs. Because term loans are negotiated directly between an institutional lender and the borrower, as opposed to being sold to the general public, formal documentation is minimized. The key provisions of the loan can be worked out much more quickly, and with more flexibility, than can those for a public issue. Furthermore, it is not necessary for a term loan to go through the Securities and Exchange Commission (SEC) registration process. Finally, after a term loan has been negotiated, changes can be renegotiated more easily than with bonds if financial circumstances so dictate.

The interest rate on a term loan can be either fixed for the life of the loan or variable. If it is *fixed*, the rate used will be close to the rate on equivalent maturity bonds issued by businesses of comparable risk. If the rate is *variable*, it is usually set at a certain number of percentage points over an index rate such as the prime rate.[1] When the index rate goes up or down, so does the interest rate that must be paid on the outstanding balance of the term loan.

Bonds

Like a term loan, a *bond* is a long-term contract under which a borrower agrees to make payments of interest and principal, on specific dates, to the holder of the bond. Although bonds are similar in many ways to term loans, a bond issue generally is registered with the SEC, advertised, offered to the public through investment bankers, and actually sold to many different investors. Indeed, thousands of individual and institutional investors may participate when a firm, such as HCA, sells a bond issue, while there is generally only one lender in the case of a term loan.

Bonds are categorized as either government (Treasury), corporate, or municipal. *Government*, or *Treasury, bonds* are issued by the U.S. Treasury and are used to raise money for the federal government.[2] Because Treasury bonds are not used by businesses, we will not discuss them here.

Corporate Bonds

Corporate bonds are issued by investor-owned firms, while *municipal bonds* are issued by governments and governmental agencies other than federal. In this section, the primary focus is on corporate bonds, but much of the discussion also is relevant to municipal bonds. The unique features of municipal bonds will be discussed in the next major section.

Although corporate bonds generally have maturities in the range of 20 to 30 years, shorter maturities, as well as longer maturities, are occasionally used. In fact, in 1995 HCA (then Columbia/HCA) issued $200 million worth of 100-year bonds, following the issuance of 100-year bonds by Disney and Coca-Cola in 1993. These ultra-long term bonds had not been used by any firm since the 1920s. Unlike term loans, bonds usually pay only interest over the life of the bond, with the entire amount of principal returned to lenders at maturity.

Most bonds have a *fixed* interest rate, which locks in the current rate for the entire maturity of the bond and hence minimizes interest payment uncertainty. However, some bonds have a *floating*, or *variable, rate* that is tied to some interest rate index, so the interest payments move up and down with the general level of interest rates.

Some bonds do not pay any interest at all but are sold at a substantial discount from face (principal) value. Such bonds, called *zero-coupon bonds*, provide the investor (lender) with capital appreciation rather than interest income. For example, a zero-coupon bond with a $1,000 face value and ten-year maturity might sell for $385.54 when issued. An investor who buys the bond would realize a 10 percent annual rate of return if the bond were held to maturity, even though he or she would receive no interest payments along the way. (Note though, for tax purposes, the difference between par value and the purchase price is amortized and treated as interest income.) Other bonds, instead of paying interest in cash, pay coupons that grant the lender additional bonds (or a proportion of an additional bond). These bonds are called *payment-in-kind (PIK)* bonds. PIK bonds usually are issued by companies that are in poor financial condition and do not have the cash to pay interest; hence, they tend to be quite risky.

In rare cases, bonds have *step-up provisions*, which mean that the interest rate paid on the bond is increased if the bond's rating is downgraded. (A downgrading means that the company's financial condition has deteriorated. Bond ratings are discussed in a later section.) A step-up provision is very risky for the issuing company because they must pay a higher interest rate at the worst possible time—when their financial condition weakens. Conversely, such a provision reduces the risk to buyers (lenders).

The bottom line here is that bonds in general, and corporate bonds in particular, come in many different flavors. In an introductory healthcare finance text, we can only scratch the surface.

Mortgage Bonds

With a *mortgage bond*, the issuer pledges certain real assets as security for the bond. To illustrate the concept, consider the following example. Mid-Texas Healthcare System recently needed $100 million to purchase land and to build a new hospital. *First mortgage bonds* in the amount of $30 million, secured by a mortgage on the property, were issued. If the firm *defaults* (fails to make the promised payments) on the bonds, the bondholders could foreclose on the hospital and sell it to satisfy their claims.

Mid-Texas could, if it so chose, also issue *second mortgage bonds* secured by the same $100 million hospital. In the event of bankruptcy and liquidation, the holders of these second mortgage bonds would have a claim against the property only after the first mortgage bondholders had been paid off in full. Thus, second mortgages are sometimes called *junior mortgages*, or *junior liens*, because they are junior in priority to claims of senior mortgages, or first mortgage bonds.

Debentures

A *debenture* is an unsecured bond, and as such, it has no lien against specific property as security for the obligation. For example, Mid-Texas Healthcare System has $5 million of debentures outstanding. These bonds are not secured by real property but are backed instead by the revenue-producing power of the corporation. Debenture holders are, therefore, general creditors whose claims, in the event of bankruptcy, are protected by property not otherwise pledged. In practice, the use of debentures depends on the nature of the firm's assets and general credit strength. If a firm's credit position is exceptionally strong, it can issue debentures because it simply does not need to pledge specific assets as security. Debentures are also issued by firms with only a small amount of assets suitable as collateral. Finally, firms that have used up their capacity to borrow in the lower-cost mortgage market may be forced to use higher-cost debentures.

Subordinated Debentures

The term *subordinate* means "below" or "inferior." Thus, *subordinated debt* has a claim on assets in the event of bankruptcy only after senior debt has been paid off. Debentures may be subordinated either to designated debt—usually bank loans—or to all other debt. In the event of liquidation, holders of subordinated debentures cannot be paid until senior debt, as named in the debenture, has been paid. Subordinated debentures are normally quite risky and hence carry interest rates that are much higher than the rate on mortgage bonds.

Municipal Bonds

Municipal, or *muni, bonds* are long-term debt obligations issued by states and their political subdivisions such as counties, cities, port authorities, toll road or bridge authorities, and so on. Short-term municipal securities are used primarily to meet temporary cash needs, while municipal bonds are usually used to finance capital projects.

There are several types of municipal bonds. For example, *general obligation bonds* are secured by the full faith and credit of the issuing municipality (i.e., they are backed by the full taxing authority of the issuer). Conversely, *special tax bonds* are secured by a specified tax such as a tax on utility services. *Revenue bonds* are bonds that are not backed by taxing power but by the revenues derived from such projects as roads or bridges, airports, and water and sewage systems. Revenue bonds are of particular interest to not-for-profit healthcare providers because they are legally entitled to issue such securities through government-sponsored healthcare financing authorities.

Not-for-profit healthcare firms issue large amounts of municipal debt. To illustrate, such providers issued more than $20 billion of municipal bonds in 2006, and the total amount of such debt outstanding is approaching $200 billion. Recently, about 20 percent of the dollar volume of healthcare muni bonds has had floating rates, while the remaining 80 percent has had fixed rates. Floating rate bonds are riskier to the issuer because interest rates could rise in the future. Conversely, floating rate bonds are less risky to buyers because rising rates will trigger an increase in the amount of each interest payment. However, virtually all such municipal debt has call provisions that permit issuers to replace the floating rate debt with fixed rate debt should interest rates rise substantially. The ability to redeem the debt should interest rates soar places a cap on the riskiness to the borrower as well as on the potential gains to floating rate bondholders. (Call provisions are discussed in more detail in the next major section.)

Municipal bonds generally are sold in *serial* form—that is, a portion of the issue comes due periodically, anywhere from six months after issue to 30 years or more. Thus, a single issue actually consists of a series of sub-issues of different maturities. In effect, the bond issue is amortized, with a portion of the issue retired every year. The purpose of structuring a bond issue in this way is to match the overall maturity of the issue to the maturity of the assets being financed. For example, a new hospital that has a predicted useful life of about 30 years might be financed with a 30-year serial issue. Over time, some of the revenues associated with the new hospital will be used to meet the *debt service requirements* (i.e., the interest and principal payments). At the end of 30 years, the entire issue will be paid off, and the issuer can plan for a replacement facility or major renovation that would be funded, at least in part, by another debt issue.

Whereas the vast majority of federal government and corporate bonds are held by institutions, close to half of all municipal bonds outstanding are held by individual investors. The primary attraction of most municipal bonds is their exemption from federal and state (in the state of issue) taxes. To illustrate, the interest rate on a AAA-rated, long-term corporate bond recently was 5.5 percent, while the rate on a similar risk healthcare muni was 4.6 percent. To an individual investor in the 40 percent federal-plus-state tax bracket, the corporate bond's after-tax yield was $5.5\% \times (1 - 0.40) = 5.5\% \times 0.6 = 3.3\%$, while the muni's after-tax yield was the same as its before-tax yield, 4.6 percent. This yield differential on otherwise similar securities illustrates why investors in high tax brackets are so enthusiastic about municipal bonds.

Most healthcare municipal bonds are issued by large hospitals in amounts of $100 million or more because the administrative costs associated with stand-alone issues make them cost-prohibitive for small hospitals needing only small amounts of debt financing. To provide the benefits associated with tax-exempt financing to small hospitals, many state hospital associations have established municipal *bond pools*. These pools raise funds by issuing municipal bonds that are then loaned to not-for-profit hospitals that are too small to "tap" the muni market directly. To avoid abuses of tax-sheltered debt, federal law requires that there be an expectation up front that at least 95 percent of the bond pool will be loaned out to individual hospitals within three years. Unfortunately, some pools, which loaned out only a small percentage of the total funds available, were unable to demonstrate that this requirement had been met and were fined for violating federal law.

Private Versus Public Placement

Most bonds, including Treasury, corporate, and municipal bonds, are sold primarily through investment bankers to the public at large. For example, the New York State Medical Care Facilities Financing Agency recently sold a $675 million municipal mortgage revenue issue for New York Hospital. The issue was marketed both to the public at large and to institutional investors by

Goldman Sachs & Co., one of the top underwriters of tax-exempt healthcare issues. However, smaller bond issues, typically $10 million or less, often are sold directly to a single buyer or a small group of buyers. Issues placed directly with lenders, or *private placements*, have the same advantages as term loans, which were discussed in a previous section.

Although the interest rate on private placements is generally higher than the interest rate set on public issues, the administrative costs of placing an issue, such as legal, accounting, printing, and selling fees, are less for private placements than for public issues. Moreover, because there is direct negotiation between the borrower and lender, the opportunity is greater to structure bond terms that are more favorable to the borrower than the terms routinely contained in public debt issues.

Self-Test Questions

1. Describe the primary features of the following long-term debt securities:
   - Term loan
   - Bond
   - First mortgage bond
   - Junior mortgage
   - Debenture
   - Subordinated debenture
   - Municipal bond
2. What are the key differences between a private placement and a public issue?
3. What is the purpose of a bond pool?

Debt Contracts

Debt contracts, which spell out the rights of the borrower and lender(s), have different names depending on the type of debt. The contract between the issuer and bondholders is called an *indenture*. Indentures tend to be long—some run several hundred pages in length. For other types of debt, a similar, but much shorter, document called a *loan agreement* or *promissory note* is used. Health services managers are most concerned about the overall cost of debt, including administrative costs, as well as any provisions that may restrict the business's future actions. In this section, some relevant debt contract features are discussed.

Restrictive Covenants

Many debt contracts include provisions, called *restrictive covenants*, which are designed to protect creditors from managerial actions that would be detrimental to their best interests. For example, the indenture for Palm Coast Medical Center's municipal bond issues contains several restrictive covenants, including the covenant that the issuer must maintain a minimum current ratio of

2.0. The current ratio is defined as current assets divided by current liabilities, so a current ratio of 2.0 indicates that current assets are twice as large as current liabilities. Because the current ratio measures a business's *liquidity*—the ability to meet cash obligations as they become due—a minimum current ratio provides some assurance to bondholders that the interest and principal payments coming due can be covered. If Palm Coast violates any of its restrictive covenants—say, by allowing its current ratio to drop below 2.0—it is said to be in *technical default*. ("Regular" default occurs when an interest or principal payment is not paid on time, which is called a *missed* payment.)

Trustees

When debt is supplied by a single creditor, there is a one-to-one relationship between the lender and borrower. However, bond issues can have thousands of lenders, so a single voice is needed to represent bondholders. This function is performed by a *trustee*, usually an institution such as a bank, which represents the bondholders and ensures that the terms of the indenture are being carried out. The trustee is responsible for monitoring the issuer and for taking appropriate action if a covenant violation occurs. What constitutes appropriate action varies with the circumstances. A trustee has the power to *foreclose* on an issue in default, which makes the full amount of principal and unpaid interest due and payable immediately. However, insisting on immediate payment may result in bankruptcy and possibly large losses on the bonds. In such a case, the trustee may decide that the bondholders would be better served by giving the issuer a chance to work out its problems, which would avoid forcing the business into bankruptcy.

Call Provisions

A *call provision* gives the issuer the right to call a bond for *redemption* prior to maturity; that is, the issuer can pay off the bond in its entirety and *redeem*, or *retire*, the issue. If it is used, the call provision generally states that the firm must pay an amount greater than the initial amount borrowed. The additional sum required is defined as the *call premium*.

Many callable bonds offer a period of call protection, which protects investors from a call just a short time after the bonds are issued. For example, the 20-year callable bonds issued by Vanguard Healthcare in 2006 are not callable until 2115, which is ten years after the original issue date. This type of call provision is known as a *deferred call*.

The call privilege is valuable to the issuer but potentially detrimental to bondholders, especially if the bond is issued during a period when interest rates are cyclically high. In general, bonds are called when interest rates have fallen because the issuer usually replaces the old, high-interest issue with a new, lower-interest issue and hence reduces annual interest expense. When this occurs, investors are forced to reinvest the principal returned in new securities at the then current (lower) rate. As readers will see later, the added risk to lenders of a call provision causes the interest rate on a new issue of callable bonds to exceed that on a similar new issue of noncallable bonds.

If a bond, or other debt security, has a call provision and interest rates drop, the issuer has to make a decision, called a *refunding decision*, as to whether or not to call the issue. In essence, the decision involves a cost/benefit analysis wherein the costs are the administrative costs associated with calling one bond and issuing another, while the benefits are lower future interest payments.[3]

Self-Test Questions

1. Describe the following debt contract features:
   • Bond indenture
   • Restrictive covenant
   • Trustee
   • Call provision
2. What is the difference between technical default and "regular" default?
3. What impact does a call provision have on an issue's interest rate?

Bond Ratings

Since the early 1900s, bonds have been assigned quality ratings that reflect their probability of going into default.[4] The three primary rating agencies are Fitch Ratings, Moody's Investors Service (Moody's), and Standard & Poor's (S&P). All three agencies rate both corporate and municipal bonds. Standard & Poor's rating designations are shown in Table 11.1, but all three have similar rating designations. Bonds with a BBB and higher rating are called *investment grade*, while double B and lower bonds, called *junk bonds*, are more speculative in nature because they have a much higher probability of going into default than do higher rated bonds.

TABLE 11.1
Standard & Poor's Bond Ratings

Credit Risk	Rating Category
Prime	AAA
Excellent	AA
Upper medium	A
Lower medium	BBB
Speculative	BB
Very speculative	B
	CCC
	CC
Default	D

Note: S&P uses plus and minus modifiers for bond ratings below triple A. Thus, A+ designates the strongest A-rated bond and A− the weakest.

Bond Rating Criteria

Although the rating assignments are subjective, they are based on both qualitative characteristics, such as quality of management, and quantitative factors, such as a business's financial strength. Analysts at the rating agencies have consistently stated that no precise formula is used to set a firm's rating—many factors are taken into account, but not in a mathematically precise manner. Statistical studies have supported this contention. Researchers who have tried to predict bond ratings on the basis of quantitative data have had only limited success, which indicates that the agencies do indeed use a good deal of judgment to establish a bond rating.

Importance of Bond Ratings

Bond ratings are important both to businesses and to investors. First, a bond's rating is an indicator of its default risk, so the rating has a direct, measurable influence on the interest rate required by investors and hence on the firm's cost of debt capital. Second, most corporate (i.e., taxable) bonds are purchased by institutional investors rather than by individuals. Many of these institutions are restricted to investment-grade securities. Also, most individual investors who buy municipal bonds are unwilling to take high risks in their bond purchases. Thus, if an issuer's bonds fall below BBB, it will be more difficult to sell new bonds because the number of potential purchasers is reduced. As a result of their higher risk and more restricted market, low-grade bonds typically carry much higher interest rates than do high-grade bonds. For example, in mid-2007, long-term BBB-rated corporate bonds had an interest rate that was 1.1 percentage points above AAA-rate bonds, BB bonds were 1.6 points above BBB bonds, B bonds were 4.5 points above BB bonds, and CCC bonds were 8.2 points above B bonds. Clearly, the interest rate penalty for having a low bond rating is significant.

Changes in Ratings

A change in a firm's bond rating will have a significant effect on the firm's ability to borrow long-term capital and on the cost of that capital. Rating agencies review outstanding bonds on a periodic basis, and occasionally they upgrade or downgrade a bond as a result of the issuer's changed circumstances. Also, an announcement that a company plans to sell a new debt issue, or to merge with another company and pay for the acquisition by exchanging bonds for the stock of the acquired company, will trigger an agency review and possibly lead to a rating change. If a firm's situation has deteriorated somewhat, but its bonds have not been reviewed and downgraded, it may choose to use a term loan or short-term debt rather than to finance through a public bond issue. This will perhaps postpone a rating agency review until the situation has improved.

Credit Enhancement

Credit enhancement, or *bond insurance*, which is available primarily for municipal bonds, is a relatively recent form of insurance that upgrades a bond's rating to AAA. Credit enhancement is offered by several credit insurers, the three largest being the Municipal Bond Investors Assurance (MBIA) Corporation, Ambac Assurance Corporation, and Financial Guaranty Insurance Company. Currently, almost half of all new healthcare municipal issues carry bond insurance.

Here is how credit enhancement works. Regardless of the inherent credit rating of the issuer, the bond insurer guarantees that bondholders will receive the promised interest and principal payments. Thus, bond insurance protects investors against default by the issuer. Because the insurer gives its guarantee that payments will be made, an insured bond carries the credit rating of the insurance company rather than that of the issuer. For example, Sabal Palms Medical Center has an A rating, so new bonds issued by the hospital without credit enhancement would be rated A. However, in 2006, Sabal Palms Medical Center issued $50 million of hospital revenue bonds with an AAA rating because of MBIA insurance.

Credit enhancement gives the issuer access to the lowest possible interest rate, but not without a cost. Bond insurers typically charge an up-front fee of about 45 to 75 basis points of the **total debt service** over the life of the bond—the lower the hospital's inherent credit rating, the higher the cost of bond insurance. Most of the newly issued insured municipal bonds have an underlying credit rating of AA or A. The remainder are still of investment grade, rated BBB.

Interest Rate Components

As we discussed previously, investors require compensation for time value, inflation, and risk. The relationship is formalized for stock investments by the Capital Asset Pricing Model (CAPM), which we discussed in Chapter 10. For debt investments, the rate of return (i.e., the interest rate) required by investors consists of several components. By understanding the components, it is possible to gain insights into why interest rates change over time, differ among borrowers, and even differ on separate issues by the same borrower.

Real Risk-Free Rate (RRF)

The base upon which all interest rates are built is the *real risk-free rate* (RRF). This is the rate that investors would demand on a debt security that is totally **riskless** when there is **no inflation**. Thus, the RRF compensates investors for the time value of money but considers no other factors. Although difficult to measure, the RRF is thought to fall somewhere in the range of 2 to 4 percent. In the real world, inflation is rarely zero, and most debt securities have some risk; thus, the actual interest rate on a given debt security will typically be higher than the real risk-free rate.

Inflation Premium (IP)

Inflation has a major impact on required interest rates because it erodes the purchasing power of the dollar and lowers the value of investment returns. Creditors, who are the suppliers of debt capital, are well aware of the impact of inflation. Thus, they build an *inflation premium* (IP) into the interest rate that is equal to the expected inflation rate over the life of the security.

For example, suppose that the real risk-free rate was RRF = 3%, and that inflation was expected to be 2 percent (and hence IP = 2%) during the next year. The rate of interest on a one-year riskless debt security would be 3% + 2% = 5%.

The rate of inflation built into interest rates is the rate of inflation **expected in the future**, not the rate experienced in the past. Thus, the latest reported figures may show an annual inflation rate of 3 percent, but that is for a past period. If investors expect a 2 percent inflation rate in the future, then 2 percent would be built into the current rate of interest. Also, the inflation rate reflected in any interest rate is the average rate of inflation expected **over the life of the security**. Thus, the inflation rate built into a one-year bond is the expected inflation rate for the next year, but the inflation rate built into a 30-year bond is the average rate of inflation expected over the next 30 years. Note that the combination of the RRF and the IP is called the *risk-free rate* (RF). Thus, the risk-free rate incorporates inflation expectations, but it does not incorporate any risk factors. In this example, RF = 5%.

Default Risk Premium (DRP)

The risk that a borrower will default (not make the promised payments) has a significant impact on the interest rate set on a debt security. This risk, along with the possible consequences of default, are captured by a *default risk premium* (DRP). Treasury securities have no default risk; thus, they carry the lowest interest rates on taxable securities in the United States. For corporate and municipal bonds, the higher the bond's rating, the lower its default risk. All else the same, the lower the default risk, the lower the DRP and interest rate.

Liquidity Premium (LP)

A *liquid asset* is one that can be sold quickly at a predictable fair market price, and thus can be converted to a known amount of cash on short notice. Active markets, which provide liquidity, exist for Treasury securities and for the stocks and bonds of larger corporations. Securities issued by small companies, including healthcare providers that issue municipal bonds, are *illiquid*—once bought they can be resold by the owner, but not quickly and not at a predictable price. Furthermore, illiquid securities are normally difficult to sell and hence have relatively high *transactions costs*. (Transactions costs include commissions, fees, and other expenses associated with selling securities.)

If a security is illiquid, investors will add a *liquidity premium* (*LP*) when they set their required interest rate. It is very difficult to measure liquidity premiums with precision, but a differential of at least 2 percentage points is thought to exist between the least liquid and the most liquid securities of similar default risk and maturity.

Price Risk Premium (PRP)

As will be demonstrated later in the bond valuation section, the market value (price) of a long-term bond declines sharply when interest rates rise. Because interest rates can and do rise, all long-term bonds, including Treasury bonds, have an element of risk called *price risk*. For example, assume an individual bought a 30-year Treasury bond for $1,000 when the long-term interest rate on Treasury securities was 7 percent. Then, if ten years later T-bond rates had risen to 14 percent, the value of the bond would have fallen to under $600. That would represent a sizable loss on the investment, which demonstrates that long-term bonds—even U.S. Treasury bonds—are not riskless.

As a general rule, the bonds of any organization, from the U.S. government to Manor Care to St. Vincent's Community Hospital, have more price risk the longer the maturity of the bond. Therefore, a *price risk premium* (*PRP*), which is tied directly to the term to maturity, must be included in the interest rate. The effect of price risk premiums is to raise interest rates on long-term bonds relative to those on short-term bonds. This premium, like the others, is extremely difficult to measure, but it seems to vary over time; it rises when interest rates are more volatile and uncertain and falls when they are more stable. In recent years, the price risk premium on 30-year T-bonds appears to have been generally in the range of 0.5 to 2 percentage points.

Call Risk Premium (CRP)

Bonds that are callable are riskier for investors than those that are noncallable because callable bonds have uncertain maturities. Furthermore, bonds typically are called when interest rates fall, so bondholders must reinvest the call proceeds at a lower interest rate. To compensate for bearing call risk, investors charge a *call risk premium* (*CRP*) on callable bonds. The amount of the premium depends on such factors as the interest rate on the bond, current interest rate levels, and time to first call (the call deferral period). Historically, call risk premiums have been in the range of 30 to 50 basis points.

Combining the Components

When all the interest rate components are taken into account, the interest rate required on any debt security can be expressed as follows:

$$\text{Interest rate} = \text{RRF} + \text{IP} + \text{DRP} + \text{LP} + \text{PRP} + \text{CRP}.$$

First consider one-year Treasury bills. Assume that RRF is 2 percent, and inflation is expected to average 3 percent in the coming year. Because T-bills have no default, liquidity, or call risk, and almost no price risk, the interest rate on a one-year T-bill would be 5 percent:

$$\text{Interest rate}_{\text{T-bill}} = \text{RRF} + \text{IP} + \text{DRP} + \text{LP} + \text{PRP} + \text{CRP}$$
$$= 2\% + 3\% + 0 + 0 + 0 + 0 = 5\%.$$

As discussed previously, the combination of RRF and IP is the risk-fee rate, so RF = 5%. In general, the rate of interest on short-term Treasury securities (T-bills) is used as a proxy for the **short-term** risk-free rate.

Consider another illustration, the callable 30-year corporate bonds issued by HealthWest Corporation. Assume that these bonds have an inflation premium of 4 percent; default risk, liquidity, and price risk premiums of 1 percent each; and a call risk premium of 40 basis points. Under these assumptions, these bonds would have an interest rate of 9.4 percent:

$$\text{Interest rate}_{\text{30-year bonds}} = \text{RRF} + \text{IP} + \text{DRP} + \text{LP} + \text{PRP} + \text{CRP}$$
$$= 2\% + 4\% + 1\% + 1\% + 1\% + 0.4\% = 9.4\%.$$

When interest rates are viewed as the sum of a base rate plus premiums for inflation and risk, it is easy to visualize the underlying economic forces that cause interest rates to vary among different issues and over time.

Self-Test Questions

1. Write out an equation for the required interest rate on a debt security.
2. What is the difference between the real risk-free rate, RRF, and the risk-free rate, RF?
3. Do the interest rates on Treasury securities include a default risk premium? A liquidity premium? A price risk premium? Explain your answer.
4. Why are callable bonds riskier for investors than similar bonds without a call provision?
5. What is price risk? What type of debt securities would have the largest price risk premium?

The Term Structure of Interest Rates

At certain times, short-term interest rates are lower than long-term rates; at other times, short-term rates are higher than long-term rates; and at yet other times, short-term and long-term rates are roughly equal. The relationship between long- and short-term rates, which is called the *term structure of interest rates*, is important to health services managers who must decide whether to borrow by issuing long- or short-term debt and to investors who must decide whether to buy long- or short-term debt. Thus, it is important to understand how interest rates on long- and short-term debt are related to one another.

To examine the current term structure, look up the interest rates on debt of various maturities by a single issuer (usually the U.S. Treasury) in a source such as the *Wall Street Journal*. For example, the tabular section of Figure 11.1 presents interest rates for Treasury securities of different maturities on two dates. The set of data for a given date, when plotted on a graph, is called a *yield curve*. As shown in the figure, the yield curve changes both in position and in shape over time. Had the yield curve been drawn during late July 2006, it would have been essentially horizontal because long-term and short-term bonds at that time had about the same rate of interest.

On average, long-term rates have been higher than short-term rates, so the yield curve usually slopes upward. An *upward-sloping curve* would be expected if the inflation premium is relatively constant across all maturities because the price risk premium applied to long-term issues will push long-term rates above short-term rates. Because an upward-sloping yield curve is most prevalent, this shape is also called a *normal yield curve*. Conversely, a yield curve that slopes downward is called an *inverted*, or *abnormal*, *yield curve*. Thus, the yield curve for March 1980 is inverted, but the one for March 2004 is normal.[5]

Figure 11.1 shows yield curves for U.S. Treasury securities, but the curves could have been constructed for similarly rated corporate or municipal (i.e., tax-exempt) debt, if the data were available. In each case, the yield curve would be approximately the same shape but would differ in vertical position. For example, had the yield curve been constructed for Beverly Enterprises, a for-profit nursing home operator, it would fall above the Treasury curve because interest rates on corporate debt include default risk premiums, while Treasury rates do not. Conversely, the curve for Baptist Medical Center, a not-for-profit hospital, would probably fall below the Treasury curve because the tax-exemption benefit, which lowers the interest rate on tax-exempt securities, generally outweighs the default risk premium. In every case, however, the riskier the issuer (i.e., the lower the debt is rated), the higher the yield curve plots on the graph.

Health services managers use yield curve information to help make decisions regarding debt maturities. To illustrate, assume for the moment that it is December 2007, and that the yield curve for March 2004 in Figure 11.1

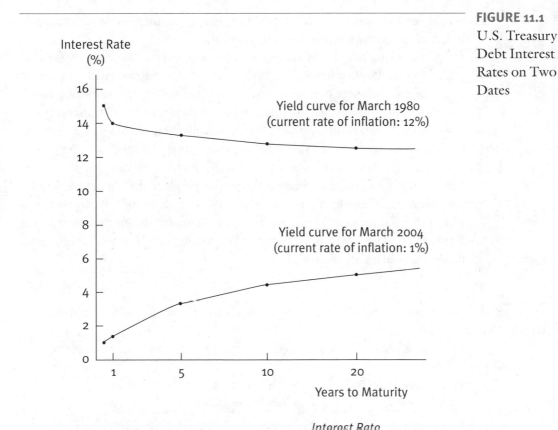

FIGURE 11.1

U.S. Treasury
Debt Interest
Rates on Two
Dates

	Interest Rate	
Term to Maturity	March 1980	March 2004
6 months	15.0%	1.0%
1 year	14.0	1.3
5 years	13.5	3.2
10 years	12.8	4.2
20 years	12.5	5.0

applies to Baptist Medical Center. Now, assume that the hospital plans to issue $10 million of debt to finance a new outpatient clinic with a 30-year life. If it borrowed in 2007 on a short-term basis—say for one year—Baptist's interest cost for that year would be 1.3 percent, or $130,000. If it used long-term (20-year) financing, its cost would be 5.0 percent, or $500,000. Therefore, at first glance, it would seem that Baptist should use short-term debt.

However, if the hospital uses short-term debt, it will have to renew the loan every year at the then current short-term rate. Although unlikely, it is possible that interest rates could soar to 1980 levels. If this happened, by 2013 or so the hospital might be paying 14 percent, or $1.4 million, per year. Conversely, if Baptist used long-term financing in 2007, its interest costs would remain constant at $500,000 per year, so an increase in interest rates in the economy would not hurt the hospital.

Financing decisions would be easy if managers could accurately forecast interest rates. Unfortunately, predicting future interest rates with consistent accuracy is somewhere between difficult and impossible—people who make a living by selling interest rate forecasts say it is difficult, but many others say it is impossible. Sound financial policy, therefore, calls for a mix of long- and short-term debt, as well as equity, in such a manner that the business can survive in all but the most severe, and hence unlikely, interest rate environments. Furthermore, the optimal financing policy depends in an important way on the maturities of the firm's assets: In general, to reduce risk, managers try to match the maturities of the financing with the maturities of the assets being financed. This issue will be addressed again in Chapter 16 when current asset financing policies are discussed.

Self-Test Questions	1. What is a yield curve, and what information is needed to create this curve?
	2. What is the difference between a normal yield curve and an abnormal one?
	3. If short-term rates are lower than long-term rates, why may a business still choose to finance with long-term debt?
	4. Explain the following statement: "A firm's financing policy depends in large part on the nature of its assets."

Economic Factors That Influence Interest Rate Levels

The general level of interest rates, as opposed to the rate set on a particular debt issue, and the shape of the yield curve are influenced by economic factors. The three most important of these factors are (1) Federal Reserve policy, (2) federal budgetary policy, and (3) the overall level of business activity.

Federal Reserve Policy

The money supply has a significant effect on both the level of economic activity and the inflation rate, and hence on the level of interest rates. In the United States, the money supply and short-term interest rates are controlled by the *Federal Reserve Board* (the "*Fed*"). If the Fed wants to stimulate the economy, it increases the growth of the money supply and lowers the short-term interest rate that banks charge one another to borrow funds. Alternatively, if the Fed believes that the economy is overheated and inflation will be a problem in the future, it tightens (reduces) the money supply and raises short-term rates. During periods when the Fed is actively intervening in the credit markets, interest rates are affected and the yield curve may be temporarily distorted— that is, short-term rates may temporarily be "too high" or "too low." Typically, the impact of Fed actions on short-term interest rates is much greater than on long-term rates.

Federal Budgetary Policy

If the federal government spends more than it receives in tax revenues, it runs a deficit. Typically the shortfall is covered by government borrowing (issuing treasury securities), which increases the demand for debt capital and hence raises the general level of interest rates. The relative impact on short-term and long-term rates depends on how the deficit is financed. Reliance on short-term debt would raise short-term rates, while reliance on long-term debt would increase long-term rates. Over the past several decades, the federal government has, except for a few years, had an annual deficit, which has pushed the national debt to over $8 trillion. Clearly, federal borrowings have exerted upward pressure on the overall level of interest rates. Because the government uses both short- and long-term borrowing to finance its deficits, the impact on the yield curve is uncertain.

Level of Economic Activity

Business conditions have a significant effect on interest rates. Consumer demand slows during recessions and low-growth periods, which means that less goods and services are sold, especially durable goods (houses, automobiles, and the like). At the same time, companies hire fewer employees and spend less on new capital assets (land, buildings, and equipment). The net result is downward pressure on inflation and on the demand for borrowed funds, and hence downward pressure on interest rates. At the same time, the Fed is trying to stimulate the economy by increasing the money supply and lowering short-term rates. In general, these conditions tend to have more of an impact on short-term rates than on long-term rates because (1) the Fed operates in the short end of the credit markets, and (2) long-term inflation expectations are not as volatile as short-term expectations. The story is reversed when the economy is booming.

1. Describe three economic factors that influence the general level of interest rates.
2. Do these factors have a greater influence on short-term or long-term rates? Explain.

Self-Test Questions

Debt Valuation

Now that the basics of long-term debt financing have been discussed, the next step is to understand how investors value debt securities. Security valuation concepts are important to health services managers for many reasons. Here are just a few:

- The lifeblood of any business is capital. In fact, one of the most common reasons for business failures is insufficient capital. Therefore, it is vital that managers understand how investors make investment decisions.
- For investor-owned firms, stock price maximization is the primary goal, so managers of for-profit firms must know how investors value the firm's stock to understand how managerial actions affect price.
- For both for-profit and not-for-profit businesses, debt financing is an important source of capital. Thus, health services managers must understand how lenders value debt securities.
- For health services managers to make financially sound decisions regarding real-asset investments (e.g., plant and equipment), it is necessary to estimate the business's cost of capital. Security valuation is a necessary skill in this process, which is covered in detail in Chapter 13.
- Real assets are valued in the same general way as securities. Thus, security valuation provides managers with an excellent foundation to learn real-asset valuation, the heart of capital investment decision making within health services organizations. The concepts presented here are crucial to a good understanding of Chapters 14 and 15.

General Valuation Model

In the financial sense, the value of any asset (investment) stems from the same source: the cash flows that the asset is expected to produce. Thus, all assets are valued financially in the same way:

- **Estimate the expected cash flow stream.** Estimating the cash flow stream involves estimating the expected cash flow in each period during the life of the asset. For some assets, such as Treasury securities, the estimation process is quite easy because the interest and principal repayment stream is specified by contract. For other assets, such as the stock of a biotechnology start-up company that is not yet paying dividends or a healthcare provider's new service line, the estimation process can be very difficult.
- **Assess the riskiness of the stream.** The next step is to assess the riskiness of the cash flows. The cash flows of most assets are not known with certainty but are best represented by probability distributions. The more uncertain these distributions, the greater the riskiness of the cash flow stream. Again, in some situations it will be fairly easy to assess the riskiness of the estimated cash flow stream; in other situations it may be quite difficult.
- **Set the required rate of return.** The required rate of return on the cash flow stream is established on the basis of the stream's riskiness and the returns available on alternative investments of similar risk. In essence, the *opportunity cost* principle discussed in Chapter 9 is applied here. By investing in one asset, the funds are no longer available for alternative investments. This opportunity cost sets the required rate of return on the asset being valued.

- **Discount and sum the expected cash flows.** Each expected cash flow is now discounted at the asset's required rate of return and the present values are summed to find the value of the asset.

The following time line formalizes the valuation process:

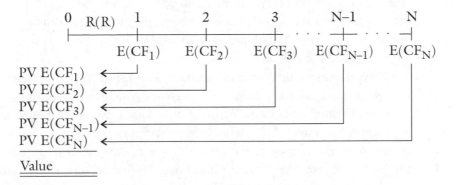

Here, $E(CF_t)$ is the expected cash flow in each Period t, $R(R)$ is the required rate of return (i.e., the opportunity cost rate) on the asset, and N is the number of periods for which cash flows are expected. The periods can be months, quarters, semiannual periods, or years, depending on the frequency of the cash flows expected from the asset.

The general valuation model can be applied to both *financial assets (securities)*, such as stocks and bonds, and *real (physical) assets*, such as buildings, equipment, and even whole businesses. Each asset type requires a somewhat different application of the general valuation model, but the basic approach remains the same. In this chapter, the general valuation model is applied to debt securities (bonds). In the chapters that follow, the model is applied to stocks and to real assets.

Definitions

We will use bonds to illustrate debt valuation, although the techniques used are applicable to most types of debt. To begin, here are some required definitions:

- **Par value.** The *par value*, also called *par*, is the stated (face) value of the bond. It is often set at $1,000 or $5,000. The par value generally represents the amount of money the business borrows (per bond) and promises to repay at some future date.
- **Maturity date.** Bonds generally have a specified *maturity date* on which the par value will be repaid. For example, Big Sky Healthcare, a for-profit hospital system, issued $50 million worth of $1,000 par value bonds on January 1, 2007. The bonds will mature on December 31, 2021, so they had a 15-year maturity at the time they were issued. The effective maturity of a bond declines each year after it was issued. Thus, at the beginning of 2008, Big Sky's bonds will have a 14-year maturity, and so on.

- **Coupon rate.** A bond requires the issuer to pay a specific amount of interest each year or, more typically, each six months. The rate of interest is called the *coupon interest rate*, or just *coupon rate*. The rate may be variable, in which case it is tied to some index, such as 2 percentage points above the prime rate. More commonly, the rate will be fixed over the life (maturity) of the bond. For example, Big Sky's bonds have a 10 percent coupon rate, so each $1,000 par value bond pays $0.10 \times \$1,000 = \$100$ in interest each year. The dollar amount of annual interest, in this case $100, is called the *coupon payment*.[6]

- **New issues versus outstanding bonds.** A bond's value is determined by its coupon payment—the higher the coupon payment, other things held constant, the higher its value. At the time a bond is issued, its coupon rate is generally set at a level that will cause the bond to sell at its par value. In other words, the coupon rate is set at the rate that investors require to buy the bond (i.e., the *going rate*). A bond that has just been issued is called a *new issue*. After the bond has been on the market for about a month it is classified as an *outstanding bond*, or a *seasoned issue*. New issues sell close to par, but because a bond's coupon payment is generally fixed, changing economic conditions (and hence interest rates) will cause a seasoned bond to sell for more or less than its par value.

- **Debt service requirement.** Firms that issue bonds are concerned with their total *debt service requirement*, which includes both interest expense and repayment of principal. For Big Sky, the debt service requirement (payment) is $0.10 \times \$50$ million $= \$5$ million per year until maturity. In 2021, the firm's debt service requirement will be $5 million in interest plus $50 million in principal repayment. Thus, the total debt service requirement on the issue is $(15 \times \$5) + \$50 = \$125$ million. In Big Sky's case, only interest is paid until maturity, so the entire principal amount must be repaid at that time. As discussed earlier, many municipal bonds are serial issues structured so that the debt service requirements are relatively constant over time. In this situation, the issuer pays back a portion of the principal during each year.

The Basic Bond Valuation Model

Bonds typically call for the payment of a specific amount of interest for a specific number of years, and for the repayment of par on the bond's maturity date. Thus, a bond represents an annuity plus a lump sum, and its value is found as the present value of this cash flow stream. Here are the cash flows from Big Sky's bonds on a time line:

0	1	2		13	14	15
	$100	$100	. . .	$100	$100	$ 100
						1,000

If the bonds had just been issued, and the coupon rate was set at the current interest rate for bonds of this risk, then the required rate of return on the bonds, $R(R_d)$, would be 10 percent. Because the value of a bond is merely the present value of the bond's cash flows, discounted to Time 0 at a 10 percent discount rate, the value of the bond at issue was $1,000:

Present value of a 15-year, $100 payment annuity at 10 percent $= \$\ 760.61$

Present value of a $1,000 lump sum discounted 15 years $=\ \underline{239.39}$

Value of bond $= \underline{\$1,000.00}$

The value of the bond can be found using a financial calculator as follows:

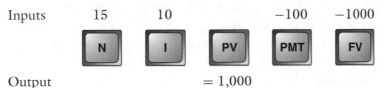

| Inputs | 15 | 10 | | −100 | −1000 |

Output $= 1,000$

Note that the cash flows were treated as outflows so that the value would be displayed as a positive number. Also, in bond valuation, all five time-value-of-money keys on a financial calculator are used because bonds involve both an annuity and a lump sum.

There are two alternative approaches to using a spreadsheet to value bonds:

	A	B	C	D
1				
2	10.0%	Rate	Interest rate	
3				
4	$ 100	Value 1	Year 1 coupon	
5	$ 100	Value 1	Year 2 coupon	
6	$ 100	Value 1	Year 3 coupon	
7	$ 100	Value 1	Year 4 coupon	
8	$ 100	Value 1	Year 5 coupon	
9	$ 100	Value 1	Year 6 coupon	
10	$ 100	Value 1	Year 7 coupon	
11	$ 100	Value 1	Year 8 coupon	
12	$ 100	Value 1	Year 9 coupon	
13	$ 100	Value 1	Year 10 coupon	
14	$ 100	Value 1	Year 11 coupon	
15	$ 100	Value 1	Year 12 coupon	
16	$ 100	Value 1	Year 13 coupon	
17	$ 100	Value 1	Year 14 coupon	
18	$ 1,100	Value 1	Year 15 coupon + Principal	
19				
20	$ 1,000.00	=NPV(A2,A4:A18) (entered into Cell A20)		

Here we listed all of the bond's cash flows and used the NPV function to value the bond. Note that Cell A18 contains $1,100 as the entry, which reflects the $100 interest payment in Year 15 plus the $1,000 return of principal.

	A		B	C	D
1					
2	15		Nper	Number of periods	
3	$	100.00	Pmt	Payment (coupon amount)	
4	$	1,000.00	Fv	Future value (principal)	
5	10%		Rate	Interest rate	
6					
7					
8	$	1,000.00	=−PV(A5,A2,A3,A4) (entered into Cell A8)		
9					
10					

Here we used the PV function to value the bond. Note that when bonds are being valued, the function requires four arguments (entries): interest rate, number of payments, payment (coupon amount), and future value. In Chapter 9, when we used this function to find the present values of annuities, no future value was entered.

The first approach has the advantage that we can easily visualize the bond's cash flows. The second approach has the advantage of being more compact and requiring fewer entries. To save space, we will use the second approach for the remainder of this chapter.

If $R(R_d)$ remained constant at 10 percent over time, what would be the value of the bond one year after it was issued? Now, the term to maturity is only 14 years—that is, $N = 14$. As seen below, the bond's value remains at $1,000:

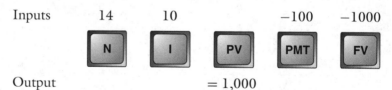

Inputs   14   10   −100   −1000

N   I   PV   PMT   FV

Output   = 1,000

	A		B	C	D
1					
2	14		Nper	Number of periods	
3	$	100.00	Pmt	Payment (coupon amount)	
4	$	1,000.00	Fv	Future value (principal)	
5	10%		Rate	Interest rate	
6					
7					
8	$	1,000.00	=−PV(A5,A2,A3,A4) (entered into Cell A8)		
9					
10					

As long as the required rate of return remains at 10 percent, the bond's value remains at par, or $1,000.

Suppose that interest rates in the economy fell after the bonds were issued, and, as a result, $R(R_d)$ decreased from 10 percent to 5 percent. The coupon rate and par value are fixed by contract, so they remain unaffected by changes in interest rates, but now the discount rate is 5 percent rather than 10 percent. At the end of the first year, with 14 years remaining, the value of the bond would be $1,494.93:

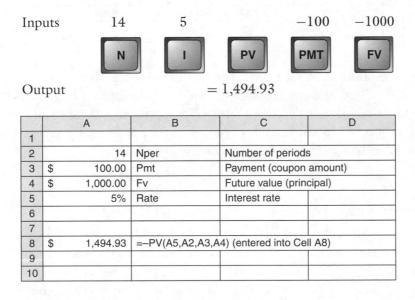

Inputs   14   5   −100   −1000

N   I   PV   PMT   FV

Output   = 1,494.93

	A	B	C	D
1				
2	14	Nper	Number of periods	
3	$ 100.00	Pmt	Payment (coupon amount)	
4	$ 1,000.00	Fv	Future value (principal)	
5	5%	Rate	Interest rate	
6				
7				
8	$ 1,494.93	=−PV(A5,A2,A3,A4) (entered into Cell A8)		
9				
10				

The arithmetic of the bond value increase should be clear (lower discount rates lead to higher present values), but what is the underlying economic logic? The fact that interest rates have fallen to 5 percent means that if an individual had $1,000 to invest, he or she could buy new bonds like Big Sky's (every day some 10 to 20 companies sell new bonds), except that these new bonds would only pay $50 in interest each year. Naturally, the individual would favor an annual payment of $100 over one of $50 and hence would be willing to pay more than $1,000 for Big Sky's bonds. All investors would recognize this; as a result, the Big Sky bonds would be bid up in price to $1,494.93, at which point they would provide the same rate of return as new bonds of similar risk—5 percent.

Assuming that interest rates stay constant at 5 percent over the next 14 years, what would happen to the value of a Big Sky bond? It would fall gradually from $1,494.93 at present to $1,000 at maturity, when the company would redeem each bond for $1,000. This point can be illustrated by calculating the value of the bond one year later, when it has only 13 years remaining to maturity:

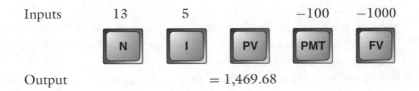

Inputs   13   5   −100   −1000

N   I   PV   PMT   FV

Output   = 1,469.68

	A	B	C	D
1				
2	13	Nper	Number of periods	
3	$ 100.00	Pmt	Payment (coupon amount)	
4	$ 1,000.00	Fv	Future value (principal)	
5	5%	Rate	Interest rate	
6				
7				
8	$ 1,469.68	=–PV(A5,A2,A3,A4) (entered into Cell A8)		
9				
10				

The value of the bond with 13 years to maturity is $1,469.68.

If an individual purchased the bond at a price of $1,494.93 and then sold it one year later with interest rates still at 5 percent, he or she would have a capital loss of $25.25. The rate of return on the bond over the year consists of an *interest*, or *current*, *yield* plus a *capital gains yield*:

Current yield	=	$100/$1,494.93	=	0.0669	=	6.69%
Capital gains yield	=	–$25.25/$1,494.93	=	–0.0169	=	–1.69%
Total rate of return, or yield	=	$74.75/$1,494.93	=	0.0500	=	5.00%

Had interest rates risen from 10 to 15 percent during the first year after issue, rather than falling as they did, the value of Big Sky's bonds would have declined to $713.78 at the end of the first year. If interest rates held constant at 15 percent, the bond would have a value of $720.84 at the end of the second year, so the total yield to investors would be:

Current yield	=	$100/$713.78	=	0.1401	=	14.01%
Capital gains yield	=	$7.06/$713.78	=	0.0099	=	0.99%
Total rate of return, or yield	=	$107.06/$713.78	=	0.1500	=	15.00%

Figure 11.2 graphs the values of the Big Sky bond over time, assuming that interest rates will remain constant at 10 percent, fall to 5 percent and remain at that level, and then rise to 15 percent and remain constant at that level. The figure illustrates the following important points:

- Whenever the required rate of return on a bond equals its coupon rate, the bond will sell at its par value.
- When interest rates, and hence required rates of return, fall after a bond is issued, the bond's value rises above its par value, and the bond sells at a *premium*.
- When interest rates, and hence required rates of return, rise after a bond is issued, the bond's value falls below its par value, and the bond sells at a *discount*.
- Bond prices on outstanding issues and interest rates are inversely related. Increasing rates lead to falling prices, and decreasing rates lead to increasing prices.
- The price of a bond will always approach its par value as its maturity date approaches, provided the issuer does not default on the bond.

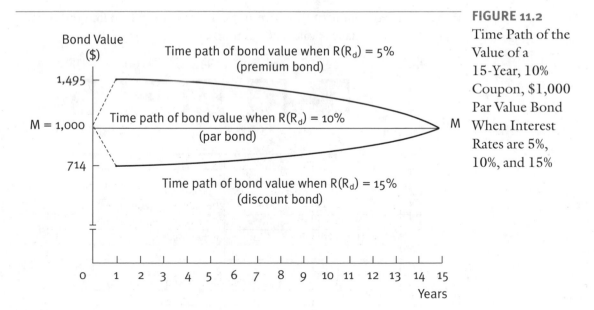

FIGURE 11.2
Time Path of the
Value of a
15-Year, 10%
Coupon, $1,000
Par Value Bond
When Interest
Rates are 5%,
10%, and 15%

| | Bond Value at a Required Rate of Return of | | |
Year	5%	10%	15%
0	—	$1,000.00	—
1	$1,494.93	1,000.00	$ 713.78
2	1,469.68	1,000.00	720.84
3	1,443.16	1,000.00	728.97
.	.	.	.
.	.	.	.
.	.	.	.
13	1,092.97	1,000.00	918.71
14	1,047.62	1,000.00	956.52
15	1,000.00	1,000.00	1,000.00

Note, however, that interest rates do **not** remain constant over time, so in reality a bond's price fluctuates both as interest rates in the economy fluctuate and the bond's term to maturity decreases. In addition, a bond's price will change if there is a change in the creditworthiness of the issuer.

Yield to Maturity on a Bond

Up to this point, a bond's required rate of return and cash flows have been used to determine its value. In reality, investors' required rates of return on securities are not observable, but security prices can be easily determined, at least on those securities that are actively traded, by looking in the *Wall Street Journal* or by using some other data source. Suppose that the Big Sky bond had 14 years remaining to maturity, and the bond was selling at a price of $1,494.93. What rate of return, or *yield to maturity* (*YTM*), would be earned if the bond was bought at this price and held to maturity? To find the answer, 5 percent, use a financial calculator as follows:

Inputs	14		1494.93	−100	−1000
	N	I	PV	PMT	FV

Output = 5.00

	A	B	C	D
1				
2	14	Nper	Number of periods	
3	$ 1,494.93	Pv	Present value (bond price)	
4	$ (100.00)	Pmt	Payment (coupon amount)	
5	$ (1,000.00)	Fv	Future value (principal)	
6				
7				
8	5.00%	=RATE(A2,A4,A3,A5) (entered into Cell A8)		
9				
10				

The YTM is the *expected rate of return* on a bond, assuming it is held to maturity and no default occurs. It is similar to the total rate of return discussed in the previous section. For a bond that sells at par, the YTM consists entirely of an interest yield, but if the bond sells at a discount or premium, the YTM consists of the current yield plus a positive or negative capital gains yield.

Bonds that are callable have both a YTM and a *yield to call (YTC)*. The YTC is the expected rate of return on the bond assuming it will be called and assuming that the probability of default is zero. The YTC is calculated like the YTM, except that N reflects the number of years until the bond will be called, as opposed to years to maturity, and M reflects the call price rather than the maturity value.

Bond Values with Semiannual Compounding

Virtually all bonds issued in the United States actually pay interest semiannually, or every six months. To apply the preceding valuation concepts to semiannual bonds, the bond valuation procedures must be modified as follows:

- Divide the annual interest payment, INT, by two to determine the dollar amount paid **each six months**.
- Multiply the number of years to maturity, N, by two to determine the number of **semiannual interest periods**.
- Divide the annual required rate of return, $R(R_d)$, by two to determine the **semiannual required rate of return**.

To illustrate the use of the semiannual bond valuation model, assume that the Big Sky bonds pay $50 every six months rather than $100 annually.

Thus, each interest payment is only half as large, but there are twice as many of them. When the going rate of interest is 5 percent annually, the value of Big Sky's bonds with 14 years left to maturity is $1,499.12:

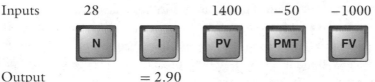

Inputs	28	2.5		−50	−1000
	N	I	PV	PMT	FV

Output   = 1,499.12

	A		B	C	D
1					
2		28	Nper	Number of periods	
3	$	50.00	Pmt	Payment (coupon amount)	
4	$	1,000.00	Fv	Future value (principal)	
5		2.5%	Rate	Interest rate	
6					
7					
8	$	1,499.12	=−PV(A5,A2,A3,A4) (entered into Cell A8)		
9					
10					

Similarly, if the bond were actually selling for $1,400 with 14 years to maturity, its YTM would be 5.80 percent:

Inputs	28		1400	−50	−1000
	N	I	PV	PMT	FV

Output   = 2.90

	A		B	C	D
1					
2		28	Nper	Number of periods	
3	$	1,400.00	Pv	Present value (bond price)	
4	$	(50.00)	Pmt	Payment (coupon amount)	
5	$	(1,000.00)	Fv	Future value (principal)	
6					
7					
8		2.90%	=RATE(A2,A4,A3,A5) (entered into Cell A8)		
9					
10					

The value for I (or rate), 2.90 percent, is the **periodic (semiannual) YTM**, so it is necessary to multiply it by two to get the **annual YTM**. It is convention in the bond markets to quote all rates on a stated annual basis, which is fine when bonds—all of which have semiannual coupons—are being compared. However, when the returns on securities that have different periodic payments are being compared, all rates of return should be expressed as effective annual rates.[7]

Interest Rate Risk

Interest rates change over time, which causes two types of risk that fall under the general classification of *interest rate risk*. First, as illustrated in our discussion of bond valuation, an increase in interest rates leads to a decline in the values of outstanding bonds. Because interest rates can increase at any time, bondholders face the risk of losses on their holdings. This risk is called *price risk*. Second, many bondholders buy bonds to build funds for future use. These bondholders reinvest the interest (and perhaps principal) cash flows as they are received. If interest rates fall, bondholders will earn a lower rate on the reinvested cash flows, which will have a negative impact on the future value of their holdings. This risk is called *reinvestment rate risk*.

An investor's exposure to price risk depends on the maturity of the bonds. To illustrate, Figure 11.3 shows the values of $1,000 par value bonds with one-year and 14-year maturities at several different market interest rates. Notice how much more sensitive the price of the 14-year bond is to changes in interest rates. In general, the longer the maturity of the bond, the greater its price change in response to a given change in interest rates. Thus, bonds with longer maturities are exposed to more price risk.

Although a one-year bond exposes the buyer to less price risk than a 14-year bond, the one-year bond carries with it more reinvestment rate risk. If the holding period is more than one year, the principal and interest will have to be reinvested after one year. If interest rates fall, the return earned during the second year will be less than the return earned during the first year. Reinvestment rate risk is the second dimension of interest rate risk.

Clearly, bond investors face both price risk and reinvestment rate risk as a result of interest rate fluctuations over time. Which risk is most meaningful to a particular investor depends on the circumstances, but in general, interest rate risk, including both price and reinvestment rate risk, is reduced by matching the maturity of the bond with the investor's *investment horizon*, or *holding period*. For example, suppose Hilldale Community Hospital received a $5 million contribution that it will use in five years to build a new neonatal care center. By investing the contribution in five-year bonds, the hospital would minimize its interest rate risk because it would be matching its investment horizon. Price risk would be minimized because the bond will mature in five years, and hence investors will receive par value regardless of the level of interest rates at that time. Reinvestment rate risk is also minimized because only the interest on the bond would have to be reinvested during the life of the bond, which is a less risky situation than if both principal and interest had to be reinvested.[8]

Self-Test Questions

1. What is the general valuation model?
2. How are bonds valued?

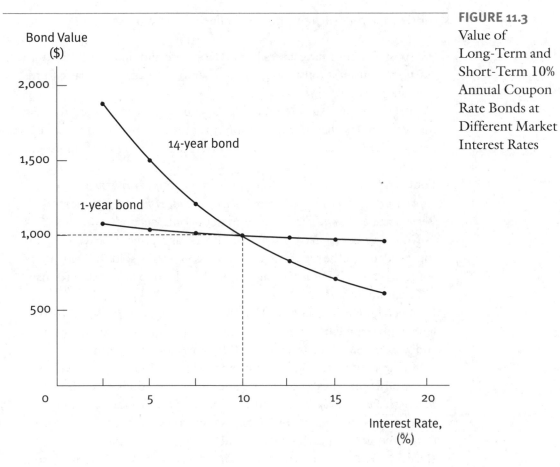

FIGURE 11.3
Value of
Long-Term and
Short-Term 10%
Annual Coupon
Rate Bonds at
Different Market
Interest Rates

Current Market	Bond Value	
Interest Rate	1-Year Bond	14-Year Bond
2.5%	$1,073.17	$1,876.82
5.0	1,047.62	1,494.93
7.5	1,023.26	1,212.23
10.0	1,000.00	1,000.00
12.5	977.78	838.45
15.0	956.52	713.78
17.5	936.17	616.25

3. What is meant by a bond's yield to maturity (YTM)? Its yield to call (YTC)?
4. Differentiate between price risk and reinvestment rate risk.

Key Concepts

This chapter provides an overview of long-term debt financing, including how interest rates are determined, the characteristics of the major types of debt securities, and how such securities are valued. The key concepts of this chapter are:

- Any business must have assets if it is to operate and, in order to acquire assets, the business must raise *capital*. Capital comes in two basic forms, *debt* and *equity* (or *fund*) capital.
- Capital is allocated through the price system; a price is charged to "rent" money. Lenders charge *interest* on funds they lend, while equity investors receive *dividends* and *capital gains* in return for letting the firm use their money.
- Four fundamental factors affect the cost of money: *investment opportunities, time preferences for consumption, risk,* and *inflation.*
- *Term loans* and *bonds* are long-term debt contracts under which a borrower agrees to make a series of interest and principal payments on specific dates to the lender. A term loan is generally sold to one (or a few) lenders, while a bond is typically offered to the public and sold to many different investors.
- In general, debt is categorized as *Treasury*, which is debt issued by the federal government; *corporate*, which is debt issued by taxable businesses; and *municipal*, which is debt issued by non-federal governmental entities, including debt issued on behalf of not-for-profit healthcare providers.
- Many different types of corporate and municipal bonds exist, including *mortgage bonds, debentures,* and *subordinated debentures.* Prevailing interest rates, the bond's riskiness, and tax consequences determine the return required on each type of bond.
- *Revenue bonds* are municipal bonds in which the revenues derived from such projects as roads or bridges, airports, water and sewage systems, and not-for-profit healthcare facilities are pledged as security for the bonds.
- A bond's *indenture* (or a term loan's *agreement*) is a legal document that spells out the rights of both lenders and borrowers.
- A *trustee* is assigned to make sure that the terms of a bond indenture are carried out.
- Bond indentures typically include *restrictive covenants*, which are provisions designed to protect bondholders against detrimental managerial actions.
- A *call provision* gives the issuer the right to redeem the bonds prior to maturity under specified terms, usually at a price greater than the maturity value (the difference is a *call premium*). A firm will call a bond issue and refund it if interest rates fall sufficiently after the bond has been issued.
- Bonds are assigned *ratings* that reflect the probability of their going into default. The higher a bond's rating, and the greater the probability of recovering bondholder capital should default occur, the lower its interest rate.
- *Credit enhancement*, or *bond insurance*, upgrades a municipal bond rating to AAA regardless of the inherent credit rating of the issuer. In essence,

the bond insurer guarantees that bondholders will receive the promised interest and principal payments, even if the issuer defaults.

- The *interest rate* required on a debt security is composed of the real risk-free rate (RRF) plus premiums that reflect inflation (IP), default risk (DRP), liquidity (LP), price risk (PRP), and call risk (CRP):

$$\text{Interest rate } = \text{RRF} + \text{IP} + \text{DRP} + \text{LP} + \text{PRP} + \text{CRP}.$$

- The relationship between the yield and the term to maturity on a security is known as the *term structure of interest rates*. The *yield curve* is a graph of this relationship.
- The general level of interest rates is influenced primarily by three factors: (1) Federal Reserve policy, (2) federal budgetary policy, and (3) the level of economic activity.
- Bonds call for the payment of a specific amount of *interest* for a specific number of years and for the *repayment of par* on the bond's maturity date. Like most assets, a bond's value is simply the present value of the expected cash flow stream.
- The annual rate of return on a bond consists of an *interest*, or *current*, *yield* plus a *capital gains yield*. Assuming constant interest rates, a bond selling at a *discount* will have a positive capital gains, while a bond selling at a *premium* will have a negative capital gains yield.
- A bond's *yield to maturity (YTM)* is the rate of return earned on a bond if it is held to maturity and no default occurs. The YTM for a bond that sells at par consists entirely of an interest yield, but if the bond sells at a discount or premium, the YTM consists of the current yield plus a positive or negative capital gains yield.
- Bondholders face *price risk* because bond values change when interest rates change. An investor's exposure to price risk depends on the maturity of the bonds.
- Bondholders face *reinvestment rate risk* when the investment horizon exceeds the maturity of the bond issue.

Long-term debt is a major source of capital for health services organizations. Thus, it is necessary for health services managers to be familiar with debt concepts. Furthermore, learning how to value long-term debt provides an excellent introduction to asset valuation. The topics covered in this chapter will be useful throughout the remainder of the book.

Questions

11.1 The four fundamental factors that affect the supply of and demand for investment capital, and hence interest rates, are productive opportunities, time preferences for consumption, risk, and inflation. Explain how each of these factors affects the cost of money.

11.2 The interest rate required by investors on a debt security can be expressed by the following equation:

$$\text{Interest rate} = RRF + IP + DRP + LP + PRP + CRP.$$

Define each term of the equation, and explain how it affects the interest rate.

11.3 a. What is a yield curve?
   b. Is the yield curve static, or does it change over time?
   c. What is the difference between a normal yield curve and an inverted yield curve?
   d. What impact does the yield curve have on debt financing decisions?

11.4 Briefly describe the following types of debt:
   a. Term loan
   b. Bond
   c. Mortgage bond
   d. Senior debt; junior debt
   e. Debenture
   f. Subordinated debenture
   g. Municipal bond

11.5 Briefly explain the following debt features:
   a. Indenture
   b. Restrictive covenant
   c. Trustee
   d. Call provision

11.6 a. • What are the three primary bond rating agencies?
      • What do bond ratings measure?
      • How do investors interpret bond ratings?
      • What is the difference between an A-rated bond and a B-rated bond?
   b. • Why are bond ratings important to investors?
      • Why are ratings important to businesses that issue bonds?

11.7 What is credit enhancement?

11.8 What three factors primarily influence the general level of interest rates?

11.9 a. What is price risk?
   b. What is reinvestment rate risk?

11.10 State whether this statement is true or false: "The values of outstanding bonds change whenever the going rate of interest changes. In general, short-term interest rates are more volatile than long-term rates, so short-term bond prices are more sensitive to interest rate changes than are long-term bond prices." Explain your answer.

Problems

11.1 Assume Venture Healthcare sold bonds that have a ten-year maturity, a 12 percent coupon rate with annual payments, and a $1,000 par value.
   a. Suppose that two years after the bonds were issued, the required interest rate fell to 7 percent. What would be the bonds' value?
   b. Suppose that two years after the bonds were issued, the required interest rate rose to 13 percent. What would be the bonds' value?
   c. What would be the value of the bonds three years after issue in each scenario above, assuming that interest rates stayed steady at either 7 percent or 13 percent?

11.2 Twin Oaks Health Center has a bond issue outstanding with a coupon rate of 7 percent and four years remaining until maturity. The par value of the bond is $1,000, and the bond pays interest annually.
   a. Determine the current value of the bond if present market conditions justify a 14 percent required rate of return.
   b. Now, suppose Twin Oaks' four-year bond had semiannual coupon payments. What would be its current value? (Assume a 7 percent semiannual required rate of return. However, the actual rate would be slightly less than 7 percent because a semiannual coupon bond is slightly less risky than an annual coupon bond.)
   c. Assume that Twin Oaks' bond had a semiannual coupon but 20 years remaining to maturity. What is the current value under these conditions? (Again, assume a 7 percent semiannual required rate of return, although the actual rate would probably be greater than 7 percent because of increased price risk.)

11.3 Tidewater Home Health Care, Inc., has a bond issue outstanding with eight years remaining to maturity, a coupon rate of 10 percent with interest paid annually, and a par value of $1,000. The current market price of the bond is $1,251.22.
   a. What is the bond's yield to maturity?
   b. Now, assume that the bond has semiannual coupon payments. What is its yield to maturity in this situation?

11.4 Pacific Homecare has three bond issues outstanding. All three bonds pay $100 in annual interest plus $1,000 at maturity. Bond S has a maturity of five years, Bond M has a 15-year maturity, and Bond L matures in 30 years.
   a. What is the value of each of these bonds when the required interest rate is 5 percent, 10 percent, and 15 percent?
   b. Why is the price of Bond L more sensitive to interest rate changes than the price of Bond S?

11.5 Minneapolis Health System has bonds outstanding that have four years remaining to maturity, a coupon interest rate of 9 percent paid annually, and a $1,000 par value.

a. What is the yield to maturity on the issue if the current market price is $829?

b. If the current market price is $1,104?

c. Would you be willing to buy one of these bonds for $829 if you required a 12 percent rate of return on the issue? Explain your answer.

11.6 Six years ago, Bradford Community Hospital issued 20-year municipal bonds with a 7 percent annual coupon rate. The bonds were called today for a $70 call premium—that is, bondholders received $1,070 for each bond. What is the realized rate of return for those investors who bought the bonds for $1,000 when they were issued?

11.7 Regal Health Plans issued a ten-year, 12 percent annual coupon bond a few years ago. The bond now sells for $1,100. The bond has a call provision that allows Regal to call the bond in four years at a call price of $1,060.

a. What is the bond's yield to maturity?

b. What is the bond's yield to call?

Notes

1. The *prime rate* is the interest rate that banks charge their very best (most creditworthy) customers. Theoretically, the prime rate is set separately by every bank, but in practice all banks follow the lead of the major New York City banks, so there usually is a single prime rate in the United States. The prime rate is changed, sometimes quite rapidly, in response to changing inflation expectations and Federal Reserve Board actions. In July 2007, after a series of interest rate increases by the Federal Reserve Board (the "Fed"), the prime rate stood at 8.25 percent, its highest level since 2001.

2. *Treasury bonds*, or *T-bonds*, have original maturities at issue greater than ten years. The Treasury also issues *notes*, called *T-notes*, which have maturities of two to ten years, and *bills*, called *T-bills*, which have maturities of one year or less. Note that the names of Treasury securities are fixed at issue even though their maturities shorten over time. Thus, a 20-year T-bond that was issued 15 years ago now has only five years remaining to maturity, but it is still classified as a bond, not a note.

3. For more information on the refunding decision, see Louis C. Gapenski, *Understanding Healthcare Financial Management* (Chicago: Health Administration Press, 2007), Chapter 7.

4. Although we focus on bond ratings here, the rating agencies also assign ratings to other types of debt as well as to entire companies.

5. For a discussion of the forces that influence the shape of the yield curve, see Eugene F. Brigham and Michael C. Ehrhardt, *Financial Management: Theory and Practice* (Fort Worth, TX: Thomson/South-Western, 2005), Chapter 1.

6. The term *coupon* goes back to the time when all bonds were *bearer bonds*. Such bonds had small coupons attached, one for each interest payment. To collect an

interest payment, bondholders would remove (i.e., "clip") a coupon and send it to the issuer or take it to a bank, where it would be exchanged for the dollar payment. Today, all bonds are *registered bonds*, and the issuer (through an *agent*) automatically sends interest payments to the registered owner.

7. The effective annual YTM on the bond is $(1.029)^2 - 1.0 = 1.0588 - 1.0 = 0.0588 = 5.88\%$, as compared with the stated rate of 5.80%.

8. Note that reinvestment rate risk could be eliminated if Hilldale purchased five-year *zero coupon bonds*, which pay no interest but sell at a discount when issued.

References

Ambrose, J., and A. Harris. 2006. "Tax-Exempt Private Placements: A New Opportunity for Not-for-Profit Providers." *Healthcare Financial Management* (August): 88–92.

Carlile, L. L., and B. M. Serchuk. 1995. "The Coming Changes in Tax-Exempt Health Care Finance." *Journal of Health Care Finance* (Fall): 1–42.

Carlson, D. A., Jr. 2005. "Catch the Eye of the Capital Markets." *Healthcare Financial Management* (May): 51–58.

Carpenter, C. E., M. J. McCue, and J. B. Hossack. 2001. "Association of Bond, Market, Operational, and Financial Factors with Multi-Hospital System Bond Issues." *Journal of Health Care Finance* (Winter): 26–34.

Carpenter, C. E., M. J. McCue, and S. Moon. 2003. "The Hospital Bond Market and the AHERF Bankruptcy." *Journal of Health Care Finance* (Summer): 17–28.

Cleverley, W. O., and S. J. Baserman. 2005. "Patterns of Financing for the Largest Hospital Systems in the United States." *Journal of Healthcare Management* (November/December): 361–365.

Culler, S. D. 1993. "Assessing Hospital Credit Risk: A Banker's View." *Topics in Health Care Financing* (Summer): 35–43.

———. 1993. "A Creditor's Perspective on the Hospital Industry." *Topics in Health Care Financing* (Summer): 12–20.

Demby, H. J. 1995. "Overcoming Financial Challenges with Bond Insurance." *Healthcare Financial Management* (March): 48–49.

Galtney, B. 2000. "Capital Financing Options for Group Practices." *Healthcare Financial Management* (May): 86–88.

Harris, J. P., and J. B. Price. 1988. "Finding Money Under Your Nose Using New Capital Techniques." *Healthcare Financial Management* (July): 24–30.

Healthcare Financial Management Association (HFMA). 2003. "How Are Hospitals Financing the Future? Access to Capital in Health Care Today." *Healthcare Financial Management* (November): 51–53.

Kaufman, K., and M. L. Hall. 1990. *The Capital Management of Health Care Organizations.* Chicago: Health Administration Press.

LeBuhn, J. 1994. "Primary Market Derivatives: Satisfying Investor Appetites." *Journal of Health Care Finance* (Winter): 11–21.

Lough, S. B. 2000. "Some Tax-Exempt Bond Issues Could Become Taxable." *Healthcare Financial Management* (December): 37–40.

Nemes, J. 1991. "Dealing with the Authorities." *Modern Healthcare* (October 14): 22–29.

O'Neil, P. S., and T. C. Cutting. 2005. "Bondholder Disclosure and Sarbanes-Oxley." *Healthcare Financial Management* (August): 68–73.

Prince, T. R., and R. Ramanan. 1994. "Bond Ratings, Debt Insurance, and Hospital Operating Performance." *Topics in Health Care Financing* (Fall): 36–50.

Rosenthal, R. A., and G. P. Nelson. 2003. "Selling Real Estate to Meet Capital Needs." *Healthcare Financial Management* (May): 50–52.

Smith, S. D. 1994. "The Use of Interest Rate Swaps in Hospital Capital Finance." *Journal of Health Care Finance* (Winter): 35–44.

Sterns, J. B. 1994. "Emerging Trends in Health Care Finance." *Journal of Health Care Finance* (Winter): 1–10.

Sussman, J. H., M. W. Louge, and R. J. McKeown. 2006. "Developing and Implementing a Comprehensive Debt Management Policy." *Healthcare Financial Management* (August): 80–86.

Wareham, T. L. 2004. "A Capital Idea: Bonds and Nontraditional Financing Options." *Healthcare Financial Management* (May): 54–62.

Woodward, M. A. 1993. "Interest Rate Swaps: Financial Tool of the '90s." *Healthcare Financial Management* (November): 56–64.

EQUITY FINANCING

Learning Objectives

After studying this chapter, readers will be able to:

- Describe the key features associated with equity financing.
- Discuss the investment banking process.
- Conduct simple valuation analyses of common stock.
- Explain the concepts of market equilibrium and efficiency.

Introduction

Long-term debt financing was discussed in Chapter 11, including how interest rates are set in the economy; the features of various long-term debt securities; and how debt securities, particularly bonds, are valued. The second primary source of capital to healthcare businesses is *equity financing*. Within investor-owned, or for-profit, firms, equity financing is obtained from shareholders through the sale of *common stock* and by retaining earnings within the business.[1] The equivalent financing in not-for-profit firms, which is sometimes called *fund capital*, is raised through contributions and grants and by retaining earnings. From a financial perspective, common stock and fund financing serve the same basic purpose, so the generic term *equity* will be used to refer to all non-debt capital, regardless of a business's ownership.

In this chapter, we cover the same general issues as in Chapter 11, but the focus here is on equity rather than debt financing. In addition, supplemental information is provided on how securities are sold to investors (the investment banking process) and market efficiency.

Equity in For-Profit Businesses

In for-profit businesses, equity financing is supplied by the owners of the business, either directly through the purchase of an equity interest in the business or indirectly through earnings retention. Because most large for-profit businesses are organized as corporations, the discussion here focuses on corporate stockholders as opposed to proprietors or partners, although many of the concepts apply to all owners.

Stockholders are the owners of for-profit corporations, and as such they have certain rights and privileges. The most important of these rights and privileges are discussed in this section.

Claim on Residual Earnings

The reason that most people buy common stock is to gain the right to a proportionate share of the *residual earnings* of the firm. A firm's net income, which is the residual earnings after all expenses have been paid, belongs to the firm's stockholders. Some portion of net income may be paid out in *dividends*, in which case stockholders receive quarterly cash payments.[2]

The portion of net income that is retained within the business will be invested in new assets, which presumably will increase the firm's earnings, and hence dividends, over time. An increasing dividend stream means that the stock will be more valuable in the future than it is today because dividends will be higher—for example, in five years—than they are now. Thus, stockholders typically expect to be able to sell their stock at some time in the future at a higher price than they paid for it and hence realize a *capital gain*. To illustrate the payment of dividends, consider Table 12.1, which lists the annual per share dividend payment and earnings, as well as the average annual stock price, for Big Sky Healthcare from 1997 through 2007. Over the ten growth periods, Big Sky's dividend grew by 275 percent, or at an average annual rate of 14.1 percent. At the same time, the firm's stock price grew by 247 percent, producing an average annual rate of return of 13.2 percent.

Although Big Sky's dividend growth **averaged** 14.1 percent annually over the period, it was not a **constant** 14.1 percent each year. Firms often hold the dividend constant for several years to allow earnings to climb to a point where it is clear that a higher dividend payment is warranted. For example, Big Sky kept its dividend at $0.23 a share from 1998 through 2000, while earnings per share were flat at about $0.55.

In general, managers are very reluctant to reduce dividends because investors interpret lower dividends as a signal that management forecasts poor earnings ahead. Thus, when Big Sky saw its earnings per share temporarily

TABLE 12.1

Big Sky Healthcare: Selected Financial Data

Year	Annual per Share Dividend	Annual per Share Earnings	Average Annual Stock Price
1997	$0.20	$0.48	$ 7.70
1998	0.23	0.55	10.95
1999	0.23	0.52	11.00
2000	0.23	0.58	10.40
2001	0.48	0.85	15.30
2002	0.52	1.10	18.70
2003	0.58	1.25	20.60
2004	0.58	0.45	19.50
2005	0.65	1.35	23.20
2006	0.70	1.50	24.40
2007	0.75	1.55	26.70

tumble from $1.25 in 2003 to $0.45 in 2004, it maintained its $0.58 per share dividend. Big Sky was able to pay a cash dividend that exceeded earnings in 2004 because the firm's cash flow, which generally exceeds net income, easily supported the dividend.[3] When earnings picked up again in 2005, Big Sky increased its dividend to $0.65.

Over the entire period, Big Sky has proved to be a good investment for stockholders. For example, assume that the stock was purchased for $7.70 in 1997, a $0.20 dividend payment was paid for the stock, and then the stock was sold one year later for $10.95. For simplicity, assume that the dividend payment, rather than occurring quarterly, was paid at the end of the one-year holding period. Thus, $7.70 was paid for the stock, and one year later $10.95 + $0.20 = $11.15 was received, for a rate of return of 44.8 percent. However, investors who bought Big Sky's stock in 1999 or 2003 and then sold it one year later would have had a capital loss rather than a capital gain on the sale, even though they would have received quarterly dividends over each one-year holding period. As we discussed earlier, holding the stock for the entire ten-year period would have resulted in dividend income plus a 13.2 percent annual capital gain. (This simple example illustrates that, in general, holding stocks for longer periods involves less risk than holding stocks for shorter periods.) We will discuss stock valuation in more detail later in the chapter.

Control of the Firm

Common stockholders have the right to elect the firm's directors, who in turn elect the officers who will manage the business. In small firms, the major stockholder often assumes the positions of chief executive officer and chairman of the board of directors. In large, publicly owned firms, managers typically own some stock, but their personal holdings are insufficient to allow them to exercise voting control. Thus, stockholders can remove the management of most publicly owned firms if they decide a management team is ineffective.

Various state and federal laws stipulate how stockholder control is to be exercised. First, corporations must hold an election of directors periodically, usually once a year, with the vote taken at the annual meeting. Frequently, one third of the directors are elected each year for a three-year term. Each share of stock has one vote; thus, the owner of 1,000 shares has 1,000 votes. Stockholders can appear at the annual meeting and vote in person, but typically they transfer their right to vote to a second party by means of a *proxy*. Management always solicits stockholders' proxies and usually gets them. However, if common stockholders are dissatisfied with current management, an outside group may solicit the proxies in an effort to overthrow management and take control of the business. Such a bid for control is known as a *proxy fight*.

A *hostile takeover* occurs when a control change takes place without approval by the managers of the firm being bought. Managers who do not have majority control are very concerned about hostile takeovers. One of the most common tactics to thwart a hostile takeover is to place a *poison pill* provision in the corporate charter. A poison pill typically permits stockholders of the firm that is taken over to buy shares of the firm that instituted the takeover at a greatly reduced price. Obviously, shareholders of the acquiring firm do not want an outside group to get bargain-priced stock, so such provisions effectively stop hostile takeovers. Although poison pill provisions of this type might appear to be illegal, they have withstood all court challenges. The ultimate effect of poison pills is to force acquiring firms to get the approval of the managers of the other firm prior to the takeover. Although the stated reason for poison pills is to protect shareholders against a hostile takeover at a price that is too low, many people believe that they protect managers more than stockholders.

The Preemptive Right

Common stockholders sometimes have the right, called the *preemptive right*, to purchase any new shares sold by the firm. The purpose of the preemptive right is twofold. First, it protects the present stockholders' power of control. If it were not for this safeguard, the management of a corporation under criticism from stockholders could secure its position by issuing a large number of additional shares and purchasing the shares themselves or selling them to a friendly party. Management would thereby gain control of the corporation and frustrate current stockholders.

The second, and more important, purpose for the preemptive right is that it protects stockholders against dilution of value should new shares be issued at less than the current market price. For example, suppose HealthOne HMO has 1,000 shares of common stock outstanding, each with a price of $100, making a total market value of $100,000. If an additional 1,000 shares were sold to friends and relatives of management at $50 a share, or for $50,000, this would presumably raise the total market value of HealthOne's stock to $150,000. When the new market value is divided by the new number of shares outstanding, a share price of $75 is obtained. HealthOne's old stockholders thus lose $25 per share, and the new stockholders have an instant profit of $25 per share. As demonstrated by this example, selling common stock at a price below the current market price dilutes value and transfers wealth from the present stockholders to those who purchase the new shares. The preemptive right, which gives current stockholders the first opportunity to buy any new shares, protects them against such dilution of value.

Self-Test Questions
1. In what forms do common stock investors receive returns?
2. How do common stockholders exercise their right of control?
3. What is the preemptive right, and what is its purpose?

Types of Common Stock

Although most for-profit corporations issue only one type of common stock, in some instances several types of stock are used to meet the special needs of the company. Generally, when special classifications of stock are used, one type is designated *Class A*, another *Class B*, and so on. For this reason, such stock is called *classified stock*.

Small, new companies that seek to obtain funds from outside sources frequently use classified stock. For example, when Genetic Research, Inc., went public in 2004, its Class A stock was sold to the public and paid a dividend but carried no voting rights for five years. Its Class B stock was retained by the organizers of the company and carried full voting rights for five years, but dividends could not be paid on the Class B stock until the company had established its earning power by building up retained earnings to a designated level. The firm's use of classified stock allowed the public to take a position in a conservatively financed growth company without sacrificing income, while the founders retained absolute control during the crucial early stages of the firm's development. At the same time, outside investors were protected against excessive withdrawals of funds by the original owners. As is often the case in such situations, the Class B stock was also called *founders' shares*.

Class A, Class B, and so on, have no standard meanings. Most firms have no classified shares, but a firm that does could designate its Class B shares as founders' shares and its Class A shares as those sold to the public. Other firms could use the A and B designations for entirely different purposes.

1. What is meant by the term *classified stock*?
2. Give one reason for using classified stock.

**Self-Test
Questions**

Procedures for Selling New Common Stock

For-profit corporations can sell new common stock in a variety of ways. In this section, we describe the most common methods.

Rights Offerings

As discussed previously, common stockholders often have the *preemptive right* to purchase any additional shares sold by the firm. If the preemptive right is contained in a particular firm's charter, the company must offer any newly issued common stock to existing stockholders. If the charter does not prescribe a preemptive right, the firm can choose to sell to its existing stockholders or to the public at large. If it sells its newly issued shares to the existing stockholders, the stock sale is called a *rights offering*. Each existing stockholder is issued an *option* giving the holder the right to buy a certain number of the new shares, typically at a price below the existing market price. The precise terms of the option are listed on a certificate called a *stock purchase right*, or simply a *right*. If the stockholder does not wish to purchase any additional shares in the company, he or she can sell the rights to another person who does want to buy the stock.

Public Offerings

If the preemptive right exists in a company's charter, it must sell new stock through a rights offering. If the preemptive right does not exist, the company may choose to offer the new shares to the general public through a *public offering*. Procedures for public offerings are discussed in detail in a later section.

Private Placements

In a *private placement*, securities are sold to one or a few investors, generally institutional investors. As discussed in Chapter 11, private placements are most common with bonds, but they also occur with stock. The primary advantages of private placements are lower administrative costs and greater speed because the shares do not have to go through the Securities and Exchange Commission (SEC) registration process.

The primary disadvantage of a private placement is that the securities, because they are unregistered, must be sold to a large, sophisticated investor— usually an insurance company, mutual fund, or pension fund. Furthermore, in the event that the original purchaser wants to sell privately placed securities, they must be sold to a similar investor. However, the SEC currently allows any institution with a portfolio of $100 million or more to buy and sell private placement securities. Because thousands of institutions have assets that exceed this limit, there is a large market for the resale of private placements, and hence they are becoming more popular with issuers.

Employee Stock Purchase Plans

Many companies have plans that allow employees to purchase stock of the employing firm on favorable terms. Such plans are generically referred to as *employee stock purchase plans*. Under executive incentive *stock option plans*, key managers are given options to purchase stock at a fixed priced. These managers generally have a direct, material influence on the company's fortunes, so if they perform well, the stock price will go up and the options will become valuable.

Also, many companies have *stock purchase plans* for lower-level employees. For example, Texas HealthPlans, Inc., a regional investor-owned HMO, permits employees who are not participants in its stock option plan to allocate up to 10 percent of their salaries to its stock purchase plan. The funds are then used to buy newly issued shares at 85 percent of the market price on the purchase date. The company's contribution, the 15 percent discount, is not *vested* in an employee until five years after the purchase date. Thus, the employee cannot realize the benefit of the company's contribution without working an additional five years. This type of plan is designed both to improve employee performance and to reduce employee turnover.

Dividend Reinvestment Plans

Many large companies have *dividend reinvestment plans (DRIPs)*, whereby stockholders can automatically reinvest their dividends in the stock of the paying corporation. There are two basic types of DRIPs: plans that involve only old stock that is already outstanding and plans that involve newly issued stock. In either case, the stockholder must pay income taxes on the dollar amount of the dividends, even though stock, rather than cash, is received.

Under both types of DRIP, stockholders must choose between continuing to receive cash dividends and using the cash dividends to buy more stock in the corporation. Under the *old stock* type of plan, a bank, acting as a trustee, takes the total funds available for reinvestment from each quarterly dividend, purchases the corporation's stock on the open market, and allocates the shares purchased to the participating stockholders on a pro rata basis. The brokerage costs of buying the shares are low because of volume purchases, so these plans benefit small stockholders who do not need cash for current consumption.

The *new stock* type of DRIP provides for dividends to be invested in newly issued stock; hence, these plans raise new capital for the firm. No fees are charged to participating stockholders, and some companies offer the new stock at a discount of 3 to 5 percent below the prevailing market price. The companies absorb these costs as a trade-off against the issuance costs that would be incurred if the stock were sold through investment bankers rather than through the DRIP.

Direct Purchase Plans

In recent years, many companies have established *direct purchase plans*, which allow individual investors to purchase stock directly from the company. Many of these plans grew out of DRIPs, which were expanded to allow participants to purchase shares in excess of the dividend amount. In direct purchase plans, investors usually pay little or no brokerage fees, and many plans offer convenient features such as fractional share purchases, automatic purchases by bank debit, and quarterly statements. Although employee purchase plans, DRIPS, and direct purchase plans are an excellent way for employees and individual investors to purchase stock, they typically do not raise large sums of new capital for the firm, so other methods must be used when equity needs are great.

Self-Test Questions

1. What is a rights offering?
2. What is a private placement, and what are its primary advantages over a public offering?
3. Briefly, what are employee stock purchase plans?
4. What is a dividend reinvestment plan?
5. What is a direct purchase plan?

The Market for Common Stock

Some for-profit corporations are so small that their common stock is not actively traded—it is owned by only a few people, usually the companies' managers. Such companies are said to be *privately held*, or *closely held*, and the stock is said to be *closely held stock*.

The stocks of some publicly owned firms are not listed on any exchange; they trade in the *over-the-counter (OTC)* market. This market is composed of brokers and dealers who belong to a trade group called the *National Association of Securities Dealers (NASD)*, which licenses brokers and oversees their trading practices. The computerized trading network that is used for the OTC market is known as the NASD Automated Quotation System, or *NASDAQ*. Thus, over-the-counter transactions are listed in the *Wall Street Journal* and other publications under the title NASDAQ. Stocks traded on the OTC market (and their companies) are said to be *unlisted*.

Most large publicly owned companies apply for listing on an exchange. These companies and their stocks are said to be *listed*. As a general rule, companies are first listed on a regional exchange, such as the *Pacific* or *Midwest*; then they move up to the *American (AMEX)*; and finally, if they grow large enough, to the "Big Board"—the *New York Stock Exchange (NYSE)*. For example, American Healthcare Management, a company based in King of Prussia, Pennsylvania, that owns or manages 16 hospitals in nine states, recently listed on the NYSE. The stock had previously traded on the AMEX, but the firm's managers believed that listing on the NYSE would increase the trading of its shares and make the company more visible to the investment community, which presumably would have a positive impact on stock price. Many more stocks are traded in the OTC market than on the NYSE, and daily trading volume in the OTC market exceeds that of the NYSE.

Institutional investors such as pension funds, insurance companies, and mutual funds own about 60 percent of all common stocks. However, the institutions buy and sell relatively actively, so they account for about 75 percent of all transactions. Thus, the institutions have a heavy influence on the prices of individual stocks.

Stock market transactions can be classified into three distinct categories:

1. **The new issue market.** A small firm typically is owned by its management and a handful of private investors. At some point, if the firm is to grow further, its stock must be sold to the general public, which is defined as *going public*. The market for stock that is in the process of going public is often called the *new issue market*, and the issue is called an *initial public offering (IPO)*. To illustrate, Community Health Systems, a Tennessee-based hospital operator, recently raised more than $200 million in an IPO by selling about 16 million shares at $13 per share. At the time, insiders held about 3 million shares, so the IPO left the company

with about 19 million shares outstanding. The share price climbed to $35 by the end of the year, giving the new public investors, as well as the original insiders, cause to celebrate.

2. **The primary market.** Pacific Eldercare, which operates 79 nursing homes in ten states, recently sold 3.1 million shares of new common stock, thereby raising $31.2 million of new equity financing. Because the shares sold were newly created, the issue was defined as a *primary market* offering, but because the firm was already publicly held, the offering was not an IPO. Corporations prefer to obtain equity by retaining earnings because of issuance costs and the tendency for a new stock issue to depress stock prices. Still, if a firm requires more equity funds than can be generated from retained earnings, a stock sale may be required.

3. **The secondary market.** If the owner of 100 shares of Tenet Healthcare sells his or her stock, the trade is said to have occurred in the *secondary market*. The market for shares that have already been issued, and hence are *outstanding*, is defined as the secondary market. More than 5 million shares of Tenet stock are bought and sold on the NYSE daily, but the company does not receive a dime from these transactions.

Self-Test Questions

1. What is an initial public offering (IPO)?
2. What is meant when a stock is listed?
3. What are the differences between Tenet Healthcare selling shares in the primary market versus its shares being sold in the secondary market?

Regulation of Securities Markets

Sales of securities are regulated by the SEC and, to a lesser extent, by the Federal Reserve Board and each of the 50 states. Here are the primary elements of SEC regulation:

- The SEC has jurisdiction over all **interstate** offerings of new securities to the public in amounts of $1.5 million or more.
- Newly issued securities must be registered with the SEC at least 20 days before they are offered to the public. The *registration statement* provides the SEC with financial, legal, and technical information about the company, and the *prospectus* summarizes this information for investors. SEC lawyers and accountants analyze both the registration statement and the prospectus; if the information is inadequate or misleading, the SEC will delay or stop the public offering.
- After the registration becomes effective, new securities may be offered, but any sales solicitation must be accompanied by the prospectus. Preliminary, or *red herring,* prospectuses may be distributed to potential buyers during the 20-day waiting period, but no sales may occur during this time. The

red herring prospectus contains all the key information that will appear in the final prospectus, except the price, which is generally set after the market closes the day before the new securities are actually offered to the public.

- If the registration statement or prospectus contains misrepresentations or omissions of material facts, any purchaser who suffers a loss may sue for damages. Severe penalties may be imposed on the issuer or its officers, directors, accountants, engineers, appraisers, underwriters, and all others who participated in the preparation of the registration statement or prospectus.

- The SEC also regulates all national stock exchanges. Companies whose securities are listed on an exchange must file annual reports with both the SEC and the exchange.

- The SEC has control over corporate *insiders*. Officers, directors, and major stockholders must file monthly reports of changes in their holdings of the stock of the corporation.

- The SEC has the power to prohibit manipulation by such devices as *pools* (i.e., large amounts of money used to buy or sell stocks to artificially affect prices) or *wash sales* (i.e., sales between members of the same group to record artificial transaction prices).

- The SEC has control over the form of the proxy and the way the company uses it to solicit votes.

Control over the use of credit to buy securities (primarily common stock) is exercised by the Federal Reserve Board through *margin requirements*, which specify the maximum percentage of the purchase price that can be financed by brokerage borrowings. The current margin requirement is 50 percent, so a stock investor can borrow up to half of the cost of a stock purchase from his or her broker. If the stock price of a stock bought on margin falls, then the margin money (50 percent of the original value) becomes more than half of the current value, and the investor is forced to put up additional personal funds. Such a demand for more personal money is known as a *margin call*. The amount of additional funds required depends on the *maintenance margin*, which is set by the broker supplying the loan. When a large proportion of trades are on margin and the stock market begins a retreat, the volume of margin calls can be substantial. Because most investors who buy on margin do not have a large reserve of personal funds, they are forced to sell some stock to meet margin calls, which, in turn, can accelerate a market decline.

States also exercise control over the issuance of new securities within their boundaries. Such control is usually supervised by a corporation commissioner or someone with a similar title. State laws that relate to security sales are called *blue sky laws* because they were put into effect to keep unscrupulous promoters from selling securities that offered the "blue sky" (something wonderful) but that actually had no assets or earnings to back up the promises.

The securities industry itself realizes the importance of stable markets, sound brokerage firms, and the absence of price manipulation. Therefore, the various exchanges, as well as other industry trade groups, work closely with the SEC to monitor transactions and to maintain the integrity and credibility of the system. These industry groups also cooperate with regulatory authorities to set net worth and other standards for securities firms, to develop insurance programs that protect the customers of brokerage houses, and the like.

In general, government regulation of securities trading, as well as industry self-regulation, is designed to ensure that investors receive information that is as accurate as possible, that no one artificially manipulates the market price of a given security, and that corporate insiders do not take advantage of their position to profit in their companies' securities at the expense of others. Neither the SEC nor state regulators nor the industry itself can prevent investors from making foolish decisions, but they can and do help investors obtain the best information possible, which is the first step in making sound investment decisions.

1. What is the purpose of securities markets regulation? 2. What agencies and groups are involved in such regulation? 3. What is a prospectus? 4. What is a margin requirement? 5. What are "blue sky" laws?	**Self-Test Questions**

The Investment Banking Process

Investment banks are the companies, such as Citigroup, J.P. Morgan, and Merrill Lynch, that help businesses sell securities to the public. When new securities will be sold to the public, the first step is to select an investment banker. This can be a difficult decision for a firm that is going public. However, an older firm that has already "been to market" will have an established relationship with an investment banker. Changing bankers is easy, though, if the firm is dissatisfied.

The procedures followed in issuing new securities are collectively known as the *investment banking process*. Generally, the following key decisions regarding the issuance of new securities are made jointly by the issuing company's managers and the investment bankers that will handle the deal:

- **Dollars to be raised.** How much new capital is needed?
- **Type of securities used.** Should common stock, bonds, another security, or a combination of securities be used? Furthermore, if common stock is

to be issued, should it be done as a rights offering, by a direct sale to the general public, or by a private placement?

- **Contractual basis of issue.** If an investment banker is used, will the banker work on a *best efforts* basis or will the banker *underwrite* the issue? In a best efforts sale, the banker guarantees neither the price nor the sale of the securities, only that it will put forth its best efforts to sell the issue. On an underwritten issue, the company does get a guarantee because the banker agrees to buy the entire issue and then resell the securities to its customers. Bankers bear significant risk in underwritten offerings because the banker must bear the loss if the price of the security falls between the time the security is purchased from the issuer and the time of resale to the public.

- **Banker's compensation and other expenses.** The investment banker's compensation (if a banker is used) must be negotiated. Also, the firm must estimate the other *issuance expenses* (often called *flotation costs*) it will incur in connection with the issue—lawyers' fees, accountants' costs, printing and engraving, and so on. In an underwritten issue, the banker will buy the issue from the company at a discount below the price at which the securities are to be offered to the public, with this spread being set to cover the banker's costs and to provide a profit. In a best efforts sale, fees to the investment banker are normally set as some percentage of the dollar volume sold. Issuance costs as a percentage of the proceeds are higher for stocks than for bonds, and costs are higher for small than for large issues. The relationship between size of issue and issuance cost primarily is a result of the existence of fixed costs—certain costs must be incurred regardless of the size of the issue, so the percentage cost is quite high for small issues. To illustrate, issuance costs for a $5 million bond issue are about 5 percent, while the costs drop to about 1 percent for issues over $50 million. For a stock issue, the costs are about 12 percent and 4 percent, respectively.

- **Setting the offering price.** Usually, the *offering price* will be based on the existing market price of the stock or the yield to maturity on outstanding bonds. On initial public offerings, however, pricing decisions are much more difficult because there is no existing market price for guidance. The investment banker will have an easier job if the issue is priced relatively low, but the issuer of the securities naturally wants as high a price as possible. Conflict of interest on price therefore arises between the investment banker and the issuer. If the issuer is financially sophisticated and makes comparisons with similar security issues, the investment banker will be forced to price the new security close to its true value.

After the company and its investment banker have decided how much money to raise, the types of securities to issue, and the basis for pricing the issue, they will prepare and file a registration statement and a prospectus (if needed). The final price of the stock or the interest rate on a bond issue is set at the close of business the day the issue clears the SEC, and the securities are offered to the public the following day.

Investors are required to pay for securities within ten days, and the investment banker must pay the issuing firm within four days of the official commencement of the offering. Typically, the banker sells the securities within a day or two after the offering begins. However, on occasion, the banker miscalculates, sets the offering price too high, and thus is unable to move the issue. At other times, the market declines during the offering period, forcing the banker to reduce the price of the stock or bonds. In either instance, on an underwritten offering, the firm receives the agreed-upon dollar amount, so the banker must absorb any losses incurred.

Because they are exposed to large potential losses, investment bankers typically do not handle the purchase and distribution of issues single-handedly unless the issue is a very small one. If the sum of money involved is large, investment bankers form *underwriting syndicates* in an effort to minimize the risk that each banker carries. The banking house that sets up the deal is called the *lead,* or *managing, underwriter.*

In addition to the underwriting syndicate, on larger offerings even more investment bankers are included in a *selling group,* which handles the distribution of securities to individual investors. The selling group includes all members of the underwriting syndicate, plus additional dealers who take relatively small percentages of the total issue from members of the underwriting syndicate. Thus, the underwriters act as *wholesalers,* while members of the selling group act as *retailers.* The number of investment banks in a selling group depends partly on the size of the issue but also on the number and types of buyers. For example, the selling group that handled a recent $92 million municipal bond issue for Adventist Health System/Sunbelt consisted of three members, while the one that sold $1 billion in B-rated junk bonds for National Medical Enterprises consisted of eight members.[4]

1. What types of decisions must the issuer and its investment banker make?
2. What is the difference between an underwritten and a best efforts issue?
3. Are there any conflicts that might arise between the issuer and the investment banker when setting the offering price on a securities issue?

Self-Test Questions

Equity in Not-for-Profit Businesses

Investor-owned businesses have two sources of equity financing: retained earnings and new stock sales. Not-for-profit businesses can and do retain earnings, but they do not have access to the equity markets—that is, they cannot sell common stock to raise equity capital.[5] Not-for-profit firms can, however, raise equity capital through *government grants* and *charitable contributions.*

Federal, state, and local governments are concerned about the provision of healthcare services to the general population. Therefore, these public entities often make grants to not-for-profit providers to help offset the costs of services rendered to patients who cannot pay for those services. Sometimes these grants are nonspecific, but often they are to provide specific services such as neonatal intensive care to needy infants.

As for charitable contributions, individuals and companies are motivated to contribute to not-for-profit health services organizations for a variety of reasons, including concern for the well-being of others, the recognition that often accompanies large contributions, and tax deductibility. Because only contributions to not-for-profit firms are tax deductible, this source of funding is, for all practical purposes, not available to investor-owned health services organizations. Although charitable contributions are not a substitute for profit retentions, charitable contributions can be a significant source of fund capital. For example, the Association for Health Care Philanthropy reported that total gifts to not-for-profit hospitals in recent years have averaged more than $5 billion per year, and about half of those gifts were immediate cash contributions (as opposed to endowments). However, many healthcare philanthropy experts believe that it will be more difficult to obtain contributions in the future than it has been in the past. The reasons given include intense competition for contribution dollars and some public concern over whether not-for-profit hospitals are truly meeting their charitable missions.

Most not-for-profit hospitals received their initial, start-up equity capital from religious, educational, or governmental entities, and today some hospitals continue to receive funding from these sources. However, since the 1970s, these sources have provided a much smaller proportion of hospital funding, forcing not-for-profit hospitals to rely more on profits and outside contributions. In addition, state and local governments, which are also facing significant financial pressures, are finding it more and more difficult to fund grants to healthcare providers.

Finally, as discussed in Chapter 2, a growing trend among legislative bodies and tax authorities is to force not-for-profit hospitals to "earn" their favorable tax treatment by providing a certain amount of charity care. Even more severe, some cities have pressured not-for-profit hospitals to make "voluntary" payments to the city to make up for lost property tax revenue. These trends tend to reduce the ability of not-for-profit health services organizations to raise equity capital by grants and contributions; hence, the result is increased reliance on making money the old fashioned way—by earning it.

On the surface, investor-owned firms may appear to have a significant advantage in raising equity capital. In theory, new common stock can be issued at any time and in any reasonable amount. Conversely, charitable contributions are much less certain. The planning, solicitation, and collection periods can take years, and pledges are not always collected. Therefore, charitable contributions that were counted on may not materialize. Also, the proceeds of new stock sales may be used for any purpose, but charitable contributions often are *restricted*, in which case they can be used only for a designated purpose.

In reality, however, managers of investor-owned firms do **not** have complete freedom to raise capital by selling new common stock. First, the issuance expenses associated with a new common stock issue are not trivial. Second, if market conditions are poor and the stock is selling at a low price, a new stock issue can dilute the value of existing shares and hence be harmful to current stockholders. Finally, new stock issues are often viewed by investors as a signal that the firm's stock is overvalued, and hence new issues often drive the stock price lower.

For all these reasons, managers of investor-owned firms would rather not issue new common stock. The key point here is that yes, for-profit health services organizations have greater access to equity capital than do not-for-profit organizations. However, the differential access to equity capital may not be as great an advantage as it initially appears. The greatest advantage is for young, growing businesses that need a great deal of new capital. More mature companies have much less flexibility in raising new equity capital.

1. What are the sources of equity (i.e., fund capital) to not-for-profit firms? 2. Are not-for-profit firms at a disadvantage when it comes to raising equity capital? Explain your answer.	**Self-Test Questions**

Common Stock Valuation

For many reasons, the valuation of common stocks is a difficult and perplexing process. To begin, the type of valuation model used depends on the characteristics of the firm being valued. In general, there are three distinct types of investor-owned businesses:

1. **Start-up businesses.** A business in its infancy generally pays no dividends because all earnings must be reinvested in the business to fund growth. To make matters worse, start-up firms often take years to make a profit, so there is no track record of positive earnings to use as a basis for a cash flow forecast. Under such conditions, the general valuation (discounted cash flow) model cannot be applied because the value of such a business stems more from potential opportunities than from the cash flows produced by existing product or service lines. Even if most of the opportunities do not materialize, one or two could turn into blockbusters and hence create a highly successful firm. With such firms, *option pricing techniques*, which are beyond the scope of this book, can be used, at least in theory, to value the stock. In reality, valuations on these firms are not much more than a shot in the dark, and hence stock prices are based mostly on qualitative

factors, including emotions. The end result is that the stock prices of such businesses usually are highly volatile.

2. **Young businesses.** If a firm successfully passes through its initial start-up phase, it often reaches a point where it has more or less predictable positive earnings but still requires reinvestment of these earnings, so no dividends are paid. In such cases, it is possible to value the entire firm, as well as the stock of the firm, on the basis of the **expected earnings stream**. In such a valuation, the expected earnings stream is discounted, or *capitalized*, to find the current value of the firm. Then, the value of the debt is stripped off to estimate the value of the common stock.

3. **Mature businesses.** Mature firms generally pay a relatively predictable dividend, and hence the future dividend stream can be forecasted with reasonable confidence. In such cases, the common stock can be valued on the basis of the present value of the **expected dividend stream**. We illustrate this approach in the following sections.

The Dividend Valuation Model

Common stocks with a predictable dividend stream can be valued using the general valuation model applied to the expected dividend stream. This approach is called the *dividend valuation model.*

Basic Definitions

Here are some definitions that will be used in the illustration:

- $E(D_t)$ = Dividend the stockholder *expects* to receive at the end of Year t. D_0 is the most recent dividend, which has already been paid and is known with certainty; $E(D_1)$ is the first dividend expected and for valuation purposes is assumed to be paid **at the end** of one year; $E(D_2)$ is the dividend expected at the end of two years; and so forth. $E(D_1)$ represents the **first** cash flow a new purchaser of the stock will receive. D_0, the dividend that has just been paid, is known with certainty, but all future dividends are expected values, so the estimate of any $E(D_t)$ may differ among investors.[6]

- P_0 = Actual *market price* of the stock today.

- $E(P_t)$ = Expected price of the stock at the end of each Year t. $E(P_0)$ is the *value* of the stock today, as seen by a particular investor based on his or her estimate of the stock's expected dividend stream and riskiness; $E(P_1)$ is the price expected at the end of one year; and so on. Thus, whereas P_0, the current stock price, is fixed and is identical for all investors, $E(P_0)$ will differ among investors depending on each investor's assessment of the stock's riskiness and dividend stream. $E(P_0)$, each investor's estimate of the value today, could be above or below P_0, but an investor would buy the stock only if his or her estimate of $E(P_0)$ were equal to or greater than P_0.

- $E(g_t)$ = Expected growth rate in dividends in each future Year t. Different investors may use different $E(g_t)$s to evaluate a firm's stock. In reality, $E(g_t)$ is normally different for each Year t. However, the valuation process will be simplified by assuming that $E(g_t)$ is constant across time.
- $R(R_e)$ = Required rate of return on the stock, considering both its riskiness and the returns available on other investments. Again, we use the subscript "e" (for equity) to identify the return as a stock return.
- $E(R_e)$ = Expected rate of return on the stock. $E(R_e)$ could be above or below $R(R_e)$, but an investor would buy the stock only if his or her $E(R_e)$ were equal to or greater than $R(R_e)$. Note that $E(R_e)$ is an **expectation**. A return of $E(R_e) = 15\%$ may be expected if Tenet Healthcare stock were purchased today. If conditions in the market or prospects at Tenet take a turn for the worse, however, the realized return may be much lower than expected, perhaps even negative.
- $E(D_1) / P_0$ = Expected *dividend yield* on a stock during the first year. If a stock is expected to pay a dividend of \$1 during the next 12 months, and if its current price is \$10, then its expected dividend yield is \$1 / \$10 = 0.10 = 10\%.
- $[E(P_1) - P_0] / P_0$ = Expected *capital gains yield* on the stock during the first year. If the stock sells for \$10 today, and if it is expected to rise to \$10.50 at the end of the year, then the expected capital gain is $E(P_1) - P_0$ = \$10.50 - \$10.00 = \$0.50; and the expected capital gains yield is $[E(P_1) - P_0] / P_0$ = \$0.50 / \$10 = 0.050 = 5\%.

Expected Dividends as the Sole Basis for Stock Values

At first blush it might appear that the value of a stock is influenced by both the dividend stream and expected capital gains. However, the value of capital gains is embedded in the dividend stream. Consider an investor who buys a stock with the intention of holding it in his or her family forever. In this situation, all the investor and his or her heirs will receive is a stream of dividends, and the value of the stock today is calculated as the present value of an infinite stream of dividends.

Now consider the more typical case in which an investor expects to hold the stock for a finite period and then sell it. What would be the value of the stock in this case? The value of the stock is again the present value of the expected dividend stream. To understand this, recognize that for any individual investor, expected cash flows consist of expected dividends plus the expected price of the stock when it is sold. However, the sale price received by the current investor will depend on the dividends some future investor expects to receive. Therefore, for all present and future investors in total, expected cash flows must be based on expected future dividends. To put it another way, unless a business is liquidated or sold to another concern, the cash flows it provides to its stockholders consist only of a stream of dividends; therefore, the value of a share of its stock must be the present value of that expected dividend stream. Occasionally, stock shares could have additional value, such as the value of a controlling interest when an investor buys 51 percent of a company's outstanding stock or the added value brought about by a takeover bid. However, in most situations, the sole value inherent in stock ownership stems from the dividends that are expected to be paid by the company to its shareholders.

Investors periodically lose sight of the long-run nature of stocks as investments and forget that in order to sell a stock at a profit, one must find a buyer who will pay the higher price. Suppose that a stock's value is analyzed on the basis of expected future dividends and the conclusion is that the stock's market price exceeded a reasonable value. If an investor buys the stock anyway, he or she would be following the "bigger fool" theory of investment: The investor may be a fool to buy the stock at its excessive price, but he or she believes that an even bigger fool will be found when the time is right to sell.

Constant Growth Stock Valuation

If the projected stream of dividends follows a systematic pattern, it is possible to develop a simplified (i.e., easier to evaluate) version of the dividend valuation model. Although only a few firms have dividends that actually grow at a constant rate, the assumption of constant growth is often made because it makes the forecasting of individual dividends over a long time period unnecessary. Furthermore, many firms come close to meeting constant growth assumptions. For a constant growth company, the expected dividend growth rate is constant for all years, so $E(g_1) = E(g_2) = E(g_3)$ and so on, which implies that $E(g_t)$ becomes merely $E(g)$. Under this assumption, the dividend in any future Year t may be forecast as $E(D_t) = D_0 \times [1 + E(g)]^t$, where D_0 is the last dividend paid and hence is known with certainty, and $E(g)$ is the constant expected rate of growth.

To illustrate, if Minnesota Health Systems, Inc. (MHS) just paid a dividend of \$1.82 (i.e., $D_0 = \$1.82$), and if investors expect a 10 percent constant dividend growth rate, the dividend expected in one year will be $E(D_1)$ = \$1.82 \times 1.10 = \$2.00$; $E(D_2)$ will be \$1.82 \times (1.10)^2 = \$2.20$, and the dividend expected in five years will be $E(D_5) = D_0 \times [1 + E(g)]^5 = \$1.82 \times (1.10)^5 = \$2.93$.

The Value of a Constant Growth Stock

When $E(g)$ is assumed to be constant, a stock can be valued using the *constant growth model*:

$$E(P_0) = \frac{D_0 \times [1 + E(g)]}{R(R_e) - E(g)} = \frac{E(D_1)}{R(R_e) - E(g)},$$

where $R(R_e)$ is the required rate of return on the stock. If $D_0 = \$1.82$, $E(g) = 10\%$, and $R(R_e) = 16\%$ for MHS, the value of its stock would be \$33.33:

$$E(P_0) = \frac{\$1.82 \times 1.10}{0.16 - 0.10} = \frac{\$2.00}{0.06} = \$33.33.$$

	A	B	C	D
1				
2	$ 1.82	D_0	Last dividend payment	
3	10.0%	E(g)	Expected growth rate	
4	16.0%	$R(R_s)$	Required rate of return	
5				
6				
7				
8	$ 33.37	=A2*(1+A3)/(A4−A3) (entered into Cell A8)		
9				
10				

Note a small rounding difference between the calculator answer (where the first expected dividend was rounded to $2.00) and the spreadsheet solution.

A necessary condition for the derivation of the constant growth model is that the required rate of return on the stock is greater than its constant dividend growth rate—that is, $R(R_e)$ is greater than E(g). If the constant growth model is used when $R(R_e)$ is not greater than E(g), the results will be meaningless. However, this problem does not affect the model's use because no company could grow **over the long run** at a rate that exceeds the required rate of return on its stock. Also, note that although the constant growth model is applied here to stock valuation, it can be used in any situation in which cash flows are growing at a constant rate.

How does an investor determine his or her required rate of return on a particular stock, $R(R_e)$? One way is to use the Security Market Line (SML) of the Capital Asset Pricing Model as discussed in Chapter 10. Assume that MHS's market beta, as reported by a financial advisory service, is 1.6. Assume also that the risk-free interest rate (the rate on long-term Treasury bonds) is 5 percent and the required rate of return on the market is 12 percent. According to the SML, the required rate of return on MHS's stock is approximately 16 percent:

$$R(R_{MHS}) = RF + [R(R_M) - RF] \times b$$
$$= 5\% + (12\% - 5\%) \times 1.6$$
$$= 5\% + (7\% \times 1.6)$$
$$= 5\% + 11.2\% = 16.2\% \approx 16\%.$$

Remember, in the SML, RF is the risk-free rate; $R(R_M)$ is the required rate of return on the market, or the required rate of return on a $b = 1.0$ stock; and b is MHS's market beta.

	A	B	C	D
1				
2	1.6	b	Beta coeficient	
3	5.0%	RF	Risk-free rate	
4	12.0%	R(R$_M$)	Required return on market	
5				
6				
7				
8	16.2%	=A3+(A4–A3)*A2 (entered into Cell A8)		
9				
10				

Growth in dividends occurs primarily as a result of growth in earnings per share (EPS). Earnings growth, in turn, results from a number of factors, including the general inflation rate in the economy and the amount of earnings the company retains and reinvests. Regarding inflation, if output in units is stable, and if both sales prices and input costs increase at the inflation rate, EPS also will grow at the inflation rate. EPS will also grow as a result of the reinvestment, or plowback, of earnings. If the firm's earnings are not all paid out as dividends (i.e., if a fraction of earnings is retained), the dollars of investment behind each share will rise over time, which should lead to growth in productive assets and hence growth in earnings and dividends.

When using the constant growth model, the most critical input is E(g)—the expected constant growth rate in dividends. Investors can make their own E(g) estimates on the basis of historical dividend growth, but E(g) estimates are also available from brokerage and investment advisory firms.

Expected Rate of Return on a Constant Growth Stock

The constant growth model can be rearranged to solve for $E(R_e)$, the *expected rate of return*. In its normal form, the required rate of return, $R(R_e)$, is an input into the model, but when it is rearranged, the expected rate of return, $E(R_e)$, is found. This transformation requires that the required rate of return equal the expected rate of return, or $R(R_e) = E(R_e)$. This equality holds if the stock is in equilibrium, a condition that will be discussed later in the chapter. After solving the constant growth model for $E(R_e)$, this expression is obtained:

$$E(R_e) = \frac{D_0 \times [1 + E(g)]}{P_0} + E(g) = \frac{E(D_1)}{P_0} + E(g).$$

If an investor buys MHS's stock today for $P_0 = \$33.33$, and expects the stock to pay a dividend $E(D_1) = \$2.00$ one year from now, and for dividends to grow at a constant rate $E(g) = 10\%$ in the future, the expected rate of return on that stock is 16 percent:

$$E(R_{MHS}) = \frac{\$2.00}{\$33.33} + 10.0\% = 6.0\% + 10.0\% = 16.0\%.$$

In this form, $E(R_e)$, the expected total return on the stock, consists of an expected dividend yield, $E(D_1) / P_0 = 6\%$, plus an expected growth rate or capital gains yield, $E(g) = 10\%$.

	A	B	C	D
1				
2	$ 33.33	P_0	Stock price	
3	$ 2.00	D_1	Next expected dividend	
4	10.0%	$E(g)$	Expected growth rate	
5				
6				
7				
8	16.0%	=A3/A2+A4 (entered into Cell A8)		
9				
10				

Suppose this analysis had been conducted on January 1, 2007, so P_0 = $33.33 is MHS's January 1, 2007, stock price and $E(D_1)$ = $2.00 is the dividend expected at the end of 2007. What is the value of $E(P_1)$, the company's stock price expected at the end of 2007 (the beginning of 2008)? The constant growth model would again be applied, but this time the 2008 dividend, $E(D_2) = E(D_1) \times [1 + E(g)] = \$2.00 \times 1.10 = \$2.20$, would be used:

$$E(P_1) = \frac{E(D_2)}{R(R_e) - E(g)} = \frac{\$2.20}{0.06} = \$36.67.$$

Notice that $E(P_1)$ = $36.67 is 10 percent greater than P_0 = $33.33: $33.33 $\times$ 1.10 = $36.67. Thus, a capital gain of $36.67 − $33.33 = $3.34 would be expected during 2007, which results in a capital gains yield of 10 percent:

$$\text{Capital gains yield} = \frac{\text{Capital gain}}{\text{Beginning price}} = \frac{\$3.34}{\$33.33} = 0.100 = 10.0\%.$$

If the analysis were extended, in each future year the expected capital gains yield would always equal $E(g)$ because the stock price would grow at the 10 percent constant dividend growth rate. The expected dividend yield in 2008 (Year 2) could be found as follows:

$$\text{Dividend yield} = \frac{E(D_2)}{E(P_1)} = \frac{\$2.20}{\$36.67} = 0.060 = 6\%.$$

The dividend yield for 2009 (Year 3) could also be calculated, and again it would be 6 percent. Thus, for a constant growth stock, the following conditions must hold:

- The dividend is expected to grow forever (or at least for a long time) at a constant rate, $E(g)$.
- The stock price is expected to grow at this same rate.

- The expected dividend yield is a constant.
- The expected capital gains yield is also a constant, and it is equal to E(g).
- The expected total rate of return in any Year t, which is equal to the expected dividend yield plus the expected capital gains yield (growth rate), is expressed by this equation: $E(R_t) = [E(D_{t+1}) / E(P_t)] + E(g)$.

The term *expected* should be clarified—it means expected in a statistical sense. Thus, if MHS's dividend growth rate is expected to remain constant at 10 percent, this means that the growth rate in each year can be represented by a probability distribution with an expected value of 10 percent and not that the growth rate is expected to be exactly 10 percent in each future year. In this sense, the constant growth assumption is reasonable for many large, mature companies.

Nonconstant Growth Stock Valuation

What happens when a company does not meet the constant growth assumption? For example, what if MHS's dividend was expected to grow at 30 percent for three years and then to settle down to a constant growth rate of 10 percent? Under these nonconstant growth conditions, the value of MHS stock would be $53.86, which is significantly higher than the $33.33 value of the stock assuming 10 percent constant growth. Dividend growth of 30 percent for three years followed by 10 percent constant growth creates a more valuable expected dividend stream than straight constant growth at 10 percent. In this situation, the constant growth model does not apply, so it is necessary to apply a nonconstant growth model to value the stock. Although nonconstant stock valuation models are not very complicated, they are beyond the scope of an introductory book on healthcare finance.[7]

Self-Test Questions

1. What are three approaches to valuing common stocks?
2. Does the holding period matter when using the dividend valuation model?
3. Write out and explain the valuation model for a constant growth stock.
4. What are the assumptions of the constant growth model?
5. Show the constant growth model in its expected rate of return form.
6. What are the key features of constant growth regarding dividend yield and capital gains yield?

Security Market Equilibrium

Investors will want to buy a security if its expected rate of return exceeds its required rate of return or, put another way, when its value exceeds its current price. Conversely, investors will want to sell a security when its required rate of return exceeds its expected rate of return (i.e., when its current price exceeds its value). When more investors want to buy a security than to sell it, its price is bid up. When more investors want to sell a security than to buy it, its price falls. In *equilibrium*, these two conditions must hold:

- The expected rate of return on a security must equal its required rate of return. This means that no investor who owns the security believes that its expected rate of return is less than its required rate of return, and no investor who does not own the security believes that its expected rate of return is greater than its required rate of return.
- The market price of a security must equal its value.

If these conditions do not hold, trading will occur until they do. Of course, security prices are not constant. A security's price can swing wildly as new information becomes available to the market that changes investors' expectations concerning the security's cash flow stream or risk or when the general level of returns (i.e., interest rates) changes. However, evidence suggests that securities prices, especially prices of securities that are actively traded, such as those issued by the U. S. Treasury or by large firms, adjust rapidly to disequilibrium situations. Thus, most people believe that the bonds of the U. S. Treasury and the bonds and stocks of major corporations are generally in equilibrium. The key to the rapid movement of securities prices toward equilibrium is informational efficiency, which is discussed in the next section.

1. What is meant by security market equilibrium?
2. What securities are most likely to be in equilibrium?

Self-Test Questions

Informational Efficiency

A securities market—say, the market for long-term U. S. Treasury bonds—is "*informationally*" *efficient* if (1) all information relevant to the values of the securities traded can be obtained easily and at low cost and (2) the market contains many buyers and sellers who act **rationally** on this information. If these conditions hold, current market prices will have embedded in them all information of possible relevance; hence, future price movements will be based solely on **new** information as it becomes known.

The *Efficient Markets Hypothesis (EMH),* which has three forms, formalizes the theory of informational efficiency:

1. The *weak form* of the EMH holds that all information contained in **past price movements** is fully reflected in current market prices. Therefore, information about recent trends in a security's price is of no value in choosing which securities will "outperform" other securities.
2. The *semistrong form* of the EMH holds that current market prices reflect all **publicly available information**. Therefore, it makes no sense to spend

hours and hours analyzing economic data and financial reports because whatever information you might find, good or bad, has already been absorbed by the market and imbedded in current prices.

3. The *strong form* of the EMH holds that current market prices reflect **all relevant information**, whether publicly available or privately held. If this form holds, then even investors with "inside information," such as corporate officers, would find it impossible to earn abnormal returns—that is, returns in excess of that justified by the riskiness of the investment.

The EMH, in any of its three forms, is merely a hypothesis, so it is not necessarily true. However, hundreds of empirical tests have been conducted to try to prove, or disprove, the EMH, and the results are surprisingly consistent. In general, the tests support the weak and semistrong forms of the EMH for well-developed markets such as the U.S. markets for large firms' stocks and bond issues and for Treasury securities. Supporters of these forms of the EMH note that there are some 100,000 or so full-time, highly trained professional analysts and traders operating in these markets. Furthermore, many of these analysts and traders work for businesses such as Citigroup, Fidelity Investments, Merrill Lynch, Prudential, and the like, which have billions of dollars available to take advantage of undervalued securities. Finally, as a result of disclosure requirements and electronic information networks, new information about heavily followed securities is almost instantaneously available. Therefore, security prices in these markets adjust almost immediately as new developments occur, and hence prices reflect all publicly available information, including information on past price movements.

Virtually no one, however, believes that the strong form of the EMH holds. Studies of legal purchases and sales by individuals with inside information indicate that insiders can make abnormal profits by trading on that information. It is even more apparent that insiders can make abnormal profits if they trade illegally on specific information that has not been disclosed to the public, such as a takeover bid, a research and development breakthrough, and the like.

The EMH has important implications both for securities investment decisions and for business financing decisions. Because security prices appear to generally reflect all public information, most actively followed and traded securities are in equilibrium and fairly valued. Being in equilibrium, however, does not mean that new information could not cause a security's price to soar or to plummet, but it does mean that most securities are neither undervalued nor overvalued. Therefore, **in the short run**—for example, a year—an investor can only expect to earn a return that is the same as the average for securities of equal risk. **Over the long run**, an investor with no inside information can only expect to earn a return on a security that compensates him or her for the amount of risk assumed. In other words, investors should not expect to "beat the market" after adjusting for risk. Also, because the EMH applies to most bond markets, bond prices, and hence interest rates, reflect all current public information. Consistently forecasting future interest rates is impossible because interest rates change in response to new information, and this information could either lower or raise rates.

For managers, the EMH indicates that managerial decisions generally should not be based on perceptions about the market's ability to properly price the firm's securities or on perceptions about the direction of future interest rates. In other words, managers should not try to time security issues to try to catch stock prices while they are high or interest rates while they are low. However, in some situations, managers may have information about their own firms that is unknown to the public. This condition is called *asymmetric information*, which can affect managerial decisions. For example, suppose a drug manufacturer has made a breakthrough in AIDS research but wants to maintain as much secrecy as possible about the new drug. During final development and testing, the firm might want to delay any new securities offerings because securities could probably be sold under more favorable terms once the announcement is made. Managers can, and should, act on inside information for the benefit of their firms, but inside information cannot legally be used for personal profit.

Are markets really efficient? If markets were not efficient, the better managers of stock and bond mutual funds and pension plans would be able to consistently outperform the broad averages over long periods of time. In fact, very few managers can consistently better the broad averages, and during most years, mutual fund managers, on average, underperform the market. In any year, some mutual fund managers will outperform the market and others will underperform the market—this is known with certainty. But for an investor to beat the market by investing in mutual funds, he or she must identify the successful managers beforehand, which seems very difficult, if not impossible, to do.

In spite of the evidence, many theorists, and even more Wall Street experts, believe that pockets of inefficiency do exist. In some cases, entire markets may be inefficient. For example, the markets for the securities issued by small firms may be inefficient because there are neither enough analysts ferreting out information on these companies nor sufficient numbers of investors trading these securities. Many people also believe that individual securities traded in efficient markets are occasionally priced inefficiently or that investor emotions can drive prices too high during good times or too low during bad times. The stock market "bubble" of the late 1990s is one example. Indeed, if investors are driven more by greed and emotion than by rational assessments of security values, it may be that markets are not really as efficient as supporters of the EMH claim.

In closing our discussion of market efficiency, let's talk a little bit more about what it means to "beat the market." First, consider the short run—say, one year. You may hold a portfolio of stocks that realizes a 20 percent return in a given year. Is that a very good return? Yes. On average over the past 80 or so years, a diversified investment in stocks averaged an annual return of roughly 11 percent. However, the 20 percent return does not mean that you beat the market in that year. To actually beat the market, your return must be higher than the average return on similar portfolios of stocks (portfolios that have the same risk as yours). If the average return on a similar-risk portfolio for that year was 25 percent, you actually did worse than the relevant benchmark (the return on similar-risk holdings). Of course, if the return on similar-risk holdings was 25 percent, some portfolios did better than average and others, including yours, did worse. But, if market efficiency holds, those that did better in one year will not be able to consistently beat the relevant benchmark.

What about the long run? Over the long run—say, ten or more years— beating the market means a return in excess of that commensurate with the riskiness undertaken. For average risk stocks, this means an average annual return of roughly 11 percent (based on historical performance).

We really don't know whether it is possible to beat the market by skill or whether it is just a matter of luck. Nevertheless, it is wise for both investors and managers to consider the implications of market efficiency when making investment and financing decisions. If investors want to believe that they can beat the market, fine, but they should at least recognize that there is a lot of evidence that tells us that most people who try will ultimately fail.

Self-Test Questions	1. What two conditions must hold for markets to be efficient?
	2. Briefly, what is the Efficient Markets Hypothesis (EMH)?
	3. What are the implications of the EMH for investors and managers?

The Risk/Return Trade-Off

Most financial decisions involve alternative courses of action. For example, should a hospital invest its excess funds in Treasury bonds that yield 5 percent or in Tenet Healthcare bonds that yield 7 percent? Should a group practice buy a replacement piece of equipment now or wait until next year? Should a joint venture outpatient diagnostic center purchase a small, limited-use MRI system or a large, and more expensive, multipurpose system?

Generally, such alternative courses of action will have different expected rates of return, and one may be tempted to automatically accept the alternative with the higher expected return. However, this approach to financial decision making would be incorrect. **In efficient markets**, those alternatives that offer higher returns will also entail higher risk. The correct question to ask when making financial decisions is not which alternative has the higher expected rate of return, but which alternative has the higher return **after adjusting for risk**. In other words, which alternative has the higher return over and above the return commensurate with that alternative's riskiness?

To illustrate the *risk/return trade-off*, suppose Tenet Healthcare stock has an expected rate of return of 11 percent, while its bonds yield 7 percent. Does this mean that investors should flock to buy the firm's stock and ignore the bonds? Of course not. The higher expected rate of return on the stock merely reflects the fact that the stock is riskier than the bonds. Those investors who are not willing to assume much risk will buy Tenet's bonds, while those who are less risk averse will buy the stock. From the perspective of Tenet's managers, financing with stock is less risky than using debt, so the firm is willing to pay the higher cost of equity to limit the firm's risk exposure.

In spite of the efficiency of major securities markets, the markets for products and services (i.e., the markets for real assets such as MRI systems) are usually not efficient; hence, returns are not necessarily related to risk. Thus, hospitals, group practices, and other healthcare businesses can make real-asset investments and achieve returns in excess of those required by the riskiness of the investment. Furthermore, the market for *innovation* (i.e., the market for ideas) is not efficient. Thus, it is possible for people like Bill Gates, the founder of Microsoft, to become multibillionaires at a relatively young age. However, when excess returns are found in the product, service, or idea markets, new entrants quickly join the innovators, and competition over time will usually force rates of return down to efficient market levels. The result is that later entrants can only expect to earn returns that are commensurate with the risks involved.

1. Explain the meaning of the term *risk/return trade-off*. 2. In what markets does this trade-off hold?	**Self-Test Questions**

Key Concepts

This chapter contains a wealth of material on equity financing, including valuation, the investment banking process, and market efficiency. The key concepts of this chapter are:

- The most important *common stockholder* rights are a claim on the firm's residual earnings, control, and the preemptive right.
- New common stock may be sold by for-profit corporations in six ways: on a pro rata basis to existing stockholders through a *rights offering*; through investment bankers to the general public in a *public offering*; to a single buyer, or small number of buyers, in a *private placement*; to employees through an *employee stock purchase plan*; to shareholders through a *dividend reinvestment plan*; and to individual investors by *direct purchase*.
- A *closely held corporation* is one that is owned by a few individuals who typically are the firm's managers.
- A *publicly owned corporation* is one that is owned by a relatively large number of individuals, most of whom are not actively involved in its management.

- Securities markets are regulated at the national level by the *Securities and Exchange Commission (SEC)* and the *Federal Reserve Board* and at the state level by state agencies that typically are called *corporation commissions* (or something similar).
- An *investment banker* assists in the issuing of securities by helping the business determine the size of the issue and the type of securities to be used, by establishing the selling price, by selling the issue, and, in some cases, by maintaining an after-market for the securities.
- Not-for-profit firms do not have access to the equity markets. However, *charitable contributions*, which are tax deductible to the donor, and *governmental grants* constitute unique equity sources for not-for-profit firms.
- The *value* of a share of stock of a dividend-paying company is found by *discounting* the stream of *expected dividends* by the stock's required rate of return.
- The value of a stock whose dividends are expected to grow at a constant rate for many years is found by applying the *constant growth model*:

$$E(P_0) = \frac{D_0 \times [1 + E(g)]}{R(R_e) - E(g)} = \frac{E(D_1)}{R(R_e) - E(g)}.$$

- The *expected rate of return* on a stock consists of an *expected dividend yield* plus an *expected capital gains yield*. For a constant growth stock, both the expected dividend yield and the expected capital gains yield are constant over time, and the expected rate of return can be found by this equation:

$$E(R_e) = \frac{D_0 \times [1 + E(g)]}{P_0} + E(g) = \frac{E(D_1)}{P_0} + E(g).$$

- The *Efficient Markets Hypothesis (EMH)* holds that (1) stocks are always in equilibrium and fairly valued, (2) it is impossible for an investor to consistently beat the market, and (3) managers should not try to forecast future interest rates or time security issues.
- In efficient markets, alternatives that offer higher returns must also have higher risk; this is called the *risk/return trade-off*. The implication is that investments must be evaluated on the basis of both risk and return.

The coverage of long-term financing continues in Chapter 13 with a discussion of how managers choose between debt and equity financing. Chapter 13 also covers the cost of capital, an important concept that provides the benchmark required rate of return used in capital investment analyses.

Questions

12.1 a. What is the preemptive right?
   b. Why is it important to shareholders?

12.2 Why might an investor-owned firm choose to issue different classes of common stock?

12.3 Describe the primary means by which investor-owned firms raise new equity capital.

12.4 What are the similarities and differences between equity capital in investor-owned firms and fund capital in not-for-profit firms?

12.5 What is the general approach for valuing a share of stock of a dividend paying company?

12.6 Two investors are evaluating the stock of Beverly Enterprises for possible purchase. They agree on the stock's risk and on expectations about future dividends. However, one investor plans to hold the stock for five years, while the other plans to hold the stock for 20 years. Which of the two investors would be willing to pay more for the stock? Explain your answer.

12.7 Evaluate the following statement: One of the assumptions of the constant growth model is that the required rate of return must be greater than the expected dividend growth rate. Because of this assumption, the constant growth model is of limited use in the real world.

12.8 a. What is the Efficient Markets Hypothesis (EMH)?
   b. What are its implications for investors and managers?

12.9 a. What is meant by the term *risk/return trade-off*?
   b. Does this trade-off hold in all markets?

Problems

12.1 A person is considering buying the stock of two home health companies that are similar in all respects except the proportion of earnings paid out as dividends. Both companies are expected to earn $6 per share in the coming year, but Company D (for dividends) is expected to pay out the entire amount as dividends, while Company G (for growth) is expected to pay out only one-third of its earnings, or $2 per share. The companies are equally risky, and their required rate of return is 15 percent. D's constant growth rate is zero and G's is 8.33 percent. What are the intrinsic values of Stocks D and G?

12.2 Medical Corporation of America (MCA) has a current stock price of $36 and its last dividend (D_0) was $2.40. In view of MCA's strong financial position, its required rate of return is 12 percent. If MCA's dividends are expected to grow at a constant rate in the future, what is the firm's expected stock price in five years?

12.3 A broker offers to sell you shares of Bay Area Healthcare, which just paid a dividend of $2 per share. The dividend is expected to grow at a constant rate of 5 percent per year. The stock's required rate of return is 12 percent.

a. What is the expected dollar dividend over the next three years?

b. What is the current value of the stock and the expected stock price at the end of each of the next three years?

c. What is the expected dividend yield and capital gains yield for each of the next three years?

d. • What is the expected total return for each of the next three years?

   • How does the expected total return compare with the required rate of return on the stock? Does this make sense? Explain your answer.

12.4 Assume the risk-free rate is 6 percent and the market risk premium is 6 percent. The stock of Physicians Care Network (PCN) has a beta of 1.5. The last dividend paid by PCN (D_0) was $2 per share.

a. What would PCN's stock value be if the dividend was expected to grow at a constant:

   • –5 percent?

   • 0 percent?

   • 5 percent?

   • 10 percent?

b. What would be the stock value if the growth rate is 10 percent, but PCN's beta falls to:

   • 1.0?

   • 0.5?

12.5 Better Life Nursing Home, Inc., has maintained a dividend payment of $4 per share for many years. The same dollar dividend is expected to be paid in future years. If investors require a 12 percent rate of return on investments of similar risk, determine the value of the company's stock.

12.6 Jane's sister-in-law, a stockbroker at Invest, Inc., is trying to get Jane to buy the stock of HealthWest, a regional HMO. The stock has a current market price of $25, its last dividend ($D_0$) was $2.00, and the company's earnings and dividends are expected to increase at a constant growth rate of 10 percent. The required return on this stock is 20 percent. From a strict valuation standpoint, should Jane buy the stock?

12.7 Lucas Clinic's last dividend (D_0) was $1.50. Its current equilibrium stock price is $15.75, and its expected growth rate is a constant 5 percent. If the stockholders' required rate of return is 15 percent, what is the expected dividend yield and expected capital gains yield for the coming year?

12.8 St. John Medical, a surgical equipment manufacturer, has been hit hard by increased competition. Analysts predict that earnings and dividends will decline at a rate of 5 percent annually into the foreseeable future. If the firm's last dividend (D_0) was $2.00, and the investors' required rate of return is 15 percent, what will be the company's stock price in **three** years?

12.9 California Clinics, an investor-owned chain of ambulatory care clinics, just paid a dividend of $2 per share. The firm's dividend is expected to grow at a constant rate of 5 percent per year, and investors require a 15 percent rate of return on the stock.

    a. What is the stock's value?

    b. Suppose the riskiness of the stock decreases, which causes the required rate of return to fall to 13 percent. Under these conditions, what is the stock's value?

    c. Return to the original 15 percent required rate of return. Assume that the dividend growth rate estimate is increased to a constant 7 percent per year. What is the stock's value?

Notes

1. Some for-profit firms use *preferred stock*, which is a form of equity financing that combines features of both debt and equity. However, few healthcare businesses use preferred stock financing, so this type of equity will not be covered here. For more information on preferred stock, see Louis C. Gapenski, *Understanding Healthcare Financial Management* (Chicago: Health Administration Press, 2007), Chapter 6.

2. Traditionally, dividend-paying corporations have paid dividends quarterly. However, some corporations are now paying dividends annually. The advantage to annual dividends is the reduction in administrative costs associated with paying dividends. For much more information about corporate dividend policy as well as other distributions, see Chapter 19 (Distributions to Owners: Bonuses, Dividends, and Repurchases), which is available from Health Administration Press at ache.org/books/HCFinance4.

3. If a firm is experiencing temporary financial difficulties, it might even borrow the funds necessary to pay the dividend expected by stockholders rather than lower or omit the payment. The folk wisdom among corporate managers is that "like diamonds, dividends are forever." The reason is that a dividend cut, or worse yet an omission, sends a signal that will trigger a sell-off that substantially lowers the firm's stock price and places management in a precarious position. Thus, dividends typically are cut only under extreme circumstances and after all other options have been exhausted.

4. Large security issues are announced in the *Wall Street Journal* and other publications by advertisements called *tombstones*. Check several recent issues of the *Journal* to see if any healthcare issues are advertised.

5. Although rare, some types of not-for-profit corporations can sell shares to raise capital. However, such "stock" does not pay dividends and cannot be sold at a profit. This form of not-for-profit corporation is used mostly to finance not-for-profit clinics, whereby the physicians who will practice in the clinic contribute the start-up capital. When a physician leaves the clinic, his or her initial capital investment is returned.

6. Stocks generally pay dividends quarterly, so theoretically they should be evaluated on a quarterly basis. However, in stock valuation, most analysts work on an

annual basis because the data are not precise enough in most situations to warrant the refinement of a quarterly model.

7. For more information on nonconstant growth stock valuation, see Louis C. Gapenski, *Understanding Healthcare Financial Management* (Chicago: Health Administration Press, 2007), Chapter 7.

References

Cleverley, W. O., and J. O. Cleverley. 2005. "Philanthropy: The Last Frontier for Capital Funding." *Journal of Healthcare Management* (September/October): 290–293.

Dunn, K. C., G. B. Shields, and J. B. Stern. 1991. "The Dynamics of Leveraged Buy-Outs, Conversions, and Corporate Reorganizations of Not-For-Profit Health Care Institutions." *Topics in Health Care Financing* (Spring): 5–20.

Flaherty, M. P. 1991. "Planned Giving Programs as a Source of Financing: Creating a 'Win-Win' Situation for a Health Care Organization and Its Donors." *Topics in Health Care Financing* (Fall): 70–81.

Healthcare Financial Management Association (HFMA). 2003. "How Are Hospitals Financing the Future? Access to Capital in Health Care Today." *Healthcare Financial Management* (November): 51–53.

Shields, G. B., and G. C. McKann. 1991. "Raising Health Care Capital Through the Public Equity Markets." *Topics in Health Care Financing* (Fall): 21–36.

Sykes, C. S., Jr. 1991. "The Role of Equity Financing in Today's Health Care Environment." *Topics in Health Care Financing* (Fall): 1–4.

Wallace, C. 1985. "Not-For-Profits Competing for Capital by Selling Stock in Alternative Ventures." *Modern Healthcare* (August 16): 32–38.

CHAPTER

13

CAPITAL STRUCTURE AND THE COST OF CAPITAL

Learning Objectives

After studying this chapter, readers will be able to:

- Explain the effects of debt financing on a business's risk and return.
- Discuss the factors that influence the choice between debt and equity financing.
- Describe the general process for estimating a business's corporate cost of capital.
- Estimate the component costs as well as the overall (corporate) cost of capital for any healthcare business.
- Explain the economic interpretation of the corporate cost of capital and how it is used in capital investment decisions.

Introduction

In previous chapters, we have noted that businesses use two inherently different sources of capital: debt and equity. In this chapter, we discuss two key issues related to financing: the choice between debt and equity and the overall cost of capital to the business.

Capital Structure Basics

The mix of debt and equity financing used by a business is called its *capital structure*, which is, in reality, the structure of the liabilities and equity side of the business's balance sheet. One of the most perplexing issues facing health services organizations is how much debt financing, as opposed to equity (or fund) financing, they should use. Is there an optimal mix of debt and equity (i.e., is there an *optimal capital structure*)? If optimal capital structures do exist, do hospitals have different optimal structures than home health agencies or ambulatory surgery centers? If so, what are the factors that lead to these differences? These questions, although difficult to answer, are important to the financial well-being of any business.[1]

Impact of Debt Financing on Accounting Risk and Return

To fully understand the consequences of capital structure decisions, it is essential to understand the effects of debt financing on a business's risk and return as reflected in its financial statements. Consider the situation that faces Super Health, Inc., a for-profit (investor-owned) company that is just being formed. Its founders have identified two financing alternatives for the business: all equity (all common stock) and 50 percent debt.

Table 13.1 contains the business's projected financial statements under the two financing alternatives. To begin, consider the balance sheets shown in the top portion of the table. Super Health requires $100,000 in current assets and $100,000 in fixed assets to begin operations. The asset requirements for any business depend on the nature and size of the business rather than on how the business will be financed, so the asset side of the balance sheet in Table 13.1 is unaffected by the financing mix. However, the type of financing does affect the liabilities and equity side. Under the all-equity alternative, Super Health's owners will put up the entire $200,000 needed to purchase the assets. If 50 percent debt financing is used, the owners will contribute only $100,000, with the remaining $100,000 obtained from creditors—say, a bank loan with a 10 percent interest rate.

What is the impact of the two financing alternatives on Super Health's projected first year's income statement? Revenues are projected to be $150,000 and operating costs are forecasted at $100,000, so the firm's operating income is expected to be $50,000. Because a business's capital structure does not affect revenues and operating costs, the operating income projection is the same under both financing alternatives.

However, interest expense must be paid if debt financing is used. Thus, the 50 percent debt alternative results in a $0.10 \times \$100,000 = \$10,000$ annual interest charge, while no interest expense occurs if the firm is all-equity financed. The result is taxable income of $50,000 under the all-equity alternative and a lower taxable income of $40,000 under the 50 percent debt alternative. Because the business anticipates being taxed at a 40 percent federal-plus-state rate, the expected tax liability is $0.40 \times \$50,000 = \$20,000$ under the all-equity alternative and $0.40 \times \$40,000 = \$16,000$ for the 50 percent debt alternative. Finally, when taxes are deducted from the income stream, the business expects to earn $30,000 in net income if it is all-equity financed and $24,000 in net income if 50 percent debt financing is used.

At first glance, the use of debt financing appears to be the **inferior** alternative. After all, if 50 percent debt financing is used, the business's projected net income will fall by $\$30,000 - \$24,000 = \$6,000$. But the conclusion that

	All Equity	50% Debt
Balance Sheets:		
Current assets	$ 100,000	$ 100,000
Fixed assets	100,000	100,000
Total assets	$200,000	$200,000
Bank loan (10% cost)	$ 0	$ 100,000
Common stock	200,000	100,000
Total liabilities and equity	$200,000	$200,000
Income Statements:		
Revenues	$ 150,000	$ 150,000
Operating costs	100,000	100,000
Operating income	$ 50,000	$ 50,000
Interest expense	0	10,000
Taxable income	$ 50,000	$ 40,000
Taxes (40%)	20,000	16,000
Net income	$ 30,000	$ 24,000
ROE	15%	24%
Total dollar return to investors	$ 30,000	$ 34,000

TABLE 13.1
Super Health, Inc.: Projected Financial Statements Under Two Financing Alternatives

debt financing is bad requires closer examination. What is most important to the owners of Super Health is not the business's net income but the return expected on their equity investment. The best measure of return to the owners of a business is the *rate of return on equity (ROE)*—defined as net income divided by the book value of equity. Under all-equity financing, the projected ROE is $30,000 / $200,000 = 0.15 = 15%, but with 50 percent debt financing, projected ROE increases to $24,000 / $100,000 = 24%. The key to the increased ROE is that although net income decreases when debt financing is used, so does the amount of equity needed, and the capital requirement decreases proportionally more than does net income.

The bottom line of this analysis is that debt financing can increase owners' expected rate of return. Because the use of debt financing increases, or leverages up, the return to equityholders, such financing is often called *financial leverage*. Hence, the use of financial leverage is merely the use of debt financing.

To view the impact of financial leverage from a different perspective, take another look at the Table 13.1 income statements. The total dollar return to all investors, including **both** the owners and the bank, is $30,000 in net income when all-equity financed but $24,000 in net income plus $10,000 of interest = $34,000 when 50 percent debt financing is used. Thus, the use of debt financing increased the projected total dollar return to investors by $34,000 − $30,000 = $4,000. Where did the extra $4,000 come from? The answer is from the taxman. Taxes are $20,000 if the business is all-equity financed but only $16,000 if debt financing is used, and $4,000 less in taxes means $4,000 more for investors. Because the use of debt financing reduces taxes, more of a firm's operating income is available for distribution to investors.[2]

At this point, it appears that Super Health's financing decision is a "no brainer." Given only these two financing alternatives, 50 percent debt financing should be used because it promises owners the higher rate of return. Unfortunately, like the proverbial no free lunch, there is a catch. The use of financial leverage not only increases owners' projected return, it also increases their risk.

To demonstrate the risk-increasing characteristics of debt financing, consider Table 13.2, which recognizes that Super Health, like all businesses, is risky. The first year's revenues and operating costs listed in Table 13.1 are *not* known with certainty but are expected values taken from probability distributions. Super Health's founders believe that operating income could be as low as zero or as high as $100,000 in the business's first year of operation. Furthermore, there is a 25 percent chance of the worst and the best cases occurring, and a 50 percent chance that the Table 13.1 forecast, with an operating income of $50,000, will be realized.

The assumptions regarding uncertainty in the future profitability of the business lead to three different ROEs for each financing alternative. The expected ROEs are the same as when uncertainty was ignored (i.e., 15 percent if the firm is all-equity financed and 24 percent when 50 percent debt financing is used). For example, the expected ROE under all-equity financing is (0.25 ×

TABLE 13.2		All Equity			50% Debt		
Super Health, Inc.: Partial Income Statements in an Uncertain World	Probability	0.25	0.50	0.25	0.25	0.50	0.25
	Operating income	$0	$50,000	$100,000	$ 0	$50,000	$100,000
	Interest expense	0	0	0	10,000	10,000	10,000
	Taxable income	$0	$50,000	$100,000	($10,000)	$40,000	$ 90,000
	Taxes (40%)	0	20,000	40,000	(4,000)	16,000	36,000
	Net income	$0	$30,000	$ 60,000	($ 6,000)	$24,000	$ 54,000
	ROE	0%	15%	30%	−6%	24%	54%
	Expected ROE		15%			24%	
	Standard deviation of ROE		10.6%			21.2%	

0%) + (0.50 × 15%) + (0.25 × 30%) = 15%. However, the uncertainty in operating income produces uncertainty, and hence risk, in the owners' return. If owners' risk is measured by the standard deviation of ROE (stand-alone risk), the return is twice as risky in the 50 percent debt financing alternative: 21.2 percent standard deviation of ROE versus 10.6 percent standard deviation in the zero-debt alternative.[3]

The increase in risk is apparent without even calculating the standard deviations. If all equity financing is used, the worst return that can occur is a ROE of zero. However, with 50 percent debt financing, a ROE of -6 percent can occur. In fact, with no operating income to pay the $10,000 interest to the bank in the worst case scenario, the owners would either have to put up additional equity capital to pay the interest due (assuming insufficient deprecation cash flow) or declare the business bankrupt. Clearly, the use of 50 percent debt financing has increased the riskiness of the owners' investment.

This simple example illustrates two key points about the use of debt financing:

1. A business's use of debt financing increases the percentage return to owners (ROE).[4]
2. At the same time that return is increased, the use of debt financing also increases owners' risk. In the Super Health example, 50 percent debt financing doubled the owners' risk as measured by standard deviation of ROE.

When risk is considered, the ultimate decision on which financing alternative should be chosen is not so clear-cut. The zero-debt alternative has a lower expected ROE but also lower risk. The 50 percent debt alternative offers a higher expected ROE but carries with it more risk. Thus, the decision is a classic risk/return trade-off: higher returns can be obtained only by assuming greater risk. What Super Health's founders need to know is whether or not the higher return is **enough** to compensate them for the higher risk assumed. To complicate the decision even more, there are an almost unlimited number of debt-level choices available, not just the 50/50 mix used in the illustration. This example vividly illustrates that health services managers face a difficult decision in setting a business's optimal capital structure.

1. What is the impact of debt financing on owners' rate of return?
2. What is the impact of debt financing on owners' risk?
3. What is the basis for choosing the optimal level of debt financing?

Self-Test Questions

Capital Structure Theory

At the end of the previous section, Super Health's founders were left in a quandary because debt financing brings with it both higher returns and higher risk. *Capital structure theory*, which was developed for **investor-owned businesses**, attempts to resolve this dilemma. If the relationship between the use of debt financing and equity value (stock price) were known, then the optimal capital structure could be identified.

There are many competing theories of capital structure, but one theory—the *trade-off theory*—is most widely accepted. In general, this theory tells managers that an optimal capital structure does exist for every business. Furthermore, the optimal structure balances the tax advantages of debt financing against the increased risk that arises when debt financing is used. The trade-off theory is summarized in Figure 13.1. Here, the proportion of debt in a firm's capital structure is plotted on the X axis, while the Y axis plots the costs of debt and equity as well as the combined cost of both financing sources. The focus in Figure 13.1 is not on the absolute level of debt financing but rather on the **proportion of debt financing used**: Larger firms have higher dollar values of debt than do smaller firms. Furthermore, growing firms add additional amounts of both debt and equity to their balance sheets on a regular basis. In Figure 13.1, we assume that the business's assets are held constant, and what changes, and hence what is shown on the X axis, is the proportion of debt: 0 percent (i.e., no debt), 10 percent, 20 percent, and so on, up to 100 percent (i.e., all debt).

To begin, consider the relationship between the cost of debt and the proportion of debt financing. As a business uses a greater proportion of debt financing, the risk to creditors increases because the greater the debt service requirement, the higher the probability that default will occur. In essence, the greater the proportion of debt financing, the riskier the lender's position. Thus, the cost of debt (i.e., the interest rate) increases as the proportion of debt increases. However, the cost of debt increases slowly at low and moderate proportions of debt because the incremental risk to lenders is relatively small, but then it increases at a faster rate as even more debt is used. Thus, in Figure 13.1 the cost-of-debt line first rises slowly and, as more and more debt is used, rises at a faster and faster rate.

As discussed in the Super Health illustration, the use of debt financing also increases the risk to equityholders. Furthermore, the greater the proportion of debt, the greater the risk. Thus, the cost of equity also increases with the proportion of debt financing, just as does the cost of debt. The primary difference between the cost of debt and the cost of equity curves is not their shape but where they are located on the graph. The cost of equity is higher than the cost of debt because owners face more risk than do creditors. (Equityholders have a residual claim on the earnings of the firm, while creditors' claims are fixed by contract.) Furthermore, the cost of debt is lowered even more relative to equity because interest payments are tax deductible while returns to equityholders are not. Thus, as shown in Figure 13.1, the cost of equity is appreciably greater than the cost of debt at any proportion of debt.

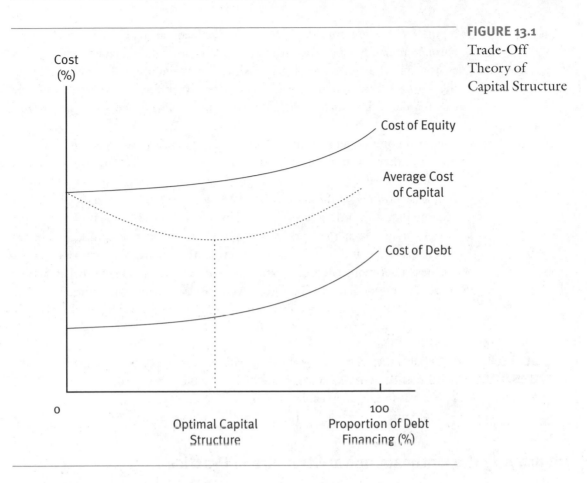

FIGURE 13.1

Trade-Off
Theory of
Capital Structure

In practice, firms tend to use some, but not all, debt financing, so firms actually use a blend of the two major sources of financing. Under these conditions, what is most relevant to financing decisions is not just the cost of debt or just the cost of equity but rather the weighted average (blended) cost of the two components. The weighted average cost is shown on the graph as a dotted line labeled "average cost of capital." At zero debt (the Y axis), the firm is all-equity financed, so its average cost of capital is simply its cost of equity. When a business first starts using debt financing, it adds a lower cost component to its capital structure, and hence the average cost of financing decreases. However, as the proportion of debt financing increases, both the cost of equity and the cost of debt increase, and at an increasing rate. At some point, the increasing component costs outweigh the fact that more of the lower-cost debt component is being used, and the average cost of capital bottoms out. Beyond this point, the average cost of capital begins to increase.

The point at which the average cost of capital is minimized defines the firm's *optimal capital structure*. At this proportion of debt financing, overall financing costs are minimized. Capital, like labor, is an input to the firm, and the firm's financial condition is maximized at any given output when its input costs are minimized. Once the optimal capital structure, or perhaps an *optimal range*, has been identified for a business, its managers will finance asset acquisitions in a way that keeps the firm at its optimal structure. Thus, the optimal capital structure becomes the target for future financing. For this reason, a firm's optimal capital structure is also called its *target capital structure*.

Although theory indicates that an optimal capital structure exists, it turns out that it is not easy in practice to identify this structure for any given business. However, there is some good news associated with Figure 13.1. Empirical studies confirm that the average cost-of-capital curve, similar to the one plotted in the figure, has a relatively shallow shape. Thus, variations in debt usage from the optimal structure do not have a significant impact on capital costs, and hence it is not essential that managers identify exactly a business's optimal structure. Furthermore, even if a precise optimal structure could be identified, relatively large movements away from this structure, which commonly occur in practice, will not materially affect financial performance.

Self-Test Questions

1. What is the relationship between a business's use of debt financing and its cost of debt? Its cost of equity? Its overall cost of capital?
2. How is the optimal capital structure defined?
3. Is it critical that the precise structure be identified and followed?

Identifying the Optimal Capital Structure in Practice

Unfortunately, capital structure theory cannot provide managers with the optimal capital structure for a given business because the component costs, particularly the cost of equity, cannot be estimated with any confidence for different capital structures. Thus, health services managers must apply judgment in making the capital structure decision. The qualitative analysis involves several different factors, and in one situation a particular factor may have great importance, while the same factor may be relatively unimportant in another situation. Here are some of the more important qualitative issues that managers consider in setting a business's target capital structure.

Business Versus Financial Risk

Businesses have a certain amount of risk, called *business risk*, inherent in operations even when no debt financing is used. This risk is associated with the ability of managers to forecast future profitability. The more difficult the forecasting process, the greater the inherent risk of the business. To illustrate, refer to Table 13.2. Super Health's business risk can be measured by the standard deviation of ROE **assuming the firm uses zero-debt financing**. Thus, the business risk of Super Health is 10.6 percent. If no debt financing is used, return on equity is equal to return on assets, so business risk is measured by the inherent uncertainty in the return on a business's assets.

When debt financing is used, equityholders must bear additional risk. In a capital structure context, the risk added when debt financing is used is called *financial risk*. For Super Health, the standard deviation of ROE when 50 percent debt financing is used is 21.2 percent. The difference between the standard deviations of ROE with and without debt financing measures the amount of financial risk. Thus, for Super Health, the financial risk at 50 percent debt financing is 21.2% − 10.6% = 10.6%. Using a mix of half debt and half equity doubles the risk to the owners of a business as measured by the standard deviation of ROE.

In general, managers will place some limit on the total amount of risk, including **both** business and financial, undertaken by a business. Thus, the greater the inherent business risk, the less "room" available for the use of financial leverage and hence the lower the optimal proportion of debt financing.

Lender and Rating Agency Attitudes

Regardless of a manager's own analysis of the proper capital structure for his or her firm, there is no question that lenders' and rating agencies' attitudes are frequently important determinants of financial structures. In the majority of situations, corporate managers discuss the business's financial structure with lenders and rating agencies and give much weight to their advice. Often, managers want to maintain some target debt rating—say, single A. Furthermore, rating agencies publish guidelines that link firms' capital structures within an industry to specific bond ratings, so guidance is readily available.

If a particular firm's management is so confident of the future that it seeks to use debt financing beyond the norms of its industry, lenders may be unwilling to accept such debt levels or may do so only at a high price. In effect, lenders and rating agencies set an absolute limit on the proportion of debt financing that can be used by any business as well as some bounds on the amount of debt that can be raised at "reasonable" interest rates.

Reserve Borrowing Capacity

Firms generally maintain a *reserve borrowing capacity* that preserves the ability to issue debt when conditions so dictate. In essence, managers want to maintain *financial flexibility*, which is defined in a capital structure context as the ability to access, at any time, alternative forms of capital under reasonable terms. For example, suppose Merck had just successfully completed an R&D program on a new drug and its internal projections forecast much higher earnings in the future. However, the new earnings are not yet anticipated by investors and hence are not reflected in the price of its stock. If Merck needed additional capital, its managers would not want to issue stock; they would prefer to finance with debt until the higher earnings materialized and were reflected in the stock price. Then they could sell an issue of common stock, retire the debt, and return the firm to its target capital structure. To maintain this reserve borrowing capacity, businesses generally use less debt than other factors may indicate should be used.

Industry Averages

Presumably, managers act rationally, so the capital structures of other firms in the industry, particularly the industry leaders, should provide insights about the optimal structure. In general, there is no reason to believe that the managers of one firm are better than the managers of another firm. Thus, if one firm has a capital structure that is significantly different from other firms in its industry, the managers of that firm should identify the unique circumstances that contribute to the anomaly. If unique circumstances cannot be identified, then it is doubtful that the firm has identified the correct target structure.

Asset Structure

Firms whose assets are suitable as security (collateral) for loans pay lower interest rates on debt financing than do other firms and hence tend to use more debt. Thus, hospitals tend to use more debt than do companies involved in technological research. Both the ability to use assets as collateral and low inherent business risk give a firm more *debt capacity*, and hence a target capital structure that includes a relatively high proportion of debt.

Self-Test Questions
1. Is the capital structure decision mostly objective or subjective?
2. What is the difference between business and financial risk?
3. What are some of the factors that managers must consider when setting the target capital structure?

Not-for-Profit Businesses

Our discussion of capital structure has focused on investor-owned businesses. What about not-for-profit corporations? The same general concepts apply—namely, some debt financing is good, but too much is bad. However, not-for-profit firms have a unique problem—they cannot go to the capital markets to raise equity capital. If an investor-owned firm has more capital investment opportunities than it can finance with retained earnings and debt financing, it can always raise the needed funds with a new stock issue. It may be costly, but it can be done. Additionally, it is quite easy for investor-owned firms to adjust their capital structures. If they are financially underleveraged (i.e., using too little debt), they can simply issue more debt and use the proceeds to repurchase stock. On the other hand, if they are financially overleveraged (i.e., using too much debt), they can issue additional equity and use the proceeds to refund debt.

Not-for-profit firms do not have access to the equity markets; their sources of equity capital consist of government grants, private contributions, and excess revenues (retained earnings). Managers of not-for-profit organizations do not have the same degree of flexibility in either capital investment or capital structure decisions as do their proprietary counterparts. Thus, it is sometimes necessary for not-for-profit firms to delay new projects, even profitable ones, because of funding insufficiencies or to use more than the theoretically optimal amount of debt because that is the only way that needed services can be financed.

Although such actions may be required in certain situations, not-for-profit managers must recognize that these strategies are suboptimal. Project delays mean that needed services are not being provided on a timely basis. Using more debt than is optimal pushes the firm beyond the point of the greatest net benefit of debt financing, and hence capital costs are increased above the minimum. If a not-for-profit firm is forced into a situation where it is using more than the optimal amount of debt financing, its managers should reduce the firm's level of debt as soon as the situation permits.

The ability of a not-for-profit business to garner governmental grants, attract private contributions, and generate earnings plays an important role in establishing its competitive position. A firm that has an adequate amount of equity (fund) capital can operate at its optimal capital structure and thus minimize capital costs. If insufficient equity capital is available, too much financial leverage is then used, and the result is higher capital costs. To illustrate this point, consider two not-for-profit hospitals that are similar in all respects, except that one has more equity capital and can operate at its optimal structure while the other has insufficient equity capital and thus must use more debt financing than is optimal. In effect, the hospital with insufficient equity must operate with an inefficient capital structure. The former has a significant competitive advantage because it can either offer more services at the same cost by using additional, nonoptimal debt financing, or it can offer matching services at lower costs.

Sufficient equity capital provides not-for-profit businesses with the flexibility to offer all of the necessary services and still operate at the lowest capital cost structure. Like companies that have low operating cost structures, not-for-profit firms that have low capital cost structures—that is, they operate at their optimal capital structures—have an advantage over their competitors that have higher capital cost structures.

1. What unique problems do managers of not-for-profit businesses face regarding capital structure decisions?
2. Why is capital structure important to the managers of not-for-profit businesses?

Self-Test Questions

Cost of Capital Basics

In the first part of this chapter, the discussion focused on choosing between debt and equity financing. Once that decision is made, the business will raise capital over time in such a way as to maintain (or move toward) its optimal (target) structure. Of course, other considerations also come into play when raising new capital, but over the long run, businesses will attempt to keep their capital structures close to the target.

Now, we turn our attention to identifying the specific costs of maintaining that structure. The ultimate goal of the cost of capital estimation process is to estimate a business's *corporate cost of capital*, which represents the blended, or average, cost of a business's financing. This cost, in turn, is used as the required rate of return, or hurdle rate, when evaluating the business's capital investment opportunities. For example, assume Bayside Memorial Hospital has a corporate cost of capital of 10 percent. If a new MRI investment, which has been judged to have average risk, is expected to return at least 10 percent, then it is financially attractive to the hospital. If the MRI is expected to return less than 10 percent, accepting it will have an adverse effect on the hospital's financial soundness. In effect, the corporate cost of capital sets the **opportunity cost rate** for new capital investment.

The corporate cost of capital is a weighted average of the *component* (i.e., debt and equity) *costs*. After the component costs have been estimated, they are combined to form the corporate cost of capital. Thus, the first step in the cost of capital estimation process is to estimate both the cost of debt and the cost of equity. However, before we discuss the mechanics of cost estimation, some other issues regarding the corporate cost of capital estimation process must be considered.

The Capital Components

The first task in estimating a business's corporate cost of capital is to determine which sources of capital on the liabilities and equity side of the balance sheet should be included in the estimate. In general, the corporate cost of capital focuses on the cost of *permanent capital* (long-term capital) because these are the sources used to finance capital asset acquisitions (land, buildings, and equipment). Thus, for most firms, the relevant capital components are equity and long-term debt. Typically, short-term debt is used only for temporary financing of current assets to support seasonal or cyclical fluctuations in volume, and hence it is not included in the cost-of-capital estimate. However, if a firm does use short-term debt as part of its permanent financing mix, then such debt should be included. As discussed in Chapter 16, the use of short-term debt to finance permanent assets is highly risky and is not common under normal conditions.

Tax Effects

In developing component costs, the issue of taxes arises for investor-owned companies. Should the component costs be estimated on a before-tax or an after-tax basis? As discussed in the previous section on capital structure, the use of debt financing creates a tax benefit because interest expense is tax deductible, while the use of equity financing has no impact on taxes. This tax benefit can be handled in several ways when working with capital costs, but the most common way is to include it in the cost-of-capital estimate. Thus, the tax benefit associated with debt financing will be recognized in the component cost of debt estimate, resulting in an after-tax cost of debt. For not-for-profit firms, the benefit that arises from the issuance of tax-exempt debt will be incorporated directly into the cost estimate because investors require a lower interest rate on tax-exempt (municipal) debt.

Historical Versus Marginal Costs

Two very different sets of capital costs can be measured: *historical*, or *embedded*, *costs*, which reflect the cost of funds **raised in the past**; and *new*, or *marginal*, *costs*, which measure the cost of funds to be **raised in the future**. Historical costs are important for many purposes. For example, payers that reimburse on a cost basis are concerned with embedded costs. However, the primary purpose of estimating a firm's corporate cost of capital is to use the estimate in making capital investment decisions, which involve future asset acquisitions and future financing. Thus, for purposes here, the relevant costs are the marginal costs of new funds to be raised during some future planning period—say, a year—and not the cost of funds raised in the past.

1. What is the basic concept of the corporate cost of capital?
2. What financing sources are typically included in a firm's cost of capital estimate?
3. Should the component costs be estimated on a before- or an after-tax basis?
4. Should the component costs reflect historical or marginal costs?

Self-Test Questions

Cost of Debt Capital

Although the cost of capital estimation process is the same, some of the details of component cost estimation differ depending on the type of business. We will begin our discussion by focusing on large businesses, primarily publicly traded for-profit businesses. Along the way, we will point out some of the differences in cost estimation between investor-owned and not-for-profit businesses. Later in the chapter, we will discuss some unique features of estimating the cost of capital for small businesses.

It is unlikely that a firm's managers will know at the start of a planning period the exact types and amounts of debt that will be issued in the future; the type of debt actually used will depend on the specific assets to be financed and on market conditions as they develop over time. However, a firm's managers do know what types of debt the firm usually issues. For example, Bayside Memorial Hospital (a not-for-profit hospital) typically uses bank debt to raise short-term funds to finance seasonal or cyclical working capital needs and uses 30-year tax-exempt bonds to raise long-term debt capital. Because Bayside does not use short-term debt to finance permanent assets, its managers include only long-term debt in their corporate cost-of-capital estimate, and they assume that this debt will consist solely of 30-year tax-exempt bonds.

Suppose that Bayside's managers are developing the hospital's corporate cost-of-capital estimate for the coming year. How should they estimate the hospital's component *cost of debt*? Bayside's managers would begin by discussing current and prospective interest rates with the firm's investment bankers, the institutions that help companies bring security issues to market. Assume that the municipal bond analyst at Suncoast Securities, Inc., Bayside's investment banker, states that a new 30-year tax-exempt healthcare issue would require semiannual interest payments of $30.50 ($61 annually) for each $1,000 par value bond issued. Thus, municipal bond investors currently require a $61 / $1,000 = 0.061 = 6.1% return on Bayside's 30-year bonds.[5]

The true cost of the issue to Bayside would be somewhat higher than 6.1 percent because the hospital must incur administrative expenses, or *flotation costs*, to sell the bonds. However, such expenses are typically small on bond issues, so their impact on the cost of debt estimate is inconsequential, especially when the uncertainty inherent in the entire cost of capital estimation process is considered. Therefore, it is common practice to ignore flotation costs when estimating debt costs. Bayside follows this practice, so its managers would estimate the component cost of debt as 6.1 percent:

$$\text{Tax-exempt component cost of debt} = R(R_d) = 6.1\%.$$

If Bayside's currently outstanding debt were actively traded, then the current **yield to maturity (YTM)** on this debt could be used to estimate the cost of new debt. Using the yield to maturity on an outstanding issue to estimate the cost of new debt works reasonably well when the remaining life of the old issue approximates the anticipated maturity of the new issue. If this is not the case, then yield curve differentials may cause the estimate to be biased. For example, if the yield curve is upward sloping in the 15- to 30-year range, the yield to maturity on a 15-year outstanding issue would understate the actual cost of new 30-year debt.

A taxable healthcare provider would use one or more of the techniques just described to estimate its before-tax cost of debt. However, the tax benefits of interest payments must then be incorporated into the estimate. To illustrate, consider Ann Arbor Health Systems, Inc., an investor-owned company that operates 16 acute care hospitals in Michigan, Indiana, and Ohio. The company's investment bankers indicate that a new 30-year taxable bond issue would require a yield of 10 percent. Because the firm's federal-plus-state tax rate is 34 percent, its component cost of debt estimate is 6.6 percent:

$$\text{Taxable component cost of debt} = R(R_d) \times (1 - T)$$

$$= 10\% \times (1 - 0.34)$$

$$= 10\% \times 0.66 = 6.6\%.$$

The component cost of debt to an investor-owned firm is an after-tax cost because the effective cost to the firm is reduced by the $(1 - T)$ term. By reducing Ann Arbor's component cost of debt from 10 percent to 6.6 percent, the cost of debt estimate has incorporated the benefit associated with interest payment tax deductibility.

In general, the **effective** cost of debt is roughly comparable between investor-owned and not-for-profit firms of similar risk. Investor-owned firms have the benefit of tax deductibility of interest payments, while not-for-profit firms have the benefit of being able to issue lower interest-rate tax-exempt debt.

---

1. What are some methods used to estimate a firm's cost of debt?
2. What is the impact of flotation costs on the cost of debt? Are these costs generally material?
3. For investor-owned firms, how is the before-tax cost of debt converted to an after-tax cost?
4. Not-for-profit businesses can issue tax-exempt debt and hence pay a lower interest rate on debt financing than for-profit businesses. Does this mean that debt financing generally is less costly for not-for-profit businesses?

Self-Test Questions

Cost of Equity Capital

Investor-owned businesses raise equity capital by selling new common stock and by retaining earnings for use by the firm rather than paying them out as dividends to shareholders. Not-for-profit businesses raise equity capital through contributions and grants, and by generating an excess of revenues over expenses, none of which can be paid out as dividends. In the following sections, we describe how to estimate the cost of equity capital both to investor-owned and not-for-profit businesses.[6]

Cost of Equity to Investor-Owned Businesses

The cost of debt is based on the return that investors require on debt securities, and the *cost of equity* to investor-owned businesses can be defined similarly: It is the rate of return that investors require on the firm's common stock. This concept is clear when new common stock is sold, but it may appear that equity raised through **retained earnings** is costless. The reason that a cost of capital must be assigned to all forms of equity financing involves the *opportunity cost principle*. An investor-owned firm's net income literally belongs to its common stockholders. Employees are compensated by wages, suppliers are compensated by cash payments for supplies, bondholders are compensated by interest payments, governments are compensated by tax payments, and so on. The residual earnings of a firm, its net income, belongs to the stockholders and serves to "pay the rent" on stockholder-supplied capital.

Management can either pay out earnings in the form of dividends or retain earnings for reinvestment in the business. If part of the earnings is retained, an opportunity cost is incurred: stockholders could have received these earnings as dividends and then invested this money in stocks, bonds, real estate, commodity futures, and so on. Thus, the firm should earn on its retained earnings at least as much as its stockholders themselves could earn on **alternative investments of similar risk**. If the firm cannot earn as much as stockholders can in similar risk investments, then the firm's net income should be paid out as dividends rather than being retained for reinvestment within the firm. What rate of return can stockholders expect to earn on other investments of equivalent risk? The answer is $R(R_e)$—the required rate of return on equity. Investors can earn this return either by buying more shares of the firm in question or by buying the stock of similar firms.

Three primary methods may be used by large, publicly traded businesses to estimate the cost of equity: the Capital Asset Pricing Model (CAPM), the discounted cash flow (DCF) model, and the debt cost plus risk premium model. These methods should **not** be regarded as mutually exclusive because no single approach dominates the estimation process. In practice, all three approaches (if applicable) should be used to estimate the cost of equity, and then the final value should be chosen on the basis of one's confidence in the data at hand.

Capital Asset Pricing Model (CAPM) Approach

The *Capital Asset Pricing Model (CAPM)*, which was introduced in Chapter 10, is a widely accepted finance model that specifies the equilibrium risk/return relationship on common stocks. Basically, the model assumes that investors consider only one risk factor when setting required rates of return—the volatility of returns on the stock compared with the volatility of returns on a well-diversified stock portfolio called the *market portfolio*, or just the *market*. The measure of risk in the CAPM is the stock's *market beta*.

Within the CAPM, the actual equation that relates risk to return is the *Security Market Line (SML)*:

$$R(R_e) = RF + [R(R_M) - RF] \times b$$
$$= RF + (RP_M \times b).$$

Managers can estimate the required rate of return on the firm's stock, $R(R_e)$, given estimates of the risk-free rate, RF, the beta of the stock, b, and the required rate of return on the market, $R(R_M)$. This estimate, in turn, can be used as the estimate for the firm's cost of equity.

The starting point for the CAPM cost of equity estimate is the risk-free rate. Unfortunately, there is no security in the United States that is truly riskless. Treasury securities are essentially free of default risk, but long-term T-bonds will suffer capital losses if interest rates rise, and a portfolio invested in short-term T-bills will provide a volatile earnings stream because the rate paid on T-bills varies over time. Because a truly riskless rate cannot be found in practice, what rate should be used? The preference shared by most finance professionals is to use the rate on long-term Treasury bonds.

There are many reasons for favoring the T-bond rate, including the fact that T-bill rates are very volatile because they are directly affected by actions taken by the Federal Reserve Board. Perhaps the most persuasive argument is that common stocks are generally viewed as long-term securities, and although a particular stockholder may not have a long investment horizon, the majority of stockholders do invest on a long-term basis. Therefore, it is reasonable to think that stock returns embody long-term inflation expectations similar to those embodied in bonds rather than the short-term inflation expectations embodied in bills. On this account, the cost of equity should be more highly correlated with T-bond rates than with T-bill rates. T-bond rates can be found in local newspapers, in the *Wall Street Journal*, and on numerous websites. Generally, the yield on ten-year T-bonds is used as the proxy for the risk-free rate.

The required rate of return on the market, and its derivative, the market risk premium, $RP_M = R(R_M) - RF$, can be estimated on the basis of either historical returns or expected returns. The most widely used set of historical market returns is provided by Ibbotson Associates. Their data, which are published annually, include annual rates of return on stocks, T-bills, T-bonds, and a set of high-grade corporate bonds.[7] In recent years, the historical market risk premium has been in the range of 4 to 6 percentage points.

The last parameter needed for a CAPM cost of equity estimate is the stock's beta coefficient. Unfortunately, beta measures how risky a stock was **in the past**, whereas investors are interested in **future** risk. It may be that a given company was judged to be quite safe in the past but that things have changed and its future risk is judged to be higher than its past risk, or vice versa. In general, is future risk sufficiently similar to past risk to warrant the use of historical betas in a CAPM framework? For individual firms, historical betas are often not very stable, so past risk is often *not* a good predictor of future risk.[8]

Furthermore, betas can be calculated over different time periods, and different measures for the market return can be used, so different financial advisory services report different betas for the same company. The choice is a matter of judgment and data availability, for there is no right beta. With luck, the betas derived from different sources will, for a given company, be close together. If they are not, confidence in the CAPM cost of equity estimate will be diminished.

To illustrate the CAPM approach, consider Ann Arbor Health Systems, which has a beta coefficient, b, of 1.50. Furthermore, assume that the current yield on T-bonds, RF, is 6 percent and that the best estimate for the current market risk premium, RP_M, is 5 percentage points. In other words, the current required rate of return on the market, $R(R_M)$, is 11 percent. All the required input parameters have been estimated, and the SML equation can be solved as follows:

$$R(R_e) = RF + [R(R_M) - RF] \times b_{AAHS}$$

$$= 6\% + (11.0\% - 6\%) \times 1.50$$

$$= 6\% + (5.0\% \times 1.50)$$

$$= 6\% + 7.5\% = 13.5\%.$$

Thus, according to the CAPM, Ann Arbor's required rate of return on equity is 13.5 percent.

What does the 13.5 percent estimate for $R(R_e)$ imply? In essence, equity investors believe that Ann Arbor's stock, with a beta of 1.50, is more risky than the average stock with a beta of 1.00. With a risk-free rate of 6 percent, and a market risk premium of 5 percentage points, an average firm, with $b = 1.0$, has a required rate of return on equity of $6\% + (5\% \times 1.00) = 6\% + 5\% = 11\%$. Thus, according to the CAPM, equity investors require 250 basis points (2.50 percentage points) more return for investing in Ann Arbor Health Systems, with $b = 1.50$, rather than an average stock, with $b = 1.00$.

There is a great deal of uncertainty in the CAPM estimate of the cost of equity. Some of this uncertainty stems from the fact that there is no assurance that the CAPM is correct—that is, that the CAPM accurately describes the risk/return choices of stock investors. Additionally, there is a great deal of uncertainty in the input parameter estimates, especially the required rate of return on the market and the beta coefficient. Because of these uncertainties, it is highly unlikely that Ann Arbor's true, but unobservable, cost of equity is 13.5 percent. Thus, instead of picking single values for each parameter, it may be better to develop high and low estimates and then to combine all of the high estimates and all of the low estimates to develop a range, rather than a point estimate, for $R(R_e)$.

Discounted Cash Flow (DCF) Approach The second approach to estimating the cost of equity is the *discounted cash flow (DCF)* approach, which uses the dividend valuation model as its basis. As we discussed in Chapter 12, if the company has an established track record of paying dividends and if the dividend is expected to grow each year at a constant rate, $E(g)$, then the *constant growth model* can be used to estimate the expected rate of return on the stock, $E(R_e)$:

$$E(R_e) = \frac{D_0 \times [1 + E(g)]}{P_0} + E(g) = \frac{E(D_1)}{P_0} + E(g).$$

Because stock prices typically are in equilibrium, the expected rate of return, $E(R_e)$, is also the required rate of return, $R(R_e)$.

As in the CAPM approach, there are three input parameters in the DCF model. Current stock price, P_0, is readily available for firms that are actively traded. Ann Arbor Health Systems' stock is traded in the over-the-counter (OTC) market, so its stock price can be determined easily. At the time of the analysis, Ann Arbor's stock price was $40.

Next year's dividend payment, $E(D_1)$, is also relatively easy to estimate. Ann Arbor's managers can obtain this estimate from the firm's five-year financial plan. For an outsider, dividend data on larger publicly traded firms are available from brokerage houses and investment advisory firms. Ann Arbor Health Systems is followed by several analysts at major brokerage houses, and their consensus estimate for next year's dividend payment is $2.50, so for purposes of this analysis, $E(D_1) = \$2.50$. If next year's dividend estimate is not available, the current dividend, D_0, along with the expected growth rate can be used to make the estimate.

The dividend growth rate is the most difficult of the DCF model parameters to estimate. Although historical earnings and dividend data can be analyzed directly to estimate growth rates, most finance professionals rely on expert analysts for growth-rate estimates. Analysts forecast and then publish growth rate estimates for most of the larger publicly owned companies. For example, *Value Line* provides such forecasts on about 1,700 companies, and all of the larger brokerage houses provide similar forecasts. Furthermore, several companies compile analysts' forecasts on a regular basis and provide summary information such as the median and range of forecasts on widely followed companies. These growth rate summaries, such as the one compiled by the *Institutional Brokers Estimate System (IBES)*, can be ordered for a fee and obtained either in hardcopy format or as online electronic data.

However, analysts' forecasts often assume nonconstant growth. For example, analysts who follow Ann Arbor Health Systems, on average, forecasted a 12 percent annual growth rate in earnings and dividends over the next five years, followed by a steady-state growth rate of 6.5 percent. A rough way to handle this situation is to use the nonconstant growth forecast to develop a proxy constant growth rate. Computer simulations indicate that dividends beyond Year 50 contribute very little to the value of any stock: The present value of dividends beyond Year 50 is virtually zero, so it is reasonable to ignore dividends beyond that point. If only a 50-year horizon is considered, a weighted average growth rate can be developed and used as a constant growth rate for cost of capital purposes. For Ann Arbor Health Systems, the growth rate of 12 percent for five years was assumed to be followed by a growth rate of 6.5 percent for 45 years, which produced an arithmetic average annual growth rate of $(0.10 \times 12\%) + (0.90 \times 6.5\%) = 7.2\%$. This figure, together with other estimates, leads to the conclusion that Ann Arbor Health Systems' expected dividend growth rate is in the range of 7 to 8 percent.[9]

To illustrate the DCF approach, consider the data developed thus far for Ann Arbor Health Systems. The company's current stock price, P_0, is $40, and its next expected annual dividend, $E(D_1)$, is $2.50. Thus, the firm's DCF estimate of $R(R_e)$, according to the DCF model, is:

$$R(R_e) = \frac{E(D_1)}{P_0} + E(g)$$

$$= \frac{\$2.50}{\$40} + E(g) = 6.3\% + E(g).$$

With an $E(g)$ estimate range of 7 to 8 percent, the midpoint, 7.5 percent, will be used as the final estimate. Thus, the DCF estimate for Ann Arbor Health Systems' cost of equity is $6.3\% + 7.5\% = 13.8\%$.

Debt Cost Plus Risk Premium Approach The *debt cost plus risk premium* approach relies on the fact that stock investments are riskier than debt investments; hence the cost of equity for any business can be thought of as the cost of debt **to that business,** plus a risk premium:

$$R(R_e) = R(R_d) + \text{Risk premium}.$$

The cost of debt is relatively easy to estimate, so the key input to this model is the risk premium.

Note that the risk premium used here is **not** the same as the market risk premium used in the CAPM. The market risk premium is the amount that investors require above the **risk-free rate** to invest in an average risk common stock. Here, we need the risk premium above the firm's own **cost of debt**. How might this new risk premium be estimated? Using the data from above, we know that the cost of equity for an average risk ($b = 1.0$) stock is 11 percent. Furthermore, the cost of debt for an average firm, which has roughly an A rating, is 7 percent. Thus, for an average firm the risk premium of the cost of equity over the cost of debt is $11\% - 7\% = 4$ percentage points.

Empirical work suggests that the risk premium for use in the debt cost plus risk premium model has ranged from 3 to 5 percentage points, so our current estimate of 4 percentage points is consistent with historical results. Perhaps the greatest weakness of this approach is that there is no assurance that the risk premium for the average firm is the same as the risk premium for the firm in question—in this case, Ann Arbor Health Systems. Thus, the risk premium method does not have the theoretical precision that the other models do. On the other hand, the input values required by the debt cost plus risk premium model are fewer and easier to estimate than in the other models, and hence it can be used in situations where the other models cannot.

With a before-tax cost of debt estimate of 10 percent and a current risk premium estimate of 4 percentage points, the debt cost plus risk premium estimate for Ann Arbor's cost of equity is 14 percent:

$$R(R_e) = R(R_d) + \text{Risk premium}$$

$$= 10\% + 4\% = 14\%.$$

We have presented three methods for estimating the cost of equity. The CAPM estimate was 13.5 percent, the DCF estimate was 13.8 percent, and the debt cost plus risk premium estimate was 14 percent. At this point, judgment is required. Most analysts would conclude that there is sufficient consistency in the three results to warrant the use of a cost of equity estimate somewhere in the range of 13.5 to 14 percent. We choose 13.9 percent as our final estimate because of our concern over the input values used in the CAPM estimate. In general, analysts must judge the relative merits of each estimate and then choose a final estimate that seems most reasonable under the circumstances. This choice typically is made on the basis of the analyst's confidence in the input parameters of each approach.

Comparison of the Three Methods

Cost of Equity to Not-for-Profit Businesses

Not-for-profit businesses raise equity (fund) capital in two basic ways: (1) by receiving contributions and grants and (2) by earning an excess of revenues over expenses (retained earnings). In this section we first discuss some views regarding the cost of fund capital, and then we illustrate how this cost might be estimated.

Our primary purpose in this chapter is to develop a corporate cost-of-capital estimate that can be used in making capital investment decisions. Thus, the estimated "costs" represent the cost of using capital to purchase fixed (capital) assets, rather than for alternative uses. What is the cost of using equity capital for real-asset investments within not-for-profit businesses? There are several positions that can be taken on this question.[10]

- **Fund capital has a zero cost.** The rationale here is that (1) contributors do not expect a monetary return on their contributions and (2) the firm's stakeholders, especially the patients who pay more for services than warranted by the firm's tangible costs, do not require an explicit return on the capital retained by the firm. With no explicit return required by the suppliers of equity capital, the cost of that capital is zero.
- **Fund capital has a cost equal to the return forgone on short-term (marketable) securities investments.** When a not-for-profit firm receives contributions or retains earnings, it can always invest these funds in marketable securities (highly liquid, safe securities) rather than purchase real assets. Thus, fund capital has a relatively low opportunity cost that

should be acknowledged; this cost is roughly equal to the return available on a portfolio of short-term, low-risk securities such as T-bills.

- **Fund capital has a cost equal to the expected growth rate of the business's assets.**[11] Assume that a hospital must increase its total assets by 8 percent per year to keep pace with an increasing patient load. To purchase the required assets without increasing its proportion of debt financing, the hospital must grow its fund capital at an 8 percent rate. In this way, it can finance asset growth by growing both debt and equity at the same 8 percent rate and hence can hold the proportion of debt at its target. If the hospital earned zero return on its existing fund capital, it would be unable to add new assets without increasing its debt ratio or relying on grants and contributions to provide the needed equity. Even if no volume growth is expected, a not-for-profit business must earn a return on its fund capital just to replace its existing asset base as assets wear out or become obsolete. New equity capital is required because new assets generally will cost more than the ones being replaced and hence depreciation cash flow in itself will not be sufficient to replace assets as needed. The bottom line here is that not-for-profit firms must earn a return on equity merely to support dollar growth in assets; and the greater the growth rate, including that caused by inflation and technology improvements, the greater the return that must be earned.

- **Fund capital has a cost equal to that required to maintain the business's creditworthiness.** One of the factors that rating agencies consider when assigning debt ratings is the profitability of the business: All else the same, the higher the profitability of the business, the better the credit rating. In general, managers of not-for-profit healthcare businesses have some target debt rating that they seek to achieve (or maintain). Furthermore, rating agencies publish profitability measures, including return on equity, that they consider to be appropriate for each debt rating. Thus, to maintain the business's desired rating, managers must achieve the return on equity recommended by the rating agencies, which in turn sets the business's cost of equity target.

- **Fund capital has a cost equal to the cost of equity to similar for-profit businesses.** Like the second position above, this position also rests on the opportunity cost concept, but the opportunity cost is now defined as the return available from investing fund capital in **alternative investments of similar risk**. To illustrate, suppose Bayside Memorial Hospital, a not-for-profit corporation, receives $500,000 in unrestricted contributions in 2008 and also retains $4.5 million in earnings, so it has $5 million of new fund capital available for investment. The $5 million could be (1) used to purchase assets related to its core business, such as an outpatient clinic; (2) temporarily invested in securities with the intent of purchasing healthcare assets some time in the future; (3) used to retire debt; (4) used to pay management bonuses; (5) placed in a non-interest-bearing account at the bank; and on and on. If it uses this capital to invest in real assets, Bayside will be deprived of the opportunity to use the capital for other purposes, so an opportunity cost must be assigned that reflects the riskiness associated with an equity investment in hospital assets. What return is available on securities with similar risk to hospital assets? The answer is the return expected from investing in the stock of an investor-owned hospital business, such as Ann Arbor Health Systems. Instead of using fund capital to purchase real healthcare assets, Bayside could always use the funds to buy the stock of a for-profit hospital corporation and delay the real-asset purchase until some time in the future.

With these five positions in mind, which one should prevail in practice? Unfortunately, the answer is not clear-cut. Here are our views on this issue. At a minimum, a not-for-profit business should require a return on its equity investments in real assets that is as large as its projected asset growth rate. In that way, the business is setting the **minimum** rate of return that will, if it is actually achieved, ensure the financial stability of the organization. Thus, the expected growth rate sets the minimum required rate of return, and hence the minimum cost of equity, for not-for-profit businesses. However, if the rating agency's target return on equity is greater than the growth rate target, the rating agency's target should be used as the required return on equity to maintain the business's creditworthiness.

But to fully recover **all opportunity costs**, including the opportunity cost of employing equity capital in healthcare assets, the real-asset investments must offer an expected return equal to the return expected on similar-risk securities investments. Thus, the "true" economic opportunity cost of equity to a not-for-profit healthcare provider is the rate that could be earned on stock investments in similar investor-owned firms. Using this cost of equity, a not-for-profit business is requiring that all costs, including full opportunity costs, be considered in the cost of capital estimate. Note that full opportunity costs do not have to be recovered on every new capital investment undertaken. Not-for-profit businesses do invest in projects that are beneficial in ways other than financial, so the cost of capital estimate does not set an absolute limit on new investment. We do believe, however, that healthcare managers should be aware of the true financial opportunity costs inherent in capital investments, and the only way this can be accomplished is to use the cost of equity to similar for-profit businesses as the cost of fund capital.

Although the "full opportunity cost" approach appears to be most correct, many would argue that the unique mission of not-for-profit businesses precludes securities investments as realistic alternatives to healthcare plant and equipment investments because securities investments do not contribute directly to the mission of providing healthcare services. If that is the case, then the cost of fund capital should be the greater of the expected growth rate and the creditworthiness-maintaining rate.

The Corporate Cost of Capital

The final step in the cost of capital estimation process is to combine the debt and equity cost estimates to form the *corporate cost of capital*. As discussed at the beginning of this chapter, each firm has a target capital structure—that is, the particular mix of debt and equity that causes its average cost of capital to be minimized. Furthermore, when a firm raises new capital, it generally tries to finance in a way that will keep the actual capital structure reasonably close to its target over time.

Here is the general formula for the corporate cost of capital (CCC) for all firms, regardless of ownership:

$$CCC = [w_d \times R(R_d) \times (1 - T)] + [w_e \times R(R_e)],$$

where w_d and w_e are the target weights for debt and equity, respectively. The cost of the debt component, $R(R_d)$, will be an average if the firm uses several types of debt for its permanent financing. Alternatively, the above equation could be expanded to include multiple debt terms. Investor-owned firms would use their marginal tax rate for T, while T would be zero for not-for-profit firms.

The corporate cost of capital represents the cost of each **new** dollar of capital raised, rather than the average cost of all the dollars raised in the past. Because the primary interest is in obtaining a cost of capital for use in capital investment analysis; a *marginal cost* is required. Furthermore, the corporate cost of capital formula implies that each new dollar of capital will consist of both debt and equity that is raised, at least conceptually, in proportion to the firm's target capital structure.

The Corporate Cost of Capital for Investor-Owned Firms

To illustrate the corporate cost of capital calculation for investor-owned firms, consider Ann Arbor Health Systems, which has a target capital structure of 60 percent debt and 40 percent equity. As previously estimated, the company's before-tax cost of debt, $R(R_d)$, is 10 percent; its tax rate, T, is 34 percent; and its cost of equity, $R(R_e)$ is 13.9 percent, so Ann Arbor's corporate cost of capital estimate is 9.5 percent:

$$CCC = [w_d \times R(R_d) \times (1 - T)] + [w_e \times R(R_e)]$$
$$= [0.60 \times 10\% \times (1 - 0.34)] + [0.40 \times 13.9\%]$$
$$= 9.5\%.$$

Conceptually, every dollar of new capital that Ann Arbor will obtain consists of 60 cents of debt with an after-tax cost of 6.6 percent and 40 cents of equity with a cost of 13.9 percent. The average cost of each new dollar is 9.5 percent. In any one year, Ann Arbor may raise all its required new capital by issuing debt, by retaining earnings, or by selling new common stock. But over the long run, Ann Arbor plans to use 60 percent debt financing and 40 percent equity financing, and these weights must be used in the corporate cost of capital estimate **regardless** of the actual financing plans for the near term.

The Corporate Cost of Capital for Not-for-Profit Firms

The corporate cost of capital for not-for-profit businesses is developed in the same way as for investor-owned firms. To illustrate, the corporate cost of capital for Bayside Memorial Hospital, assuming a target capital structure of 50 percent debt and 50 percent equity, and using the estimates for the component costs that were developed earlier, is 10 percent:

$$CCC = [w_d \times R(R_d) \times (1 - T)] + [w_e \times R(R_e)]$$
$$= [0.50 \times 6.1\% \times (1 - 0)] + [0.50 \times 13.9\%]$$
$$= 10.0\%.$$

Note that we have assigned the full opportunity cost of equity capital to Bayside, which is the cost of equity to similar for-profit businesses (13.9 percent).

Businesses, regardless of ownership, cannot raise unlimited amounts of new capital in any given year at a constant cost. Eventually, for several reasons, as more new capital is raised, investors will require higher returns on debt and equity capital, even though the capital is raised in accordance with the firm's target structure. Thus, the corporate costs of capital, as estimated here for Ann Arbor and Bayside, are only valid when the amount required for capital investment falls within the firm's normal range. If capital is required in amounts that far exceed those normally raised, the corporate cost of capital must be subjectively adjusted upward to reflect the higher costs involved.

1. What is the general formula for the corporate cost of capital?
2. What weights should be used in the formula? Why?
3. What is the primary difference between the corporate costs of capital for investor-owned and not-for-profit firms?

Self-Test Questions

4. Is the corporate cost of capital affected by short-term financing plans? Explain your answer.
5. Is the corporate cost of capital constant regardless of the amount of new capital required? Explain your answer.

Cost of Capital Estimation for Small Businesses

The guidance given thus far in the chapter focuses on the cost of capital estimation process for large healthcare businesses. But what if the business is small, such as a solo practice, a small group practice, or a small, free-standing hospital? The estimation process is the same as described, but the manner in which the component costs are estimated must be handled differently.

Estimating the Cost of Debt

Small businesses typically obtain the bulk of their debt financing from commercial banks, so a business's commercial loan officer will be able to provide some insights into the cost of future debt financing. Alternatively, managers of small businesses can look to marketplace activity for guidance; that is, the interest rate currently being set on the debt issues of similar-risk firms can be used as an estimate of the cost of debt. Here, similar risk can be judged by subjective analysis (same industry, similar size, similar use of debt, and so on). Alternatively, the prime rate gives small businesses a benchmark for bank loan rates. If the business has borrowed from commercial banks in the past, its managers will know the historical premium charged above the prime rate for the business's bank debt. An awareness of the current interest rate environment generally permits managers to make a reasonable estimate for their own business's cost of debt, even when the business is quite small.

Estimating the Cost of Equity

Although estimating the cost of debt for a small business is relatively easy, the cost-of-equity estimate is more problematic. Here are some points to note:

Debt Cost Plus Risk Premium Approach Perhaps the easiest way to estimate the cost of equity of a small business is to use the debt cost plus risk premium method. Because the cost of debt is relatively easy to estimate, it is equally easy to add some risk premium—say, 4 percentage points—to the business's before-tax cost of debt to obtain its cost of equity estimate. However, this can only be considered a starting point estimate because the risk premiums that are applicable to small businesses may be much larger than those estimated for large firms.

Pure Play Approach As an alternative to the debt cost plus risk premium approach, a proxy publicly traded firm in the same line of business can be identified and its beta used to estimate the equity risk of the small business. This technique is called the *pure play* approach. To illustrate, suppose the beta for a publicly traded practice management firm is 0.88. **Assuming the risk inherent in the stock of a practice management company is the same as the risk involved in the ownership of a small group practice**, then a beta of 0.88 can be used to proxy the ownership risk. Then, the CAPM approach can be used to estimate the small business's cost of equity.

To use the pure play approach for a small business, the assumption must be made that the risk to the owners of the publicly traded proxy firm is the same as the risk to the owners of the small business. However, there are several important differences between the ownership of stock in a large corporation and the ownership of a small group practice. First, the geographic and business line diversification of a large business typically makes ownership less risky than a similar position in a small, localized single-line business. Second, most stockholders of large businesses hold that stock as part of a well-diversified investment portfolio that has returns that are not highly correlated with the stockholders' employment earnings. With a small group practice, the employment returns and equity returns typically are one and the same. Third, stock owned in an investment portfolio is highly liquid; the owner can sell it quickly at a fair market price with a single phone call. Conversely, an ownership position in a small group practice is very difficult to sell.

All of these factors suggest that the cost of equity to a small owner-managed business is higher, perhaps much higher, than that calculated using the CAPM and a proxy company.

When estimating the cost of equity for small businesses, it is common to use an approach called the *build-up method*. Here, the cost of equity of a similar large business is used as the base, or starting point. This base cost may be estimated by the debt cost plus risk premium method, by the pure play method, or by some blend of the two methods. Then, various adjustments, or premiums, are added to account for the differences between large and small businesses. **Build-Up Method**

Size Premium. Although returns data on businesses as small as a group practice are not readily available, studies using historical returns data indicate that the cost of equity for the smallest stocks listed on the New York Stock Exchange—those in the bottom decile of market value—is about 4 percentage points higher than the cost of equity for large businesses—those in the S&P 500. This added premium to compensate for the additional risk inherent in the ownership of small, as opposed to large, businesses is called the *size premium*. It can be argued that the size premium is even larger than 4 percentage points for firms so small that their equity is not publicly traded. The bottom line here is that when the cost of equity of a small business is estimated on the basis of equity costs to similar large businesses, an additional premium must be added just to account for the size differential.

Liquidity Premium. Because an ownership position in a small business is less liquid than the stock of a large corporation, it is common to add a liquidity premium when estimating the cost of equity for a small business.

This premium is generally thought to be about 2 percentage points. Note, however, that if an investor has a control position (more than 50 percent ownership), then some of the risk associated with small business ownership is reduced.

Unique Risk Premium. Some small businesses have unique risk. For example, the success of a start-up business might depend on new, unproven technology. Or the success of a small business might depend on the intellectual capital or managerial prowess of one person. In such situations, an equity investment is **very** risky, and it is not uncommon to add a premium of 5 percentage points or more to account for such unique risk.

To illustrate the build-up method, consider a small medical practice. The cost of equity to a large practice management company is found as follows:

$$R(R_e) = RF + [R(R_M) - RF] \times b$$

$$= 6\% + (11\% - 6\%) \times 0.88$$

$$= 6\% + (5\% \times 0.88) = 10.4\%.$$

Here we used a pure play beta of 0.88 along with the market data used in previous examples to obtain a base cost of equity of 10.4 percent.

Now, using the build-up method, and assuming a size premium of 4 percentage points and a liquidity premium of 2 percentage points, we obtain the following cost of equity estimate:

$$\text{Cost of equity} = 10.4\% + 4\% + 2\% = 16.4\%.$$

If any unique risk is identified for this practice, the cost of equity estimate could be even higher.

Although the estimation process clearly is more difficult for small businesses, it may be even more important for small businesses to recognize their corporate costs of capital than it is for large businesses. The reason is that in small businesses, owners often have their livelihoods as well as their equity investment tied to the business. With the techniques described in this section, even a small business owner can take a stab at estimating his or her business's corporate cost of capital.

Self-Test Questions

1. What are the problems faced by small businesses when estimating the corporate cost of capital?
2. What is the size premium? Liquidity premium? Unique risk premium?
3. Describe the build-up method for estimating a small business's cost of equity.

An Economic Interpretation of the Corporate Cost of Capital

Thus far, the focus of the cost of capital discussion has been on the mechanics of the estimation process. In closing, it is worthwhile to step back from the mathematics of the process and examine the corporate cost of capital's economic interpretation.

The component cost estimates (the costs of debt and equity) that make up a firm's corporate cost of capital are based on the returns that investors require to supply capital to the business. In turn, investors' required rates of return are based on the opportunity costs borne by investing in the debt and equity of the firm in question, rather than in alternative investments of similar risk. These opportunity costs to investors, when combined into the firm's corporate cost of capital, establish the **opportunity cost** to the business; that is, the corporate cost of capital is the return that the business could earn by investing in alternative investments that have the same risk as its own real assets. From a purely financial perspective, if a business (especially one that is investor owned) cannot earn its corporate cost of capital on new capital investments, no new investments should be made and no new capital should be raised. If existing investments are not earning the corporate cost of capital, they should be terminated, the assets liquidated, and the proceeds returned to investors for reinvestment elsewhere.

However, the corporate cost of capital is not the appropriate minimum rate of return for all new real-asset investments. The required rates of return set by investors on the business's debt and equity are based on perceptions regarding the riskiness of their investments, which in turn are based on two factors: (1) the inherent riskiness of the business (i.e., business risk) and (2) the amount of debt financing used (i.e., financial risk). Thus, the firm's inherent business risk and capital structure are embedded in its corporate cost of capital estimate.

Because different firms have different business risk and use different proportions of debt financing, different firms have different corporate costs of capital. Differential capital costs are most pronounced for firms in different industries. Still, even firms in the same industry can have different business risk, and capital structure differences among such firms can compound corporate cost of capital differences.

The primary purpose of estimating a business's corporate cost of capital is to help make capital budgeting decisions; that is, the cost of capital will be used as the benchmark capital budgeting *hurdle rate*, or minimum return necessary for a project to be attractive financially. The firm can always earn its cost of capital by investing in selected stocks and bonds that in the aggregate have the same risk as the firm's assets, so it should not invest in real assets unless it can earn at least as much. However, remember that the corporate cost of capital reflects opportunity costs based on the aggregate risk of the firm (i.e., the riskiness of the firm's average project). Thus, the corporate cost of capital can be applied without modification only to those projects under consideration that have average risk, where average is defined as that applicable to the firm's currently held assets in the aggregate. If a project under consideration has risk that differs significantly from that of the firm's average asset, then the corporate cost of capital must be adjusted to account for the differential risk when the project is being evaluated.

To illustrate the concept, Bayside Memorial Hospital's corporate cost of capital, 10 percent, is probably appropriate for use in evaluating a new outpatient clinic that has risk similar to the hospital's average project, which involves the provision of healthcare services. Clearly, it would **not** be appropriate to apply Bayside's 10 percent corporate cost of capital without adjustment to a new project that involves establishing a managed care subsidiary; this project does not have the same risk as the hospital's average asset.

As discussed in Chapter 10, investors require higher returns for riskier investments. Thus, a high-risk project must have a higher *project cost of capital* than a low-risk project. Figure 13.2 illustrates the relationship between project risk, the corporate cost of capital, and project costs of capital. The figure illustrates that Bayside's 10 percent corporate cost of capital is the appropriate hurdle rate **only** for an **average risk** project (Project A), where average means

FIGURE 13.2
Bayside
Memorial
Hospital:
Corporate and
Project Costs of
Capital

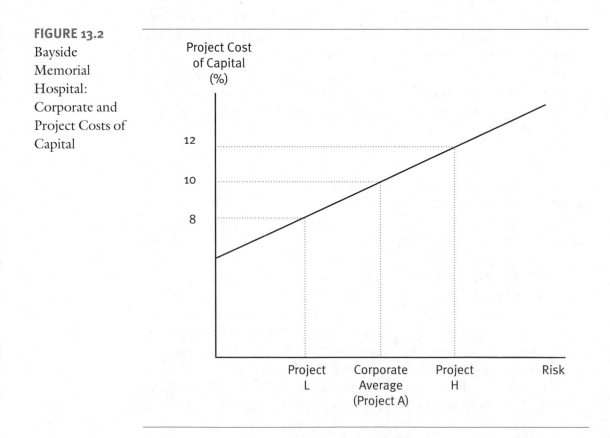

a project that has the same risk as the aggregate business. Project L, which has less risk than Bayside's average project, has a project cost of capital of 8 percent, which is less than the corporate cost of capital. Conversely, Project H, with more risk than the average project, has a higher project cost of capital of 12 percent.

The key point here is that the corporate cost of capital is merely a **benchmark** that will be used as the basis for estimating project costs of capital. It is not a one-size-fits-all rate that can be used with abandon whenever an opportunity cost is needed in a financial analysis. This point will be revisited in Chapter 15 when capital investment risk considerations are addressed.

Finally, note that large businesses often have subsidiaries that operate in diverse lines of business. When this situation exists, for capital investment purposes it is best to estimate *divisional costs of capital* in addition to the corporate cost of capital. Whereas the overall cost of capital reflects the aggregate risk of the business, the divisional costs of capital reflect the unique risk (and perhaps unique capital structure) of each division. (In Chapter 15, we explore the concept of divisional costs of capital in more detail.)

1. Explain the economic interpretation of the corporate cost of capital.
2. Is the corporate cost of capital the appropriate opportunity cost for all projects that a business evaluates?
3. Draw a graph similar to the one shown in Figure 13.2, and explain its implications.
4. Should large businesses estimate divisional costs of capital? Explain your answer.

Self-Test Questions

Key Concepts

This chapter discusses optimal capital structure and the corporate cost of capital—two very important concepts in healthcare finance. The key concepts in this chapter are:

- The choice between debt and equity financing is one type of risk/return trade-off. The use of debt financing can *leverage up* the return to owners or, in not-for-profit firms, the return on fund capital, but it also *increases the riskiness* of the business.
- The *optimal*, or *target, capital structure* is that structure that minimizes the average cost of capital to the business.
- Unfortunately, finance theory is of limited help in actually setting a firm's target structure. Thus, in making the capital structure decision, health services managers must consider a wide range of factors, including the following: business risk, lender and rating agency attitudes, reserve borrowing capacity, industry averages, and asset structure.

- Managers of not-for-profit businesses must grapple with the same capital structure decisions as the managers of investor-owned firms. However, not-for-profit firms do not have the same flexibility in making financing decisions because they cannot issue common stock.
- In estimating a firm's corporate cost of capital, the *component cost of debt* is the *after-tax* cost of new debt. For taxable firms, it is found by multiplying the before-tax cost of new debt by $(1 - T)$, where T is the firm's marginal tax rate, so the component cost of debt is $R(R_d) \times (1 - T)$. For not-for-profit firms, the debt is often tax-exempt, but no other tax effects apply, so the component cost of debt is merely the tax-exempt $R(R_d)$.
- The *cost of equity* to investor-owned firms is the return that its stockholders could obtain by investing in the stocks of similar-risk companies. For large, publicly traded companies, it usually is estimated by using three methods: the *Capital Asset Pricing Model (CAPM)* approach, the *discounted cash flow (DCF)* approach, and the *debt cost plus risk premium* approach.
- For not-for-profit firms, the *cost of equity (fund capital)* can be estimated in two ways. First, the full opportunity cost approach uses the *cost of equity* of similar investor-owned firms. Second, the minimum cost of equity approach uses the *expected growth rate* of the business (or the return on equity target set by *rating agencies.*
- Each firm has a *target capital structure,* and the target weights are used to estimate the firm's *corporate cost of capital (CCC)*:

$$CCC = [w_d \times R(R_d) \times (1 - T)] + [w_e \times R(R_e)].$$

- The corporate cost of capital for small businesses is estimated using the same techniques that are used for large businesses. However, the estimation of the component costs, particularly the cost of equity, becomes more difficult.
- The *build-up method* is used to estimate the cost of equity for a small business. This method uses the *pure play method* (cost of equity of a similar large business) or the debt cost plus risk premium method to establish a starting point, and then adds (1) a *size premium*, (2) a *liquidity premium*, and (3) any *unique risk premium*.
- When making *capital investment decisions,* a business will use the corporate cost of capital as the *hurdle rate* for **average risk** projects. A firm with divisions that operate in diverse lines of business should use divisional costs of capital for the same purpose.

The concepts developed in this chapter play a vital role in making capital investment decisions and hence will be revisited in Chapters 14 and 15.

Questions

13.1 Critique this statement: "The use of debt financing lowers the net income of the firm, and hence debt financing should be used only as a last resort."

13.2 Discuss some factors that health services managers must consider when setting a firm's target capital structure. Consider both investor-owned and not-for-profit firms in your answer.

13.3 Is the corporate cost of capital estimate based on historical or marginal costs? Why?

13.4 What capital components are typically included when estimating a firm's corporate cost of capital?

13.5 How may a firm's cost of debt be estimated?

13.6 a. Why is there a cost to retained earnings in investor-owned businesses?

   b. What are the three methods commonly used to estimate the cost of equity?

   c. Is the risk premium in the CAPM the same as the risk premium in the debt cost plus risk premium model?

   d. How would you estimate the cost of equity (fund capital) for a not-for-profit business?

   e. How would you estimate the cost of equity for a small investor-owned business?

13.7 What is the economic interpretation of the corporate cost of capital?

13.8 Is the corporate cost of capital the same for all firms? Explain your answer.

13.9 For any given firm, can the corporate cost of capital be used as the hurdle rate for all projects under consideration? Explain your answer.

Problems

13.1 Seattle Health Plans currently uses zero-debt financing. Its operating income (EBIT) is $1 million, and it pays taxes at a 40 percent rate. It has $5 million in assets and, because it is all-equity financed, $5 million in equity. Suppose the firm is considering replacing half of its equity financing with debt financing bearing an interest rate of 8 percent.

   a. What impact would the new capital structure have on the firm's net income, total dollar return to investors, and ROE?

   b. Redo the analysis, but now assume that the debt financing would cost 15 percent.

   c. Return to the initial 8 percent interest rate. Now, assume that EBIT could be as low as $500,000 (with a probability of 20 percent) or as high as $1.5 million (with a probability of 20 percent). There remains a 60 percent chance that EBIT would be $1 million. Redo the analysis for each level of EBIT, and find the expected values for the firm's net income, total dollar return to investors, and ROE. What lesson about capital structure and risk does this illustration provide?

    d. Repeat the analysis required for Part a, but now assume that Seattle Health Plans is a not-for-profit corporation and hence pays no taxes. Compare the results with those obtained in Part a.

13.2 Calculate the after-tax cost of debt for the Wallace Clinic, a for-profit healthcare provider, assuming that the coupon rate set on its debt is 11 percent and its tax rate is:

    a. 0 percent

    b. 20 percent

    c. 40 percent

13.3 St. Vincent's Hospital has a target capital structure of 35 percent debt and 65 percent equity. Its cost of equity (fund capital) estimate is 13.5 percent and its cost of tax-exempt debt estimate is 7 percent. What is the hospital's corporate cost of capital?

13.4 Richmond Clinic has obtained the following estimates for its costs of debt and equity at various capital structures:

Percent Debt	After-Tax Cost of Debt	Cost of Equity
0%	—	16%
20	6.6	17
40	7.8	19
60	10.2	22
80	14.0	27

What is the firm's optimal capital structure? (Hint: Calculate its corporate cost of capital at each structure. Also, note that data on component costs at alternative capital structures are not reliable in real-world situations.)

13.5 Medical Associates is a large for-profit group practice. Its dividends are expected to grow at a constant rate of 7 percent per year into the foreseeable future. The firm's last dividend (D_0) was $2, and its current stock price is $23. The firm's beta coefficient is 1.6; the rate of return on 20-year T-bonds currently is 9 percent; and the expected rate of return on the market, as reported by a large financial services firm, is 13 percent. The firm's target capital structure calls for 50 percent debt financing, the interest rate required on the business's new debt is 10 percent, and its tax rate is 40 percent.

    a. What is Medical Associates' cost of equity estimate according to the DCF method?

    b. What is the cost of equity estimate according to the CAPM?

    c. On the basis of your answers to Parts a and b, what would be your final estimate for the firm's cost of equity?

    d. What is your estimate for the firm's corporate cost of capital?

13.6 Morningside Nursing Home, a not-for-profit corporation, is estimating its corporate cost of capital. Its tax-exempt debt currently requires an interest rate of 6.2 percent and its target capital structure calls for 60 percent debt financing and 40 percent equity (fund capital) financing. The estimated costs of equity for selected investor-owned healthcare companies are given below:

Glaxo Wellcome	15.0%
Beverly Enterprises	16.4
HEALTHSOUTH	17.4
Humana	18.8

   a. What is the best estimate for Morningside's cost of equity?
   b. What is the firm's corporate cost of capital?

13.7 Golden State Home Health, Inc., is a large, California-based for-profit home health agency. Its dividends are expected to grow at a constant rate of 5 percent per year into the foreseeable future. The firm's last dividend (D_0) was $1, and its current stock price is $10. The firm's beta coefficient is 1.2; the rate of return on 20-year T-bonds currently is 8 percent; and the expected rate of return on the market, as reported by a large financial services firm, is 14 percent. Golden State's target capital structure calls for 60 percent debt financing, the interest rate required on its new debt is 9 percent, and the firm's tax rate is 30 percent.
   a. What is the firm's cost of equity estimate according to the DCF method?
   b. What is the cost of equity estimate according to the CAPM?
   c. On the basis of your answers to Parts a and b, what would be your final estimate for the firm's cost of equity?
   d. What is your estimate for the firm's corporate cost of capital?

Notes

1. In this book, we present only an overview of the capital structure decision. For more information, see Louis C. Gapenski, *Understanding Healthcare Financial Management* (Chicago: Health Administration Press, 2007), Chapter 10.
2. Our illustration does not address the impact of debt financing on not-for-profit firms. Here are the income statements assuming zero taxes:

	Stock	Stock/Debt
Revenues	$150,000	$150,000
Operating costs	100,000	100,000
Operating income	$ 50,000	$ 50,000
Interest expense	0	10,000
Net income	$ 50,000	$ 40,000
ROE	25%	40%

We see here that the use of debt also leverages up the return on ownership capital in not-for-profit firms. Note, however, that the interest rate on tax-exempt debt would be lower than the rate we used here, so the advantage of debt financing is actually greater than this illustration suggests.

3. If we examined the impact of debt financing on portfolio (market) risk, as opposed to stand-alone risk, we would get the same result. Namely, the use of debt financing increases the beta of the stock and hence the riskiness seen by equity investors.

4. For the use of debt financing to increase owners' rate of return, the inherent return on the business must be greater than the interest rate on the debt. The basic return on the business in the Super Health illustration is 25 percent ($50 in operating income divided by $200 in assets), and debt financing costs only 10 percent, so the use of debt financing increases ROE.

5. A question arises here as to whether the stated rate or the effective annual rate should be used in the cost of debt estimate. In general, the difference will be inconsequential, so most firms opt for the easier approach, which is simply to use the stated rate. (The effective annual rate in this example is $[1.0305]^2 - 1.0 = 6.19\%$ versus a 6.1 percent stated rate.) More importantly, most capital budgeting analyses use end-of-year cash flows to proxy cash flows that occur throughout the year, in effect creating nominal cash flows. For consistency, we prefer to use a nominal (stated) cost of capital—the cash flows will be understated but so will the cost of capital.

6. Only a few firms in the health services industry use preferred stock financing, so we will not include preferred stock in our cost-of-capital examples. If preferred stock is used as a source of permanent financing, it should be included in the cost of capital estimate, and its cost would be estimated using procedures similar to those discussed for the cost of debt.

7. See *Stocks, Bonds, Bills and Inflation: 2007 Yearbook* (Chicago: Ibbotson Associates, 2007).

8. Because historical betas may not be good predictors of future risk, researchers have sought ways to improve them. This has led to the development of two other types of betas: adjusted betas and fundamental betas. *Adjusted betas* recognize the fact that true betas tend to move toward 1.0 over time. Therefore, one can begin with a firm's pure historical statistical beta, make an adjustment for the expected future movement toward 1.0, and produce an adjusted beta that on average will be a better predictor of the future beta than would the unadjusted historical beta. *Fundamental betas* extend the adjustment process to include such fundamental risk variables as the use of debt financing, sales volatility, and the like. These betas are constantly adjusted to reflect changes in a firm's operations and capital structure, whereas with historical betas (including adjusted ones) such changes might not be fully reflected until several years after the company's "true" beta has changed.

9. The *retention growth method* is another method for estimating the growth rate in dividends:

$$E(g) = \text{Retention ratio} \times E(ROE).$$

To illustrate the retention growth model, suppose Ann Arbor Health Systems has had an average return on equity of about 14 percent over the past ten years. The ROE has been relatively steady, but even so it has ranged from a low of 8.9 percent to a high of 17.6 percent during this period. In addition, the firm's dividend payout ratio has averaged 0.45 over the past ten years, so its retention ratio has averaged $1.0 - 0.45 = 0.55$. Using these data, the retention growth method gives an E(g) estimate of 7.7 percent:

$$E(g) = 0.55 \times 14\% = 7.7\%.$$

10. For one of the classic works on this topic, see Douglas A. Conrad, "Returns on Equity to Not-For-Profit Hospitals: Theory and Implementation," *Health Services Research* (April 1984): 41–63. Also, see the follow-up articles by Pauly, Conrad, and Silvers and Kauer in the April 1986 issue of *Health Services Research*.

11. For an excellent discussion of this position, see William O. Cleverley, "Return on Equity in the Hospital Industry: Requirement or Windfall?" *Inquiry* (Summer 1982): 150–159.

References

Boles, K. E. 1986. "Implications of the Method of Capital Cost Payment on the Weighted Average Cost of Capital." *Health Services Research* (June): 191–211.

———. 1986. "What Accounting Leaves Out of Hospital Financial Management." *Hospital & Health Services Administration* (March/April): 8–27.

Cleverley, W. O., and J. O. Cleverley. 2005. "The Link Between a Formal Debt Policy and Replacement Reserves." *Journal of Healthcare Management* (May/June): 148–150.

Gapenski, L. C. 1993. "Hospital Capital Structure Decisions: Theory and Practice." *Health Services Management Research* (November): 237–247.

Harris, J. P., and V. E. Schimmel. 1987. "Market Value: An Underused Financial Planning Tool." *Healthcare Financial Management* (April): 40–46.

Messinger, S. F., and P. B. Stevenson. 1999. "Practice Financing Strategies Should Match Investors' Objectives." *Healthcare Financial Management* (May): 72–76.

McCue, M. J., and Y. A. Ozcan. 1992. "Determinants of Capital Structure." *Hospital & Health Services Administration* (Fall): 333–346.

Sloan, F. A., J. Valvona, and M. Hassan. 1988. "Cost of Capital to the Hospital Sector." *Journal of Health Economics* (March): 25–45.

Smith, D. G., and J. R. C. Wheeler. 1989. "Accounting Based Risk Measures for Not-for-Profit Hospitals." *Health Services Management Research* (November): 221–226.

Smith, D. G., J. R. C. Wheeler, H. L. Rivenson, and K. L. Reiter. 2000. "Sources of Project Financing in Health Care Systems." *Journal of Health Care Finance* (Summer): 53–58.

Sterns, J. B., and T. K. Majidzadeh. 1995. "A Framework for Evaluating Capital Structure." *Journal of Health Care Finance* (Winter): 80–85.

Valvona, J., and F. A. Sloan. 1988. "Hospital Profitability and Capital Structure: A Comparative Analysis." *Health Services Research* (August): 343–357.

Vaughan, J., and J. Wise. 1996. "How to Choose the Right Capitalization Option." *Healthcare Financial Management* (December): 72–74.

Wedig, G. J., M. Hassan, and M. A. Morrisey. 1996. "Tax-Exempt Debt and the Capital Structure of Nonprofit Organizations: An Application to Hospitals." *Journal of Finance* (September): 21–40.

Wedig, G. J., F. A. Sloan, M. Hassan, and M. A. Morrisey. 1988. "Capital Structure, Ownership, and Capital Payment Policy: The Case of Hospitals." *Journal of Finance* (March): 21–40.

Wheeler, J. R. C., and D. G. Smith. 1988. "The Discount Rate for Capital Expenditure Analysis in Health Care." *Health Care Management Review* (Spring): 43–51.

Wheeler, J. R. C., D. G. Smith, H. L. Rivenson, and K. L. Reiter. 2000. "Capital Structure Strategy in Health Care Systems." *Journal of Health Care Finance* (Summer): 42–52.

Capital Investment Decisions

In Part V, we focused on capital acquisition (long-term financing), including cost of capital and capital structure—in other words, how businesses raise the funds used to buy needed land, plant, and equipment. Now we turn our attention to the capital investment decision, or how those funds can be deployed (spent) in the most economically efficient manner. The overall process of choosing the fixed asset investments to be undertaken by a business is called *capital budgeting*.

The first chapter in this section covers the basic concepts of project analysis, such as how to estimate a project's cash flows and how to measure its expected financial impact. The second chapter discusses how to assess the riskiness of a project and, equally important, how to incorporate that assessment into the decision process.

THE BASICS OF CAPITAL BUDGETING

Learning Objectives

After studying this chapter, readers will be able to:

- Explain how managers use project classifications and post-audits in the capital budgeting process.
- Discuss the role of financial analysis in health services capital budgeting decisions.
- Discuss the key elements of cash flow estimation, breakeven analysis, and profitability analysis.
- Conduct basic capital budgeting analyses.

Introduction

This chapter focuses on fixed asset acquisition decisions, which involve the expenditure of capital funds. Thus, decisions of this type are called *capital investment*, or *capital budgeting*, *decisions*. Capital budgeting decisions are among the most critical decisions that health services managers must make. First and most importantly, the results of capital budgeting decisions generally affect the business for an extended period. If a business invests too heavily in fixed assets, it will have too much capacity and its costs will necessarily be too high. On the other hand, a business that invests too little in fixed assets may face two problems: technological obsolescence and inadequate capacity. A healthcare provider without the latest in technology will lose patients to its more up-to-date competitors and, further, will deprive its patients of the best healthcare diagnostics and treatments available.

Effective capital budgeting procedures provide several benefits to businesses. A business that forecasts its needs for capital assets well in advance will have the opportunity to plan the acquisitions carefully, and thus will be able to negotiate the highest quality assets at the best prices. Additionally, asset expansion typically involves substantial expenditures, and because large amounts of funds are not usually at hand, they must be raised externally. Good capital budgeting practices permit a business to identify its financing needs and sources well in advance, which ensures both the lowest possible procurement costs and the availability of funds as they are needed.

Project Classifications

Although benefits can be gained from the careful analysis of capital investment proposals, such efforts can be costly. For certain projects, a relatively detailed analysis may be warranted, along with senior management involvement; for others, simpler procedures should be used. Accordingly, healthcare businesses generally classify projects into categories, and by cost within each category, and then analyze each project on the basis of its category and cost. For example, Bayside Memorial Hospital uses the following classifications:

- **Category 1: Mandatory replacement.** Category 1 consists of expenditures necessary to replace worn-out or damaged equipment necessary to the operations of the hospital. In general, these expenditures are mandatory, so they are usually made with only very limited analyses and decision processes.
- **Category 2: Discretionary replacement.** This category includes expenditures needed to replace serviceable but obsolete equipment. The purpose of these projects generally is to lower costs or to provide more clinically effective services. Because Category 2 projects are not mandatory, a more detailed decision process is generally required to support the expenditure than that needed for Category 1 projects.
- **Category 3: Expansion of existing services or markets.** Expenditures to increase capacity, or to expand within markets currently being served by the hospital, are included here. These decisions are more complex, so still more detailed analysis is required, and the final decision is made at a higher level within the organization.
- **Category 4: Expansion into new services or markets.** These are projects necessary to provide new services or to expand into geographical areas not currently being served. Such projects involve strategic decisions that could change the fundamental nature of the hospital, and they normally require the expenditure of large sums of money over long periods of time. Invariably, a particularly detailed analysis is required, and the board of trustees generally makes the final decision as part of the hospital's strategic plan.
- **Category 5: Environmental projects.** This category consists of expenditures necessary to comply with government orders, labor agreements, accreditation requirements, and so on. Unless the expenditures are large, Category 5 expenditures are treated like Category 1 expenditures.
- **Category 6: Other.** This category is a catchall for projects that do not fit neatly into another category. The primary determinant of how Category 6 projects are evaluated is the amount of funds required.

In general, relatively simple analyses and only a few supporting documents are required for replacement decisions and safety/environmental projects, especially those that are mandatory. A more detailed analysis is required for expansion and other projects.

Note that, within each category, projects are classified by size: Larger projects require increasingly detailed analyses and approval at a higher level within the hospital. Thus, department heads can authorize spending up to $25,000 on discretionary replacement projects, while the full board of directors must approve expansion projects that cost more than $5 million.

1. What is the primary advantage of classifying capital projects?
2. What are some typical classifications?
3. What role does project size (cost) play in the classifications?

Self-Test Questions

The Role of Financial Analysis in Healthcare Capital Budgeting

For investor-owned businesses, with shareholder wealth maximization as the primary goal, the role of financial analysis in capital investment decisions is clear. Those projects that contribute to shareholder wealth should be undertaken, while those that do not should be ignored. However, what about not-for-profit firms, which do not have shareholder wealth maximization as a goal? In such businesses, the appropriate goal is providing high-quality, cost-effective service to the communities served. (A strong argument could be made that this should also be the goal of investor-owned businesses in the health services industry.) In this situation, capital budgeting decisions must consider many factors besides a project's financial implications. For example, the needs of the medical staff and the good of the community must be taken into account. Indeed, in many instances, noneconomic factors will outweigh financial considerations.

Nevertheless, good decision making, and hence the future viability of healthcare businesses, requires that the financial impact of capital investments be fully recognized. If a business takes on a series of highly unprofitable projects that meet nonfinancial goals, and such projects are not offset by profitable ones, the firm's financial condition will deteriorate. If this situation persists over time, the business will eventually lose its financial viability and could even be forced into bankruptcy and closure.[1]

Because bankrupt firms cannot meet a community's needs, even managers of not-for-profit businesses must consider a project's potential impact on the firm's financial condition. Managers may make a conscious decision to accept a project with a poor financial prognosis because of its nonfinancial virtues, but it is important that managers know the financial impact up front, rather than be surprised when the project drains the firm's financial resources. Financial analysis provides managers with the relevant information about a project's financial impact and hence helps managers make better decisions, including those decisions based primarily on nonfinancial considerations.

Overview of Capital Budgeting Financial Analysis

The financial analysis of capital investment proposals typically involves the following four steps:

1. Estimate the project's expected cash flows, which consist of the following:
   a. The capital outlay, or cost
   b. The operating cash flows
   c. The terminal (ending) cash flow
   Cash flow estimation is discussed in the next section.
2. The riskiness of the estimated cash flows must be assessed. Risk assessment will be discussed in Chapter 15.
3. Given the riskiness of the project, the project's cost of capital (opportunity cost or discount rate) is estimated. As discussed in Chapter 13, a business's corporate cost of capital reflects the aggregate risk of the business's assets—that is, the riskiness inherent in the average project. If the project being evaluated does not have average risk, the corporate cost of capital must be adjusted.
4. Finally, the financial impact of the project, including profitability, is assessed. Several measures can be used for this purpose; we will discuss four in this chapter.

Cash Flow Estimation

The most critical and most difficult step in evaluating capital investment proposals is *cash flow estimation*. This step involves estimating the investment outlays, the annual net operating flows expected when the project goes into operation, and the cash flows associated with project termination. Many variables are involved in cash flow estimation, and many individuals and departments participate in the process. Making accurate projections of the costs and revenues associated with a large, complex project is difficult, so forecast errors can be quite large.[2] Thus, it is essential that risk analyses be performed on prospective projects.

Neither the difficulty nor the importance of cash flow estimation can be overstated. However, if the principles discussed in the next section are observed, errors that often arise in the next sections can be minimized.

Incremental Cash Flows

The relevant cash flows to consider when evaluating a new capital investment are the project's *incremental cash flows*, which are defined as the firm's cash flows in each period if the project is undertaken minus the firm's cash flows if the project is not undertaken:

$$\text{Incremental CF}_t = \text{CF}_{t(\text{Firm with project})} - \text{CF}_{t(\text{Firm without project})}.$$

Here the subscript t specifies a time period—often years. CF_0 is the incremental cash flow during Year 0, which is generally assumed to end when the first cash flow occurs; CF_1 is the incremental cash flow during the first year; CF_2 is the incremental cash flow during Year 2; and so on. In practice, the early incremental cash flows, and Year 0 in particular, are usually cash outflows—the costs associated with getting the project up and running. As the project begins to generate revenues, the incremental cash flows normally turn positive.

In practice, it typically is not feasible to forecast the cash flows of a business with and without a new project. Thus, the actual estimation process focuses on the cash flows unique to the project being evaluated. However, if a doubt ever arises as to whether or not a particular cash flow is relevant to the analysis, it is often useful to fall back on the basic definition given above.

Cash Flow Versus Accounting Income

As discussed in Chapters 3 and 4, accounting income statements define revenues and costs in terms that do not reflect the actual movement of cash. In capital investment decisions, the decision must be based on the actual dollars that flow into and out of the business. A firm's true profitability, and hence its future financial condition, depends more on its cash flows than on income as reported in accordance with GAAP.

Cash Flow Timing

Financial analysts must be careful to account properly for the timing of cash flows. Accounting income statements are for periods such as years or quarters, so they do not reflect exactly when during the period any revenues and expenses occur. In theory, capital budgeting cash flows should be analyzed exactly as they are expected to occur. Of course, there must be a compromise between accuracy and simplicity. A time line with daily cash flows would in theory provide the most accuracy, but daily cash flow estimates would be costly to construct, unwieldy to use, and probably no more accurate than annual cash flow estimates. Thus, in most cases, analysts simply assume that all cash flows occur at the end of each year. However, for some projects, it may be useful to assume that cash flows occur every six months or to forecast quarterly or monthly cash flows.

Project Life

Perhaps the first decision that must be made in forecasting a project's cash flows is the life of the project. Does the forecast for cash flows need to be for 20 years or is five years sufficient? Many projects, such as a new hospital wing or an ambulatory care clinic, have very long productive lives. In theory, a cash flow forecast should extend for the full life of a project, yet most managers would have very little confidence in any cash flow forecasts beyond the near term. Thus, most organizations set an arbitrary limit on the project life assumed in capital budgeting analyses—often five or ten years. If the forecasted life is less than the arbitrary limit, the forecasted life is used to develop the cash flows, but if the forecasted life exceeds the limit, project life is *truncated* and the operating cash flows beyond the limit are ignored.

Although cash flow truncation is a practical solution to a difficult problem, it does create another problem; the value inherent in the cash flows beyond the truncation point is lost to the project. This problem can be addressed either objectively or subjectively. The standard procedure at some organizations is to estimate the project's *terminal value*, which is the estimated value of the cash flows beyond the truncation point. Sometimes, the terminal value is estimated as the *liquidation value* of the project at that point in time. If the terminal value is too difficult to estimate, the fact that some portion of the project's cash flow value is being ignored should, at a minimum, be subjectively recognized by decision makers. The saving grace in all of this is that cash flows forecasted to occur well into the future typically contribute a relatively small amount to a project's initial profitability estimate. For example, a $100,000 terminal value projected ten years in the future contributes only about $38,500 to the project's value when the project cost of capital (discount rate) is 10 percent.

Some projects have short lives, and hence the analysis can extend over the project's entire life. In such situations, the assets associated with the project may still have some value remaining when the project is terminated. The cash flow expected to be realized from selling the project's assets at termination is called *salvage value*. Even if a project is being terminated for "old age," any cash flow that will arise by virtue of scrap value must be included in the project's cash flows. For investor-owned businesses, such asset sales typically will trigger tax consequences, which are discussed in the cash flow estimation example presented in the next major section.

Sunk Costs

A *sunk cost* refers to an outlay that has already occurred or has been irrevocably committed, so it is an outlay that is unaffected by the current decision to accept or reject a project. To illustrate, suppose that in 2008 Bayside Memorial Hospital is evaluating the purchase of a lithotripter system. To help in the decision, the hospital hired and paid $10,000 to a consultant in 2007 to conduct a marketing study. This cash flow is **not** relevant (*nonincremental*) to the capital investment decision; Bayside cannot recover it whether or not the lithotripter is purchased. Sometimes a project appears to be unprofitable when **all** of its associated costs, including sunk costs, are considered. However, on an *incremental* basis, the project may be profitable and should be undertaken. Thus, the correct treatment of sunk costs may be critical to the decision.

Opportunity Costs

All relevant *opportunity costs* must be included in a capital investment analysis. To illustrate, one opportunity cost involves the use of the funds required to finance the project. If the firm uses its capital to invest in Project A, it cannot use the capital to invest in Project B or for any other purpose. The opportunity cost associated with capital use is accounted for in the project cost of capital, which represents the return that the business could earn by investing in alternative investments of similar risk. The mathematics of the discounting process forces the opportunity cost of capital to be considered in the analysis.

In addition to the opportunity cost of capital, there are other types of opportunity costs that arise in capital budgeting analyses. For example, assume that Bayside's lithotripter would be installed in a freestanding facility and that the hospital currently owns the land on which the facility would be constructed. In fact, the hospital purchased the land ten years ago at a cost of $50,000, but the current market value of the property is $130,000, after subtracting both legal and real estate fees. When evaluating the lithotripter, the value of the land cannot be disregarded merely because no cash outlay is necessary. There is an opportunity cost inherent in the use of the property because using the property for the lithotripter facility deprives Bayside of its use for other purposes. The property might be used for a walk-in clinic or ambulatory surgery center or parking garage rather than sold, but the best measure of its value to Bayside, and hence the opportunity cost inherent in its use, is the cash flow that could be realized from selling the property.

By considering the property's current market value, Bayside is letting market forces assign the value for the land's best alternative use. Thus, the lithotripter project should have a $130,000 opportunity cost charged against it. The opportunity cost is the property's $130,000 net market value, irrespective of whether the property was acquired for $50,000 or $200,000.

Effects on Existing Business Lines

Capital budgeting analyses must consider the effects of the project under consideration on the firm's existing business lines. Such effects can be either positive or negative; when negative, it is often called *cannibalization*. To illustrate, assume that some of the patients who are expected to use Bayside's new lithotripter would have been treated surgically at Bayside, so these surgical revenues will be lost if the lithotripter facility goes into operation. Thus, the incremental cash flows to Bayside are the flows attributable to the lithotripter, **less** those lost from forgone surgery services.

On the other hand, new patients that who use the lithotripter may use ancillary services provided by the hospital. In this situation, the incremental cash flows generated by the lithotripter patients' utilization of other services should be credited to the lithotripter project. If possible, both positive and negative effects on other projects should be quantified, but at a minimum they should be noted, so that these effects are subjectively considered when the final decision regarding the project is made.

Shipping, Installation, and Related Costs

When a business acquires new equipment, it often incurs substantial costs for shipping and installation or for other related activities. These charges must be added to the invoice price of the equipment to determine the overall cost of the project. Also, the full cost of the equipment, *including* such costs, typically is used as the basis for calculating depreciation charges. Thus, if Bayside Memorial Hospital purchases intensive care monitoring equipment that costs $800,000, but another $200,000 is required for shipping and installation, the full cost of the equipment would be $1 million, and this amount would be the starting point for both tax (when applicable) and book depreciation calculations.

Changes in Net Working Capital

Normally, expansion projects require additional inventories, and expanded patient volumes also lead to additional accounts receivable. The increase in these current assets must be financed, just as an increase in fixed assets must be financed. (Increases on the asset side of the balance sheet must be offset by matching increases on the liabilities and equity side.) However, accounts payable and accruals will probably also increase as a result of the expansion, and these current liability funds will reduce the net cash needed to finance the increase in inventories and receivables.

Current assets are often referred to as *working capital*, and the difference between current assets and current liabilities is called *net working capital*. Thus, projects that have an impact on current assets and current liabilities create *changes in net working capital*. If this change is positive (i.e., if the increase in current assets exceeds the increase in current liabilities), this amount is as much a cash cost to the project as is the dollar cost of the asset itself. Such projects must be charged an additional amount above the dollar cost of the new fixed asset to reflect the net financing needed for current asset accounts. Similarly, if the change in net working capital is negative, the project is generating a positive working capital cash flow because the increase in liabilities exceeds the project's current asset requirements, and this cash flow partially offsets the cost of the asset being acquired.

As the project approaches termination, inventories will be sold off and not replaced, and receivables will be converted to cash without new receivables being created. In effect, the business will recover its investment in net working capital when the project is terminated. This will result in a cash flow that is equal but **opposite** in sign to the change in net working capital cash flow that arises at the beginning of a project.

For healthcare providers, where inventories often represent a very small part of the investment in new projects, the change in net working capital often can be ignored without materially affecting the results of the analysis. However, when a project requires a large positive change in net working capital, failure to consider the net investment in current assets will result in an overstatement of the project's profitability.

Inflation Effects

Because inflation effects can have a considerable influence on a project's profitability, inflation must be considered in any sound capital budgeting analysis. As we discussed in Chapter 13, a firm's corporate cost of capital is a weighted average of its costs of debt and equity. These costs are estimated on the basis of investors' required rates of return, and investors incorporate an inflation premium into such estimates. For example, a debt investor might require a 5 percent return on a ten-year bond in the absence of inflation. However, if inflation is expected to average 4 percent over the coming ten years, the investor would require a 9 percent return. Thus, investors add an inflation premium to their required rates of return to help protect them against the loss of purchasing power that stems from inflation.

Because inflation effects are already imbedded in the corporate cost of capital, and because this cost will be used as the starting point to discount the cash flows in the profitability measures, inflation effects must also be built into the project's estimated cash flows. If cash flow estimates do not include inflation effects, but a discount rate is used that includes inflation effects, the profitability of the project will be understated.

The most effective way to deal with inflation is to apply inflation effects to each cash flow component using the best available information about how each component will be affected. Because it is impossible to estimate future inflation rates with much precision, errors will probably be made. Often, inflation is assumed to be neutral (i.e., it is assumed to affect all revenue and cost components, except depreciation, equally). However, it is common for costs to be rising faster than revenues or vice versa. Thus, in general, it is better to apply different inflation rates to each cash flow component. For example, net revenues might be expected to increase at a 3 percent rate, while labor costs might be expected to increase at a 5 percent rate. Inflation adds to the uncertainty, and hence risk, of a project under consideration as well as to the complexity of the capital budgeting analysis. Fortunately, computers and spreadsheet programs can easily handle the mechanics of inflation analysis.

Strategic Value

Sometimes a project will have value in addition to that inherent in its cash flows. A major source of hidden value, called *strategic value*, stems from future investment opportunities that can be undertaken only if the project currently under consideration is accepted.

To illustrate this concept, consider a hospital management company that is analyzing a management contract for a hospital in Hungary, which is its first move into Eastern Europe. On a stand-alone basis, this project might be unprofitable, but the project might provide entry into the Eastern European market, which could unlock the door to a whole range of highly profitable new projects. Or consider Bayside Memorial Hospital's decision to start a kidney transplant program. The financial analysis of this project showed the program to be unprofitable, but Bayside's managers considered kidney transplants to be the first step in an aggressive transplant program that would not only be profitable in itself but would enhance the hospital's reputation for technological and clinical excellence and thus would contribute to the hospital's overall profitability.

In theory, the best approach to dealing with strategic value is to forecast the cash flows from the follow-on projects, estimate their probabilities of occurrence, and then add the expected cash flows from the follow-on projects to the cash flows of the project under consideration. In practice, this is usually impossible to do because either the follow-on cash flows are too nebulous to forecast or the potential follow-on projects are too numerous to quantify.[3] At a minimum, decision makers must recognize that some projects have strategic value, and this value should be qualitatively considered when making capital budgeting decisions.

Self-Test Questions

1. Briefly discuss the following concepts associated with cash flow estimation:
   - Incremental cash flow
   - Cash flow versus accounting income
   - Cash flow timing
   - Project life
   - Terminal value
   - Salvage value
   - Sunk costs
   - Opportunity costs
   - Effects on current business lines
   - Shipping and installation costs
   - Changes in net working capital
   - Inflation effects
   - Strategic value

2. Evaluate the following statement: Ignoring inflation effects and strategic value can result in **overstating** a project's financial attractiveness.

Cash Flow Estimation Example

Up to this point, several critical aspects of cash flow estimation have been discussed. In this section, we illustrate some of the concepts already covered and introduce several others that are important to good cash flow estimation.

The Basic Data

Consider the situation faced by Bayside Memorial Hospital in its evaluation of a new MRI system. The system costs $1.5 million, and the not-for-profit hospital would have to spend another $1 million for site preparation and installation. Because the system would be installed in the hospital, the space to be used has a very low, or zero, market value to outsiders. Furthermore, its value to Bayside for other projects is very difficult to estimate, so no opportunity cost has been assigned to account for the value of the site.

The MRI system is estimated to have weekly utilization (i.e., volume) of 40 scans, and each scan on average would cost the hospital $15 in supplies. The system is expected to be operated 50 weeks a year, with the remaining two weeks devoted to maintenance. The estimated average charge per scan is $500, but 25 percent of this amount, on average, is expected to be lost to indigent patients, contractual allowances, and bad debt losses. Bayside's managers developed the project's forecasted revenues by conducting the revenue analysis contained in Table 14.1.

The MRI system would require two technicians, resulting in an incremental increase in annual labor costs of $50,000, including fringe benefits. Cash overhead costs would increase by $10,000 annually if the MRI is activated. The equipment would require maintenance, which would be furnished by the manufacturer for an annual fee of $150,000, payable at the end of each year of operation. For book purposes, the MRI will be depreciated by the straight-line method over a five-year life.

The MRI system is expected to be in operation for five years, at which time the hospital's master plan calls for a new imaging facility. The hospital plans to sell the MRI at that time for an estimated $750,000 salvage value, net of removal costs. The inflation rate is estimated to average 5 percent over the period, and this rate is expected to affect all revenues and costs except depreciation. Bayside's managers initially assume that projects under evaluation have average risk, and thus the hospital's 10 percent corporate cost of capital is the appropriate project cost of capital (opportunity cost discount rate). In Chapter 15, a risk assessment of the project may indicate that a different cost of capital is appropriate.

Although the MRI project is expected to take away some patients from the hospital's other imaging systems, the new MRI patients are expected to generate revenues for some of the hospital's other departments. On net, the two effects are expected to balance out—that is, the cash flow loss from other imaging systems is expected to be offset by the cash flow gain from other

TABLE 14.1
Bayside
Memorial
Hospital: MRI
System Revenue
Analysis

Payer	Number of Scans per Week	Charge per Scan	Total Charges	Basis of Payment	Net Payment per Scan	Total Payments
Medicare	10	$500	$ 5,000	Fixed fee	$370	$ 3,700
Medicaid	5	500	2,500	Fixed fee	350	1,750
Private insurance	9	500	4,500	Full charge	500	4,500
Blue Cross	5	500	2,500	Percent of charge	420	2,100
Managed care	7	500	3,500	Percent of charge	390	2,730
Self-pay	4	500	2,000	Full charge	55	220
Total	40		$20,000			$15,000
Average			$ 500			$ 375

services utilized by new MRI patients. Also, the project is estimated to have negligible net working capital implications, so changes in net working capital will be ignored in the analysis.

Cash Flow Analysis (Not-for-Profit Businesses)

The first step in the financial analysis is to estimate the MRI site's net cash flows. This analysis is presented in Table 14.2. Here are the key points of the analysis by line number:

- **Line 1.** Line 1 contains the estimated cost of the MRI system. In general, capital budgeting analyses assume that the first cash flow, normally an outflow, occurs at the end of Year 0. Expenses, or cash outflows, are shown in parentheses.
- **Line 2.** The related site construction expense, $1,000,000, is also assumed to occur at Year 0.
- **Line 3.** Annual gross revenues = Weekly volume × Weeks of operation per year × Charge per scan = 40 × 50 × $500 = $1,000,000 in the first year. The 5 percent inflation rate is applied to all charges and costs that would likely be affected by inflation, so the gross revenue amount shown on Line 3 increases by 5 percent over time. Although most of the operating revenues and costs would occur more or less evenly over the year, it is very difficult to forecast exactly when the flows would occur. Furthermore, there is significant potential for large errors in cash flow estimation. For these reasons, operating cash flows are often assumed to occur at the end of each year. Also, the assumption is that the MRI system could be placed in operation quickly. If this were not the case, then the first year's operating flows would be reduced. In some situations, it might take several years from the first investment cash flow to the point when the project is operational and begins to generate revenues.

TABLE 14.2
Bayside Memorial Hospital: MRI Site Cash Flow Analysis

	0			Cash Revenues and Costs		
		1	2	3	4	5
1. System cost	($1,500,000)					
2. Related expenses	(1,000,000)					
3. Gross revenues		$1,000,000	$1,050,000	$1,102,500	$1,157,625	$1,215,506
4. Deductions		250,000	262,500	275,625	289,406	303,877
5. Net revenues		$ 750,000	$ 787,500	$ 826,875	$ 868,219	$ 911,630
6. Labor costs		50,000	52,500	55,125	57,881	60,775
7. Maintenance costs		150,000	157,500	165,375	173,644	182,326
8. Supplies		30,000	31,500	33,075	34,729	36,465
9. Incremental overhead		10,000	10,500	11,025	11,576	12,155
10. Depreciation		350,000	350,000	350,000	350,000	350,000
11. Operating income		$ 160,000	$ 185,500	$ 212,275	$ 240,389	$ 269,908
12. Taxes		0	0	0	0	0
13. Net operating income		$ 160,000	$ 185,500	$ 212,275	$ 240,389	$ 269,908
14. Depreciation		350,000	350,000	350,000	350,000	350,000
15. Net salvage value						750,000
16. Net cash flow	($2,500,000)	$ 510,000	$ 535,500	$ 562,275	$ 590,389	$1,369,908

Note: Totals are rounded.

- **Line 4.** Deductions from charges are estimated to average 25 percent of gross revenues, so in Year 1, $0.25 \times \$1,000,000 = \$250,000$ of gross revenues would be uncollected. This amount increases each year by the 5 percent inflation rate.
- **Line 5.** Line 5 contains the net revenues in each year, Line 3 − Line 4.
- **Line 6.** Labor costs are forecasted to be $50,000 during the first year, and they are assumed to increase over time at the 5 percent inflation rate.
- **Line 7.** Maintenance fees must be paid to the manufacturer at the end of each year of operation. These fees are assumed to increase at the 5 percent inflation rate.
- **Line 8.** Each scan uses $15 of supplies, so supply costs in the first year total $40 \times 50 \times \$15 = \$30,000$, and they are expected to increase each year by the inflation rate.
- **Line 9.** If the project is accepted, overhead cash costs will increase by $10,000 in the first year. Note that the $10,000 expenditure is a **cash cost** that is related directly to the acceptance of the MRI project. Existing overhead costs that are arbitrarily allocated to the MRI project are **not** incremental cash flows and thus should not be included in the analysis. Overhead costs are also assumed to increase over time at the inflation rate.
- **Line 10.** Book depreciation in each year is calculated by the straight-line method, assuming a five-year depreciable life. For book purposes, the depreciable basis is equal to the capitalized cost of the project, which includes the cost of the asset and related construction, less the estimated salvage value. Thus, the depreciable basis is ($1,500,000 + $1,000,000) − $750,000 = $1,750,000, and the straight-line depreciation in each year of the project's five-year depreciable life is $1,750,000 / 5 = $350,000. Note that depreciation is based solely on acquisition costs, so it is unaffected by inflation. Also, note that the Table 14.2 cash flows are presented in a generic format that can be used by both investor-owned and not-for-profit hospitals. Depreciation expense is not a cash flow but an accounting convention that amortizes the cost of a fixed asset over its revenue-producing life. Because Bayside Memorial Hospital is tax exempt, and hence depreciation will not affect taxes, and because depreciation is added back to the cash flows on Line 14, **depreciation could be totally omitted from the cash flow analysis.**
- **Line 11.** Line 11 shows the project's operating income in each year, which is merely net revenues less all operating expenses.
- **Line 12.** Line 12 contains zeros because Bayside is not-for-profit and hence does not pay taxes.
- **Line 13.** Bayside pays no taxes, so the project's net operating income equals its operating income.
- **Line 14.** Because depreciation, a noncash expense, was included on Line 10, it must be added back to the project's net operating income in each year to obtain each year's net cash flow.

- **Line 15.** The project is expected to be terminated after five years, at which time the MRI system would be sold for an estimated $750,000. This salvage value cash flow is shown as an inflow at the end of Year 5 on Line 15.
- **Line 16.** The project's net cash flows are shown on Line 16. The project requires a $2,500,000 investment at Year 0 but then generates cash inflows over its five-year operating life.

The Table 14.2 cash flows do not include any allowance for interest expense. On average, Bayside Memorial Hospital will finance new projects in accordance with its target capital structure, which consists of 50 percent debt financing and 50 percent equity (i.e., fund) financing. The costs associated with this financing mix, including both interest costs and the opportunity cost of equity capital, are incorporated into the firm's 10 percent corporate cost of capital. Because the cost of debt financing is included in the discount rate that will be applied to the cash flows, recognition of interest expense in the cash flows would be double counting.

Cash Flow Analysis (For-Profit Businesses)

The Table 14.2 cash flow analysis can be easily modified to reflect tax implications if the analyzing firm is a for-profit business. To illustrate, assume that the MRI project is being evaluated by Ann Arbor Health Systems, an investor-owned hospital chain. Assume also that all of the project data presented earlier apply to Ann Arbor, except that the MRI falls into the MACRS five-year class for tax depreciation and the firm has a 40 percent tax rate.

Table 14.3 contains Ann Arbor's cash flow analysis. Note the following differences from the not-for-profit analysis performed in Table 14.2:

- **Line 10.** Depreciation expense must be modified to reflect **tax depreciation** rather than **book depreciation**. Tax depreciation is calculated using the *Modified Accelerated Cost Recovery System (MACRS)* as specified in current tax laws. Each year's tax depreciation is found by multiplying the asset's depreciable basis, **without reduction by the estimated salvage value**, by the appropriate depreciation factor. In this illustration, the depreciable basis is $2,500,000, and the MRI system falls into the MACRS five-year class, so the MACRS factors specified by the tax code are 0.20, 0.32, 0.19, 0.12, 0.11, and 0.06, in Years 1 to 6, respectively. Thus, the tax depreciation in Year 1 is $0.20 \times \$2,500,000 = \$500,000$, in Year 2 the depreciation is $0.32 \times \$2,500,000 = \$800,000$, and so on.[4]
- **Line 12.** Taxable firms must reduce the operating income on Line 11 by the amount of taxes. Taxes, which appear on Line 12, are computed by multiplying the Line 11 pretax operating income by the firm's marginal tax rate. For example, the project's taxes for Year 1 are $0.40 \times \$10,000 =$

TABLE 14.3
Ann Arbor Health Systems: MRI Site Cash Flow Analysis

	0	1	2	3	4	5
			Cash Revenues and Costs			
1. System cost	($1,500,000)					
2. Related expenses	(1,000,000)					
3. Gross revenues		$1,000,000	$1,050,000	$1,102,500	$1,157,625	$1,215,506
4. Deductions		250,000	262,500	275,625	289,406	303,877
5. Net revenues		$ 750,000	$ 787,500	$ 826,875	$ 868,219	$ 911,630
6. Labor costs		50,000	52,500	55,125	57,881	60,775
7. Maintenance costs		150,000	157,500	165,375	173,644	182,326
8. Supplies		30,000	31,500	33,075	34,729	36,465
9. Incremental overhead		10,000	10,500	11,025	11,576	12,155
10. Depreciation		500,000	800,000	475,000	300,000	275,000
11. Operating income		$ 10,000	($ 264,500)	$ 87,275	$ 290,389	$ 344,908
12. Taxes		4,000	(105,800)	34,910	116,156	137,963
13. Net operating income		$ 6,000	($ 158,700)	$ 52,365	$ 174,233	$ 206,945
14. Depreciation		500,000	800,000	475,000	300,000	275,000
15. Net salvage value						510,000
16. Net cash flow	($2,500,000)	$ 506,000	$ 641,300	$ 527,365	$ 474,233	$ 991,945

Note: Totals are rounded.

$4,000. The taxes shown for Year 2 are a negative $105,800. In this year, the project is expected to lose $264,500, and hence Ann Arbor's taxable income, assuming that its existing projects are profitable, will be reduced by this amount if the project is undertaken. This reduction in Ann Arbor's overall taxable income would lower the firm's tax bill by T × Reduction in taxable income = 0.40 × $264,500 = $105,800.[5]

- **Line 14.** The MACRS depreciation is added back in Line 14.
- **Line 15.** Investor-owned firms will normally incur a tax liability on the sale of a capital asset at the end of the project's life. According to the IRS, the value of the MRI system at the end of Year 5 is the *tax book value*, which is the depreciation that remains on the tax books. For the MRI, five years worth of depreciation would be taken, so only one year of depreciation remains. The MACRS factor for Year 6 is 0.06, so by the end of Year 5, Ann Arbor has expensed 0.94 of the MRI's depreciable basis and the remaining tax book value is 0.06 × $2,500,000 = $150,000. Thus, according to the IRS, the value of the MRI system is $150,000. When Ann Arbor sells the system for its estimated salvage value of $750,000, it realizes a "profit" of $750,000 − $150,000 = $600,000, and it must repay the IRS an amount equal to 0.4 × $600,000 = $240,000. The $240,000 tax bill recognizes that Ann Arbor took too much depreciation on the MRI system, so it represents a *recapture* of the excess tax benefit taken over the five-year life of the system. The $240,000 in taxes reduces the cash flow received from the sale of the MRI equipment, so the salvage value net of taxes is $750,000 − $240,000 = $510,000.

As can be seen by comparing Line 16 in Tables 14.2 and 14.3, all else the same, the taxes paid by investor-owned firms tend to reduce a project's net operating cash flows and net salvage value and hence reduce the project's financial attractiveness.

Replacement Analysis

Bayside's MRI project was used to illustrate how the cash flows from an *expansion project* are analyzed. All firms, including Bayside Memorial Hospital, also make *replacement decisions*, in which a new asset is being considered to replace an existing asset that could, if not replaced, continue in operation. The cash flow analysis for a replacement decision is somewhat more complex than for an expansion decision because the cash flows from the existing asset must be considered.

Again, the key to cash flow estimation is to focus on the **incremental cash flows**. If the new asset is acquired, the existing asset can be sold, so the current market value of the existing asset is a cash inflow in the analysis. When considering the operating flows, the incremental flows are the cash flows expected from the replacement asset less the flows that the existing asset would produce if not replaced. By applying the incremental cash flow concept, the correct cash flows can be estimated for replacement decisions.

Breakeven Analysis

Breakeven analysis was first introduced in Chapter 5 in conjunction with breakeven volume in an accounting profit analysis. Now, the breakeven concept is reapplied in a project analysis setting. In project analyses, many different types of breakeven can be determined. Rather than discuss all the possible types of breakeven, the focus here is on one type—time breakeven.

Payback is defined as the expected number of years required to recover the investment in a project, so *payback*, or *payback period*, measures time breakeven. To illustrate, consider the net cash flows for the MRI project contained in Table 14.2. The best way to determine the MRI's payback is to construct the project's *cumulative cash flows* as shown in Table 14.4. The cumulative cash flow at any point in time is merely the sum of all the cash flows (with proper sign indicating an inflow or outflow) that have occurred up to that point. Thus, in Table 14.4, the cumulative cash flow at Year 0 is -$2,500,000; at Year 1 it is -$2,500,000 + $510,000 = -$1,990,000; at Year 2 it is -$2,500,000 + $510,000 + $535,500 = -$1,990,000 + $535,500 = -$1,454,500; and so on.

As shown in the rightmost column of Table 14.4, the $2,500,000 investment in the MRI project will be recovered at the end of Year 5 if the cash flow forecasts are correct. Furthermore, if the cash flows are assumed to

TABLE 14.4
Bayside Memorial Hospital: MRI Site Annual and Cumulative Cash Flows

Year	Annual Cash Flows	Cumulative Cash Flows
0	($2,500,000)	($2,500,000)
1	510,000	(1,990,000)
2	535,500	(1,454,500)
3	562,275	(892,225)
4	590,389	(301,836)
5	1,369,908	1,068,072

come in evenly during the year, breakeven will occur $301,836 / $1,369,908 = 0.22 years into Year 5, so the MRI project's payback is 4.22 years.

Initially, payback was used by managers as the primary financial evaluation tool in project analyses. For example, a business might accept all projects with paybacks of five years or less. However, payback has two serious deficiencies when it is used as a project selection criterion. First, payback ignores all cash flows that occur after the payback period. To illustrate, Bayside might be evaluating a competing project that has the same cash flows as the MRI project in Years 0 through 5. However, the alternative project might have a cash inflow of $2 million in Year 6. Both projects would have the same payback, 4.22 years, and hence be ranked the same, even though the alternative project clearly is better from a financial perspective. Second, payback ignores the opportunity costs associated with the capital employed. For these reasons, payback generally is no longer used as the primary evaluation tool.[6]

However, payback is useful in capital investment analysis. The shorter the payback, the more quickly the funds invested in a project will become available for other purposes and hence the more *liquid* the project. Also, cash flows expected in the distant future are generally regarded as being riskier than near-term cash flows, so shorter payback projects generally are less *risky* than those with longer paybacks. Therefore, payback is often used as a rough measure of a project's liquidity and risk.

Self-Test Questions

1. What is payback?
2. What are the benefits of payback?
3. What are its deficiencies when used as the primary evaluation tool?

Return on Investment (Profitability) Analysis

Up to this point, the chapter has focused on cash flow estimation and breakeven analysis. Perhaps the most important element in a project's financial analysis is its expected profitability, which generally is expressed by *return on investment (ROI)* measured either in dollars or in percentage rate of return. In the next sections, we discuss one dollar measure and two rate of return ROI measures.

Net Present Value (NPV)

Net present value (NPV), which was first discussed in Chapter 9, is a dollar ROI measure that uses discounted cash flow (DCF) techniques, so it is often referred to as a *DCF profitability measure*. To apply the NPV method:

• Find the present (Time 0) value of each net cash flow, including both inflows and outflows, when discounted at the project's cost of capital.

- Sum the present values. This sum is defined as the project's net present value.
- If the NPV is positive, the project is expected to be profitable, and the higher the NPV, the more profitable the project. If the NPV is zero, the project just breaks even in an economic sense. If the NPV is negative, the project is expected to be unprofitable.

With a project cost of capital of 10 percent, the NPV of Bayside's MRI project is calculated as follows:

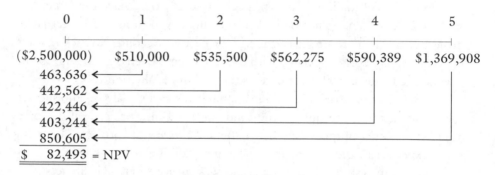

Financial calculators and spreadsheets have NPV functions that easily perform the mathematics if given the cash flows and cost of capital. Here is the spreadsheet solution:

	A	B	C	D
1				
2	10.0%		Project cost of capital	
3	$ (2,500,000)		Cash flow 0	
4	510,000		Cash flow 1	
5	535,500		Cash flow 2	
6	562,275		Cash flow 3	
7	590,389		Cash flow 4	
8	1,369,908		Cash flow 5	
9				
10	$ 82,493	=NPV(A2,A4:A8)+A3 (entered into Cell A10)		

Note that we have merely entered the net cash flows into the spreadsheet. In a typical project analysis, the spreadsheet would be used for the cash flow analysis, with the "bottom line" being the net cash flows. The project's NPV is calculated in Cell A10 using the NPV function. The first entry in the function (A2) is the discount rate (project cost of capital), while the second entry (A4:A8) designates the range of cash inflows from Years 1 through 5. Because the NPV function calculates NPV one period before the first cash flow entered in the range, it is necessary to start the range with Year 1 rather than Year 0. Finally, to complete the calculation in Cell A10, A3 (the initial outlay) is added to the NPV function. The end result, $82,493, is displayed in Cell A10.

The rationale behind the NPV method is straightforward. An NPV of zero signifies that the project's cash inflows are just sufficient to (1) return the capital invested in the project and (2) provide the required rate of return on that capital (meet the opportunity cost of capital). If a project has a positive NPV, it is generating excess cash flows, and these excess cash flows are available to management to reinvest in the business and, for investor-owned firms, to pay bonuses (if a proprietorship or partnership) or dividends. If a project has a negative NPV, its cash inflows are insufficient to compensate the firm for the capital invested or perhaps even insufficient to recover the initial investment, so the project is unprofitable and acceptance would cause the financial condition of the firm to deteriorate. For investor-owned firms, NPV is a direct measure of the contribution of the project to shareholder wealth, so NPV is considered by many academics and practitioners to be the best measure of project profitability.

The NPV of the MRI project is $82,493, so on a present value basis, the project is expected to generate a cash flow excess of over $80,000 after all costs, including the opportunity cost of capital, have been considered. Thus, the project is economically profitable and its acceptance would have a positive impact on Bayside's financial condition.

Internal Rate of Return (IRR)

Like NPV, *internal rate of return (IRR)* is also a discounted cash flow (DCF) ROI measure. However, whereas NPV measures a project's dollar profitability, IRR measures a project's percentage profitability (i.e., its expected rate of return).

Mathematically, IRR is defined as the discount rate that equates the present value of the project's expected cash inflows to the present value of the project's expected cash outflows, so the IRR is simply that discount rate that forces the NPV of the project to equal **zero**. Financial calculators and spreadsheets have IRR functions that calculate IRRs very rapidly. Simply input the project's cash flows, and the computer or calculator computes the IRR.

For Bayside's MRI project, the IRR is that rate that causes the sum of the present values of the cash inflows to equal the $2,500,000 cost of the project:

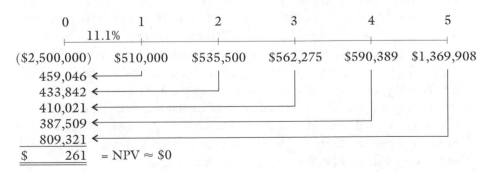

When all of the MRI project's cash flows are discounted at 11.1 percent, the NPV of the project is approximately zero. Thus, the MRI project's IRR is 11.1 percent. Put another way, the project is expected to generate an 11.1 percent rate of return on its $2,500,000 investment. Note that the IRR is like a bond's yield to maturity: it is the rate of return expected on the investment assuming that all the cash flows anticipated actually occur.

Here is the spreadsheet solution:

	A	B	C	D
1				
2	10.0%		Project cost of capital	
3	$ (2,500,000)		Cash flow 0	
4	510,000		Cash flow 1	
5	535,500		Cash flow 2	
6	562,275		Cash flow 3	
7	590,389		Cash flow 4	
8	1,369,908		Cash flow 5	
9				
10	11.1%	=IRR(A2,A3:A8) (entered into Cell A10)		

Note that we have placed the IRR function in Cell A10. The first entry in the function (A2) gives a starting value for the spreadsheet calculation, while the next entry (A3:A8) specifies the range of cash flows to be used in the calculation. The answer, 11.1%, is displayed in Cell A10.

If the IRR exceeds the project cost of capital, a surplus is projected to remain after recovering the invested capital and paying for its use, and this surplus accrues to the firm's stockholders (in Bayside's case, to its stakeholders). If the IRR is less than the project cost of capital, however, taking on the project imposes an expected financial cost on the firm's stockholders or stakeholders. The MRI project's 11.1 percent IRR exceeds its 10 percent project cost of capital. Thus, as measured by IRR, the MRI project is profitable and its acceptance would enhance Bayside's financial condition.

Comparison of the NPV and IRR Methods

Consider a project with a zero NPV. In this situation, the project's IRR must equal its cost of capital. The project has zero expected profitability, and acceptance would neither enhance nor diminish the firm's financial condition. To have a positive NPV, the project's IRR must be greater than its cost of capital, and a negative NPV signifies a project with an IRR less than its cost of capital. Thus, projects that are deemed profitable by the NPV method will also be deemed profitable by the IRR method. In the MRI example, the project would have a positive NPV for all costs of capital less than 11.1 percent. If the cost of capital were greater than 11.1 percent, the project would have a negative NPV. In effect, the NPV and IRR are perfect substitutes for each other in measuring whether or not a project is profitable.[7]

Modified Internal Rate of Return (MIRR)

In general, academics prefer the NPV profitability measure. This preference stems from two factors: (1) NPV measures profitability in dollars, which is a direct measure of the contribution of the project to the value of the business, and (2) both the NPV and the IRR, because they are discounted cash flow techniques, require an assumption about the rate at which project cash flows can be reinvested, and the NPV method has the better assumption.

To further explain the second point, consider the MRI project's Year 2 net cash flow of $535,500. In effect, the discounting process inherent in the NPV and IRR methods automatically assigns a reinvestment rate to this cash flow; that is, both the NPV and IRR methods assume that Bayside has the opportunity to reinvest the $535,500 Year 2 cash flow in other projects, and each method automatically assigns a reinvestment rate to this flow for Years 3, 4, and 5. The NPV method assumes reinvestment at the project cost of capital, 10 percent, while the IRR method assumes reinvestment at the IRR rate, 11.1 percent. Which is the better assumption—reinvestment at the cost of capital or reinvestment at the IRR rate? In this situation, it does not make much difference. But in general, a business will take on all projects that exceed its cost of capital. Thus, at the margin, the returns from capital reinvested within the firm are more likely to be at or close to the cost of capital than at the project's IRR, especially for projects with exceptionally high or low IRRs. Furthermore, a business can obtain outside capital at a cost roughly equal to the cost of capital, so cash flows generated by a project could be replaced by capital having this cost. So, in general, reinvestment at the cost of capital is a better assumption than reinvestment at the IRR rate, and hence NPV is a theoretically better measure of profitability than IRR.

Even though academics strongly favor the NPV method, practicing managers prefer the IRR method because it is more intuitive for most people to analyze investments in terms of percentage rates of return than dollars of NPV. Thus, an alternative rate of return measure has been developed that eliminates the primary problem with IRR. This method is the *modified IRR (MIRR)*, and it is calculated as follows:

- Discount all the project's net cash **outflows** back to Year 0 at the project cost of capital.
- Compound all the project's net cash **inflows** forward to the last (terminal) year of the project, at the project cost of capital. This value is called the *inflow terminal value*.
- The discount rate that forces the present value of the inflow terminal value to equal the present value of costs is defined as the MIRR.

Applying these steps to Bayside's MRI project produces a MIRR of about 10.7 percent:

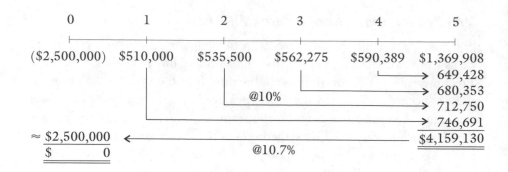

Here is the spreadsheet solution for the IRR:

	A	B	C	D
1				
2	10.0%		Project cost of capital	
3	$ (2,500,000)		Cash flow 0	
4	510,000		Cash flow 1	
5	535,500		Cash flow 2	
6	562,275		Cash flow 3	
7	590,389		Cash flow 4	
8	1,369,908		Cash flow 5	
9				
10	10.7%	=MIRR(A3:A8,A2,A2) (entered into Cell A10)		

The MIRR function was placed in Cell A10. The first entry in the function (A3:A8) is the range of cash flows, while the next two entries (A2,A2) are the project cost of capital. (The MIRR function allows the reinvestment rate to differ from the project cost of capital: the first of the two entries is the project cost of capital and the second is the reinvestment rate. For our purposes, the two rates are the same). The resulting MIRR, 10.7%, is displayed in Cell A10.

The MIRR method, by compounding the cash inflows forward at 10 percent, forces the reinvestment rate to equal 10 percent, which is the project cost of capital. Note that the MIRR for the MRI project is less than the project's IRR because the cash inflows are reinvested at only 10 percent rather than at the project's 11.1 percent IRR. In general, the MIRR is less than the IRR when the IRR is greater than the cost of capital, but it is greater than the IRR when the IRR is less than the cost of capital. In effect, the IRR overstates the profitability of profitable projects and understates the profitability of unprofitable projects. By forcing the correct reinvestment rate, the MIRR method provides decision makers with a theoretically better measure of a project's expected rate of return than does the IRR.

In closing our discussion, note that the MIRR has other advantages over the IRR besides the proper reinvestment rate. Primarily, it avoids potential problems when a project has *nonnormal* cash flows. A project with normal cash flows has one or more outflows followed by one or more inflows, while one with nonnormal cash flows has outflows occurring after one or more in-flows have occurred. In the nonnormal situation, it is possible for a project to have two IRRs or even to have no IRR. These unusual results occur be-cause of the mathematics of the IRR calculation. The MIRR overcomes these problems, so it is the only rate of return measure available for some projects.

Self-Test Questions

1. Briefly describe how to calculate net present value (NPV), internal rate of return (IRR), and modified IRR (MIRR).
2. What is the rationale behind each method?
3. Do the three methods lead to the same conclusions regarding project profitability? Explain your answer.

Some Final Thoughts on Breakeven and Profitability Analyses

Although we have discussed one breakeven and three profitability measures, there are many other measures commonly used in project financial analyses.[8] Today, virtually all capital budgeting decisions of financial consequence are analyzed by computer, and hence the mechanics of calculating and listing numerous breakeven and profitability measures is easy. Because each measure contributes slightly different information about the financial consequences of a project, managers should not focus on only one or two financial measures. A thorough financial analysis of a new project includes numerous financial measures, and capital budgeting decisions are enhanced if all information inherent in all measures is considered in the process.

Self-Test Questions

1. Evaluate the following statement: The difficulty in calculating nu-merous breakeven and profitability measures restricts the amount of information available in capital budgeting analyses.
2. Should capital budgeting analyses look at only one breakeven or profitability measure? Explain your answer.

Capital Budgeting in Not-for-Profit Businesses

Although the capital budgeting techniques discussed to this point are appro-priate for use by all businesses when assessing the financial impact of a pro-posed project, a not-for-profit firm has the additional consideration of meet-ing its charitable mission. In this section, two models that extend the capital budgeting decision to include the charitable mission are discussed.

Net Present Social Value (NPSV) Model[9]

The financial analysis techniques discussed so far have focused exclusively on the cash flow implications of a proposed project. Some healthcare businesses, particularly not-for-profit providers, have the goal of producing social services along with commercial services. For such firms, the proper analysis of proposed projects must, at least in theory, systematically consider the *social value* of a project along with its pure financial, or cash flow, value.

When social value is considered, the *total net present value (TNPV)* of a project can be expressed as follows:

$$TNPV = NPV + NPSV.$$

Here, NPV represents the conventional NPV of the project's cash flow stream and *NPSV* is the *net present social value* of the project. The NPSV term, which represents managers' assessment of the social value of a project, clearly differentiates capital budgeting in not-for-profit firms from that in investor-owned firms. In evaluating each project, a project is acceptable if its TNPV is greater than or equal to zero. This means that the sum of the project's financial and social values is at least zero, so when both facets of value are considered, the project has positive, or at least non-negative, worth. Probably not all projects will have social value, but if a project does, it is considered formally in this decision model. However, no project should be accepted if its NPSV is negative, even if its TNPV is positive. Furthermore, to ensure the financial viability of the firm, the sum of the conventional NPVs of all projects initiated in a planning period must equal or exceed zero.[10] If this restriction were not imposed, social value could displace financial value over time, and a business cannot continue to provide social value without financial integrity.

NPSV is the sum of the present (Year 0) values of each year's social value. In essence, the suppliers of fund capital to a not-for-profit firm never receive a cash return on their investment. Instead, they receive a return on their investment in the form of social dividends. These dividends take the form of services with social value to the community such as charity care, medical research and education, and a myriad of other services that, for one reason or another, do not pay their own way. Services provided to patients at a price equal to or greater than the full cost of production do not create social value. Similarly, if governmental entities purchase care directly for beneficiaries of a program or support research, the resulting social value is created by the funding organization as opposed to the service provider.

In estimating a project's NPSV, first it is necessary to estimate in dollar terms the social value of the services provided in each year. When a project produces services to individuals who are willing and able to pay for those services, the value of those services is captured by the amount that they actually pay. Thus, the value of the services provided to those who cannot pay, or to those who cannot pay the full amount, can be estimated by the average net price paid by those individuals who are able to pay. Next, a discount rate must be applied to the social value cash flows. In general, providers should require a return on their social value stream that approximates the return available on the equity investment in for-profit firms that offer the same services.

This approach to valuing social services has intuitive appeal, but certain implementation problems merit further discussion.

- Price is a fair measure of value only if the payer has the capacity to judge the true value of the service provided. Many observers of the health services industry would argue that information asymmetries between the provider and the purchaser inhibit the ability of the purchaser to judge true value.
- The fact that most payments for healthcare services are made by third-party payers may result in price distortions. For example, insurers may be willing to pay more for services than an individual would pay in the absence of insurance, or the market power of some insurers, such as Medicare, may result in a price that is less than individuals would be willing to pay.
- A great deal of controversy exists over the true value of treatment in many situations. Suppose that some people are entitled to whatever healthcare is available, regardless of cost, and are not required to personally pay for the care. Even though society as a whole must cover the cost, people may demand a level of care that is of questionable value. For example, should large sums be spent to keep a comatose 92-year old alive for a few more days? If the true value to society of such an expenditure is zero, assigning a high social value just because that is its cost makes little sense.

Although the NPSV model formalizes the capital budgeting decision process applicable to not-for-profit healthcare firms, few organizations actually attempt to quantify NPSV. However, not-for-profit providers should, at a minimum, subjectively consider the social value inherent in projects under consideration.

Project Scoring

Managers of not-for-profit firms, as well as many managers of investor-owned firms, recognize that nonfinancial factors should be considered in any capital budgeting analysis. The NPSV model examines only one other factor, and it is difficult to implement in practice. Thus, many firms use a quasi-subjective *project scoring* approach to capital budgeting decisions that attempts to capture both financial and nonfinancial factors. Table 14.5, which is used by Bayside Memorial Hospital, illustrates one such approach.

Bayside ranks projects on three dimensions: stakeholder, operational, and financial. Within each dimension, multiple factors are examined and assigned scores that range from two points for very favorable impact to minus one point for negative impact. The scores within each dimension are added

TABLE 14.5

Bayside Memorial Hospital: Project Scoring Matrix

Criteria	Relative Score			
	2	1	0	−1
Stakeholder Factors				
Physicians	Strongly support	Support	Neutral	Opposed
Employees	Greatly helps morale	Helps morale	No effect	Hurts morale
Visitors	Greatly enhances visit	Enhances visit	No effect	Hurts image
Social value	High	Moderate	None	Negative
Operational Factors				
Outcomes	Greatly improves	Improves	No effect	Hurts outcomes
Length of stay	Documented decrease	Anecdotal decrease	No effect	Increases
Technology	Breakthrough	Improves current	Adds to current	Lowers
Productivity	Large decrease in FTEs	Decrease in FTEs	No change in FTEs	Adds FTEs
Financial Factors				
Life cycle	Innovation	Growth	Stabilization	Decline
Payback	Less than 2 years	2–4 years	4–6 years	Over 6 years
IRR	Over 20%	15–20%	10–15%	Less than 10%
Correlation	Negative	Uncorrelated	Somewhat positive	Highly positive
Stakeholder factor score	_____			
Operational factor score	_____			
Financial factor score	_____			
Total score	_____			

together to obtain scores for each of the three dimensions, and then the dimension scores are summed to obtain a total score for the project. The total score gives Bayside's managers a feel for the relative values of projects under consideration when all factors, including financial, are taken into account.

Bayside's managers recognize that the scoring system is completely arbitrary, so a project with a score of ten, for example, is not necessarily twice as good as a project that scores five. Nevertheless, Bayside's project scoring approach forces its managers to address multiple issues when making capital budgeting decisions and it does provide a relative ranking of projects under consideration. Although Bayside's approach should not be used at other organizations without modification for firm- and industry-unique circumstances, it does provide insights into how a firm-unique matrix might be developed.

Self-Test Questions

1. Describe the net present social value (NPSV) model of capital budgeting.
2. Describe the construction and use of a project-scoring matrix.

The Post-Audit

Capital budgeting is not a static process. If there is a long lag between a project's acceptance and its implementation, any new information concerning either capital costs or the project's cash flows should be analyzed before the final start-up occurs. Furthermore, the performance of each project should be monitored throughout the project's life. The process of formally monitoring project performance over time is called the *post-audit*. It involves comparing actual results with those projected, explaining why differences occur, and analyzing potential changes to the project's operations, including replacement or termination.

The post-audit has several purposes:

- **Improve forecasts.** When managers systematically compare projections to actual outcomes, there is a tendency for estimates to improve. Conscious or unconscious biases that occur can be identified and, one hopes, eliminated; new forecasting methods are sought as the need for them becomes apparent; and managers tend to do everything better, including forecasting, if they know that their actions are being monitored.
- **Develop historical risk data.** Post-audits permit managers to develop historical data on new project analyses regarding risk and expected rates of return. These data can then be used to make judgments about the relative risk of future projects as they are evaluated.
- **Improve operations.** Managers run businesses, and they can perform at higher or lower levels of efficiency. When a forecast is made, for example, by the surgery department, the department director and medical staff are, in a sense, putting their reputations on the line. If costs are above predicted levels and volume is below expectations, the managers involved will strive, within ethical bounds, to improve the situation and to bring results into line with forecasts. As one hospital CEO put it: "You academics worry only about making good decisions. In the health services industry, we also have to worry about making decisions good."
- **Reduce losses.** Post-audits monitor the performance of projects over time, so the first indication that termination or replacement should be considered often arises when the post-audit indicates that a project is performing poorly.

1. What is a post-audit?
2. Why are post-audits important to the efficiency of a business?

Self-Test Questions

Using Capital Budgeting Techniques in Other Contexts

The techniques developed in this chapter can help health services managers make a number of different types of decisions in addition to project selection.

One example is the use of NPV and IRR to evaluate corporate merger opportunities. Healthcare companies often acquire other companies to increase capacity or expand into other service areas, or for other reasons. A key element of any merger analysis is the valuation of the target company. Although the cash flows in such an analysis may be structured differently than in project analysis, the same evaluation tools are applied. We will discuss business valuation in more detail in Chapter 18.

Managers also use capital budgeting techniques when deciding whether or not to divest assets or reduce staffing. Like capital budgeting, these actions require an analysis of the impact of the decision on the firm's cash flows. When eliminating personnel, businesses typically spend money up-front in severance payments but then receive benefits in the form of lower wages and benefits in the future. When assets are sold, the pattern of cash flows is reversed—that is, cash inflows occur when the asset is sold, but any future cash inflows associated with the asset are sacrificed. (If future cash flows are negative, the decision, at least from a financial perspective, should be easy.) In both situations, the techniques discussed in this chapter, perhaps with modifications, can be applied to assess the financial consequences of the action.

Self-Test Question

1. Can capital budgeting tools be used in different settings? Explain your answer.

Key Concepts

This chapter discussed the basics of capital budgeting. The key concepts of this chapter are:

- *Capital budgeting* is the process of analyzing potential expenditures on fixed assets and deciding whether the firm should undertake those investments.
- A capital budgeting financial analysis consists of four steps: (1) estimate the expected cash flows, (2) assess the riskiness of those flows, (3) estimate the appropriate cost of capital discount rate, and (4) determine the project's profitability and breakeven characteristics.
- The most critical and most difficult step in analyzing a project is estimating the *incremental cash flows* that the project will generate.
- In determining incremental cash flows, *opportunity costs* (i.e., the cash flows forgone by using an asset) must be considered, but *sunk costs* (i.e., cash outlays that cannot be recouped) are not included. Furthermore, any impact of the project on the firm's *other projects* must be included in the analysis.
- *Tax laws* generally affect investor-owned firms in three ways: (1) taxes reduce a project's operating cash flows, (2) tax laws prescribe the

depreciation expense that can be taken in any year, and (3) taxes affect a project's salvage value cash flow.

- Capital projects often require an investment in *net working capital* in addition to the investment in fixed assets. Such increases represent a cash outlay that, if material, must be included in the analysis. The investment in net working capital is recovered when the project is terminated.

- A project may have some *strategic value* that is not accounted for in the estimated cash flows. At a minimum, strategic value should be noted and considered qualitatively in the analysis.

- The *effects of inflation* must be considered in project analyses. The best procedure is to build inflation effects directly into the component cash flow estimates.

- Time breakeven, which is measured by the *payback period,* provides managers with insights concerning a project's liquidity and risk.

- Project profitability is assessed by *return on investment (ROI)* measures. The two most commonly used ROI measures are net present value and internal rate of return.

- *Net present value (NPV)*, which is simply the sum of the present values of all the project's net cash flows when discounted at the project's cost of capital, measures a project's expected dollar profitability. An NPV greater than zero indicates that the project is expected to be profitable after all costs, including the opportunity cost of capital, have been considered. Furthermore, the higher the NPV, the more profitable the project.

- *Internal rate of return (IRR)*, which is the discount rate that forces a project's NPV to equal zero, measures a project's expected rate of return. If a project's IRR is greater than its cost of capital, the project is expected to be profitable; and the higher the IRR, the more profitable the project.

- The NPV and IRR profitability measures provide identical indications of profitability; that is, a project that is judged to be profitable by its NPV will also be profitable by its IRR. However, when mutually exclusive projects are being evaluated, NPV might rank a different project higher than IRR. This difference can occur because the two measures have different *reinvestment rate assumptions*—IRR assumes that cash flows can be reinvested at the project's IRR, while NPV assumes that cash flows can be reinvested at the project's cost of capital.

- The *modified internal rate of return (MIRR)*, which forces a project's cash flows to be reinvested at the project's cost of capital, is a better measure of a project's percentage rate of return than the IRR.

- The *net present social value (NPSV) model* formalizes the capital budgeting decision process for not-for-profit firms.

- Firms often use *project scoring* to subjectively incorporate a large number of factors, including financial and nonfinancial, into the capital budgeting decision process.

- The *post-audit* is a key element in capital budgeting. By comparing actual results with predicted results, managers can improve both operations and the cash flow estimation process.
- Capital budgeting techniques are used in a wide variety of settings in addition to project evaluation.

The discussion of capital investment decisions will continue in Chapter 15, which focuses on risk assessment and incorporation.

Questions

14.1 a. What is capital budgeting? Why are capital budgeting decisions so important to businesses?
   b. What is the purpose of placing capital projects into categories such as mandatory replacement, or expansion of existing products, services, or markets?
   c. Should financial analysis play the dominant role in capital budgeting decisions? Explain your answer.
   d. What are the four steps of capital budgeting analysis?

14.2 Briefly define the following cash flow estimation concepts.
   a. Incremental cash flow
   b. Cash flow versus accounting income
   c. Sunk cost
   d. Opportunity cost
   e. Net working capital
   f. Strategic value
   g. Inflation effects

14.3 Describe the following project breakeven and profitability measures. Be sure to include each measure's economic interpretation.
   a. Payback
   b. Net present value (NPV)
   c. Internal rate of return (IRR)
   d. Modified internal rate of return (MIRR)

14.4 Critique this statement: NPV is a better measure of project profitability than IRR because it leads to better capital investment decisions.

14.5 a. Describe the net present social value (NPSV) model.
   b. What is a project scoring matrix?

14.6 What is a post-audit? Why is the post-audit critical to good investment decision making?

14.7 From a purely financial perspective, are there situations in which a business would be better off choosing a project with a shorter payback over one that has a larger NPV?

Problems

14.1 Winston Clinic is evaluating a project that costs $52,125 and has expected net cash inflows of $12,000 per year for eight years. The first inflow occurs one year after the cost outflow, and the project has a cost of capital of 12 percent.

a. What is the project's payback?

b. What is the project's NPV? Its IRR? Its MIRR?

c. Is the project financially acceptable? Explain your answer.

14.2 Better Health, Inc., is evaluating two investment projects, each of which requires an up-front expenditure of $1.5 million. The projects are expected to produce the following net cash inflows:

Year	Project A	Project B
1	$ 500,000	$2,000,000
2	1,000,000	1,000,000
3	2,000,000	600,000

a. What is each project's IRR?

b. What is each project's NPV if the cost of capital is 10 percent? 5 percent? 15 percent?

14.3 Capitol Healthplans, Inc., is evaluating two different methods for providing home health services to its members. Both methods involve contracting out for services, and the health outcomes and revenues are not affected by the method chosen. Therefore, the incremental cash flows for the decision are all outflows. Here are the projected flows:

Year	Method A	Method B
0	($300,000)	($120,000)
1	(66,000)	(96,000)
2	(66,000)	(96,000)
3	(66,000)	(96,000)
4	(66,000)	(96,000)
5	(66,000)	(96,000)

a. What is each alternative's IRR?

b. If the cost of capital for both methods is 9 percent, which method should be chosen? Why?

14.4 Great Lakes Clinic has been asked to provide exclusive healthcare services for next year's World Exposition. Although flattered by the request, the clinic's managers want to conduct a financial analysis of the project. There will be an up-front cost of $160,000 to get the clinic in operation. Then, a net cash inflow of $1 million is expected from operations in each of the two years of the exposition. However, the clinic has to pay the organizers of the exposition a fee for the marketing value of the opportunity. This fee, which must be paid at the end of the second year, is $2 million.

a. What are the cash flows associated with the project?

b. What is the project's IRR?

c. Assuming a project cost of capital of 10 percent, what is the project's NPV?

d. What is the project's MIRR?

14.5 Assume that you are the chief financial officer at Porter Memorial Hospital. The CEO has asked you to analyze two proposed capital investments—Project X and Project Y. Each project requires a net investment outlay of $10,000, and the cost of capital for each project is 12 percent. The projects' expected net cash flows are:

Year	Project X	Project Y
0	($10,000)	($10,000)
1	6,500	3,000
2	3,000	3,000
3	3,000	3,000
4	1,000	3,000

a. Calculate each project's payback period, net present value (NPV), and internal rate of return (IRR).

b. Which project (or projects) is financially acceptable? Explain your answer.

14.6 The director of capital budgeting for Big Sky Health Systems, Inc., has estimated the following cash flows in thousands of dollars for a proposed new service:

Year	Expected Net Cash Flow
0	($100)
1	70
2	50
3	20

The project's cost of capital is 10 percent.

a. What is the project's payback period?

b. What is the project's NPV?

c. What is the project's IRR? Its MIRR?

14.7 California Health Center, a for-profit hospital, is evaluating the purchase of new diagnostic equipment. The equipment, which costs $600,000, has an expected life of five years and an estimated pretax salvage value of $200,000 at that time. The equipment is expected to be used 15 times a day for 250 days a year for each year of the project's life. On average, each procedure is expected to generate

$80 in collections, which is net of bad debt losses and contractual allowances, in its first year of use. Thus, net revenues for Year 1 are estimated at $15 \times 250 \times \$80 = \$300,000$.

Labor and maintenance costs are expected to be $100,000 during the first year of operation, while utilities will cost another $10,000 and cash overhead will increase by $5,000 in Year 1. The cost for expendable supplies is expected to average $5 per procedure during the first year. All costs and revenues, except depreciation, are expected to increase at a 5 percent inflation rate after the first year.

The equipment falls into the MACRS five-year class for tax depreciation and hence is subject to the following depreciation allowances:

Year	Allowance
1	0.20
2	0.32
3	0.19
4	0.12
5	0.11
6	0.06
	1.00

The hospital's tax rate is 40 percent, and its corporate cost of capital is 10 percent.

a. Estimate the project's net cash flows over its five-year estimated life. (Hint: Use the following format as a guide.)

	Year					
	0	1	2	3	4	5
Equipment cost						
Net revenues						
Less: Labor/maintenance costs						
Utilities costs						
Supplies						
Incremental overhead						
Depreciation						
Operating income						
Taxes						
Net operating income						
Plus: Depreciation						
Plus: Equipment salvage value						
Net cash flow						

b. What are the project's NPV and IRR? (Assume for now that the project has average risk.)

14.8 You have been asked by the president and CEO of Kidd Pharmaceuticals to evaluate the proposed acquisition of a new labeling machine for one of the firm's production lines. The machine's price is $50,000, and it would cost another $10,000 for transportation and installation. The machine falls into the MACRS three-year class, and hence the tax depreciation allowances are 0.33, 0.45, and 0.15 in Years 1, 2, and 3, respectively. The machine would be sold after three years because the production line is being closed at that time. The best estimate of the machine's salvage value after three years of use is $20,000. The machine would have no effect on the firm's sales or revenues, but it is expected to save Kidd $20,000 per year in before-tax operating costs. The firm's tax rate is 40 percent and its corporate cost of capital is 10 percent.

a. What is the project's net investment outlay at Year 0?

b. What are the project's operating cash flows in Years 1, 2, and 3?

c. What are the terminal cash flows at the end of Year 3?

d. If the project has average risk, is it expected to be profitable?

14.9 The staff of Jefferson Memorial Hospital has estimated the following net cash flows for a satellite food services operation that it may open in its outpatient clinic:

Year	Expected Net Cash Flow
0	($100,000)
1	30,000
2	30,000
3	30,000
4	30,000
5	30,000
5 (salvage value)	20,000

The Year 0 cash flow is the investment cost of the new food service, while the final amount is the terminal cash flow. (The clinic is expected to move to a new building in five years.) All other flows represent net operating cash flows. Jefferson's corporate cost of capital is 10 percent.

a. What is the project's IRR? Its MIRR?

b. Assuming the project has average risk, what is its NPV?

c. Now, assume that the operating cash flows in Years 1–5 could be as low as $20,000 or as high as $40,000. Furthermore, the salvage value cash flow at the end of Year 5 could be as low as $0 or as high as $30,000. What are the worst case and best case IRRs? The worst case and best case NPVs?

Notes

1. Within not-for-profit providers, project losses can be offset by contributions and grants. However, long-run financial sustainability is best ensured by striving for operating profitability.

2. To emphasize the difficulties involved, one manager with a good sense of humor developed the following principles of capital budgeting cash flow estimation:

   - It is very difficult to forecast cash flows, especially those that occur in the future.
   - Those who live by the crystal ball soon learn how to eat ground glass.
   - The moment someone forecasts cash flows, they know that they are wrong—they just don't know by how much and in what direction.
   - If someone makes a correct forecast, never let the bosses forget.
   - An expert in cash flow estimation is someone who has been right at least once.

   Neither the difficulty nor the importance of cash flow estimation can be overstated. However, if the principles discussed in the text are observed, errors that often arise in the process can be minimized.

3. In most situations, the strategic value of a project stems from *managerial (real) options* brought about by the project that may or may not be used (exercised). One way to assess the value of these options is to use option pricing techniques that were first developed to value stock options, which confer upon their holders the right, but not the obligation, to buy or sell a particular stock at a specified price. For more information, see Louis C. Gapenski, *Understanding Healthcare Financial Management* (Chicago: Health Administration Press, 2007), Chapter 12.

4. As stated in Chapter 2, tax laws are complex and they change often. Therefore, this book does not include a complete discussion of the MACRS system. For more information, see either the IRS publication pertaining to depreciation or any of the tax guidebooks available at local bookstores.

5. If Ann Arbor did not have taxable income to offset in Year 2, and had no taxable income to offset in the three previous years, the loss would have to be carried forward, and hence the tax benefit would not be immediately realized. In this situation, the *tax shield* value of the loss would be reduced because it would be pushed into the future rather than recognized immediately.

6. The *discounted payback* is a breakeven measure similar to the conventional payback, except that the cash flows in each year are discounted to Year 0 by the project's cost of capital (but kept at their original positions on the time line) prior to calculating the payback. Thus, the discounted payback solves the conventional payback's problem of not considering the project's cost of capital in the payback calculation.

7. However, when mutually exclusive projects are being analyzed (i.e., two or more projects are being investigated but only one can be chosen), NPV and IRR rankings can conflict—that is, Project A could have the higher NPV, but Project

B could have the higher IRR. In such situations, the NPV method is generally considered to be the best measure of profitability.

8. For example, the *profitability index* (*PI*) gives decision makers information about a project's cost effectiveness (i.e., the project's bang for the buck). For more information on the PI, see Louis C. Gapenski, *Understanding Healthcare Financial Management* (Chicago: Health Administration Press, 2007), Chapter 11.

9. This section is drawn primarily from J. R. C. Wheeler and J. P. Clement, "Capital Expenditure Decisions and the Role of the Not-for-Profit Hospital: An Application of the Social Goods Model," *Medical Care Review* (Winter 1990): 467–486.

10. Not-for-profit providers can use contributions to offset some, or even all, of any aggregate negative NPV created by the acceptance of projects with positive social value.

References

Allen, R. J. 1989. "Proper Planning Reduces Risk in New Technology Acquisitions." *Healthcare Financial Management* (December): 48–56.

Bergman, J. T., and B. J. McIntyre. 1989. "Valuation Analysis." *Topics in Health Care Financing* (Summer): 32–40.

Campbell, C. 1994. "Hospital Plant and Equipment Replacement Decisions: A Survey of Hospital Financial Managers." *Hospital & Health Services Administration* (Winter): 538–556.

Chow, C. W., and A. H. McNamee. 1991. "Watch for Pitfalls of Discounted Cash Flow Techniques." *Healthcare Financial Management* (April): 34–43.

Chow, C. W., K. M. Haddad, and A. Wong-Boren. 1991. "Improving Subjective Decision Making in Health Care Administration." *Hospital & Health Services Administration* (Summer): 191–210.

Clarke, R. L., and R. Wolfert. 2003. "Capital Allocation: Three Cases of Financing for the Future." *Healthcare Financial Management* (October): 58–62.

Cleverley, W. O., and J. G. Felkner. 1984. "The Association of Capital Budgeting Techniques with Hospital Financial Performance." *Health Care Management Review* (Summer): 45–55.

Gapenski, L. C. 1989. "A Better Approach to Internal Rate of Return." *Healthcare Financial Management* (April): 93–99.

———. 1989. "Analysis Provides Test for Profitability of New Services." *Healthcare Financial Management* (November): 48–58.

———. 1993. "Capital Investment Analysis: Three Methods." *Healthcare Financial Management* (August): 60–66.

Gordon, D. C., and D. F. Londal. 1989. "Guidelines to Capital Investment." *Topics in Health Care Financing* (Summer): 9–17.

Henley, R. J., and M. A. Zimmerman. 2005. "10 Proven Strategies for Reducing Equipment Costs." *Healthcare Financial Management* (May): 78–81.

Healthcare Financial Management Association (HFMA). 2004. "Inside the Real World of Capital Allocation." *Healthcare Financial Management* (December): 81–86.

Horowitz, J. L., and P. F. Straley. 1988. "Developing Investment Criteria: There Is More To It Than Financial Criteria Alone." *Topics in Health Care Financing* (Fall): 23–31.

Horowitz, J. L. 1993. "Contribution Margin Analysis: A Case Study." *Healthcare Financial Management* (June): 129–133.

Kamath, R. R., and J. Elmer. 1989. "Capital Investment Decisions in Hospitals: Survey Results." *Health Care Management Review* (Spring): 45–56.

Kennedy, W. F., and D. A. Plath. 1994. "A Return-Based Alternative to IRR Evaluations." *Healthcare Financial Management* (March): 38–49.

Manecke, S. R. 1993. "Practice Acquisition: Buy or Build." *Healthcare Financial Management* (December): 33–41.

Mellen, C. M. 1992. "Valuing a Long-Term Care Facility." *Healthcare Financial Management* (October): 20–25.

Meyer, A. D. 1985. "Hospital Capital Budgeting: Fusion of Rationality, Politics and Ceremony." *Health Care Management Review* (Spring): 17–27.

Reiter, K. L., D. G. Smith, J. R. C. Wheeler, and H. L. Rivenson. 2000. "Capital Investment Strategies in Health Care Systems." *Journal of Health Care Finance* (Summer): 31–41.

Ryan, J. B., M. E. Ward, and D. S. Kolb. 1990. "Capital Management Balances Charitable, Financial Goals." *Healthcare Financial Management* (March): 32–40.

Ryan, J. B., and M. E. Ward (eds). 1992. "Capital Management." *Topics in Health Care Financing* (Fall) 1–88.

Schramm, C. J., and G. D. Pillari. 1987. "Investing in the Wrong Future for Hospitals." *Health Care Management Review* (Fall): 31–37.

Smith, D. G., J. R. Wheeler, H. L. Rivenson, and K. L. Reiter. 2000. "Sources of Project Financing in Health Care Systems." *Journal of Health Care Finance* (Summer): 53–58.

Straley, P. F., and C. R. Swaim. 1993. "Financial Analysis of Medical Office Buildings." *Topics in Health Care Financing* (Spring): 76–85.

Watts, D., D. L. Finney, and B. Louie. 1993. "Integrating Technology Assessment into the Capital Budgeting Process." *Healthcare Financial Management* (February): 21–29.

Weitzner, W. M., and T. Kurmel. 2004. "The Cost of Staying Young." *Healthcare Financial Management* (May): 93–96.

PROJECT RISK ASSESSMENT AND INCORPORATION

Learning Objectives

After studying this chapter, readers will be able to:

- Describe the three types of risk relevant to capital budgeting decisions.
- Discuss the techniques used in project risk assessment.
- Conduct a project risk assessment.
- Incorporate risk into the capital budgeting decision process.

Introduction

Chapter 14 covered the basics of capital budgeting, including cash flow estimation, breakeven analysis, and ROI (profitability) measures. This chapter extends the discussion of capital budgeting to include risk analysis, which is composed of three elements: defining the type of risk relevant to the project, measuring the project's risk, and incorporating that risk assessment into the capital budgeting decision process. Although risk analysis is a key element in all financial decisions, the importance of capital investment decisions to a healthcare business's success or failure makes risk analysis vital in such decisions.

The higher the risk associated with an investment, the higher its required rate of return. This principle is just as valid for healthcare businesses that make capital expenditure decisions as it is for individuals who make personal investment decisions. Thus, the ultimate goal in project risk analysis is to ensure that the cost of capital used as the discount rate in a project's ROI analysis properly reflects the riskiness of that project. The corporate cost of capital, which was covered in detail in Chapter 13, reflects the cost of capital to the organization based on its aggregate risk—that is, based on the riskiness of the firm's average project. In project risk analysis, a project's risk is assessed relative to the firm's average project: Does the project have average risk, below-average risk, or above-average risk? The corporate cost of capital is then adjusted to reflect any differential risk, resulting in a *project cost of capital*. In general, above-average-risk projects are assigned a project cost of capital that is higher than the corporate cost of capital, average risk projects are evaluated at the corporate cost of capital, and below-average-risk projects are assigned a discount rate that is less than the corporate cost of capital. (Note that when capital budgeting is conducted at the divisional level, the adjustment process is handled in a similar manner, but the starting value is the divisional cost of capital.)

Types of Project Risk

Three separate and distinct types of financial risk can be defined in a capital budgeting context:

1. **Stand-alone risk.** Stand-alone risk assumes the project is held in isolation and hence ignores portfolio effects both within the firm and among equity investors.
2. **Corporate risk.** This type of risk views the risk of a project within the context of the firm's portfolio of projects.
3. **Market risk.** Market risk views the project from the perspective of a shareholder who holds a well-diversified portfolio of stocks.[1]

The type of risk that is most relevant to a particular capital budgeting decision depends on the number of projects the business holds and its form of ownership.

Stand-Alone Risk

Stand-alone risk is present in a project whenever there is a chance of a return that is less than the expected return. In effect, **a project is risky whenever its cash flows are not known with certainty**, because uncertain cash flows mean uncertain profitability. Furthermore, the greater the probability of a return far below the expected return, the greater the risk. Stand-alone risk can be measured by the *standard deviation* (or *coefficient of variation*) of the project's profitability (ROI), often measured by net present value (NPV), internal rate of return (IRR), or modified internal rate of return (MIRR). Because standard deviation measures the dispersion of a distribution around its expected value, the larger the standard deviation, the greater the probability that the project's ROI will be far below that expected.

Conceptually, *stand-alone risk* is only relevant in one situation: when a not-for-profit firm is evaluating its first project. In this situation, the project will be operated in isolation, so no portfolio diversification is present—the business does not have a collection of different projects, nor does the firm have stockholders who hold diversified portfolios of stocks.

Corporate Risk

In reality, businesses usually offer many different products or services and thus can be thought of as having a large number (perhaps even hundreds or thousands) of individual projects. For example, MinuteMan Healthcare, a

New England not-for-profit managed care company, offers healthcare services to a large number of diverse employee groups in numerous service areas, and each different group can be considered to be a separate project. In this situation, the stand-alone risk of a project under consideration by MinuteMan is not relevant because the project will not be held in isolation. The relevant risk of a new project to MinuteMan is its contribution to the HMO's overall risk (the impact of the project on the variability of the overall profitability of the business). This type of risk, which is relevant when the project is part of a not-for-profit business's portfolio of projects, is called *corporate risk*.

A project's corporate risk, which is measured by its corporate beta, depends on the context (i.e., the firm's other projects), so a project may have high corporate risk to one business but low corporate risk to another, particularly when the two businesses operate in widely different industries.

Market Risk

Market risk is generally viewed as the relevant risk for projects being evaluated by investor-owned businesses. The goal of shareholder (owner) wealth maximization implies that a project's returns, as well as its risk, should be defined and measured from the shareholders' perspective. The riskiness of an individual project, as seen by a well-diversified shareholder, is not the riskiness of the project as if it were owned and operated in isolation, which is defined as stand-alone risk, nor is it the contribution of the project to the riskiness of the business, which is defined as corporate risk. Most shareholders hold a large diversified portfolio of stocks of many firms, which can be thought of as a very large diversified portfolio of individual projects. Thus, the risk of any single project as seen by a business's stockholders is its contribution to the riskiness of their well-diversified stock portfolios.

A project's absolute market risk, as measured by its market beta, is independent of the context; that is, a project's market beta does not depend on the characteristics of the business, assuming the project's cash flows are the same to all firms. However, the market risk of a project, **relative to the market risk of the firm's other projects**, depends on the aggregate market risk of the business.

1. What are the three types of project risk?	**Self-Test**
2. How is each type of project risk measured, both in absolute and relative terms?	**Questions**

Relationships Among Stand-Alone, Corporate, and Market Risk

After discussing the three different types of project risk, and the situations in which each is relevant, it is tempting to say that stand-alone risk is almost never important because not-for-profit firms should focus on a project's corporate risk and investor-owned firms should focus on a project's market risk. Unfortunately, the situation is not quite that simple.

First, it is almost impossible in practice to quantify a project's corporate or market risk. Fortunately, as will be demonstrated in the next section, it is possible to get a rough idea of the relative stand-alone risk of a project. Thus, managers can make statements such as Project A has above-average risk, Project B has below-average risk, or Project C has average risk, all in the stand-alone sense. After a project's stand-alone risk has been assessed, the primary factor in converting stand-alone risk to either corporate or market risk is *correlation*. If a project's returns are expected to be highly positively correlated with the firm's returns, high stand-alone risk translates to high corporate risk. Similarly, if the firm's returns are expected to be highly correlated with the stock market's returns, high corporate risk translates to high market risk. The same analogies hold when the project is judged to have average or low stand-alone risk.

Most projects will be in a firm's primary line of business. Because all projects in the same line of business are generally affected by the same economic factors, such projects' returns are usually highly correlated. When this situation exists, a project's stand-alone risk is a good proxy for its corporate risk. Furthermore, most projects' returns are also positively correlated with the returns on other assets in the economy—most assets have high returns when the economy is strong and low returns when the economy is weak. When this situation holds, a project's stand-alone risk is a good proxy for its market risk.

Thus, for most projects, the stand-alone risk assessment also gives good insights into a project's corporate and market risk. The only exception is when a project's returns are expected to be independent of or negatively correlated to the firm's average project. In these situations, considerable judgment is required because the stand-alone risk assessment will overstate the project's corporate risk. Similarly, if a project's returns are expected to be independent of or negatively correlated to the market's returns, the project's stand-alone risk overstates its market risk.[2]

| **Self-Test Questions** | 1. Name and define the three types of risk relevant to capital budgeting. |
| | 2. How are these risks related? |

Risk Analysis Illustration

To illustrate project risk analysis, consider Bayside Memorial Hospital's evaluation of a new MRI system that was first presented in Chapter 14. Table 15.1 contains the project's cash flow analysis. If all of the project's component cash flows were known with certainty, the project's projected profitability would be known with certainty, and hence the project would have no risk. However,

TABLE 15.1
Bayside Memorial Hospital: MRI Site Cash Flow Analysis

	0	1	2	3	4	5
				Cash Revenues and Costs		
1. System cost	($1,500,000)					
2. Related expenses	(1,000,000)					
3. Gross revenues		$1,000,000	$1,050,000	$1,102,500	$1,157,625	$1,215,506
4. Deductions		250,000	262,500	275,625	289,406	303,877
5. Net revenues		$ 750,000	$ 787,500	$ 826,875	$ 868,219	$ 911,630
6. Labor costs		50,000	52,500	55,125	57,881	60,775
7. Maintenance costs		150,000	157,500	165,375	173,644	182,326
8. Supplies		30,000	31,500	33,075	34,729	36,465
9. Incremental overhead		10,000	10,500	11,025	11,576	12,155
10. Depreciation		350,000	350,000	350,000	350,000	350,000
11. Operating income		$ 160,000	$ 185,500	$ 212,275	$ 240,389	$ 269,908
12. Taxes		0	0	0	0	0
13. Net operating income		$ 160,000	$ 185,500	$ 212,275	$ 240,389	$ 269,908
14. Depreciation		350,000	350,000	350,000	350,000	350,000
15. Net salvage value						750,000
16. Net cash flow	($2,500,000)	$ 510,000	$ 535,500	$ 562,275	$ 590,389	$1,369,908

Profitability Measures:
Net present value (NPV) = $82,493.
Internal rate of return (IRR) = 11.1%.

in virtually all project analyses, future cash flows and hence profitability are uncertain—and in many cases highly uncertain—so risk is present.

The starting point for analyzing a project's risk involves estimating the uncertainty inherent in the project's cash flows. Most of the individual cash flows in Table 15.1 are subject to uncertainty. For example, volume was projected at 40 scans per week. However, utilization would almost certainly be higher or lower than the 40-scan forecast. In effect, the volume estimate is really an expected value taken from some probability distribution of potential utilization, as are many of the other values listed in Table 15.1.

The nature of the component cash flow distributions and their correlations with one another determine the nature of the project's profitability distribution and thus the project's risk. In the following sections, two quantitative techniques for assessing a project's risk are discussed: sensitivity analysis and scenario analysis.[3] Then we discuss a qualitative approach to risk assessment. Remember that our focus here is on the stand-alone risk of the project. After the stand-alone risk is assessed, we will use judgment to translate that assessment into corporate and market risk (if relevant).

Self-Test Questions

1. What condition creates project risk?
2. What makes one project riskier than another?
3. What type of risk is being assessed initially?

Sensitivity Analysis

Historically, *sensitivity analysis* has been classified as a risk assessment tool. In reality, it is not very useful in assessing a project's risk. However, it does have significant value in project analysis, so we will discuss it in some detail here.

Many of the variables that determine a project's cash flows are subject to some type of probability distribution and are not known with certainty. If the realized value of such a variable is different from its expected value, the project's profitability will differ from its expected value. Sensitivity analysis shows exactly how much a project's profitability (NPV or IRR or MIRR) will change in response to a given change in a single input variable, with other things held constant.

Sensitivity analysis begins with a *base case* developed using **expected values** (in the statistical sense) for all uncertain variables. To illustrate, assume that Bayside's managers believe that all of the MRI project's component cash flows are known with certainty except for weekly volume and salvage value. The expected values for these variables (volume = 40 and salvage value = $750,000) were used in Table 15.1 to obtain the base case NPV of $82,493. Sensitivity analysis is designed to provide managers the answers to such questions as these: What if volume is more or less than the expected level? What if salvage value is more or less than expected?

In a typical sensitivity analysis, each uncertain variable is changed by a fixed percentage amount above and below its expected value, while all other variables are held constant at their expected values. Thus, all input variables except one are held at their base case values. The resulting NPVs (or IRRs or MIRRs) are recorded and plotted. Table 15.2 contains the NPV sensitivity analysis for the MRI project, assuming that there are two uncertain variables: volume and salvage value.

Note that the NPV is a constant $82,493 when there is no change in any of the variables. This situation occurs because a zero percent change recreates the base case. Managers can examine the Table 15.2 values to get a feel for which input variable has the greatest impact on the MRI project's NPV—the larger the NPV change for a given percentage input change, the greater the impact. Such an examination shows that the MRI project's NPV is affected by changes in volume more than by changes in salvage value. This result should be somewhat intuitive because salvage value is a single cash flow in the analysis, whereas volume influences the cash flow in each year of operation.

Often, the results of sensitivity analyses are shown in graphical form. For example, the Table 15.2 sensitivity analysis is graphed in Figure 15.1. Here, the slopes of the lines show how sensitive the MRI project's NPV is to changes in each of the two uncertain input variables—the steeper the slope, the more sensitive NPV is to a change in the variable. Note that the sensitivity lines intersect at the base case values—0 percent change from base case level and $82,493. Also, spreadsheet models are ideally suited for performing sensitivity analyses because such models both automatically recalculate NPV when an input value is changed and facilitate graphing.[4]

Figure 15.1 vividly illustrates that the MRI project's NPV is very sensitive to volume but only mildly sensitive to changes in salvage value. If a sensitivity plot has a negative slope, it indicates that **increases** in the value of that input variable **decrease** the project's NPV. If two projects were being compared, the one with the steeper sensitivity lines would be regarded as riskier because a relatively small error in estimating a variable—for example,

Change from Base Case Level	Net Present Value (NPV)	
	Volume	Salvage Value
−30%	($814,053)	($ 57,215)
−20	(515,193)	(10,646)
−10	216,350	35,923
0	82,493	82,493
+10	381,335	129,062
+20	680,178	175,631
+30	979,020	222,200

TABLE 15.2
MRI Project Sensitivity Analysis

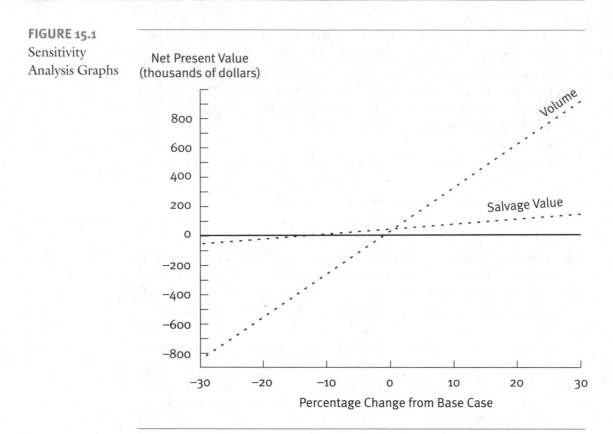

FIGURE 15.1
Sensitivity
Analysis Graphs

volume—would produce a large error in the project's projected NPV. If information was available on the sensitivity of NPV to input changes for Bayside's average project, similar judgments regarding the riskiness of the MRI project could be made relative to the firm's average project.

Although sensitivity analysis is considered to be a risk assessment tool, it does have severe limitations in this role. For example, suppose that Bayside Memorial Hospital had a contract with an HMO that guaranteed a minimum MRI usage at a fixed reimbursement rate. In that situation, the project would not be very risky at all, in spite of the fact that the sensitivity analysis showed the NPV to be highly sensitive to changes in volume. In general, a project's **stand-alone** risk, which is what is being measured in a sensitivity analysis, depends on both the sensitivity of its profitability to changes in key input variables and the ranges of likely values of these variables. Because sensitivity analysis considers only the first factor, it can give misleading results. Furthermore, sensitivity analysis does not consider any interactions among the uncertain input variables; it considers each variable independently of the others.

In spite of the shortcomings of sensitivity analysis as a risk assessment tool, it does provide managers with valuable information. First, it provides profitability breakeven information for the project's uncertain variables. For example, Table 15.2 and Figure 15.1 show that a decrease of just a few percent in expected volume makes the project unprofitable, whereas the project remains profitable even if salvage value falls by more than 10 percent. Although somewhat rough, this breakeven information is clearly of value to Bayside's managers.

Second, and perhaps more important, sensitivity analysis identifies those input variables that are are **most critical** to the analysis. By most critical, we mean those variables that have the largest impact on profitability when their realized values differ from their forecasted values. In this example, volume is clearly the most critical input variable of the two being examined, so Bayside's managers should ensure that the volume estimate is the best possible. A small overestimate in volume can make the project seem very attractive financially when evaluated, yet the actual results could easily be disappointing. The concept here is that Bayside's managers have a limited amount of time to spend on analyzing the MRI project, so the resources expended should be as productive as possible.

In addition, sensitivity analysis can be useful after a project has been initiated. For example, assume Bayside's MRI project was accepted and the first post-audit indicates that the project is not meeting its financial expectations. Bayside's managers must take actions to try to improve the project's financial results. But what actions should they take? Sensitivity analysis identifies the variables that have the greatest impact on profitability. Thus, managers can try to influence those variables that have the greatest potential for improving financial performance, such as volume, rather than those variables that have little impact on profitability.

1. Briefly describe sensitivity analysis?
2. What type of risk does it attempt to measure?
3. Is sensitivity analysis a good risk assessment tool? If not, what is its value in the capital budgeting process?

Self-Test Questions

Scenario Analysis

Scenario analysis is a stand-alone risk analysis technique that considers the sensitivity of NPV to changes in key variables, the likely range of variable values, and the interactions among variables. To conduct a scenario analysis, the managers pick a "bad" set of circumstances (i.e., low volume, low salvage value, and so on), an average or "most likely" set, and a "good set." The resulting input values are then used to create a probability distribution of NPV.

To illustrate scenario analysis, assume that Bayside's managers regard a drop in weekly volume below 30 scans as very unlikely and a volume above 50 as also improbable. On the other hand, salvage value could be as low as $500,000 or as high as $1 million. The most likely (and expected) values are 40 scans per week for volume and $750,000 for salvage value. Thus, a volume of 30 and a $500,000 salvage value define the lower bound, or worst case scenario, while a volume of 50 and a salvage value of $1 million define the upper bound, or best case scenario.

Bayside can now use the *worst, most likely,* and *best case* values for the input variables to obtain the NPV that corresponds to each scenario. Bayside's managers used a spreadsheet model to conduct the analysis, and Table 15.3 summarizes the results. The most likely (base) case results in a positive NPV; the worst case produces a negative NPV; and the best case results in a very large, positive NPV. These results can now be used to determine the expected NPV and standard deviation of NPV. For this, an estimate is needed of the probabilities of occurrence of the three scenarios. Suppose that Bayside's managers estimate that there is a 20 percent chance of the worst case occurring, a 60 percent chance of the most likely case, and a 20 percent chance of the best case. Of course, it is very difficult to estimate scenario probabilities with any confidence.

Table 15.3 contains a discrete distribution of returns, so the expected NPV can be found as follows:

$$\text{Expected NPV} = (0.20 \times [-\$819,844]) + (0.60 \times \$82,493) + (0.20 \times \$984,829)$$

$$= \$82,493.$$

The expected NPV in the scenario analysis is the same as the base case NPV, $82,493. The consistency of results occurs because the values of the uncertain variables used in the scenario analysis—30, 40, and 50 scans for volume and $500,000, $750,000, and $1,000,000 for salvage value—when coupled with the scenario probabilities produce the same expected values that were used in the Table 15.1 base case analysis. If inconsistencies exist between the base case NPV and the expected NPV in the scenario analysis, the two analyses have inconsistent input value assumptions.

Using the distribution of NPVs, we can calculate the standard deviation:

$$\sigma_{\text{NPV}} = [0.20 \times (-\$819,844 - \$82,493)^2 + 0.60 \times (\$82,493 - \$82,493)^2$$

$$+ 0.20 \times (\$984,829 - \$82,493)^2]^{1/2}$$

$$= \$570,688.$$

The standard deviation of NPV measures the MRI project's stand-alone risk. Bayside's managers can compare the standard deviation of NPV of this project with the uncertainty inherent in Bayside's aggregate cash flows, or average project. Often, the coefficient of variation (CV) is used to measure the stand-alone risk of a project: $\text{CV} = \sigma_{\text{NPV}} / \text{E(NPV)} = \$570,688 / \$82,493 = 6.9$ for the MRI project. The CV measures the risk per unit of return and hence is a better measure of comparative risk than the standard deviation, especially when projects have widely differing NPVs. If Bayside's average project has

Scenario	Probability of Outcome	Volume	Salvage Value	NPV
Worst case	0.20	30	$ 500,000	($819,844)
Most likely case	0.60	40	750,000	82,493
Best case	0.20	50	1,000,000	984,829
Expected value		40	$ 750,000	$ 82,493
Standard deviation				$570,688

TABLE 15.3
MRI Project
Scenario Analysis

a CV of 4.0, the MRI project would be judged to be riskier than the firm's average project, so it would be classified as having above-average risk. (We used NPV as the ROI measure is this scenario analysis, but we could have focused on either IRR or MIRR.)

Scenario analysis can also be interpreted in a less mathematical way. The worst case NPV, a loss of about $800,000 for the MRI project, represents an estimate of the worst possible financial consequences of the project. If Bayside can absorb such a loss in value without much impact on its financial condition, the project does not represent a significant financial danger to the hospital. Conversely, if such a loss would mean financial ruin for the hospital, its managers might be unwilling to undertake the project, regardless of its profitability under the most likely and best case scenarios. Note that the risk of the project is **not** changing in these two situations. The difference is in the ability of the organization to **bear** the risk inherent in the project.

While scenario analysis provides useful information about a project's stand-alone risk, it is limited in two ways. First, it only considers a few states of the economy and hence provides information on only a few potential profitability outcomes for the project. In reality, an almost infinite number of possibilities exist. Although the illustrative scenario analysis contained only three scenarios, it could be expanded to include more states of the economy— say, five or seven. However, there is a practical limit to how many scenarios can be included in a scenario analysis.

Second, scenario analysis, at least as normally conducted, implies a very definite relationship among the uncertain variables; that is, the analysis assumed that the worst value for volume (30 scans per week) would occur at the same time as the worst value for salvage value ($500,000) because the worst case scenario was defined by combining the worst possible value of each uncertain variable. Although this relationship (all worst values occurring together) may hold in some situations, it may not hold in others. For example, if volume is low, maybe the MRI will have less wear and tear and hence be worth more after five years of use. The worst value for volume, then, should be coupled with the best salvage value. Conversely, poor volume may be symptomatic of poor medical effectiveness of the MRI and hence lead to limited demand for used equipment and a low salvage value. Scenario analysis tends to create extreme profitability values for the worst and best cases because it automatically combines all worst and best input values, even if these values actually have only a remote chance of occurring together.[5]

A **word of warning** regarding the relationship between profitability and risk analyses is in order here. When conducting a scenario analysis, it is natural to consider both the resulting profitability (NPV in the illustration) and risk. However, it is possible for inconsistencies in the input variable assumptions to cause the expected NPV from the scenario analysis to differ from the base case NPV. A scenario analysis is conducted for the **sole purpose of assessing a project's stand-alone risk**. A scenario analysis is **not** conducted to estimate a project's profitability. Thus, once the risk determination has been made (for example, the MRI project was judged to have high risk), the scenario analysis plays no further role in the project evaluation. As we will discuss in a later section, the project risk determination feeds back into the base case analysis to make the final judgment regarding the project's financial worthiness.

Self-Test Questions	1. Briefly describe scenario analysis.
	2. What type of risk does it attempt to measure?
	3. What are its strengths and weaknesses?

Qualitative Risk Assessment

In some situations, perhaps in many, it is very difficult to conduct a quantitative risk assessment—the numbers are just too difficult to predict. In such situations, rather than ignore differential risk, some healthcare businesses use a more subjective approach. For example, one large healthcare clinic uses the following questions to qualitatively assess project risk.

- Does the project require additional market share or represent a new service initiative?
- Is the project outside of the scope of current management expertise?
- Does the project require technical specialists, who will be difficult to recruit?
- Will the project place us in competition with a strong competitor?
- Does the project require the use of new, unproven technology?

To assess project risk, each yes answer is assigned one point. If the project has zero points, it is judged to have below-average risk. If it has one or two points, it is judged to have average risk, while a score of three or more points indicates above-average risk.

Although such a subjective approach initially appears to have little theoretical foundation, a closer examination reveals that each question in the above list is tied to cash flow uncertainty. Thus, the greater the number of "yes" answers, the greater the cash flow uncertainty and hence the greater the stand-alone risk of the project.

Even when a quantitative risk assessment is feasible, a separate qualitative assessment is a good idea. The value of using the qualitative risk assessment approach in conjunction with a quantitative risk assessment is that it forces managers to think about project risk in alternative frameworks. If the quantitative and qualitative assessments do not agree, then it is clear that the project's risk assessment requires more consideration.

After some discussion, Bayside's managers concluded that the MRI project's qualitative risk assessment score was 3. Thus, both the quantitative and the qualitative assessments reached the same conclusion: the project has above-average risk.

1. Describe qualitative risk assessment.
2. Why does it work?
3. Assume a quantitative risk assessment has been conducted on a project. Is a qualitative risk assessment necessary?

Self-Test Questions

Incorporating Risk into the Decision Process

Thus far, the MRI illustration has demonstrated that it is difficult to quantify a project's riskiness. It may be possible to reach the general conclusion that one project is more or less risky than another or to compare the riskiness of a project with the firm as a whole, but it is difficult to develop a good measure of project risk. This lack of precision in measuring project risk adds to the difficulties involved in incorporating differential risk into the capital budgeting decision.

There are two methods for incorporating project risk into the capital budgeting decision process: (1) the certainty equivalent method, in which a project's expected cash flows are adjusted to reflect project risk, and (2) the risk-adjusted discount rate method, in which differential risk is dealt with by changing the cost of capital. Although the risk-adjusted discount rate method is used by most businesses, the certainty equivalent method does have some theoretical advantages. Furthermore, it raises some interesting issues related to the risk-adjustment process.

The Certainty Equivalent Method

The *certainty equivalent (CE) method* follows directly from the economic concept of *utility*.[6] Under the CE approach, managers must first evaluate a cash flow's risk, and then specify how much money, with certainty, would be required to be indifferent between the riskless (certain) sum and the risky cash flow's expected value. To illustrate, suppose that a rich eccentric offered someone the following two choices:

1. **Flip a coin.** If it's a head, the individual wins $1 million; if it's a tail, he or she gets nothing. The expected value of the gamble is $(0.5 \times \$1,000,000) + (0.5 \times \$0) = \$500,000$, but the actual outcome will be either zero or $1 million, so the gamble is quite risky.
2. **Do not flip the coin.** Simply pocket $400,000 in cash.

If the individual is indifferent to the two alternatives, $400,000 is defined to be his or her *certainty equivalent* because the riskless $400,000 provides that individual with the same satisfaction (utility) as the risky $500,000 expected return. In general, investors are risk averse, so the certainty equivalent amount for this gamble will be something less than the $500,000 expected value. But each individual would have his or her own certainty equivalent value— the greater the individual's degree of risk aversion, the lower the certainty equivalent amount.

The CE concept can be applied to capital budgeting decisions, at least in theory, in this way:

- Convert each net cash flow of a project to its certainty equivalent value. Here, the riskiness of **each cash flow** is assessed, and a certainty equivalent cash flow is chosen on the basis of that risk. The greater the risk, the greater the difference between the cash flow's expected value and its lower certainty equivalent value. (If a cash outflow is being adjusted, the certainty equivalent value is higher than the expected value. The unique risk adjustments required on cash outflows will be discussed in a later section.)
- Once each cash flow is expressed as a certainty equivalent, discount the project's certainty equivalent cash flow stream by the **risk-free rate** to obtain the project's *differential risk-adjusted* NPV.[7] Here, the term "differential risk-adjusted" implies that the unique riskiness of the project, as compared to the overall riskiness of the business, has been incorporated into the decision process. The risk-free rate is used as the discount rate because certainty equivalent cash flows are analogous to risk-free cash flows.
- A positive differential risk-adjusted NPV indicates that the project is profitable even after adjusting for differential project risk.

The CE method is simple and neat. Furthermore, it can easily handle differential risk among the **individual** net cash flows. For example, the final year's certainty equivalent cash flow might be adjusted downward an additional amount to account for salvage value risk if that risk is considered to be greater than the risk inherent in the operating cash flows.

Unfortunately, there is no practical way to estimate a risky cash flow's certainty equivalent value. There is no benchmark available to help make the estimate, so each individual would have his or her own estimate, and these could vary significantly. Also, the risk assessment techniques—for example, scenario analysis—focus on profitability and hence measure the stand-alone risk of a project in its entirety. This process provides no information about the riskiness of individual cash flows, so there is no basis for adjusting each cash flow for its own unique risk.

The Risk-Adjusted Discount Rate Method

In the *risk-adjusted discount rate (RADR) method*, expected cash flows are used in the valuation process, and the risk adjustment is made to the discount rate (the opportunity cost of capital). All average-risk projects are discounted at the firm's corporate cost of capital, which represents the opportunity cost of capital for average-risk projects; high-risk projects are assigned a higher cost of capital; and low-risk projects are discounted at a lower cost of capital.

One advantage of the RADR method is that the process has a starting benchmark—the firm's corporate cost of capital. This discount rate reflects the riskiness of the business in the aggregate, or the riskiness of the firm's average project. Another advantage is that project risk assessment techniques identify a project's aggregate risk—the combined risk of all of the cash flows—and the RADR applies a single adjustment to the cost of capital rather than attempting to adjust individual cash flows. However, the disadvantage is that there typically is no theoretical basis for setting the size of the RADR adjustment, so the amount of adjustment remains a matter of judgment.

The RADR method has one additional disadvantage. It combines the factors that account for time value (the risk-free rate) and the adjustment for risk (the risk premium): Project cost of capital = Differential risk-adjusted discount rate = Risk-free rate + Risk premium. The CE approach, on the other hand, keeps risk adjustment and time value separate: time value is accounted for in the discount rate and risk is accounted for in the cash flows. By lumping together risk and time value, the RADR method compounds the risk premium over time—just as interest compounds over time, so does the risk premium. This compounding of the risk premium means that the RADR method automatically assigns more risk to cash flows that occur in the distant future, and the farther into the future, the greater the implied risk. Because the CE method assigns risk to each cash flow individually, it does not impose any assumptions regarding the relationship between risk and time.

The RADR method, with a constant discount rate applied to all cash flows of a project, implies that risk increases with time. This imposes a greater burden on long-term projects, so all else the same, short-term projects will tend to look better financially than long-term projects. For most projects, the assumption of increasing risk over time is probably reasonable because cash flows are more difficult to forecast the farther one moves into the future. However, managers should be aware that the RADR approach automatically penalizes distant cash flows, and an additional explicit penalty based solely on cash flow timing is probably not warranted unless some specific additional source of risk can be identified.

Making the Final Decision

In most project risk analyses, it is impossible to assess quantitatively the project's corporate or market risk, so managers are left with only an assessment of the project's stand-alone risk. However, like Bayside's MRI project, most projects being evaluated are in the same line of business as the firm's other projects. Furthermore, the profitability of most businesses is driven by the national economy. Thus, stand-alone, corporate, and market risk are usually highly correlated. This suggests that managers can get a feel for the relative risk of most projects on the basis of the scenario analysis conducted to assess the project's stand-alone risk. In Bayside's case, its managers concluded that the MRI project has above-average risk, and hence the project was categorized as a high-risk project.

The business's corporate cost of capital provides the basis for estimating a project's differential risk-adjusted discount rate—average-risk projects are discounted at the corporate cost of capital, above-average-risk projects are discounted at a higher cost of capital, and below-average-risk projects are discounted at a rate less than the corporate cost of capital. Unfortunately, there is no good way of specifying exactly how much higher or lower these discount rates should be. Given the present state of the art, risk adjustments are necessarily judgmental and somewhat arbitrary.

Bayside's standard procedure is to add 4 percentage points to its 10 percent corporate cost of capital when evaluating higher-risk projects, and to subtract 2 percentage points when evaluating lower-risk projects. Thus, to estimate the above-average-risk MRI project's differential risk-adjusted NPV, the project's expected (base case) cash flows shown in Table 15.1 are discounted at 10% + 4% = 14%. This rate is called the *project cost of capital*, as opposed to the corporate cost of capital, because it reflects the risk characteristics of a specific project rather than the aggregate risk characteristics of the business (or average project). The resultant NPV is -$200,017, so the project becomes unprofitable when the analysis is adjusted to reflect its high risk. Bayside's managers may still decide to go ahead with the MRI project for other reasons, but at least they know that its expected profitability is not sufficient to make up for its riskiness.

1. How do most firms incorporate differential risk into the capital budgeting decision process?
2. Is the risk adjustment objective or subjective?
3. What is a *project cost of capital*?

Self-Test Questions

Adjusting Cash Outflows for Risk

Some projects are evaluated on the basis of minimizing the present value of future costs rather than on the basis of the project's NPV. This is done because it is often impossible to allocate revenues to a particular project, and it is easier to focus on comparative costs when two projects will produce the same revenue stream. For example, suppose that Bayside Memorial Hospital must choose one of two ways for disposing of its medical wastes. There is no question about the need for the project, and the hospital's revenue stream is unaffected by which method is chosen. In this case, the decision will be based on the present value of expected future costs—the method with the lower present value of costs will be chosen.

Table 15.4 contains the projected annual costs associated with each method. The in-house system would require a large expenditure at Year 0 to upgrade the hospital's current disposal system, but the yearly operating costs are relatively low. Conversely, if Bayside contracts for disposal services with an outside contractor, it will have to pay only $25,000 up-front to initiate the contract. However, the annual contract fee would be $200,000 a year.[8]

If both methods were judged to have average risk, then Bayside's corporate cost of capital, 10 percent, would be applied to the cash flows to obtain the present value (PV) of costs for each method. Because the PVs of costs for the two waste disposal systems ($784,309 for the in-house system and $783,157 for the contract method) are roughly equal, on the basis solely

Year	In-House System	Outside Contract
0	($500,000)	($ 25,000)
1	(75,000)	(200,000)
2	(75,000)	(200,000)
3	(75,000)	(200,000)
4	(75,000)	(200,000)
5	(75,000)	(200,000)
Present Value of Costs at a Discount Rate of:		
10%	($784,309)	($783,157)
14%	—	($711,616)
6%	—	($867,473)

TABLE 15.4 Bayside Memorial Hospital: Waste Disposal Analysis

of financial considerations, Bayside's managers are indifferent as to which method should be chosen.

However, Bayside's managers believe that the contract method is much riskier than the in-house method. The cost of modifying the current system is known almost to the dollar, and operating costs can be predicted fairly well. Furthermore, with the in-house system, operating costs are under the control of Bayside's management. Conversely, if Bayside relies on the contractor for waste disposal, the hospital is more or less stuck with continuing the contract because it will not have the in-house capability. Because the contractor was only willing to guarantee the price for one year, perhaps the bid was low-balled, and large price increases will occur in future years. The two methods have about the same PV of costs when both are considered to have average risk, so which method should be chosen if the contract method is judged to have higher risk? Clearly, if the costs are the same under a common discount rate, the lower-risk in-house project should be chosen.

Now, try to incorporate this intuitive differential risk conclusion into the quantitative analysis. Conventional wisdom is to increase the corporate cost of capital for higher-risk projects, so the contract cash flows would be discounted using a project cost of capital of 14 percent, which is the rate that Bayside applies to above-average-risk projects. But at a 14 percent discount rate, the contract method has a PV of costs of only $711,616, which is about $70,000 lower than that for the in-house method. If the discount rate was increased to 20 percent on the contract method, it would appear to be $161,000 cheaper than the in-house method. Thus, the riskier the contract method is judged to be, the better it looks.

Something is obviously wrong here. To penalize a cash outflow for higher-than-average risk, that outflow must have a *higher* present value, not a **lower** one. Therefore, a cash outflow that has higher-than-average risk must be evaluated with a lower-than-average cost of capital. Recognizing this, Bayside's managers actually applied a $10\% - 4\% = 6\%$ discount rate to the high-risk contract method's cash flows. This produces a PV of costs for the contract method of $867,473, which is about $83,000 more than the PV of costs for the average-risk in-house method.

The appropriate risk adjustment for cash outflows is also applicable to other situations. For example, the City of Detroit offered Ann Arbor Health Systems the opportunity to use a city-owned building in one of the city's blighted areas for a walk-in clinic. The city offered to pay to refurbish the building, and all profits made by the clinic would accrue to Ann Arbor. However, after ten years, Ann Arbor would have to buy the building from the city at the then-current market value. The market value estimate that Ann Arbor used in its analysis was $1,000,000, but the realized cost could be much greater, or much less, depending on the economic condition of the neighborhood at that time. The project's other cash flows were of average risk, but this single outflow had higher risk, so Ann Arbor lowered the discount rate that it applied to this one cash flow. This action created a higher present value on a cost (outflow) and hence lowered the project's NPV.

The bottom line here is that the risk adjustment for cash outflows is the opposite of the adjustment for cash inflows. When cash outflows are being evaluated, higher risk leads to a lower discount rate.

1. Why are some projects evaluated on the basis of present value of costs?
2. Is there any difference between the risk adjustments applied to cash inflows and cash outflows? Explain your answer.
3. Can differential risk adjustments be made to single cash flows or must the same adjustment be made to all of a project's cash flows?

Self-Test Questions

Divisional Costs of Capital

In theory, project costs of capital should reflect both a project's differential risk and its differential *debt capacity*. The logic here is that if a project's optimal financing mix is significantly different from the business in the aggregate, then the weights used in estimating the corporate cost of capital do not reflect the weights appropriate to the project. Because of the difficulties encountered in estimating a project's debt capacity (its optimal capital structure), such adjustments are rarely made in practice.

Even though it is not common to make capital structure adjustments for individual projects, firms often make both capital structure and risk adjustments when developing divisional costs of capital. To illustrate, a for-profit healthcare system might have one division that invests primarily in real estate for medical uses and another division that runs an HMO. Clearly, each division has its own unique business risk and optimal capital structure. The low-risk, high debt capacity real estate division could have a cost of capital of 10 percent, while the high-risk, low debt capacity HMO division could have a cost of capital of 14 percent. The health system itself, which consists of 50 percent real estate assets and 50 percent HMO assets, would have a corporate cost of capital of 12 percent.

If all capital budgeting decisions within the system were made on the basis of the overall system's 12 percent cost of capital, the process would be biased in favor of the higher-risk HMO division. The cost of capital would be too low for the HMO division and too high for the real estate division. Over time, this cost of capital bias would result in too many HMO projects being accepted and too few real estate projects, which would skew the business line mix toward HMO assets and hence increase the overall riskiness of the firm. The solution to the cost of capital bias problem is to use *divisional costs of capital*, rather than the overall corporate cost of capital, in the capital budgeting decision process.

Unlike individual project costs of capital, divisional costs of capital often can be estimated with some confidence because it is usually possible to identify publicly traded firms that are predominantly in the same line of business as the subsidiary. For example, the cost of capital for the HMO division could be estimated by looking at the debt and equity costs and capital structures of the major for-profit HMOs such as Humana and UnitedHealth Group. With such market data at hand, it is relatively easy to develop divisional costs of capital. As a final check, the weighted average of the divisional costs of capital should equal the firm's corporate cost of capital.

Self-Test Questions

1. In theory, should project cost of capital estimates include capital structure effects?
2. Should all divisions of a firm use the firm's corporate cost of capital as the benchmark rate in making capital budgeting decisions?
3. How might a business go about estimating its divisional costs of capital?

An Overview of the Capital Budgeting Decision Process

Our discussion of capital budgeting thus far has focused on how managers evaluate individual projects. For capital planning purposes, health services managers also need to forecast the total number of projects that will be undertaken and the dollar amount of capital needed to fund the projects. The list of projects to be undertaken is called the *capital budget*, and the optimal selection of new projects is called the *optimal capital budget*.

While every healthcare provider estimates its optimal capital budget in its own unique way, some procedures are common to all firms. The procedures followed by Seattle Health System are used to illustrate the process:

- The chief financial officer (CFO) estimates the system's corporate cost of capital. As discussed in Chapter 13, this estimate depends on market conditions, the business risk of the system's assets in the aggregate, and its optimal capital structure.
- The CFO then scales the corporate cost of capital up or down to reflect the unique risk and capital structure features of each division. To illustrate, assume that the system has three divisions. For simplicity, the divisions are identified as LRD, ARD, and HRD, which stand for low-risk, average-risk, and high-risk divisions.
- Managers within each of the divisions evaluate the riskiness of the proposed projects within their divisions, categorizing each project as having low risk (LRP), average risk (ARP), or high risk (HRP). These project risk classifications are based on the riskiness of each project relative to the **other projects in the division**, not to the system in the aggregate.
- Each project is then assigned a project cost of capital that is based on the **divisional cost of capital** and the project's relative riskiness within that

division. As discussed previously, this *project cost of capital* is then used to discount the project's expected net cash flows. From a financial standpoint, all projects with positive NPVs are acceptable, while those with negative NPVs should be rejected. Subjective factors are also considered, and these factors may result in an optimal capital budget that differs from the one established solely on the basis of financial considerations.

Figure 15.2 summarizes Seattle Health System's overall capital budgeting process. It uses the same adjustment amounts as does Bayside: 4 percentage points for high risk and 2 percentage points for low risk. Thus, the corporate cost of capital is adjusted upward to 14 percent in the high-risk division and downward to 8 percent in the low-risk division. The same adjustment—4 percentage points upward for high-risk projects and 2 percentage points downward for low-risk projects—is applied to differential risk projects within each division. The end result is a range of project costs of capital within the system that runs from 18 percent for high-risk projects in the high-risk division to 6 percent for low-risk projects in the low-risk division.

This process creates a capital budget that incorporates each project's debt capacity (at least at the divisional level) and riskiness. However, managers also must consider other possible risk factors that may not have been included in the quantitative analysis. For example, could a project under consideration significantly increase the system's liability exposure? Conversely, does the

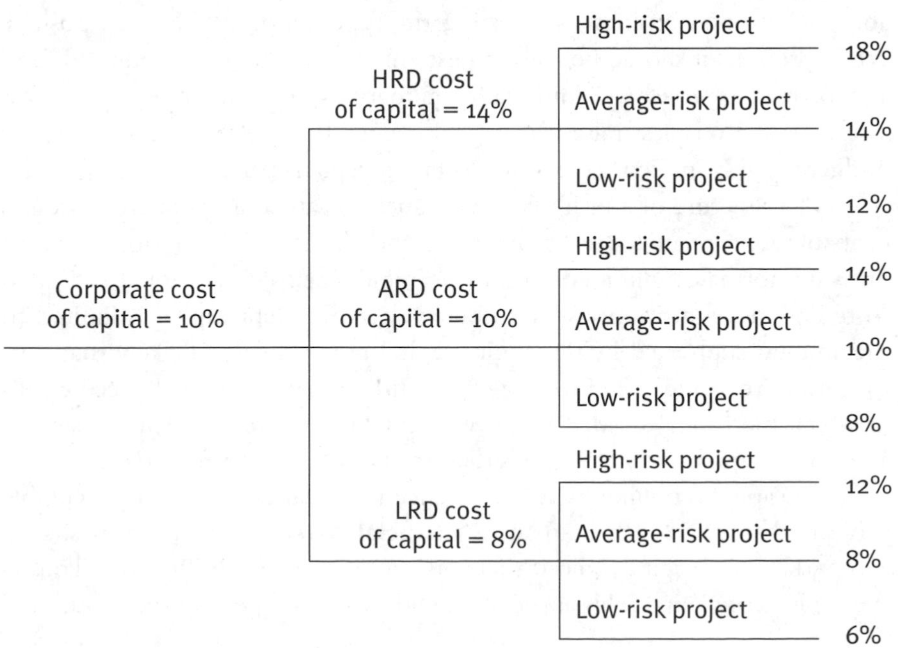

FIGURE 15.2
Seattle Health System: Project Costs of Capital

project have any strategic value or social value or other attributes that could affect its profitability? Such additional factors must be considered, at least subjectively, before a final decision can be made. Typically, if the project involves new products or services and is large (in capital requirements) relative to the size of the firm's average project, then the additional subjective factors will be very important to the final decision; one large mistake can bankrupt a firm, and "bet the company" decisions are not made lightly. On the other hand, the decision on a small replacement project would be made mostly on the basis of numerical analysis.

Ultimately, capital budgeting decisions require an analysis of a mix of objective and subjective factors such as risk, debt capacity, profitability, medical staff needs, and social value. The process is not precise, and often there is a temptation to ignore one or more important factors because they are so nebulous and difficult to measure. Despite the imprecision and subjectivity, a project's risk, as well as its other attributes, should be assessed and incorporated into the capital budgeting decision process.

Self-Test Questions	1. Describe a typical capital budgeting decision process.
	2. Are decisions made solely on the basis of quantitative factors? Explain your answer.

Capital Rationing

Standard capital budgeting procedures assume that businesses can raise virtually unlimited amounts of capital to meet capital budgeting needs. Presumably, as long as a business is investing the funds in profitable (i.e., positive NPV) projects, it should be able to raise the debt and equity needed to fund all worthwhile projects. Additionally, standard capital budgeting procedures assume that a business raises the capital needed to finance its optimal capital budget roughly in accordance with its target capital structure.

This picture of a firm's capital financing/capital investment process is probably appropriate for most investor-owned firms. However, not-for-profit firms do not have unlimited access to capital. Their equity capital is limited to retentions, contributions, and grants, and their debt capital is limited to the amount supported by the equity capital base. Thus, it is likely that not-for-profit firms, and even investor-owned firms on occasion, will face periods in which the capital needed for investment in new projects will exceed the amount of capital available. This situation is called *capital rationing*.

If capital rationing exists, and hence the business has more acceptable projects than capital, then, **from a financial perspective**, the firm should accept that set of capital projects that maximizes aggregate NPV and still meets the capital constraint. This approach could be called "getting the most bang for the buck" because it picks those projects that have the most positive impact on the firm's financial condition.

Another ROI measure, the *profitability index (PI)*, is useful under capital rationing. The PI is defined as the present value (PV) of cash inflows divided by the PV of cash outflows. Thus, for Bayside's MRI project discussed earlier in the chapter, PI = $2,582,493 / $2,500,000 = 1.03. The PI measures a project's dollars of profitability per dollar of investment, all on a present value basis. In other words, it measures the "bang for the buck." The MRI project promises three cents of profit for every dollar invested, which indicates it is not very profitable. (The PI of 1.03 is before adjusting for risk. After adjusting for risk, the project's PI is less than 1.00, indicating that the project is unprofitable.) Under capital rationing, the optimal capital budget is determined by first listing all profitable projects in descending order of PI. Then, projects are selected from the top of the list downward until the available capital is used up.

Of course, in healthcare businesses, priority may be assigned to some low or even negative NPV projects, which is fine as long as these projects are offset by the selection of profitable projects that prevent the low-profitability priority projects from eroding the business's financial condition.

Self-Test Questions

1. What is capital rationing?
2. From a financial perspective, how are projects chosen when capital rationing exists?
3. What is the profitability index, and why is it useful under capital rationing?

Key Concepts

This chapter, which continued the discussion of capital budgeting started in Chapter 14, focused on risk assessment and incorporation. The key concepts of this chapter are as follows:

- Three separate and distinct types of *project risk* can be identified and defined: (1) stand-alone risk, (2) corporate risk, and (3) market risk.
- A project's *stand-alone risk* is the relevant risk if the project were the sole project of a not-for-profit firm. It is a function of the project's profit uncertainty and is generally measured by the *standard deviation* of NPV. Stand-alone risk is often used as a proxy for both corporate and market risk because (1) corporate and market risk are often impossible to measure and (2) the three types of risk are usually highly correlated.
- *Corporate risk* reflects the contribution of a project to the overall riskiness of the business. Corporate risk ignores stockholder diversification, so it is the relevant risk for most not-for-profit firms.

- *Market risk* reflects the contribution of a project to the overall riskiness of stockholders' well-diversified portfolios. In theory, market risk is the relevant risk for investor-owned firms, but many people argue that corporate risk is also relevant to stockholders, and it is certainly relevant to a firm's other stakeholders.
- Two techniques are commonly used to *assess* a project's stand-alone risk: (1) sensitivity analysis and (2) scenario analysis.
- *Sensitivity analysis* shows how much a project's profitability—for example, as measured by NPV—changes in response to a given change in an input variable such as volume, with other things held constant.
- *Scenario analysis* defines a project's best, most likely, and worst cases and then uses these data to measure its stand-alone risk.
- In many situations, it is impractical to conduct a quantitative project risk assessment. In such situations, many healthcare businesses use a *qualitative approach* to risk assessment.
- Projects are generally classified as high risk, average risk, or low risk on the basis of their stand-alone risk assessment. High-risk projects are evaluated at a *project cost of capital* that is greater than the firm's corporate cost of capital. Average-risk projects are evaluated at the firm's corporate cost of capital, while low-risk projects are evaluated at a rate less than the corporate cost of capital.
- If a large organization has several divisions that operate in different business lines, it is best to estimate and use *divisional costs of capital* as the starting point in a project analysis.
- When evaluating *risky cash outflows*, the risk adjustment process is reversed—that is, lower rates are used to discount more risky cash flows.
- *Capital rationing* occurs when a business does not have access to sufficient capital to fund all profitable projects, so the best financial outcome results from accepting the set of projects that has the highest aggregate NPV. In such situations, the profitability index (PI) is a useful profitability (ROI) measure.
- Ultimately, capital budgeting decisions require an analysis of a mix of objective and subjective factors such as risk, debt capacity, profitability, medical staff needs, and service to the community. The process is not precise, but good managers do their best to ensure that none of the relevant factors are ignored.

This chapter concludes our discussion of capital investment decisions. The next chapter examines current asset management and financing.

Questions

15.1 a. Why is risk analysis so important to the capital budgeting process?

b. Describe the three types of project risk. Under what situation is each of the types most relevant to the capital budgeting decision?

c. Which type of risk is easiest to measure in practice?

d. Are the three types of project risk usually highly correlated? Explain your answer.

e. Why is the correlation among project risk measures important?

15.2 a. Briefly describe sensitivity analysis.

b. What are its strengths and weaknesses?

15.3 a. Briefly describe scenario analysis.

b. What are its strengths and weaknesses?

15.4 a. How is project risk incorporated into a capital budgeting analysis?

b. Suppose that two mutually exclusive projects are being evaluated on the basis of cash costs. How would risk adjustments be applied in this situation?

15.5 What is the difference between the corporate cost of capital and a project cost of capital?

15.6 What is meant by the term *capital rationing*? From a purely financial standpoint, what is the optimal capital budget under capital rationing?

15.7 Santa Roberta Clinic has estimated its corporate cost of capital to be 11 percent. What are reasonable values for the project costs of capital for low risk, average risk, and high-risk projects?

15.8 Under what conditions should a business estimate divisional costs of capital?

15.9 Describe the qualitative approach to risk assessment. Why does this approach, which does not rely on numerical data, work?

Problems

15.1 The managers of Merton Medical Clinic are analyzing a proposed project. The project's most likely NPV is $120,000, but as evidenced by the following NPV distribution, there is considerable risk involved:

Probability	NPV
0.05	($700,000)
0.20	(250,000)
0.50	120,000
0.20	200,000
0.05	300,000

a. What are the project's expected NPV and standard deviation of NPV?

b. Should the base case analysis use the most likely NPV or the expected NPV? Explain your answer.

15.2 Heywood Diagnostic Enterprises is evaluating a project with the following net cash flows and probabilities:

Year	Prob = 0.2	Prob = 0.6	Prob = 0.2
0	($100,000)	($100,000)	($100,000)
1	20,000	30,000	40,000
2	20,000	30,000	40,000
3	20,000	30,000	40,000
4	20,000	30,000	40,000
5	30,000	40,000	50,000

The Year 5 values include salvage value. Heywood's corporate cost of capital is 10 percent.

a. What is the project's expected (i.e., base case) NPV assuming average risk? (Hint: The base case net cash flows are the expected cash flows in each year.)

b. What are the project's most likely, worst, and best case NPVs?

c. What is the project's expected NPV on the basis of the scenario analysis?

d. What is the project's standard deviation of NPV?

e. Assume that Heywood's managers judge the project to have lower-than-average risk. Furthermore, the company's policy is to adjust the corporate cost of capital up or down by 3 percentage points to account for differential risk. Is the project financially attractive?

15.3 Consider the project contained in Problem 14.7 in Chapter 14.

a. Perform a sensitivity analysis to see how NPV is affected by changes in the number of procedures per day, average collection amount, and salvage value.

b. Conduct a scenario analysis. Suppose that the hospital's staff concluded that the three most uncertain variables were number of procedures per day, average collection amount, and the equipment's salvage value. Furthermore, the following data were developed:

Scenario	Probability	Number of Procedures	Average Collection	Equipment Salvage Value
Worst	0.25	10	$ 60	$100,000
Most likely	0.50	15	80	200,000
Best	0.25	20	100	300,000

c. Finally, assume that California Health Center's average project has a coefficient of variation of NPV in the range of 1.0–2.0. (Hint: The coefficient of variation is defined as the standard deviation of NPV divided by the expected NPV.) The hospital adjusts for risk by adding or subtracting 3 percentage points to its 10 percent

corporate cost of capital. After adjusting for differential risk, is the
project still profitable?

d. What type of risk was measured and accounted for in Parts b and c?
Should this be of concern to the hospital's managers?

15.4 The managers of United Medtronics are evaluating the following four
projects for the coming budget period. The firm's corporate cost of
capital is 14 percent.

Project	Cost	IRR
A	$15,000	17%
B	15,000	16
C	12,000	15
D	20,000	13

a. What is the firm's optimal capital budget?

b. Now, suppose Medtronics's managers want to consider differential
risk in the capital budgeting process. Project A has average risk, B
has below-average risk, C has above-average risk, and D has average
risk. What is the firm's optimal capital budget when differential
risk is considered? (Hint: The firm's managers **lower** the IRR of
high-risk projects by 3 percentage points and **raise** the IRR of
low-risk projects by the same amount.)

15.5 Allied Managed Care Company is evaluating two different computer
systems for handling provider claims. There are no incremental
revenues attached to the projects, so the decision will be made on the
basis of the present value of costs. Allied's corporate cost of capital is 10
percent. Here are the net cash flow estimates in thousands of dollars:

Year	System X	System Y
0	($500)	($1,000)
1	(500)	(300)
2	(500)	(300)
3	(500)	(300)

a. Assume initially that the systems both have average risk. Which one
should be chosen?

b. Assume that System X is judged to have high risk. Allied accounts
for differential risk by adjusting its corporate cost of capital up or
down by 2 percentage points. Which system should be chosen?

15.6 University Health System has three divisions: Real Estate, with an
8 percent cost of capital; Health Services, with a 10 percent cost of
capital; and Managed Care, with a 12 percent cost of capital. The
system's risk adjustment procedures call for adding 3 percentage points
to adjust for high risk and subtracting 2 percentage points for low risk.
Construct a diagram such as the one in Figure 15.2 that illustrates the
range of project costs of capital for the system.

Notes

1. The three types of risk relevant to capital budgeting decisions were first discussed in Chapter 10. A review of the applicable sections might be useful for some readers.
2. For an algebraic representation of the relationships among stand-alone, corporate, and market risk, see Louis C. Gapenski, "Project Risk Definition and Measurement in a Not-For-Profit Setting," *Health Services Management Research* (November 1992): 216–224.
3. Two other methods, *decision tree analysis* and *Monte Carlo simulation*, also are used to assess project risk. Decision tree analysis is particularly useful when a project is structured with a series of decision points (i.e., stages) that allow cancellation prior to full implementation. For more information on both methods, see Louis C. Gapenski, *Understanding Health Care Financial Management* (Chicago: Health Administration Press, 2007), Chapter 12.
4. Spreadsheet programs have Data Table functions that automatically perform sensitivity analyses. After the table is roughed in, the spreadsheet automatically calculates and records the NPV (or some other profitability measure) values in the appropriate locations on the table.
5. *Monte Carlo* simulation overcomes the deficiencies inherent in scenario analysis, but it has some deficiencies of its own.
6. *Utility theory* is used by economists to explain how individuals make choices among risky alternatives.
7. The risk-free rate does **not** incorporate the tax advantages of debt financing, so it must be adjusted by using the corporate cost of capital equation.
8. For the sake of simplicity, inflation effects are ignored in this illustration.

References

Allen, R. J. 1989. "Proper Planning Reduces Risk in New Technology Acquisitions." *Healthcare Financial Management* (December): 48–56.

Ang, J. S., and W. G. Lewellen. 1982. "Risk Adjustment in Capital Investment Project Evaluations." *Financial Management* (Summer): 5–14.

Capettini, R., C. W. Chow, and J. E. Williamson. 1990. "Breakdown Approach Helps Managers Select Projects." *Healthcare Financial Management* (November): 48–56.

Gapenski, L. C. 1992. "Accuracy of Investment Risk Models Varies." *Healthcare Financial Management* (April): 40–52.

———. 1992. "Project Risk Definition and Measurement in a Not-for-Profit Setting." *Health Services Management Research* (November): 216–224.

———. 1990. "Using Monte Carlo Simulation to Help Make Better Capital Investment Decisions." *Hospital & Health Services Administration* (Summer): 207–219.

Gup, B. E., and S. W. Norwood, III. 1981. "Divisional Cost of Capital: A Practical Approach." *Financial Management* (Spring): 20–24.

Hastie, K. L. 1974. "One Businessman's View of Capital Budgeting." *Financial Management* (Winter): 36–43.

Hertz, D. B. 1964. "Risk Analysis in Capital Investments." *Harvard Business Review* (January-February): 96–106.

Holmes, R. L., R. E. Schroeder, and L. F. Harrington. 1999. "Using Microcomputers to Improve Capital Decision Making." *Journal of Health Care Financing* (Spring): 52–59.

———. 2000. "Objective Risk Adjustment Improves Calculated ROI for Capital Projects." *Healthcare Financial Management* (December): 49–52.

Lewellen, W. G., and M. S. Long. 1972. "Simulation Versus Single-Value Estimates in Capital Expenditure Analysis." *Decision Sciences* (October): 19–33.

Ryan, J. B., and J. L. Gocke. 1988. "Incorporating Risk Into the Investment Decision." *Topics in Health Care Financing* (Fall): 49–65.

Ryan, J. B., and M. E. Ward (eds). 1992. "Capital Management." *Topics in Health Care Financing* (Fall): 1–88.

Weaver, S. C., P. J. Clemmens, III, J. A. Gunn, and B. D. Danneburg. 1989. "Divisional Hurdle Rates and the Cost of Capital." *Financial Management* (Spring): 18–25.

Other Topics

Up to this point, the financial management chapters have primarily focused on long-term, or strategic, management decisions. In Part VII, we move first to more immediate, short-term decision making. Then, in the final chapter, we focus on two topics that are of secondary importance to an introductory course in healthcare finance, but which some instructors may elect to cover.

Chapter 16 focuses on managing short-term assets, including their financing, a very important activity at all health services organizations. Chapter 17 discusses how to assess the financial condition of a business. If managers are to plan for the future, they must know the current financial status of the business. Chapter 18 covers two topics: (1) the nature of lease financing and how leases are evaluated and (2) the valuation of entire businesses, as opposed to individual projects.

In addition to the chapters in the text, two chapters are available online. Chapter 19 focuses on how for-profit businesses return capital to owners, while Chapter 20 discusses reimbursement topics, including capitation and risk sharing. These two chapters are available online from the Health Administration Press book companion website at ache.org/books/HCFinance4.

CURRENT ASSET MANAGEMENT AND FINANCING

Learning Objectives

After studying this chapter, readers will be able to:

- Describe alternative current asset investment and financing policies.
- Discuss in general terms how businesses manage cash and marketable securities.
- Discuss the key elements of receivables and supply chain management.
- Explain the alternatives available for short-term financing, including the use of security.

Introduction

In our discussion of financial management leading up to this chapter, the general focus has been on long-term, strategic decisions. This chapter covers another important element of healthcare finance—the management of short-term (current) assets and their financing. Unlike long-term financial management, the management of current assets is highly dependent on the specific type of provider organization (i.e., hospital versus medical practice versus nursing home). Thus, our treatment of this topic is somewhat basic and generic in nature. The discussion begins with an overview of short-term financial management and the policy decisions that health services managers must make regarding the level of current assets and their financing. A brief discussion of the management of each current asset account is then provided. The chapter closes with a discussion of the various types of short-term financing used by healthcare providers.

An Overview of Short-Term Financial Management

Short-term financial management involves all current assets and most current liabilities. The primary goal of short-term financial management is to support the operations of the business at the lowest possible cost. Clearly, a business must have the level of current assets necessary to meet its operational requirements. However, it is imprudent to hold too high a level because of the costs of carrying the assets.

To both illustrate the requirement for short-term financing and to review the current asset and current liability accounts, consider the situation facing Sun Coast Clinics, a for-profit operator of four ambulatory care clinics in South Florida. Table 16.1 contains the firm's December 2007 and April 2008 balance sheets. The provision of ambulatory care services in this part of Florida is a seasonal business. The peak season for Sun Coast is December through April, when the population of the area soars because of winter tourism and the arrival of the "snow birds" (i.e., retired individuals who typically live in the north during the summer and fall months but move to residences in Florida for the winter).

In December of each year, Sun Coast has just finished its slow season and is preparing for its busy season. Thus, the firm's accounts receivable are relatively low, but its cash and inventories are relatively high. By the end of April, Sun Coast has completed its busy season, so its accounts receivable are relatively high, but its cash and inventories are relatively low in preparation for the slow summer season. On the current liabilities side, Sun Coast's accounts payable and accruals are relatively high at the end of April, just after the busy season.

Consider what happens to Sun Coast's total current assets and total current liabilities over the December to April period. Current assets increase from $200,000 to $240,000, so the firm must increase its capital by $40,000—an increase on the assets side of the balance sheet must be financed by an increase on the liabilities and equity side. However, the higher volume of both purchases and labor expenditures associated with increased services causes accounts payable and accruals to increase *spontaneously* by $20,000,

TABLE 16.1
Sun Coast Clinics, Inc.: End-of-Month Balance Sheets (in thousands)

	December 2007	April 2008
Cash	$ 30	$ 20
Accounts receivable	155	210
Inventories	15	10
Total current assets	$200	$240
Net fixed assets	500	500
Total assets	$700	$740
Accounts payable	$ 30	$ 40
Accruals	15	25
Notes payable	105	125
Total current liabilities	$150	$190
Long-term debt	150	140
Common equity	400	410
Total liabilities and equity	$700	$740

from $30,000 + $15,000 = $45,000 in December to $40,000 + $25,000 = $65,000 in April. The net result is an additional $40,000 − $20,000 = $20,000 current asset financing requirement in April, which Sun Coast obtained from the bank as a short-term loan (notes payable). Therefore, at the end of April, Sun Coast showed notes payable of $125,000, up from $105,000 in December.

These fluctuations for Sun Coast result from seasonal factors. Similar fluctuations in current asset requirements, and hence in financing needs, can occur because of business cycles; typically, current asset requirements and financing needs contract during recessions and expand during boom times. In the next section, two policy issues regarding current assets and financing are discussed.

1. What is the goal of short-term financial management? 2. Describe how seasonal volume fluctuations influence both current asset levels and financing requirements.	**Self-Test Questions**

Current Asset Investment and Financing Policies

Current asset financial policy involves two basic questions:

1. What is the appropriate level for current assets, both in total and by specific accounts?
2. How should current assets be financed?

In this section, these two questions are discussed in detail.

Current Asset Investment Policies

Figure 16.1 shows three alternative policies for a single hospital regarding the total amount of current assets carried. Essentially, *current asset investment policies* differ in that different amounts of current assets are carried to support a given volume level. The line with the steepest slope represents a *high* current asset investment policy. Here, relatively large amounts of cash, marketable securities, and inventories are carried, and utilization is stimulated by the use of a credit policy that provides liberal financing to patients and a corresponding high level of receivables. Conversely, with the *low* current asset investment policy, the holdings of cash, securities, inventories, and receivables are minimized at each volume level.

Under conditions of certainty (i.e., when utilization, operating costs, collection times, and so on are known) all healthcare providers would hold only minimal levels of current assets and hence follow a low current asset investment policy. Any larger amounts would increase the need for current asset financing, and hence increase costs, without a corresponding increase

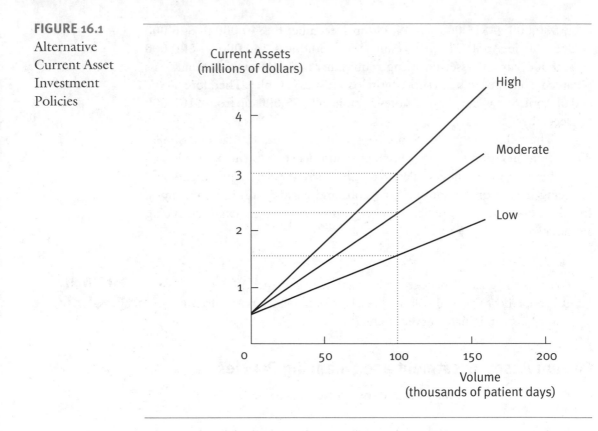

in profits. Any smaller holdings would involve late payments to labor and suppliers, operating inefficiencies because of inventory shortages, and lower utilization because of an overly restrictive credit policy.

However, the situation changes when uncertainty is introduced. Now the provider must carry the minimum amounts of cash and inventories to meet expected needs, **plus additional amounts**, or *safety stocks*, to enable the business to deal with realizations that differ from expectations. Similarly, accounts receivable levels are determined by credit terms (i.e., payer mix and collections policy), and the tougher the credit terms, the lower the receivables for any given level of sales. With a low current asset investment policy, the business would hold minimal levels of safety stocks for cash and inventories, and it would have a tight credit policy. A low policy generally provides the highest expected return on the business's investment in current assets, but it entails the greatest risk, while the converse is true under a high current asset investment policy. The moderate policy falls in between the two extremes in terms of expected risk and return.

The profit penalty for holding excess current assets is very much dependent on the cost of financing current asset holdings. Therefore, corporate policy regarding the level of current assets is never set in isolation. It is always established on the basis of current financing costs and in conjunction with the firm's current asset financing policy. In addition, current asset holdings are influenced by the amount of business risk (primarily volume uncertainty). The more difficult it is to predict utilization, the greater the amount of safety stocks held.

Current Asset Financing Policies

Most businesses experience seasonal fluctuations, as illustrated previously with Sun Coast Clinics. Similarly, most businesses must build up current assets when the economy is strong, but they then sell off inventories and reduce receivables when the economy slacks off. Still, current assets **never** drop to zero, and this realization forces us to introduce a concept of *asset maturities* that differs from the short-term/long-term categories used in financial accounting.

To illustrate the new concept, which classifies assets as either permanent or temporary, consider Sun Coast Clinics. Table 16.1 suggests that, at this stage in its life, seasonality causes the firm's total assets to fluctuate between $700,000 and $740,000. Thus, Sun Coast has $700,000 in *permanent assets,* defined as the amount of total assets required to sustain operations during seasonal (or cyclical) lows. Sun Coast's permanent assets are composed of $500,000 of *permanent fixed assets* and $200,000 in *permanent current assets*. In addition, Sun Coast carries *seasonal,* or *temporary, current assets* that fluctuate from zero to a maximum of $40,000 during the high season. No additional fixed assets are needed during the high season because the business has sufficient fixed assets to accommodate peak volume. The manner in which the permanent and temporary current assets are financed defines the firm's *current asset financing policy.*

The proper framework for evaluating current asset financing policies requires the use of the concept of permanent and temporary assets. Thus, for financing purposes, assets are **not** classified by their accounting definitions of current and long term but as either permanent or temporary. The key here is that each dollar of cash, each individual receivable, and each dollar of inventory may well be short term in the sense that these items will be quickly turned over or converted to cash. However, as each individual current asset item is converted, it will be replaced by a like item if it is permanent in nature, and hence the dollar amounts of such short-term assets are carried permanently over the long term. The implication is that the accounting definition of current assets, although useful for many purposes, does not provide managers with the correct guidance regarding the financing of such assets.

One financing policy, *maturity matching,* which is sometimes called a *moderate financing policy,* calls for a business to match asset and liability maturities as shown in Panel (a) of Figure 16.2—that is, permanent assets are financed with permanent capital (i.e., equity and long-term debt), and temporary assets are financed with temporary capital (i.e., short-term debt). This strategy limits the risk that a business will be unable to pay off its maturing

FIGURE 16.2
Alternative
Current Asset
Financing
Policies

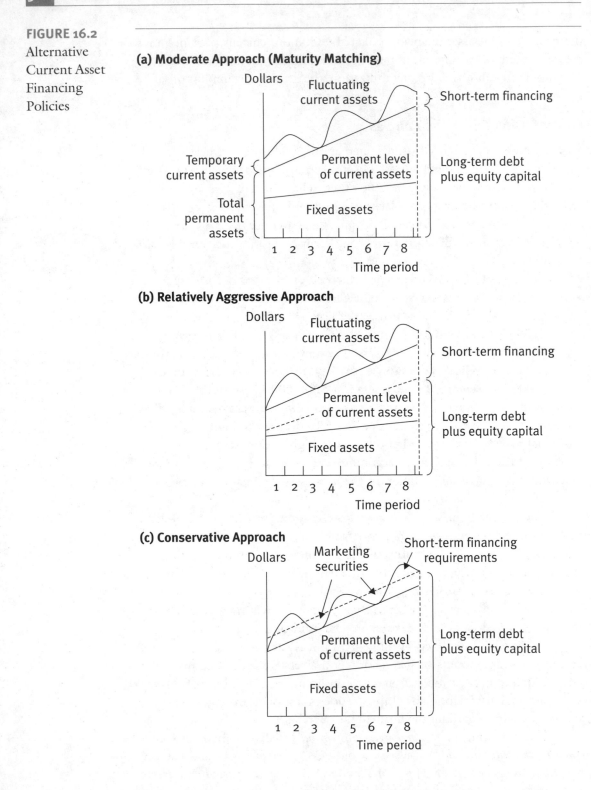

obligations. For example, suppose Sun Coast borrows on a one-year basis and uses the funds obtained to build and equip a new clinic. Cash flows from the clinic (i.e., profits plus depreciation) would almost never be sufficient to pay off the loan at the end of only one year, so the loan must be renewed at that time. If interest rates increase during the year, Sun Coast's new debt would cost more. Even worse, if the lender refused to renew the loan, Sun Coast would have problems. Had the clinic been financed with long-term financing, however, the required loan payments would have been better matched with cash flows from profits and depreciation, and the problem of loan renewal would not have arisen.[1]

Panel (b) of Figure 16.2 illustrates an *aggressive financing policy*. Here, the firm finances all of its fixed assets with long-term capital but part of its permanent current assets with short-term, nonspontaneous credit. A look back at Table 16.1 will show that Sun Coast actually follows this strategy. Assuming that the $20,000 current portion of long-term debt will be refinanced with new long-term debt, Sun Coast has $500,000 in net fixed assets and $570,000 of long-term capital, leaving only $70,000 of long-term capital to finance $200,000 in permanent current assets. Additionally, Sun Coast has a minimum of $45,000 of costless, spontaneous short-term credit (accounts payable and accruals). Thus, Sun Coast uses $85,000 of short-term notes payable to help finance its permanent level of current assets.

Returning to Figure 16.2, the term *relatively* is used in the title for Panel (b) because there can be different *degrees* of aggressiveness. For example, the dashed line in Panel (b) could have been drawn *below* the line that designates fixed assets, indicating that all of the permanent current assets and part of the fixed assets were financed with short-term credit. Such a policy would be highly aggressive, and the business would be very much subject to dangers from rising interest rates as well as to loan renewal problems. However, short-term debt usually is cheaper than long-term debt, and some managers are willing to sacrifice safety for the chance of higher profits.

As shown in Panel (c) of Figure 16.2, the dashed line could also be drawn above the line that designates permanent current assets, indicating that permanent capital is being used to finance all permanent asset requirements and also to meet some, or all, of the temporary credit demands. In the situation depicted in the graph, the firm uses a small amount of short-term, nonspontaneous credit to meet its peak requirements, but it also meets a part of its seasonal needs by storing liquidity in the form of marketable securities during the off-season. The humps above the dashed line represent short-term financing, and the troughs below the dashed line represent short-term security holdings. Panel (c) represents a very safe, *conservative financing policy*.

As with current asset investment policy, the choice among alternative financing policies involves a risk/return trade-off. The aggressive policy, with its high use of generally lower-cost short-term debt, has the highest expected return but the highest risk, while the conservative policy has the lowest expected return and lowest risk. The maturity matching policy falls between the extremes. Unfortunately, there is no underlying finance theory that managers can use to pick the "correct" financing policy. Often, firms that have low business risk elect to take on higher-than-average financial risk. Thus, such firms tend to have more debt in their target capital structures and are more likely to use an aggressive current asset financing policy. Conversely, firms with high business risk usually take a conservative view regarding added financial risk, whether that risk arises from a high level of debt or an aggressive current asset financing policy.

Self-Test Questions	1. What two key issues does current asset policy involve?
	2. What factors influence the current asset investment decision?
	3. What is meant by the term *permanent assets*?
	4. What is meant by the term *temporary assets*?
	5. What factors influence the current asset financing decision?

Cash Management

Businesses need *cash*, which includes both actual cash in hand and that held in commercial checking accounts, to pay for labor and materials, to buy fixed assets, to pay taxes, to service debt, and so on. However, cash is a *nonearning asset*—it provides no return. Thus, the goal of cash management is to minimize the amount of cash the business must hold to conduct its normal activities, but at the same time, have sufficient cash on hand to support operations. Maintaining sufficient cash ensures that a business is *liquid*, which means that it can meet its cash obligations as they become due. Conversely, a business that is illiquid cannot easily generate the cash needed to meet its obligations, and thus its operations suffer.[2]

A key element in a business's cash management process is the *cash budget*, which we discussed in Chapter 8. In essence, the cash budget tells managers how effective they are in applying the cash management techniques discussed in the following sections.

Managing Float

A well-run business has more money in its checking account than the balance shown on its checkbook. *Net float*, or just *float*, is defined as the difference between the balance shown on the bank's records and the balance on the business's checkbook. Alternatively, float can be thought of as the sum of the business's two component floats: disbursement and collections.

To illustrate net float and its components, assume that Gainesville Clinic writes, on average, checks in the amount of $5,000 each day. (As the checks are written, the amounts are deducted from the checkbook balance.) It takes six days for these checks to be mailed, delivered, deposited, and cleared, and hence for the amounts to be deducted from the clinic's bank account. This will cause the clinic's own checkbook to show a balance that is 6 × $5,000 = $30,000 less than the balance on the bank's records. Considering only disbursements, the clinic's actual balance at the bank is $30,000 greater than the amount shown on its checkbook, so it has a positive $30,000 *disbursement float*.

Now assume that the clinic receives checks in the amount of $5,000 daily, but it loses four days while they are being deposited and cleared. This difference will result in 4 × $5,000 = $20,000 of *collections float*. Because of the delay in depositing and clearing checks, the clinic's balance at the bank is $20,000 less than that on its checkbook, which represents a negative collections float of $20,000.

The clinic's net float, which is the sum of the positive $30,000 disbursement float and negative $20,000 collections float, is $10,000. On average, the clinic's balance at the bank is $10,000 larger than the balance on its checkbook. Some businesses are so good at managing float that they carry a negative checkbook balance but have a positive balance at the bank. For example, one medical equipment manufacturer stated that its bank's records show an average cash balance of about $200,000, while its own checkbook balance is *minus* $200,000—it has $400,000 of net float.

A firm's net float is a function of its ability to speed up collections on checks received and to slow down collections on checks written. Efficient businesses go to great lengths to speed up the processing of incoming checks, thus putting the funds to work faster, and they try to stretch their own payments out as long as possible (without engaging in unethical or illegal practices).

Note, however, that recent changes in check-clearing procedures have made it more difficult for businesses to create substantial floats. In 2004 a new law, called "Check Clearing for the 21st Century," gave banks greater flexibility in using electronic check clearing, which reduces disbursement float. Still, well-run businesses recognize the value inherent in float and, as we explain in the following sections, continue to do whatever is possible to maximize it.

Acceleration of Receipts

Managers have searched for ways to collect receivables faster since the day that credit transactions began. Although cash collection is the responsibility of a firm's managers, the speed with which checks are cleared is dependent on the banking system. Several techniques are now used both to speed collections and to get funds where they are needed, but the three most popular are lockbox services, concentration banking, and electronic claims processing. Here are some points to note about lockbox services and concentration banking. The discussion of electronic claims processing occurs later in this chapter.

Lockboxes are one of the oldest cash management tools, and virtually all banks that offer cash management services also offer lockbox services.

In a lockbox system, incoming checks are sent to post office boxes rather than to corporate headquarters. For example, Health SouthWest, a regional HMO headquartered in Oklahoma City, has its Texas members send their payments to a box in Dallas, its New Mexico members send their checks to Albuquerque, and so on, rather than have all checks sent to Oklahoma City. A local bank collects the contents of each lockbox and deposits the checks into the company's local account. The bank then provides the HMO with daily records of the receipts collected, usually via an electronic data transmission system in a format that permits online updating of the firm's receivables accounts.

A lockbox system reduces the time required for a business to receive incoming checks, deposit them, and get them cleared through the banking system, so the funds are available for use more quickly. This time reduction occurs because mail time and check collection time are both reduced if the lockbox is located in the geographic area where the customer is located. Lockbox services can often increase the availability of funds by one to four days over the regular system for firms with customers over a large geographical area.

Lockbox systems, although efficient in speeding up collections, result in the firm's cash being spread around among many banks. The primary purpose of *concentration banking* is to mobilize funds from decentralized receiving locations, whether they are lockboxes or decentralized company locations, into one or more central cash pools. In a typical concentration system, the firm's collection banks record deposits received each day. Based on disbursement needs, the funds are then transferred from these collection points to a concentration bank. Concentration accounts allow firms to take maximum advantage of economies of scale in cash management and investment. Health SouthWest uses an Oklahoma City bank as its concentration bank. The HMO cash manager then uses this pool for short-term investing or reallocation among its other banks.

One of the keys to concentration banking is the ability to quickly transfer funds from collecting banks to concentration banks, and electronic systems make such transfers easy. *Automated clearinghouses* are communications networks that provide a means of sending data from one financial institution to another. Instead of using paper checks, computer files are created, and all entries for a particular bank are placed on a single file that is sent to that bank. Some banks send and receive their data on tapes, while others have direct computer links to the clearinghouse.

Disbursement Control

Accelerated collections represent one side of using float, and controlling funds outflows is the flip side of the coin. Efficient cash management can only result if both inflows and outflows are effectively managed.

No single action controls disbursements more effectively than *payables centralization*. This permits the firm's managers to evaluate the payments coming due for the entire business and to meet those needs in an organized and controlled manner. Centralized disbursement also permits more efficient monitoring of payables and float balances. However, centralized disbursement does have a downside—centralized offices may have difficulty in making all payments promptly, which can create ill will with suppliers and potentially lose prompt-payment discounts.

Zero-balance accounts (ZBAs) are special disbursement accounts that have a zero-dollar balance on which checks are written. Typically, a firm establishes several ZBAs in the concentration bank and funds them from a *master account*. As checks are presented to a ZBA for payment, funds are automatically transferred from the master account. If the master account goes negative, it is replenished by borrowing from the bank against a line of credit or by selling some securities from the firm's marketable securities portfolio. Zero-balance accounts simplify the control of disbursements and cash balances and hence reduce the amount of idle (i.e., noninterest-bearing) cash.

Whereas zero-balance accounts are typically established at concentration banks, *controlled disbursement accounts* can be set up at any bank. In fact, controlled disbursement accounts were initially used only in relatively remote banks, so this technique was originally called *remote disbursement*. The basic technique is simple: Controlled disbursement accounts are not funded until the day's checks are presented against the account. The key to controlled disbursement is the ability of the bank that has the account to report the total amount of checks received for clearance each morning. This early notification gives a firm's managers sufficient time to wire funds to the controlled disbursement account to cover the checks presented for payment.

Matching the Costs and Benefits of Cash Management

Although a number of techniques have been discussed to reduce cash balance requirements, implementing these procedures is not a costless operation. How far should a firm go in making its cash operations more efficient? As a general rule, the firm should incur these expenses only so long as the marginal returns exceed the marginal costs.

The value of careful cash management depends on the opportunity costs of funds invested in cash, which in turn depends on the current level of interest rates. For example, in the early 1980s, with interest rates at relatively high levels, businesses were devoting a great deal of care to cash management. Today, with interest rates much lower, the value of cash management is reduced. Clearly, larger businesses, with larger cash balances, can better afford to hire the personnel necessary to maintain tight control over their cash positions.

Because cash management is an element of business operations in which economies of scale are present, banks have placed considerable emphasis on developing and marketing these services. Thus, banks can generally provide cash management services to smaller companies at lower costs than companies can achieve by operating in-house cash management systems.

Marketable Securities Management

Many businesses hold temporary portfolios of securities called *marketable securities* (or *short-term investments* or *near-cash*). Although cash and marketable securities management are discussed in separate sections, they cannot be separated in practice because management of one implies management of the other. There are two primary reasons for these holdings: (1) they serve as an interest-earning substitute for cash balances, and (2) they are used to hold funds that are being accumulated to meet a specific large, near-term obligation, such as a tax payment or capital expenditure. In addition to marketable securities holdings, not-for-profit hospitals tend to hold portfolios of long-term securities (as explained in the next section).

In general, the key characteristic sought in marketable securities investments is safety. Thus, most health services managers are willing to give up some return to ensure that funds are available, in the amounts expected, when needed. Large businesses, with large amounts of surplus cash, often directly own securities such as Treasury bills, commercial paper, and negotiable certificates of deposit. In addition, large taxable firms often hold preferred stock because of its 70 percent dividend exclusion from federal income taxes.

Conversely, smaller businesses are more likely to invest with a bank or with a money market or preferred stock mutual fund because a small firm's volume of investment simply does not warrant its hiring specialists to manage a marketable securities portfolio. Small businesses often use a mutual fund and then literally write checks on the fund to bolster the cash account as the need arises.[3] Interest rates on mutual funds are somewhat lower than rates on direct investments of equivalent risk because of management fees. However, for smaller companies, net returns may well be higher on mutual funds because no in-house management expense is required.

Long-Term Securities Management

Not-for-profit providers, and hospitals in particular, often have large portfolios of long-term security holdings, which is something that is not common in for-profit businesses. These holdings are listed on the balance sheet as *long-term investments*. The reasons that not-for-profit hospitals typically carry large amounts of long-term securities are as follows:

- Not-for-profit hospitals often set aside funds for future fixed asset replacement rather than obtain the funds at the time the assets are acquired. Because funds for this purpose generally stem from depreciation-generated cash flow, as opposed to net income, they are called *funded depreciation*.
- Many hospitals self-insure at least part of their professional liability exposure and hence establish an investment pool to meet actuarial needs.
- Many hospitals have defined benefit pension plans, which require a firm-sponsored pension fund.
- Not-for-profit hospitals receive endowment gifts that must be managed over time. If a separate foundation is not established to hold and administer the endowment, such funds must be carried on the hospital's balance sheet.

The selection of securities for long-term investment obviously is quite different from those selected for marketable securities. With time now on their side, managers are more willing to take risks to gain a return edge. For example, the typical hospital's funded depreciation account (portfolio) consists of roughly 30 percent domestic stocks, 45 percent domestic bonds, 20 percent cash equivalents, and 5 percent international stocks and bonds. Furthermore, the typical endowment fund consists of roughly 50 percent domestic stock, 30 percent domestic bonds, 10 percent cash equivalents, 5 percent international investments, and 5 percent alternative investments. *Alternative investments* include nontraditional investments such as hedge funds, commodities, real estate, venture capital, and private equity.

It is clear that hospital managers, especially those at big hospital systems with large amounts of money to invest for the **long term**, are willing to create riskier portfolios in the search for higher returns. The most recent trend in long-term investment portfolio management at not-for-profit hospitals has been the willingness to include more and more alternative investments. The trend may continue, but it brings significant risk, especially to smaller systems and stand-alone hospitals. Because such investments are less liquid than traditional investments, they make most sense for large, financially stable systems that can afford to invest for long periods of time.

Receivables Management

Generally, businesses would rather sell for cash than on credit, but competitive pressure forces most firms to offer credit. The problem is most acute in the health services industry, where the third-party payment system forces providers to extend credit to most patients. In a credit sale, goods are shipped or services are provided, inventories are reduced, and an account receivable is created. Eventually, the customer or third party payer will pay the account, at which time the business will receive cash and its receivables will decline.

The Accumulation of Receivables

The total amount of accounts receivable outstanding at any given time is determined by two factors: the volume of credit sales and the average length of time between sales and collections. For example, suppose Home Infusion provides an average of ten home health visits a day at an average net charge of $100 per visit, for $1,000 in *average daily billings (ADB)*. Assuming 250 workdays a year, the company's annual billings total $1,000 × 250 = $250,000. Furthermore, assume that all services are paid by two third-party payers: one pays for half of the billings 15 days after the service is provided and the second pays for the other half of billings in 25 days. Home Infusion's *average collection period (ACP)*, also called *days in patient accounts receivable*, is 20 days.

$$ACP = (0.5 \times 15 \text{ days}) + (0.5 \times 25 \text{ days}) = 20 \text{ days.}$$

Assuming a constant uniform rate of services provided, and hence billings, the accounts receivable balance will at any point in time be equal to ABD × ACP. Thus, Home Infusion's receivable balance would be $20,000:

$$\text{Receivables balance} = ADB \times ACP = \$1,000 \times 20 = \$20,000.$$

What is the cost implication of carrying $20,000 in receivables? The $20,000 on the left side of the balance sheet must be financed by a like amount on the right side.[4] Home Infusion uses a bank loan to finance its receivables, which has an interest rate of 8 percent. Thus, over a year, the firm must pay the bank 0.08 × $20,000 = $1,600 in interest to carry its receivables balance. The cost associated with carrying other current assets can be thought of in a similar way.

Monitoring the Receivables Position

If a service is provided for cash, the resulting revenue is collected "on the spot," but if payment for the service is billed to a third-party payer, the revenue is not actually received until the account is collected. If the account is never collected, the revenue is never received. Thus, health services managers must closely monitor receivables to ensure that they are being collected in a timely manner and to uncover any deterioration in the "quality" of receivables. Early detection can help managers take corrective action before the situation has a significant negative impact on the organization's financial condition.

The ACP, which is a measure of the average length of time it takes patients (or third-party payers) to pay their bills, often is compared to the industry average ACP. For example, if the home health industry average ACP is 22 days, versus Home Infusion's 20-day ACP, then its collections department is doing a better-than-average job.

Note however, that even though Home Infusion's payers are, on average, paying faster than the 22-day industry average, its two payers are paying in 15 days and 25 days. Thus, the firm's collections department should take a hard look to see if the ACP of the 25-day payer can be reduced to the industry average, or even to the 15 days of the other payer.

Why is it so important to minimize a business's average collection period? To illustrate, assume that Home Infusion's ACP was 25 days, and hence its receivables balance was $25,000. Assuming an 8 percent cost of financing (carrying) its receivables, the annual carrying cost to Home Infusion is $0.08 \times \$25,000 = \$2,000$. But, at its actual ACP of 20 days, its carrying costs are only $0.08 \times \$20,000 = \$1,600$. Thus, by reducing its ACP by 5 days, Home Infusion reduced its receivables carrying costs by $400 annually. "No big deal," you say. True, but now consider a 500-bed hospital with $100 million in receivables and a 60-day ACP, which implies average daily billings (ADB) of $100 / 60 = \$1.67$ million. A reduction of ACP by five days would reduce the receivables balance to $1.67 \times 55 = \$91.85$ million, or by about $8 million. Assuming the same 8 percent cost of carrying receivables, the savings amounts to a substantial $0.08 \times \$8 = \$0.64$ million $= \$640,000$. In addition, the hospital would receive a one-time cash flow of $8 million as the receivables balance is reduced. It should be apparent that immediate cash flow as well as large savings can be obtained by reducing a business's ACP, and hence its receivables balance.

Aging Schedules

An *aging schedule* breaks down a firm's receivables by age of account. To illustrate, Table 16.2 contains the December 31, 2007, aging schedules of two home health companies: Home Infusion and Home Care. Both firms offer the same services and show the same total receivables balance. However, Home

TABLE 16.2
Aging Schedules
for Two Firms

Age of Account (Days)	Home Infusion		Home Care	
	Value of Account	Percentage of Total Value	Value of Account	Percentage of Total Value
0–10	$10,000	50%	$ 9,000	45%
11–20	7,500	38	5,000	25
21–30	2,500	12	3,000	15
31–40	0	0	2,000	10
Over 40	0	0	1,000	5
Total	$20,000	100%	$20,000	100%

Infusion's aging schedule indicates that it is collecting its receivables faster than does Home Care. Only 50 percent of Home Infusion's receivables are more than ten days old, while Home Care shows 55 percent of its receivables fall into the more than ten—days-old categories. More importantly, Home Care has receivables that are more than 30 days old and even some that are more than 40 days old. Based on an industry average ACP of 22 days, Home Care's managers should be concerned both about the efficiency of the firm's collections effort and about the ability of the late payers to actually make the payments due.

Aging schedules cannot be constructed from the type of summary data that are reported in a firm's financial statements; they must be developed from the firm's accounts receivable ledger. However, well-run businesses have computerized accounts receivable records. Thus, it is easy to determine the age of each invoice, sort electronically by age categories, and thus generate an aging schedule.

Unique Problems Faced by Healthcare Providers

Although the general principles of receivables management discussed up to this point are applicable to all businesses, healthcare providers face some unique problems. The most obvious problem is the complexities in billing created by the third-party-payer system. For example, rather than have a single billing system that applies to all customers, providers have to deal with the rules and regulations of many different governmental and private insurers that use different payment methodologies. Thus, providers have to maintain large staffs of specialists that operate under the firm's *patient accounts manager*.

To illustrate the problem, consider Table 16.3, which contains the receivables mix for the hospital industry. There are multiple payers within many of the categories listed in the table, so the actual number of different payers can easily run into the hundreds.

Table 16.4 provides information on how long it takes hospitals to collect receivables. Because of the large number of payers, and the complexities

TABLE 16.3
Hospital
Industry's
Receivables Mix

Payer	Percentage of Total Accounts Receivable
Managed care	34.3%
Medicare	27.2
Self-pay	15.8
Medicaid	10.8
Commercial insurers	8.3
Other	3.6
	100.0%

Source: Aspen Publishers, *Hospital Accounts Receivable Analysis (HARA)*. Updated quarterly.

TABLE 16.4
Hospital
Industry's
Collection
Performance

Aggregate Aging Schedule

Age of Account (Days)	Percentage of Total Accounts Receivable
0–30	50.5%
31–60	16.0
61–90	9.5
91–120	6.2
Over 120	17.8
	100.0%

Average Collection Period
(Days in Patient Accounts Receivable)

Percentile Values	Average Collection Period (Days)
10th	33.9 days
25th	41.8
Median	51.0
75th	61.5
90th	77.4

Sources: a. Aspen Publishers, *Hospital Accounts Receivable Analysis (HARA)*. Updated quarterly.
 b. Ingenix, *Almanac of Hospital Financial and Operating Indicators*. Published annually.

involved with billing and follow-up actions, which lead to high error rates, hospitals clearly have a great deal of difficulty in collecting bills in a timely manner. On average, collecting a receivable takes about 50 days. However, this number has decreased in recent years as hospital managers have become increasingly aware of the costs associated with carrying receivables. In spite of the positive trend, almost 25 percent of receivables still were more than 90 days old. In addition, about 5 percent of patient bills were never paid at all, with about 3 percent being charged off as bad debt losses and 2 percent going to charity care.

To help providers collect from managed care plans in a timely fashion, many states have enacted "prompt payment" laws, which require payers to pay within a mandated time period or face penalties. For example, New York

State requires that all undisputed claims by providers be paid by managed care plans within 45 days of receipt. If prompt payment is not made, fines are assessed.

The Revenue Cycle

One of the current "hot" topics in healthcare finance, especially among hospitals, is the *revenue cycle*. The concept is not new, but it is gaining increased emphasis as it becomes harder and harder to maintain profitability in today's healthcare environment. Generically, the revenue cycle is defined as the set of recurring business activities and related information processing associated with billing and collecting for goods or services provided to customers. More pragmatically, the revenue cycle at provider organizations should ensure that patients are **properly** categorized regarding payment obligation, that *correct* billing takes place, and that the *correct* payment is received, all in a timely fashion.

For analysis at individual businesses, revenue cycle activities typically are broken down into three parts: (1) those that occur before the service is provided, (2) those that are simultaneous with the service, and (3) those that occur afterward. Here are some examples of revenue cycle activities:

Before-Service Activities
- **Preinsurance verification.** The payer status of the patient is identified immediately after the appointment (stay) is scheduled.
- **Precertification of managed care patients.** If the verification indicates that the payer requires precertification, it should be done immediately.
- **Preservice patient financial counseling.** The patient should be counseled before the service regarding both the payer's and the patient's responsibilities regarding payment for services.

Service Activities
- **Time of service verification.** The patient's insurance status should be checked at time of service to ensure that there have been no changes. The verification should be done both with the patient and with the payer.
- **Claims production.** The services provided should be documented in a way that facilitates correct claims submission. The documentation process should ensure that (1) the services provided are coded in accordance with the payer's claim system and (2) the code reflects the highest legitimate reimbursement amount.

After-Service Activities
- **Claims submission.** The claim should be submitted to the payer as quickly as possible after the service is rendered. However, speed should not take precedence over accuracy because incomplete and inaccurate billing accounts for a large proportion of late payments.
- **Third-party follow-up.** If payment is not received within 30 days, a follow-up should be sent.

- **Denials management.** Claim denials by third-party payers are one of the major impediments to prompt reimbursement. Most claim denials are caused by improper precertification and incomplete or erroneous claims data. Prompt claims resubmission is essential to good revenue cycle management.
- **Payment receipt and posting.** This activity ends the revenue cycle.
- **Monitoring and reporting.** Once the revenue cycle activities are identified and timing goals are set for each activity, the patient accounts manager should implement a system of key performance indicators to ensure that these goals are being met.

The revenue cycle requires constant attention because the external factors that influence the cycle are constantly changing. Also, problems that occur at any point in the cycle tend to have "ripple" effects. That is, a problem that occurs early in the cycle can create additional problems at later points in the cycle. For example, failure to obtain required precertification can lead to a denial and, at best, payment delay or, at worst, no payment at all.

Electronic Claims Processing

One development of note in provider billing and collections is the move to *electronic claims processing*. In this system, claims and reimbursement information is electronically transmitted in a standard format that can be processed without human intervention. Although the *electronic data interchange (EDI)* of payer information has been around for many years, its implementation has tended to be fragmented and payer-unique. However, one portion of the Health Insurance Portability and Accountability Act (HIPAA) of 1996 requires that all providers and insurers adhere to specific electronic data transaction standards. This initiative has provided the impetus to fully automate the exchange of all billing and collections data between providers and payers, which helps ensure the shortest possible revenue cycle.

1. Explain how a firm's receivables balance is built up over time and why there are costs associated with carrying receivables.
2. Briefly discuss two means by which a firm can monitor its receivables position.
3. What are some of the unique problems faced by healthcare providers in managing receivables?
4. What is the revenue cycle and how does electronic data interchange (EDI) fit in?

Self-Test Questions

Supply Chain Management

Supply chain management involves the requisitioning, ordering, receipt, and payment for supplies. Historically, supply chain management was called *inventory management.* Inventories are an essential part of virtually all business operations. As is the case with accounts receivable, inventory levels depend heavily on volume. However, whereas receivables build up after services have been provided, inventories must be acquired **ahead** of time. This is a critical difference, and the necessity of forecasting volume before establishing target inventory levels makes inventory management a difficult task. Also, because errors in inventory levels can lead either to catastrophic consequences for patients or to excessive carrying costs, supply chain management in health services organizations is as important as it is difficult.

Proper supply chain management requires close coordination among the marketing, purchasing, patient services, and finance departments. The marketing department is generally the first to spot changes in demand. These changes must be worked into the company's purchasing and operating schedules, and the financial manager must arrange any financing that will be needed to support inventory buildups. Improper communication among departments, poor volume forecasts, or both can lead to disaster.

The key to cost-effective supply chain management is information technology. Without information systems that support supply chain management, the control system will become bogged down with slow-moving hardcopy data. To illustrate, most healthcare businesses now employ *computerized inventory control systems.* The computer starts with an inventory count in memory. As withdrawals are made, they are recorded in the computer, and the inventory balance is revised. When the order point is reached, the computer automatically places an order, and when the order is received, the recorded balance is increased.[5]

A good supply chain management system must be dynamic. A large provider may stock thousands of different items of inventory. The usage of these various items can rise or fall quite separately from rising or falling aggregate utilization of services. As the usage rate for an individual item begins to rise or fall, the supply chain manager must adjust its balance to avoid running short or ending up with obsolete items. If the change in the usage rate appears to be permanent, then the *base inventory* level should be recomputed, the *safety stock* should be reconsidered, and the computer model used in the control process should be reprogrammed.

A relatively new approach to supply chain management, called *just-in-time (JIT),* is gaining popularity in all industries, including health services. To illustrate the use of just-in-time systems among providers, consider Bayside Memorial Hospital, which consumes large quantities of medical supplies each year. A few years ago, the hospital maintained a 25,000 square foot warehouse to hold its medical supplies. However, as cost pressures mounted, the hospital closed its warehouse and sold the inventory to a major hospital supplier. Now the supplier is a full-time partner of Bayside in ordering and delivering the products of some 400 hospital supply companies.

The supply chain streamlining process began with daily deliveries to the hospital's loading dock but soon expanded to a JIT system called *stockless inventory*. Now the supplier fills orders in exact, sometimes small, quantities and delivers them directly to departments inside the hospital, including the operating rooms and nursing floors. Bayside's managers estimate that the stockless system has saved the hospital about $1.5 million a year since it was instituted, including $350,000 from staff reductions and $650,000 from inventory reductions. Additionally, the hospital has converted space that was previously used as storerooms to patient care and other cash-generating uses. The distributors that offer stockless inventory systems typically add 3 to 5 percent service fees, but many hospitals still can realize savings on total inventory costs.

However, the stockless inventory concept has its own set of problems. The major concern is that a *stock-out*, which occurs when a needed inventory item is not available, will cause a serious problem. In addition, some hospital managers are concerned that such systems create too much dependence on a single supplier, and eventually the cost savings will disappear as prices increase because of the sole-supplier relationship.

As stockless inventory systems become more prevalent in hospitals, more and more hospitals are relying on outside contractors who assume both inventory management and supplier roles. In effect, hospitals are beginning to outsource supply chain management. For example, some hospitals are experimenting with an inventory management program known as *point-of-service distribution*, which is one generation ahead of stockless systems. Under point-of-service programs, the supplier delivers supplies, intravenous solutions, medical forms, and so on to the supply rooms. The supplier owns the products in the supply rooms until they are used by the hospital, at which time the hospital pays for the items.

In addition to reducing inventories, outside supply chain managers are often better at ferreting out waste than are their in-house counterparts. For example, an inventory management company recently found that one hospital was spending $600 for products used in open heart surgery, while another was spending only $420. Because there was no meaningful difference in the procedure or outcomes, the higher-cost hospital was able to change the medical devices used in the surgery and pocket the difference.

In an even more advanced form of supply chain management, some hospitals are just beginning to negotiate with suppliers to furnish materials on the basis of how much medical care is delivered, rather than the type and number of products used. In such agreements, providers pay suppliers a set fee for each unit of patient service provided—for example, $125 for each case-mix-adjusted patient day. Under this type of system, a hospital ties its supplies expenditures to its revenues, which, at least for now, are for the most part tied to the number of units of patient service. The end of the evolution of inventory management techniques for healthcare providers is expected to be some form of capitated payment, whereby providers will pay suppliers a previously agreed-upon fee, regardless of actual future patient volume and hence regardless of the amount of materials actually consumed.

Self-Test Questions

1. Why is good supply chain management important to a firm's success?
2. Describe some recent trends in supply chain management by healthcare providers.

Short-Term Financing

Chapters 11, 12, and 13 focus on long-term financing decisions. However, as pointed out in the introduction to Chapter 11, on average healthcare providers use 5 percent short-term debt in their total financing mix, typically to fund short-term (current) assets. This section provides some of the details associated with short-term financing.

Advantages and Disadvantages of Short-Term Debt

Short-term debt has three primary advantages over long-term debt. First, a short-term loan can be obtained much faster than long-term credit. Lenders will insist on a more thorough financial examination before extending long-term credit, and the loan agreement (or bond indenture) will have to be spelled out in considerable detail because a lot can happen during the life of a 10- or 20-year loan (or bond). Thus, if a business requires funds in a hurry, it should look to the short-term credit markets.

Second, if needs for funds are seasonal or cyclical, a firm may not want to commit itself to long-term debt for three reasons:

1. Administrative costs are generally high when raising long-term debt but trivial for short-term debt. Although long-term debt can be repaid early, provided the loan agreement includes a prepayment provision, prepayment penalties can be expensive. Accordingly, if a firm thinks its need for funds may diminish in the near future, it should choose short-term debt for the flexibility it provides.
2. Long-term loan agreements always contain restrictive covenants that constrain the firm's future actions. Short-term debt agreements are generally much less onerous in this regard.
3. The interest rate on short-term debt generally is lower than the rate on long-term debt because the yield curve normally is upward sloping. Thus, when coupled with lower administrative costs, short-term debt can have a significant total cost advantage over long-term debt.

In spite of these advantages, short-term debt has one serious disadvantage: it subjects the firm to more risk than does long-term financing. The increased risk occurs for two reasons. First, if a firm borrows on a long-term basis, its interest costs will be relatively stable over time, but if it uses short-term debt, its interest expense can fluctuate widely, at times possibly going quite high. For example, the short-term rate that banks charge large corporations (the prime rate) more than tripled over a two-year period in the early 1980s, rising from 6.25 to 21 percent.[6] Many firms that had borrowed heavily on a short-term basis simply could not meet their rising interest costs, and as a result, bankruptcies hit record levels during that period.

Second, the principal amount on short-term debt comes due on a regular basis. If the financial condition of a business temporarily deteriorates, it may find itself unable to repay this debt when it matures. Furthermore, the business may be in such a weak financial position that the lender will not extend the loan. Such a scenario can result in severe problems for the borrower, which, like unexpectedly high interest rates, could force the business into bankruptcy.

Sources of Short-Term Financing

Statements about the flexibility, cost, and riskiness of short-term versus long-term debt depend to a large extent on the type of short-term financing that is actually used. Three major types of short-term financing—accruals, accounts payable, and bank loans—are discussed in the following sections.[7]

Accruals

Firms generally pay employees on a weekly, biweekly, or monthly basis, so the balance sheet will typically show some accrued wages. Similarly, the firm's own estimated income taxes (if applicable); the social security and income taxes withheld from employee payrolls; and any required sales, workers' compensation, and unemployment taxes are generally paid on a weekly, monthly, or quarterly basis. Thus, as discussed in Chapter 4, the balance sheet accruals account typically includes both taxes and wages.

Accruals increase automatically, or spontaneously, as a firm's operations expand. Furthermore, this type of short-term debt is free in the sense that no explicit interest is paid on funds raised through accruals. However, a firm cannot ordinarily control the amount of accruals on its balance sheet because the timing of wage payments is set by economic forces and industry custom, and tax payment dates are established by law. Because accruals represent free financing, businesses should use all of the accrual financing they can obtain, but managers have little control over the levels of such accounts.

Accounts Payable (Trade Credit)

Firms often make purchases from other firms on credit. Such debt is recorded on the balance sheet as an *account payable*. Accounts payable, or *trade credit,* is the largest single category of short-term debt for many businesses. Because very small companies typically do not qualify for financing from other sources, they rely especially heavily on trade credit.[8]

Trade credit is another spontaneous source of financing in the sense that it arises from ordinary business transactions. For example, suppose that a hospital purchases an average of $2,000 a day of supplies on terms of net 30 days—meaning that it must pay for goods 30 days after the invoice date. On average, the hospital will owe 30 times $2,000, or $60,000, to its suppliers, assuming that the hospital's managers act rationally and do not pay before the credit is due. If the hospital's volume, and consequently its purchases, were to double, its accounts payable would also double to $120,000. Simply by growing, the hospital would have spontaneously generated an additional $60,000 of financing. Similarly, if the terms under which it bought supplies were extended from 30 to 40 days, the hospital's accounts payable would expand from $60,000 to $80,000. Thus, a supplier lengthening the credit period, as well as expanding volume, and hence purchases, generates additional financing for a business.

Firms that sell on credit have a *credit policy* that includes certain *terms of credit*. For example, Midwestern Medical Supply Company sells on terms of 2/10, net 30—meaning that a 2 percent discount is given if payment is made within ten days of the invoice date, with the full invoice amount being due and payable within 30 days if the discount is not taken. Suppose that Chicago Health System buys an average of $12 million of medical and surgical supplies from Midwestern each year, less a 2 percent discount, for net purchases of $11,760,000 / 360 = $32,666.67 per day. For the sake of simplicity, suppose that Midwestern is Chicago Health System's only supplier. If Chicago Health System takes the discount, paying at the end of the tenth day, its payables will average 10 × $32,666.67 = $326,667, so Chicago Health System will, on average, be receiving $326,667 of credit from its only supplier, Midwestern Medical Supply Company.

Suppose now that the system's managers decide not to take the discount. What effect will this decision have on the system's financial condition? First, Chicago Health System will begin paying invoices after 30 days, so its accounts payable will increase to 30 × $32,666.67 = $980,000.[9] Midwestern will now be supplying Chicago Health System with $980,000 − $326,667 = $653,333 of **additional** trade credit. The health system could use this additional credit to pay off bank loans, to expand inventories, to increase fixed assets, to build up its cash account, or even to increase its own accounts receivable.

Note that we used $32,666.67 for average daily sales, which is based on the discounted price of the surgical supplies, regardless of **whether or not** Chicago Health System takes the discount. In general, businesses treat the discounted price of supplies as the "true" cost when reporting expenses on the income statement. If the business does not take the discount, the cost difference is reported separately on the income statement as an expense called "discounts lost." Thus, we used the discounted price to reflect the cost of the supplies in both instances.

Chicago Health System's additional credit from Midwestern has a cost: it is foregoing a 2 percent discount on its \$12 million of purchases, so its costs will rise by \$240,000 per year. Dividing this \$240,000 dollar cost by the amount of additional credit provides the implicit approximate percentage cost of the added trade credit:

$$\text{Approximate \% cost} = \frac{\$240,000}{\$653,333} = 36.7\%.$$

Assuming that Chicago Health System can borrow from its bank or from other sources at an interest rate less than 36.7 percent, it should not expand its payables by foregoing discounts.

The following equation can be used to calculate the approximate percentage cost, on an annual basis, of not taking discounts:

$$\text{Approximate \% cost} = \frac{\text{Discount percent}}{100 - \text{Discount percent}}$$
$$\times \frac{360}{\text{Days credit received} - \text{Discount period}}.$$

The numerator of the first term, Discount percent, is the cost per dollar of credit, while the denominator in this term, $100 - \text{Discount percent}$, represents the funds made available by not taking the discount. Thus, the first term is the periodic cost rate of the trade credit—in this example, Chicago Health System must spend \$2 to gain \$98 of credit, for a cost rate of $2 / 98 = 0.0204 = 2.04\%$. The second term shows how many times each year this cost is incurred; in this example, $360 / (30 - 10) = 360 / 20 = 18$ times. Putting the two terms together, the approximate cost of not taking the discount when the terms are 2/10, net 30, is computed as follows:[10]

$$\text{Approximate \% cost} = \frac{2}{98} \times \frac{360}{20} = 0.0204 \times 18$$
$$= 0.367 = 36.7\%.$$

The cost of trade credit can be reduced by paying late—that is, by paying beyond the date that the credit terms allow. Such a strategy is called *stretching*. If Chicago Health System could get away with paying Midwestern in 60 days rather than in the specified 30, the effective credit period would become $60 - 10 = 50$ days, and the approximate cost would drop from 36.7 percent to $(2 / 98) \times (360 / 50) = 14.7\%$. In recessionary periods, businesses may be able to get away with late payments to suppliers, but they will also suffer a variety of problems associated with stretching accounts payable and being branded as a slow payer.

On the basis of the preceding discussion, it is clear that trade credit usually consists of two distinct components:

1. **Free trade credit.** This credit consists of the free credit received during the discount period. For Chicago Health System, the free trade credit amounts to ten days' net purchases, or $326,667.
2. **Costly trade credit.** The costly trade credit is that in excess of the free credit, and whose cost is an implicit one based on the foregone discount. For Chicago Health System, the amount of costly trade credit is $653,333.

From a finance perspective, managers should view trade credit in this way. First, the actual price of supplies is the discounted price—that is, the price that would be paid on a cash purchase. Any credit that can be taken without an increase in price is free credit that should be taken. Second, if the discounted price is the actual price, then the added amount that must be paid if the discount is not taken is, in reality, a *finance charge* for granting additional credit. A business should take the additional credit only if the finance charge is less than the cost of alternative credit sources.

In the example, Chicago Health System should take the $326,667 of free credit offered by Midwestern Medical Supply Company. Free credit is good credit. However, the cost rate of the additional $653,333 of costly trade credit is approximately 37 percent. The system has access to bank loans at a 9.5 percent rate, so it does not take the additional credit. Under the terms of trade found in most industries, the costly component will involve a relatively high percentage cost, so stronger firms will avoid using it.

Bank Loans

Commercial banks, whose short-term loans generally appear on firms' balance sheets as *notes payable*, are another important source of short-term financing.[11] The banks' influence is actually greater than it appears from the dollar amounts they lend because banks provide *nonspontaneous* funds. As a business's financing needs increase, it requests its bank to provide the additional funds. If the request is denied, the firm may be forced to abandon attractive growth opportunities.

Although banks make longer-term loans, the bulk of their lending is on a short-term basis (about two-thirds of all bank loans mature in a year or less). Bank loans to businesses are frequently written as 90-day notes, so the loan must be repaid or renewed at the end of 90 days. When a bank loan is approved, the agreement is executed by signing a *promissory note*, which is similar to a bond indenture or loan agreement but much less detailed. When the note is signed, the bank credits the borrower's checking account with the amount of the loan, while both cash and notes payable increase on the borrower's balance sheet.

Banks sometimes require borrowers to maintain a checking account balance equal to 10 to 20 percent of the face amount of the loan. This requirement is called a *compensating balance*, and such balances raise the effective interest rate on the loan. For example, suppose that Pine Garden nursing home needs an $80,000 bank loan to pay off maturing obligations. If the loan requires a 20 percent compensating balance, then the nursing home must borrow $100,000 to obtain a usable $80,000, assuming that the business does not have an "extra" $20,000 around to use as a compensating balance. If the stated interest rate is 8 percent, the effective cost rate is actually 10 percent: $0.08 \times \$100,000 = \$8,000$ in interest expense divided by $80,000 of usable funds equals 10 percent.

A *line of credit*, sometimes called a *revolving credit agreement* or just *revolver*, is a formal understanding between the bank and the borrower, which indicates the maximum credit the bank will extend to the borrower over some specified period of time. For example, on December 31 a bank loan officer might indicate to Pine Garden's manager that the bank regards the nursing home as being good for up to $80,000 during the forthcoming year. If on January 10, Pine Garden borrows $15,000 against the line, this would be called *taking down* $15,000 of the credit line. This take-down would be credited to the nursing home's checking account at the bank, and before repayment of the $15,000, Pine Garden could borrow additional amounts up to a total of $80,000 outstanding at any one time. Lines of credit are generally for one year or less, and borrowers typically have to pay an up-front commitment fee of about 0.5 to 1 percent of the total amount of the line. Interest is paid only on the amount of the credit line that is actually used. As a general rule, the rate of interest on credit lines is pegged to the prime rate, so the cost of the loan can vary over time if interest rates change. Pine Garden's rate was set at prime plus 0.5 percentage points.

Secured Short-Term Debt

Thus far, the question of whether or not short-term debt is *secured* has not been addressed. Given a choice, it is ordinarily better to borrow on an unsecured basis because the administrative costs associated with secured loans are often high. However, weak businesses may find that they can borrow only if they put up some form of security to protect the lender or that they can borrow at a much lower rate by using security.

Several kinds of *collateral*, or security, can be employed, including marketable securities, land or buildings, equipment, inventory, and accounts receivable. Marketable securities make excellent collateral, but businesses that need short-term credit generally do not hold large marketable securities portfolios. Both real property (i.e., land and buildings) and equipment are good forms of collateral. However, because of maturity matching, such assets are generally used as security for long-term loans rather than for short-term credit. Therefore, most secured short-term business borrowing involves the use of accounts receivable or inventories as collateral.[12]

Accounts receivable financing involves either the pledging of receivables or the selling of receivables. The *pledging* of accounts receivable is characterized by the fact that the lender not only has a claim against the dollar amount of the receivables but also has recourse against the pledging firm. This means that if the person or firm that owes the receivable does not pay, the business that borrows against the receivable must take the loss. Therefore, the risk of default on the accounts receivable pledged remains with the borrowing firm. When receivables are pledged, the payer is not ordinarily notified about the pledging, and payments are made on the receivables in the same way as when receivables are not used as loan security.

The second form of receivables financing is *factoring,* or *selling accounts receivable*. In this type of secured financing, the receivables account is actually "purchased" by the capital supplier, generally without recourse to the selling business. In a typical factoring transaction, the buyer of the receivables pays the seller about 90 to 95 percent of the face value of the receivables. When receivables are factored, the person or business that owes the receivable is often notified of the transfer and is asked to make payment directly to the company that bought the receivables. Because the factoring firm assumes the risk of default on bad accounts, it must perform a credit check on the receivables prior to the purchase. Accordingly, *factors*, which are the firms that buy receivables, can provide not only money but also a credit department for the borrower. Incidentally, the same financial institutions that make loans against pledged receivables also serve as factors. Thus, depending on the circumstances and the wishes of the borrower, a financial institution will provide either form of receivables financing.

Because healthcare providers tend to carry relatively large amounts of receivables, such businesses are prime candidates for receivables financing. For example, hospitals alone have accounts receivables that total nearly $15 billion. The selling of these receivables, especially by hospitals that are experiencing liquidity problems, represents one way to reduce carrying costs and stimulate cash flow.[13]

To illustrate receivables financing for hospitals, consider the program recently instituted between Chase Manhattan Bank and City Hospital, a large urban hospital. This program provides $15 million in advance funding of receivables over a three-year period. The hospital sells its accounts receivable to Chase for cash. The payers of the receivables technically make payments directly to Chase, although Chase actually pays the hospital a fee to service the receivables accounts. Chase charges an up-front fee for the program and then charges an interest rate of about 1 to 1.5 percent above the prime rate on the amount advanced.

Although receivables financing is a way to reduce current assets, and hence financing costs, critics contend that such programs are too expensive. Because of the costs involved, most receivables financing programs are used by providers that have serious liquidity problems, although programs are being developed that can provide benefits even to well-run businesses that are not facing a liquidity crunch.

Receivables financing dominates healthcare providers' use of secured financing, but other healthcare businesses, such as equipment manufacturers and pharmaceutical firms, are more likely to obtain credit secured by *business inventories*. If a firm is a relatively good credit risk, the mere existence of the inventory may be sufficient to obtain an unsecured loan. However, if the firm is a relatively poor risk, the lending institution may insist on security, which can take the form of a *blanket lien* against all inventory or a *trust receipt* against specific inventory items.

Self-Test Questions

1. What are accruals and what is their role in short-term financing?
2. What is the difference between free and costly trade credit?
3. How might a hospital that expects to have a cash shortage sometime during the coming year make sure that needed funds will be available?
4. What are some types of current assets that might be pledged as security for short-term loans?

Key Concepts

This chapter examines current asset management and financing. The key concepts of this chapter are:

- The goal of current asset management and financing is to *support the business's operations* at the lowest possible cost without taking undue risks.
- Under a *high current asset investment policy,* a firm holds relatively large amounts of each type of current asset. A *low policy* entails holding minimal amounts of these items, whereas a *moderate policy* falls between the two extremes.
- *Permanent assets* are those assets that businesses hold even during slack times, whereas *temporary assets* are the additional assets, usually current assets, that are needed to meet seasonal or cyclical peaks. The method used to finance permanent and temporary assets defines the firm's *current asset financing policy*.
- A *moderate* approach to current asset financing involves matching the maturities of assets and liabilities so that temporary current assets are financed with temporary financing and permanent assets are financed with permanent financing. Under an *aggressive* approach, some permanent current assets and perhaps some fixed assets are financed with short-term debt. A *conservative* approach would be to use long-term capital to finance all permanent assets and some temporary current assets.
- The *primary goal of cash management* is to reduce the amount of cash held to the minimum necessary to conduct business.

- *Float management techniques* include *accelerating collections* and *controlling disbursements.*
- *Lockboxes* are used to accelerate collections. A *concentration banking system* consolidates the collections into a centralized pool that can be managed more efficiently than a large number of individual accounts.
- Three techniques for controlling disbursements are *payables centralization, zero-balance accounts,* and *controlled disbursement accounts.*
- The implementation of a sophisticated cash management system is costly, and all cash management actions must be evaluated to ensure that the benefits exceed the costs.
- Businesses can reduce their cash balances by holding *marketable securities.* Marketable securities serve both as a *substitute for cash* and as a *temporary investment* for funds that will be needed in the near future. Safety is the primary consideration when selecting marketable securities.
- When a business sells goods to a customer on credit, an *account receivable* is created.
- Businesses can use an *aging schedule* and the *average collection period (ACP)* to help keep track of their receivables position and to help avoid the buildup of possible bad debts.
- The *revenue cycle* includes all activities associated with billings and collections for services provided.
- Proper *supply chain (inventory) management* requires close coordination among the marketing, purchasing, patient services, and finance departments. Because the cost of holding inventory can be high and stockouts can be disastrous, inventory management is very important.
- *Just-in-time (JIT)* systems are used to minimize inventory costs and, simultaneously, to improve operations.
- The advantages of short-term debt are the *speed* with which short-term loans can be arranged, increased *flexibility,* and the fact that short-term *interest rates* are generally *lower* than long-term rates. The principal disadvantage of short-term credit is the *extra risk* that borrowers must bear because lenders can demand payment on short notice, and the cost of the loan will increase if interest rates rise.
- *Accruals,* which are continually recurring short-term liabilities, represent free spontaneous credit.
- *Accounts payable,* or *trade credit,* arises spontaneously as a result of purchases on credit. Businesses should use all the *free trade credit* they can obtain, but they should use *costly trade credit* only if it is less expensive than alternative sources of short-term debt.
- *Bank loans* are an important source of short-term credit. When a bank loan is approved, a *promissory note* is signed.
- Banks sometimes require borrowers to maintain *compensating balances,* which are deposit requirements set at between 10 and 20 percent of the

loan amount. Compensating balances raise the effective rate of interest on bank loans.

- *Lines of credit*, or *revolving credit agreements*, are formal understandings between the bank and the borrower in which the bank agrees to extend some maximum amount of credit to the borrower over some specified period.
- Sometimes a borrower will find that it is necessary to borrow on a *secured basis*, in which case the borrower uses assets such as real estate, securities, equipment, inventories, or accounts receivable as collateral for the loan.

This chapter focuses on short-term financial management rather than the long-term topics that were covered in earlier chapters. In Chapter 17 we will cover financial performance analysis, while in Chapter 18 we will discuss two unrelated but interesting financial management topics: leasing and business valuation.

Questions

16.1 Describe three alternative current asset investment policies. Explain each policy's risk and return characteristics.

16.2 a. What is the difference between permanent assets and temporary assets?

b. If a firm uses the maturity matching approach to current asset financing, how will its temporary assets be financed?

c. Describe three alternative current asset financing policies. Explain each policy's risk and return characteristics.

16.3 a. What is the goal of cash management?

b. Briefly describe float and the following associated cash management techniques:
- Receipt acceleration
- Disbursement control

16.4 a. Give two reasons why businesses hold marketable securities.

b. Which types of securities are most suitable for holding as marketable securities?

c. Suppose Southwest Regional Medical Center has just raised $6 million in new capital that it plans to use to build three freestanding clinics, one each year over the next three years. (For the sake of simplicity, assume that equal payments have to be made at the end of each of the next three years.) What securities should be bought for the firm's marketable securities portfolio, assuming that the firm has no other excess cash? (Hint: Consider both the type and maturity of the securities.)

d. Now consider the situation faced by the Huntsville Physical Therapy Group. It has accumulated $20,000 in cash above its target cash balance, and it has no immediate needs for this excess cash. However, the firm may at any time need some part or all of the $20,000 to meet unforeseen cash needs. What securities should be bought for the firm's marketable securities portfolio?

16.5 a. Define average collection period.
   b. How is it used to monitor a firm's accounts receivable?
   c. What is an aging schedule?
   d. How is it used to monitor a firm's accounts receivable?

16.6 a. What is a just-in-time (JIT) inventory system?
   b. What are the advantages and disadvantages of JIT systems?
   c. Can JIT inventory systems be used by healthcare providers? Explain your answer.

16.7 Describe the three major sources of short-term financing.

16.8 a. What is the difference between free trade credit and costly trade credit?
   b. Should businesses use all the free trade credit that they can get? Explain your answer.
   c. Should businesses use all the costly trade credit they can get? Explain your answer.

16.9 Explain briefly how businesses can obtain secured short-term financing.

Problems

16.1 On a typical day, Park Place Clinic writes $1,000 in checks. It generally takes four days for those checks to clear. Each day the clinic typically receives $1,000 in checks that take three days to clear. What is the clinic's average net float?

16.2 Drugs 'R Us operates a mail order pharmaceutical business on the West Coast. The firm receives an average of $325,000 in payments per day. On average, it takes four days for the firm to receive payment, from the time customers mail their checks to the time the firm receives and processes them. A lockbox system that consists of ten local depository banks and a concentration bank in San Francisco would cost $6,500 per month. Under this system, customers' checks would be received at the lockbox locations one day after they are mailed, and the daily total would be wired to the concentration bank at a cost of $9.75 each. Assume that the firm could earn 10 percent on marketable securities and that there are 260 working days and hence 260 transfers from each lockbox location per year.
   a. What is the total annual cost of operating the lockbox system?
   b. What is the dollar benefit of the system to Drugs 'R Us?
   c. Should the firm initiate the lockbox system?

16.3 Suppose one of the suppliers to Seattle Health System offers terms of 3/20, net 60.
   a. When does the system have to pay its bills from this supplier?
   b. What is the approximate cost of the costly trade credit offered by this supplier? (Assume 360 days per year.)

16.4 Langley Clinics, Inc., buys $400,000 in medical supplies each year (at gross prices) from its major supplier, Consolidated Services, which offers Langley terms of 2.5/10, net 45. Currently, Langley is paying the supplier the full amount due on Day 45, but it is considering taking the discount, paying on Day 10, and replacing the trade credit with a bank loan that has a 10 percent annual cost.
   a. What is the amount of free trade credit that Langley obtains from Consolidated Services? (Assume 360 days per year throughout this problem.)
   b. What is the amount of costly trade credit?
   c. What is the approximate annual cost of the costly trade credit?
   d. Should Langley replace its trade credit with the bank loan? Explain your answer.
   e. If the bank loan is used, how much of the trade credit should be replaced?

16.5 Milwaukee Surgical Supplies, Inc., sells on terms of 3/10, net 30. Gross sales for the year are $1,200,000 and the collections department estimates that 30 percent of the customers pay on the tenth day and take discounts, 40 percent pay on the thirtieth day, and the remaining 30 percent pay, on average, 40 days after the purchase. (Assume 360 days per year.)
   a. What is the firm's average collection period?
   b. What is the firm's current receivables balance?
   c. What would be the firm's new receivables balance if Milwaukee Surgical toughened up on its collection policy, with the result that all nondiscount customers paid on the 30th day?
   d. Suppose that the firm's cost of carrying receivables was 8 percent annually. How much would the toughened credit policy save the firm in annual receivables carrying expense? (Assume that the entire amount of receivables had to be financed.)

16.6 Fargo Memorial Hospital has annual net patient service revenues of $14,400,000. It has two major third-party payers, plus some of its patients are self-payers. The hospital's patient accounts manager estimates that 10 percent of the hospital's paying patients (its self-payers) pay on Day 30, 60 percent pay on Day 60 (Payer A), and 30 percent pay on Day 90 (Payer B). (Five percent of total billings end up as bad debt losses, but that is not relevant for this problem.)
   a. What is Fargo's average collection period? (Assume 360 days per year throughout this problem.)

b. What is the firm's current receivables balance?

c. What would be the firm's new receivables balance if a newly proposed electronic claims system resulted in collecting from third-party payers in 45 and 75 days, instead of in 60 and 90 days?

d. Suppose the firm's annual cost of carrying receivables was 10 percent. If the electronic claims system costs $30,000 a year to lease and operate, should it be adopted? (Assume that the entire receivables balance has to be financed.)

Notes

1. At the limit, a business could attempt to match exactly the maturity structure of its assets and liabilities. Inventory expected to be sold in 30 days could be financed with a 30-day bank loan, a machine expected to last for five years could be financed by a five-year loan, a 20-year building could be financed by a 20-year mortgage bond, and so forth. Actually, three factors make this exact maturity matching strategy both unpractical and wrong: (1) there is uncertainty about the lives of assets; (2) some common equity (or fund capital) must be used, and this capital has no maturity; and (3) to develop a meaningful current asset financing policy it is necessary to consider whether an asset is permanent or temporary.

2. This discussion of cash management is necessarily brief. For a much more detailed discussion of cash management within the health services industry, see A. G. Seidner and W. O. Cleverley, *Cash and Investment Management for the Health Care Industry* (Rockville, MD: Aspen, 1990), and D. H. Zimmerman, *Cash is King* (Rockville, MD: Aspen, 1995).

3. Mutual funds cannot be used as a replacement for commercial checking accounts because the number of checks that can be written against such accounts is normally limited to a few per month.

4. To be precise, the full amount of the receivables account does **not** require financing. The cash costs associated with producing the $20,000 in revenues do need to be financed, but the profit component does not. For example, assume that Home Infusion has cash costs of $800 to support each day's sales of $1,000. Then, 20 days of receivables would actually require financing of 20 × $800 = $16,000. The remaining $4,000 in the receivables account would be offset on the balance sheet by $4,000 profit placed in the equity account.

5. It is estimated that average cost for hospitals to process a purchase order manually is $75, while the same order handled electronically would cost only $20.

6. The *prime rate* is the interest rate charged to a bank's very best customers. Each bank sets its own prime rate, but because of competition, most banks' prime rates are identical. Furthermore, most banks follow the lead of the large New York City banks.

7. The fourth major type of short-term financing is *commercial paper*, which is a type of unsecured business debt sold primarily to other businesses, insurance companies, pension funds, and money market mutual funds. Commercial paper is issued with maturities less than 270 days and generally carries an interest rate below the prime rate but above the rate on short-term Treasury securities. The

catch is that commercial paper can be issued only by very large companies with excellent credit standing, so most healthcare providers cannot use this source of financing.

8. In a credit sale, the seller records the transaction as a receivable, while the buyer records it as a payable. If a firm's payables exceed its receivables, it is said to be *receiving net trade credit*, whereas if its receivables exceed its payables, it is *extending net trade credit*. Smaller firms frequently receive net credit, while larger firms generally extend it.

9. A question arises here as to whether accounts payable should reflect gross purchases or purchases net of discounts. Although the GAAP permit either treatment on the grounds that the difference is not material, most accountants prefer to record payables net of discounts, and then to report the higher payments that result if the discounts are not taken as an additional expense, called "discounts lost."

10. This cost has purposely been labeled as the **approximate** percentage cost. The true effective cost, which recognizes intra-year compounding, is 43.8 percent, found as follows:

$$(1 + 0.0204)^{18} - 1.0 = (1.0204)^{18} - 1.0 = 0.438 = 43.8\%.$$

11. Although commercial banks remain the primary source of short-term loans, other sources are available. For example, GE Commercial Finance has over $2 billion in commercial loans outstanding. Firms such as GE Commercial Finance, which was initially established to finance consumers' purchases of GE's appliances, often find business loans to be more profitable than consumer loans.

12. In addition to business assets, owners of small businesses, such as medical practices, often are required to pledge personal assets as collateral (make personal guarantees) for bank business loans.

13. For more information on the use of receivables financing by healthcare providers, see T. J. Kincaid, "Selling Accounts Receivable to Fund Working Capital," *Healthcare Financial Management* (May 1993): 27–32.

References

Adams, W. T., G. M. Snow, and P. M. Helmick. 2000. "Automated Charge Processing Streamlines Data Entry." *Healthcare Financial Management* (May): 50–53.

Anderson, A. M. 1993. "Enhancing Hospital Cash Reserves Management." *Healthcare Financial Management* (July): 91–95.

Atchison, K. 2003. "Surefire Strategies to Reduce Claim Denial." *Healthcare Financial Management* (May): 54–58.

Bruch, N. M., and L. L. Lewis. 1994. "Using Control Charts to Help Manage Accounts Receivable." *Healthcare Financial Management* (July): 44–48.

Brody, P. 2007. "The Time Is Right for Supply Chain Synchronization." *Healthcare Financial Management* (February): 94–98.

Calvello, A. A. 2003. "Investment Management: Eight Steps to Improve Performance." *Healthcare Financial Management* (June): 45–50.

Cantone, L., and A. Bullock. 2000. "Getting Tough with Home Health Receivables." *Healthcare Financial Management* (April): 44–49.

Cathey, R. 2003. "5 Ways to Reduce Claims Denials." *Healthcare Financial Management* (August): 44–48.

Clarkin, J. F. 1990. "Managing Accounts Receivable." *Topics in Health Care Financing* (Fall): 1–93.

Coyne, J. S. 1987. "Corporate Cash Management in Health Care: Can We Do Better?" *Healthcare Financial Management* (September): 76–79.

D'Eramo, M., and L. Umbreit. 2005. "Thinking Inside the (Lock)Box: Using Banking Technology to Improve the Revenue Cycle." *Healthcare Financial Management* (August): 90–93.

Dias, K., and D. Stockamp. 1992. "Nursing Process Approach Improves Receivables Management." *Healthcare Financial Management* (September): 55–64.

Dixon, L. H., and S. K. Bossert. 1993. "The Commercial Bank as Investment Advisor for Hospital Investable Assets." *Topics in Health Care Financing* (Summer): 58–68.

Doody, D. 2007. "Measuring Up: Investment Policies and Practices in Not-for-Profit Health Care." *Healthcare Financial Management* (January): 124–128.

Edwards, D. E., W. C. Hamilton, and R. Hauser. 1991. "Financial Reserve: Hospitals Leery of Credit Lines, Factoring Receivables." *Healthcare Financial Management* (October): 82–88.

Ferconio, S., and M. R. Lane. 1991. "Financing Maneuvers: Two Opportunities to Boost a Hospital's Working Capital." *Healthcare Financial Management* (October): 74–80.

Folk, M. D., and P. R. Roest. 1995. "Converting Accounts Receivable into Cash." *Healthcare Financial Management* (September): 74–78.

Frohlich, R. M., Jr. 1994. "Effective Reassignment of Accounts Can Decrease Bad Debt." *Healthcare Financial Management* (July): 37–42.

Funsten, R. S. 1993. "Accounts Receivable Management." *Topics in Health Care Financing* (Fall): 1–91.

Green, L. A. 1993. "Cash Management: Acceleration and Information Strategies." *Topics in Health Care Financing* (Summer): 44–57.

Gapenski, L. C. 1999. "Debt Maturity Structures Should Match Risk Preferences." *Healthcare Financial Management* (December): 56–59.

Groenevelt, C. J. 1990. "Applying Japanese Management Tips to Patient Accounts." *Healthcare Financial Management* (April): 46–55.

Guyton, E. M., and C. Lund. 2003. "Transforming the Revenue Cycle." *Healthcare Financial Management* (March): 72–78.

Guyton, E., and J. Poats. 2004. "Are You Getting the Most from Your Revenue-Cycle Management System?" *Healthcare Financial Management* (April): 48–51.

Haavik, S. 2000. "Building a Demand-Driven, Vendor Managed Supply Chain." *Healthcare Financial Management* (February): 56–61.

Hammer, D. C. 2005. "Performance is Reality: How is Your Revenue Cycle Holding UP?" *Healthcare Financial Management* (July): 49–56.

Hauser, R. C., D. E. Edwards, and J. T. Edwards. 1991. "Cash Budgeting: An Underutilized Resource Management Tool in Not-for-Profit Health Care Entities." *Hospital & Health Services Administration* (Fall): 439–446.

Healthcare Financial Management Association (HFMA). 2004. "Linking Supply Costs and Revenue: The Time Has Come." *Healthcare Financial Management* (May): 97–98.

HFMA Roundtable. 2004. "No Nonsense Tactics for Revenue-Cycle Improvement." *Healthcare Financial Management* (February): 68–74.

Hoagland, C., N. Zar, and H. Nelson. 2007. "Leveraging Technology to Drive Revenue Cycle Results." Healthcare Financial Management (February): 70–76.

Kapel, A. S., et al. 2004. "Increasing Up-Front Collections." *Healthcare Financial Management* (March): 82–88.

Kelly, V. K. 1993. "Banks As a Source of Capital." *Topics in Health Care Financing* (Summer): 21–34.

Kincaid, T. J. 1993. "Selling Accounts Receivable to Fund Working Capital." *Healthcare Financial Management* (May): 27–32.

Kowalski, J. C. 1991. "Inventory to Go: Can Stockless Deliver Efficiency." *Healthcare Financial Management* (November): 21–34.

———. 1991. "Materials Management Crucial to Overall Efficiency." *Healthcare Financial Management* (January): 40–44.

Ladewig, T. L., and B. A. Hecht. 1993. "Achieving Excellence in the Management of Accounts Receivable." *Healthcare Financial Management* (September): 25–32.

Malin, J. H. 2006. "Knowing the SCOR: Using Business Metrics to Gain Measurable Improvements." *Healthcare Financial Management* (July): 54–59.

Marshall, S. 1993. "Cost Justifying the Electronic Billing Decision." *Healthcare Financial Management* (June): 68–72.

Maronson, L. N. 1992. "Banks Aggressively Marketing Cash Management Services." *Healthcare Financial Management* (December): 59–60.

McGinnis, M., E. Stark, and K. O'Leesky. 2005. "Supply and Conquer." *Healthcare Financial Management* (March): 82–86.

Moynihan, J. J. 1993. "Improving the Claims Process with EDI." *Healthcare Financial Management* (January): 48–52.

Neumann, L. 2003. "Streamlining the Supply Chain." *Healthcare Financial Management* (July): 56–62.

Newton, R. L. 1993. "Measuring Accounts Receivable Performance: A Comprehensive Method." *Healthcare Financial Management* (May): 33–36.

Palmer, D. 2004. "Key Tools for Turning Receivables into Cash." *Healthcare Financial Management* (February): 62–67.

Phillips, B. 2003. "Navigating Payment Pitfalls in Managed Care." *Healthcare Financial Management* (February): 40–43.

Prince, T. R., and R. Ramanan. 1992. "Collection Performance: An Empirical Analysis of Not-for-Profit Community Hospitals." *Hospital & Health Services Administration* (Summer): 181–196.

Reiss, J. B., and S. J. Di Cioccio. 1991. "Where There's a Will: How to Finance Medicare Receivables—Legally." *Healthcare Financial Management* (October): 90–96.

Rivenson, H. L., J. R. C. Wheeler, D. G. Smith, and K. L. Reiter. 2000. "Cash Management in Health Care Systems." *Journal of Health Care Finance* (Summer): 56–69.

Robinson, E. F. 1989. "Automated Collection Systems Improve Cash Flow." *Healthcare Financial Management* (December): 31–40.

Scotti, D. J., et al. 2003. "Best Practices for Preempting Payment Denials." *Healthcare Financial Management* (April): 72–82.

Seidner, A. G. 1987. "Reviewing the Basics of Investment Management." *Healthcare Financial Management* (October): 68–72.

Sen, S., and J. P. Lawler. 1995. " Securitizing Receivables Offers Low-Cost Financing Option." *Healthcare Financial Management* (May): 32–37.

Slater, R. M., R. Corti, and J. Privitera. 1991. "Giving Receivables an 'Outside' Chance." *Healthcare Financial Management* (October): 56–66.

Solberg, T. 2003. "How Have Hospital Investments Navigated Troubled Waters?" *Healthcare Financial Management* (September): 78–83.

Souders, R. V. 1990. "Electronic Claims Can be a Remedy for Cash Flow Troubles." *Healthcare Financial Management* (June): 62–68.

Spiegel, M. 1989. "Selling Accounts Receivable Can Improve Cash Flow." *Healthcare Financial Management* (September): 40–46.

Spradling, M. 2003. "Structuring a Sound Securitization of Healthcare Receivables." *Healthcare Financial Management* (February): 58–64.

Swarzman, G. F. 1994. "Does Your Patient Accounting System Pass the Systems Test?" *Healthcare Financial Management* (July): 27–34.

Tobe, C. 2003. "Rx for Low Cash Yields." *Healthcare Financial Management* (October): 76–82.

Waymack, P. M. 2004. "Light at the End of the Tunnel for Denials Management." *Healthcare Financial Management* (August): 57–65.

Zimmerman, D. 1993. *Cash is King.* Franklin, WI: Eagle Press.

FINANCIAL CONDITION ANALYSIS

Learning Objectives

After studying this chapter, readers will be able to:

- Explain the purposes of financial statement and operating indicator analyses.
- Describe the primary techniques used in financial statement and operating indicator analyses.
- Conduct basic financial statement and operating indicator analyses to assess the financial condition of a business.
- Describe the problems associated with financial statement and operating indicator analyses.
- Explain the Economic Value Added (EVA) model and its relevance to healthcare businesses.
- Describe how Key Performance Indicators (KPIs) and dashboards can be used to monitor financial condition.

Introduction

One of the most important characteristics of a business is its *financial condition*: Does the business have the financial capacity to perform its mission? Often, judgments about financial condition are made on the basis of *financial statement analysis*, which focuses on the data contained in a business's financial statements. Financial statement analysis is applied both to historical data, which reflect the results of past managerial decisions, and to forecasted data, which comprise the roadmap for the business's future. Therefore, managers use financial statement analysis both to assess current condition and to plan for the future.

Although financial statement analysis provides a great deal of important information regarding financial condition, it often fails to provide much insight into the operational causes of that condition. Thus, financial statement analysis is often supplemented by *operating indicator analysis*, which uses operating data not usually found in a business's financial statements, such as occupancy, patient mix, length of stay, and productivity measures, to help identify those factors that contributed to the assessed financial condition. Through operating indicator analysis, managers are better able to identify and implement strategies that ensure a sound financial condition in the future.

Financial condition analysis involves a number of techniques that extract information contained in a business's financial statements and elsewhere and combine it in a form that facilitates making judgments about the business's financial condition and operations. Often, the end result is a list of corporate strengths and weaknesses. In this chapter, several analytical techniques used in financial condition analyses, some related topics, and the problems inherent in such analyses are discussed. Along the way, you will discover that financial condition analysis generates a great deal of data. A significant problem in assessing financial condition is separating the important from the unimportant and presenting the results in a simple, easy to monitor format. Thus, we close the chapter with some ideas about data presentation.

Financial Statements

As you learned in the earlier chapters of this text, accounting standards require businesses to prepare several *financial statements,* including three basic financial statements: (1) the *income statement,* (2) the *balance sheet,* and (3) the *statement of cash flows.* Taken together, these statements give an accounting picture of the firm's operations and its financial position. Detailed data are provided for the two or three most recent periods, and brief historical summaries of key operating statistics for longer periods often are included.

In much of this chapter, Riverside Memorial Hospital, a 450-bed not-for-profit facility, is used to illustrate financial condition analysis. Although a hospital is being used to illustrate the techniques, they can be applied to any health services setting. Simplified versions of Riverside's primary financial statements are contained in Tables 17.1, 17.2, and 17.3. Riverside's income statements and balance sheets (Tables 17.1 and 17.2) will be examined in later sections when we discuss ratio analysis and other tools that are used to help interpret the data. For now, our focus is on the statement of cash flows, which can be interpreted without the need for additional data manipulation.

The statement of cash flows (Table 17.3), first described in Chapter 4, tells such things as whether or not the firm's core operations are profitable, how much capital the firm raised and how this capital was used, and what impact operating and financing decisions had on the firm's cash position.

The top part shows cash generated by and used in operations during 2007. For Riverside, operations provided $11,196,000 in net cash flow. The income statement reported net income plus depreciation of $8,572,000 + $4,130,000 = $12,702,000, but as part of its operations Riverside invested $1,297,000 in current assets (receivables and inventories) and reduced its spontaneous liabilities (payables and accruals) balances by $209,000. The end result, *net cash flow from operations,* is $12,702,000 − $1,297,000 − $209,000 = $11,196,000.

	2007	2006
Net patient service revenue	$108,600	$ 97,393
Premium revenue	5,232	4,622
Other revenue	3,644	6,014
Total revenues	$117,476	$108,029
Expenses:		
Nursing services	$ 58,285	$ 56,752
Dietary services	5,424	4,718
General services	13,198	11,655
Administrative services	11,427	11,585
Employee health and welfare	10,250	10,705
Provision for uncollectibles	3,328	3,469
Provision for malpractice	1,320	1,204
Depreciation	4,130	4,025
Interest expense	1,542	1,521
Total expenses	$108,904	$105,634
Net income	$ 8,572	$ 2,395

TABLE 17.1
Riverside Memorial Hospital: Statements of Operations (Income Statements) Years Ended December 31, 2007 and 2006 (in thousands)

The next section of the statement of cash flows focuses on investments in fixed assets. Riverside spent $4,293,000 on capital expenditures in 2007. Is that a large or small amount? The top part of the statement of cash flows reports a depreciation expense for 2007 of $4,130,000, so the hospital spent only slightly more than its depreciation on new fixed assets. Thus, it is likely that the capital expenditures were more to replace worn out and obsolete assets than to add a significant amount of new assets.

Riverside's financing activities, as shown in the third section, highlight the fact that the hospital used cash to pay off previously incurred debt and to invest in marketable securities. The net effect of the hospital's financing activities is a *net cash outflow from financing* of $7,735,000.

When the three major sections are totaled, Riverside had a $11,196,000 − $4,293,000 − $7,735,000 = $832,000 *net decrease in cash* (i.e., net cash outflow) during 2007. The very bottom of Table 17.3 reconciles the 2007 net cash flow with the ending cash balance shown on the balance sheet. Riverside began 2007 with $5,095,000; experienced a cash outflow of $832,000 during the year; and ended the year with $5,095,000 − $832,000 = $4,263,000 in its cash account, as verified by the value reported on Table 17.2.

Riverside's statement of cash flows shows nothing unusual or alarming. It does show that the hospital's operations are inherently profitable, at least in 2007. Had the statement showed an operating cash drain, Riverside's managers would have had something to worry about; if it continued, such

TABLE 17.2
Riverside
Memorial
Hospital:
Balance Sheets
December 31,
2007 and 2006
(in thousands)

	2007	2006
Cash	$ 4,263	$ 5,095
Short-term investments	2,000	0
Accounts receivable	21,840	20,738
Inventories	3,177	2,982
Total current assets	$ 31,280	$ 28,815
Gross plant and equipment	$ 145,158	$140,865
Accumulated depreciation	25,160	21,030
Net plant and equipment	$ 119,998	$ 119,835
Total assets	$ 151,278	$148,650
Accounts payable	$ 4,707	$ 5,145
Accrued expenses	5,650	5,421
Notes payable	2,975	6,237
Total current liabilities	$ 13,332	$ 16,803
Long-term debt	$ 30,582	$ 33,055
Net assets (equity)	$107,364	$ 98,792
Total liabilities and net assets	$ 151,278	$148,650

a drain could bleed the hospital to death. The statement of cash flows also provides easily interpreted information about Riverside's financing and fixed asset investing activities for the year. For example, Riverside's cash flow from operations was used primarily to purchase replacement fixed assets, to invest in short-term securities, and to pay off notes payable and long-term debt. Again, such uses of operating cash flow do not raise any red flags regarding the hospital's financial actions.

Managers and investors must pay close attention to the statement of cash flows. Financial condition is driven by cash flows, and the statement gives a good picture of the annual cash flows generated by the business. An examination of Table 17.3 (or better yet, a series of such tables going back the last five years and projected five years into the future) would give Riverside's managers and creditors an idea of whether or not the hospital's operations are self-sustaining—that is, does the business generate the cash flows necessary to pay its bills, including those associated with the capital employed? Although the statement of cash flows is filled with valuable information, the bottom line tells little about the business's financial condition because operating losses can be covered by financing transactions such as borrowing or selling new common stock (if investor-owned), at least in the short run.

Cash Flows from Operating Activities		**TABLE 17.3**
Change in net assets (net income)	$ 8,572	Riverside
Adjustments:		Memorial
Depreciation	4,130	Hospital:
Increase in accounts receivable	(1,102)	Statement of
Increase in inventories	(195)	Cash Flows
Decrease in accounts payable	(438)	Year Ended
Increase in accrued expenses	229	December 31,
Net cash flow from operations	$11,196	2007 (in
		thousands)
Cash Flows from Investing Activities		
Investment in plant and equipment	($ 4,293)	
Cash Flows from Financing Activities		
Investment in short-term securities	($ 2,000)	
Repayment of long-term debt	(2,473)	
Repayment of notes payable	(3,262)	
Net cash flow from financing	($ 7,735)	
Net increase (decrease) in cash	($ 832)	
Beginning cash and equivalents	$ 5,095	
Ending cash and securities	$ 4,263	

Self-Test Questions

1. What are the three primary financial statements?
2. What type of financial performance information is provided in the statement of cash flows?
3. What is the difference between net income and cash flow, and which is more meaningful to a business's financial condition?
4. Does the fact that a business's cash position has improved provide much insight into the year's financial results?

Financial Ratio Analysis

The first step in most financial condition analyses is to examine the business's financial statements. Thus, in the last section we analyzed Riverside's statement of cash flows. This was done first because this statement is formatted in a way that facilities interpretation without further data manipulation. Now we examine the income statement and balance sheet. Although these statements contain a wealth of financial information, it is difficult to make meaningful judgments about financial condition by merely examining the statements' raw data. To illustrate, one managed care plan may have $5,248,760 in long-term debt and interest charges of $419,900, while another may have $52,647,980 in debt and interest charges of $3,948,600. The true burden of these debts, and each managed care plan's ability to pay the interest and principal due on them, cannot be easily assessed without additional comparisons, such as those provided by *ratio analysis*.

In essence, ratio analysis combines data to create single numbers that have easily interpreted significance (for our purposes, numbers that measure various aspects of financial condition). *Financial ratio analysis* is ratio analysis applied to the data contained in a business's income statement and balance sheet. In the case of the debt and interest payments described above, ratios could be constructed that relate each plan's debt to its assets and the interest it pays to the income it has available for payment.

Unfortunately, an almost unlimited number of financial ratios can be constructed, and the choice of ratios depends in large part on the nature of the business being analyzed, the purpose of the analysis, and the availability of comparative data. Generally, ratios are grouped into categories to make them easier to interpret. In the paragraphs that follow, the data presented in Tables 17.1 and 17.2 are used to calculate an illustrative sampling of 2007 financial ratios for Riverside Memorial Hospital, which are then compared with hospital industry average ratios.[1] Note that in a real analysis, many more ratios would be calculated and analyzed. Also, although a hospital is used to illustrate ratio analysis, the specific ratios used in any analysis depend on the type of healthcare provider. Some ratios are more meaningful for hospitals, some for managed care organizations, some for group practices, and so on.[2]

Profitability Ratios

Profitability is the net result of a large number of managerial policies and decisions, so *profitability ratios* provide one measure of the aggregate financial performance of a business.

Total Margin

The *total margin*, often called the *total profit margin* or just *profit margin*, is defined as net income divided by total revenues:

$$\text{Total margin} = \frac{\text{Net income}}{\text{Total revenues}} = \frac{\$8,572}{\$117,476} = 0.073 = 7.3\%.$$

Industry average = 5.0%.

Riverside's total margin of 7.3 percent shows that the hospital makes 7.3 cents on every dollar of total revenues. The total margin measures the ability of the organization to control expenses. With all else the same, the higher the total margin, the lower the expenses relative to revenues. Riverside's total margin is above the industry average of 5 percent, indicating relatively good expense control. How good? The industry data source also reports quartiles; for total margin, the upper quartile was 8.4 percent, meaning that 25 percent of hospitals had total margins higher than 8.4 percent. Thus, although Riverside's total margin was better than average, it was not as good as the top 25 percent of hospitals.

Although industry average figures are discussed in detail later in the chapter, it should be noted here that the industry average is not a magic number that all businesses should strive to achieve. In fact, some very well-managed businesses will be above the average, while other good firms will be below it. However, if a business's ratios are far removed from the average for the industry, its managers should be concerned about why this difference occurs.

Riverside's relatively high total margin could mean that the hospital's charges are relatively high, its allowances are relatively low, its costs are relatively low, it has relatively high nonoperating (other) revenue, or a combination of these factors. A thorough operating indicator analysis would help pinpoint the cause, or causes, of Riverside's high total margin.

When data are available, another useful margin ratio is the *operating margin*, defined as operating income divided by operating revenues. (Operating revenues are defined here as patient service revenue plus premium revenue.) The advantage of this margin measure is that it focuses on core business operations and hence removes the influence of nonoperating gains and losses, which often are transitory and unrelated to core operations. However, the format of many healthcare organizations' financial statements makes this ratio difficult to determine without additional information.

With only the data given in the financial statements, Riverside's operating margin can be estimated as follows: First, Riverside's operating revenue for 2007 was $108,600,000 + $5,232,000 = $113,832,000. If the assumption is made that all expenses were operating expenses, Riverside's 2007 operating margin would be ($113,832 − $108,904) / $113,832 = $4,928 / $113,832 = 0.043 = 4.3%. Removing nonoperating (other) revenue from the calculation lowers the profit margin.

Return on Assets (ROA)

The ratio of net income to total assets measures the *return on total assets*, often just called *return on assets* (*ROA*):

$$\text{Return on assets} = \frac{\text{Net income}}{\text{Total assets}} = \frac{\$8,572}{\$151,278} = 0.057 = 5.7\%.$$

Industry average = 4.8%.

Riverside's 5.7 percent ROA, which means that each dollar of assets generated 5.7 cents in profit, is well above the 4.8 percent average for the hospital industry. ROA tells managers how productively, in a financial sense, a business is using its assets. The higher the ROA, the greater the net income for each dollar invested in assets and hence the more productive the assets. ROA measures both a business's ability to control expenses, as expressed by the total margin, and its ability to use its assets to generate revenue.

Return on Equity (ROE)

The ratio of net income to total equity (net assets) measures the *return on equity (ROE)*:

$$\text{Return on equity} = \frac{\text{Net income}}{\text{Total equity}} = \frac{\$8,572}{\$107,364} = 0.080 = 8.0\%.$$

Industry average $= 8.4\%$.

Riverside's 8 percent ROE is slightly below the 8.4 percent industry average. The hospital was able to generate 8 cents of income for each dollar of equity investment, while the average hospital produced 8.4 cents. ROE is especially meaningful for investor-owned businesses because owners are concerned with how well the business's managers are utilizing owner-supplied capital, and ROE gives the answer to this question. For not-for-profit businesses such as Riverside, ROE tells its board of trustees and managers how well, in **financial terms**, its community-supplied capital is being used.

Riverside's 2007 total margin and return on assets were above the industry averages, yet the hospital's ROE is below the average. As we will explain later in the section on Du Pont analysis, this seeming inconsistency is a result of the hospital's relatively low use of debt financing.

Liquidity Ratios

One of the first concerns of most managers, and the major concern of a firm's creditors, is the business's *liquidity*. Will the business be able to meet its obligations as they become due? Riverside has debts totaling more than $13 million (i.e., its current liabilities) that must be paid off within the coming year. Will the hospital be able to make these payments? A full liquidity analysis requires the use of a *cash budget*, which was discussed in Chapter 8. However, by relating the amount of cash and other current assets to current obligations, ratio analysis provides a quick, easy-to-use, rough measure of liquidity.

Current Ratio

The *current ratio* is calculated by dividing current assets by current liabilities:

$$\text{Current ratio} = \frac{\text{Current assets}}{\text{Current liabilities}} = \frac{\$31,280}{\$13,332} = 2.3, \text{ or } 2.3 \text{ times.}$$

Industry average $= 2.0$.

The current ratio tells managers that the liquidation of Riverside's current assets at book value would provide $2.30 of cash for every $1 of current liabilities. If a business is getting into financial difficulty, it will begin paying its accounts payable more slowly, building up short-term bank loans (i.e., notes payable), and so on. If these current liabilities rise faster than current assets, the current ratio will fall, and this could spell trouble. Because the current ratio is an indicator of the extent to which short-term claims are covered by assets that are expected to be converted to cash in the near term, it is one commonly used measure of liquidity.

Riverside's current ratio is slightly above the average for the hospital industry. Because current assets should be converted to cash in the near future, it is highly probable that these assets could be liquidated at close to their stated values. With a current ratio of 2.3, the hospital could liquidate current assets at only 43 percent of book value and still pay off current creditors in full.[3]

Days Cash on Hand

The current ratio measures liquidity on the basis of balance sheet accounts, and hence is a static measure of liquidity. However, the true measure of a business's liquidity is whether or not it can meet its payments as they become due, and so liquidity is more related to cash flows than it is to assets and liabilities. The *days-cash-on-hand ratio* moves closer to those factors that truly determine liquidity:

$$\text{Days cash on hand} = \frac{\text{Cash} + \text{Marketable securities}}{(\text{Expenses} - \text{Depreciation} - \text{Provision for uncollectibles})/365}$$

$$= \frac{\$4,263 + \$2,000}{(\$108,904 - \$4,130 - \$3,328)/365} = \frac{\$6,263}{\$277.93} = 22.5 \text{ days.}$$

Industry average = 30.6 days.

The denominator of the equation *estimates* average daily cash expenses by stripping out noncash expenses from reported total expenses. The numerator is the cash and securities that are available to make those cash payments. Because Riverside's days cash on hand is lower than the industry average, its liquidity position as measured by days cash on hand is worse than that of the average hospital.

For Riverside, the two measures of liquidity, current ratio and days cash on hand, give conflicting results. Perhaps the average hospital has a greater proportion of cash and marketable securities in its current assets than does Riverside. More analysis would be required to make a supportable judgment concerning Riverside's liquidity position. Remember, though, that the cash budget is the primary tool used by managers to ensure liquidity.

Debt Management (Capital Structure) Ratios

The degree to which a firm uses debt financing, or *financial leverage,* is an important measure of financial performance for several reasons. First, by raising funds through debt, owners of for-profit firms can maintain control of the firm with a limited investment. For not-for-profit firms, debt financing allows the organization to provide more services than it could if it were solely financed with contributed and earned capital. Next, creditors look to equity capital to provide a margin of safety; if the owners (or community) have provided only a small proportion of total financing, the risks of the enterprise are borne mainly by its creditors. Finally, if a firm earns more on investments financed with borrowed funds than it pays in interest, its return on equity capital is magnified, or leveraged up.

Two types of ratios are used to assess debt management:

1. **Capitalization ratios.** These ratios use balance sheet data to determine the extent to which borrowed funds have been used to finance assets.
2. **Coverage ratios.** Here, income statement data are used to determine the extent to which fixed financial charges are covered by reported profits.

The two sets of ratios are complementary, so most financial statement analyses examine both types.

Capitalization Ratio 1: Total Debt to Total Assets (Debt Ratio) The ratio of total debt to total assets (total liabilities and equity), generally called the *debt ratio*, measures the percentage of total capital provided by creditors:

$$\text{Debt ratio} = \frac{\text{Total debt}}{\text{Total assets}} = \frac{\$43,914}{\$151,278} = 0.290, \text{ or } 29.0\%.$$

Industry average = 42.3%.

For our purposes, debt is defined as **all debt**, including current liabilities and long-term debt—everything but equity. However, as illustrated by the next ratio discussed, capitalization ratios have many variations, many of which use different definitions of what constitutes debt.

Creditors prefer low debt ratios because the lower the ratio, the greater the cushion against creditors' losses in the event of bankruptcy and liquidation. Conversely, owners of for-profit firms may seek high leverage either to leverage up returns or because selling new stock would mean giving up some degree of control. In not-for-profit firms, managers may seek high leverage to offer more services.

Riverside's debt ratio is 29 percent. This means that its creditors have supplied somewhat less than one-third of the business's total financing. Put another way, each dollar of assets was financed with 29 cents of debt, and consequently, 71 cents of equity. (The *equity ratio* is 1 − Debt ratio, so Riverside's equity ratio is 71 percent.) Because the average debt ratio for the hospital industry is over 40 percent, Riverside uses significantly less debt than the average hospital. The low debt ratio indicates that the hospital would find it relatively easy to borrow additional funds, presumably at favorable rates.

The *debt-to-equity ratio*, which is defined as Total debt/Total equity, is a close relative of the debt ratio. These ratios are transformations of one another, and hence provide the same information, but with a slightly different twist. Both the debt ratio and debt-to-equity ratio increase as a business uses a greater proportion of debt financing, but the debt ratio rises linearly and approaches a limit of 100 percent, while the debt-to-equity ratio rises exponentially and approaches infinity. Lenders, in particular, prefer the debt-to-equity ratio to the debt ratio. Their preference is based on the fact that it tells them how much capital creditors have provided to the business **per dollar of equity capital**. The higher this ratio, the riskier the creditors' position. Other analysts tend to prefer the debt ratio because it makes it easier to visualize the liabilities and equity portion of the balance sheet.

The *debt-to-capitalization ratio*, which is defined as long-term debt divided by long-term capital (long-term debt plus equity), focuses on the proportion of debt used in a business's permanent (long-term) capital. This ratio is also called the *long-term-debt-to-capitalization ratio* or just *capitalization ratio*.

Capitalization Ratio 2: Debt-to-Capitalization Ratio

$$\text{Debt-to-capitalization ratio} = \frac{\text{Long-term debt}}{\text{Long-term debt} + \text{Equity}}$$

$$= \frac{\$30,582}{\$30,582 + \$107,364} = 0.222, \text{ or } 22.2\%.$$

Industry average = 34.6%.

Many analysts believe that the debt-to-capitalization ratio best reflects the capital structure of a business. This belief is based on the fact that most businesses use as much spontaneous free credit (current liabilities less short-term bank loans) as they can get. Furthermore, short-term interest-bearing debt typically is used only to fund **temporary** current asset needs. Thus, the "true" capital structure of a business—the one that reflects its target structure—is best reflected by the debt-to-capitalization ratio, which focuses on permanent (long-term) financing.

Riverside's debt-to-capitalization ratio is 22.2 percent, compared to the industry average of 34.6 percent. This low use of debt financing in Riverside's permanent capital mix confirms the conclusion made earlier that the hospital has unused debt capacity.

The *times interest earned (TIE) ratio* is determined by dividing earnings before interest and taxes (EBIT) by interest charges. EBIT is used in the numerator because it represents the amount of income that is available to pay interest expense. For a not-for-profit business, which does not pay taxes, EBIT = Net income + Interest expense. For Riverside:

Coverage Ratio 1: Times Interest Earned Ratio

$$\text{TIE ratio} = \frac{\text{EBIT}}{\text{Interest expense}} = \frac{\$8,572 + \$1,542}{\$1,542} = \frac{\$10,114}{\$1,542} = 6.6 \text{ times.}$$

Industry average = 4.0.

The TIE ratio measures the number of dollars of income (as opposed to cash flow) available to pay each dollar of interest expense. In essence, it is an indicator of the extent to which income can decline before it is less than annual interest costs. Failure to pay interest can bring legal action by the firm's creditors, possibly resulting in bankruptcy.

Riverside's interest is covered 6.6 times, so it has $6.60 of accounting income to pay each dollar of interest expense. Because the industry average TIE ratio is four times, the hospital is covering its interest charges by a relatively high margin of safety. Thus, the TIE ratio reinforces the previous conclusions based on the debt and debt-to-capitalization ratios—namely, that the hospital could easily expand its use of debt financing.

Coverage ratios are often better measures of a firm's debt utilization than capitalization ratios because coverage ratios discriminate between low-interest rate debt and high-interest rate debt. For example, a group practice might have $10 million of 4 percent debt on its balance sheet, while another might have $10 million of 8 percent debt. If both practices have the same income and assets, both would have the same debt ratio. However, the group that pays 4 percent interest would have lower interest charges and hence would be in better financial condition than the group that pays 8 percent. This difference in financial condition is captured by the TIE ratio.

Coverage Ratio 2: Cash Flow Coverage Ratio

Although the TIE ratio is easy to calculate, it has two major deficiencies. First, leasing has become widespread in recent years, and the TIE ratio ignores lease payments, which like debt payments, are contractual obligations. Also, many debt contracts require that principal payments be made over the life of the loan, rather than only at maturity. Thus, most businesses must meet fixed financial charges other than interest payments. Second, the TIE ratio ignores the fact that accounting income, whether measured by EBIT or net income, does not reflect the actual cash flow available to meet a business's fixed payments. These deficiencies are corrected in the *cash flow coverage (CFC) ratio,* which shows the amount by which cash flow covers fixed financial requirements. Here is Riverside's 2007 CFC ratio assuming the hospital had $1,368,000 of lease payments and $2,000,000 of required debt principal repayments:

$$\text{CFC ratio} = \frac{\text{EBIT} + \text{Lease payments} + \text{Depreciation expense}}{\text{Interest expense} + \text{Lease payments} + \text{Debt principal}/(1-T)}$$

$$= \frac{\$10,114 + \$1,368 + \$4,130}{\$1,542 + \$1,368 + \$2,000/(1-0)} = \frac{\$15,612}{\$4,910} = 3.2 \text{ times.}$$

Industry average = 2.3.

What is the purpose of the $(1 - T)$ term applied to the debt principal? For investor-owned firms, the debt principal repayments, because they are paid with **after-tax dollars**, must be *grossed up* by dividing by $1 - T$. This gives the amount of pretax dollars, contained in the numerator, that are required to cover the required principal repayments.

Like its TIE ratio, Riverside's CFC ratio exceeds industry standard, indicating that Riverside is better at covering total fixed payments with cash flow than is the average hospital. This fact should be reassuring both to creditors and to management, and it reinforces the view that Riverside has untapped debt capacity.

Asset Management (Activity) Ratios

The next group of ratios, the *asset management ratios,* is designed to measure how effectively a business's assets are being utilized. These ratios help to answer whether or not the amount of each type of asset reported on the balance sheet seems reasonable, too high, or too low in view of current (or projected) operating levels. Riverside and other hospitals must borrow or raise equity capital to acquire assets. If they have too many assets, then their capital costs will be too high and their profits will be depressed. Conversely, if the level of assets is too low, then volume may be lost or vital services not offered.

The *fixed asset turnover ratio*, also called the *fixed asset utilization ratio,* measures the utilization of plant and equipment, and it is the ratio of total revenues to net fixed assets:

Fixed Asset Turnover Ratio

$$\text{Fixed asset turnover} = \frac{\text{Total revenues}}{\text{Net fixed assets}} = \frac{\$117,476}{\$119,998} = 0.98 \text{ times.}$$

Industry average = 2.2.

Riverside's ratio of 0.98 indicates that each dollar of fixed assets generated 98 cents in revenue. This value compares poorly with the industry average of 2.2 times, indicating that Riverside is not using its fixed assets as productively as the average hospital. (The lower quartile value for the industry is 1.1; thus, Riverside falls in the bottom 25 percent of all hospitals in its fixed asset utilization.)

Before condemning Riverside's management for poor performance, it should be pointed out that a major problem exists with the use of the fixed asset turnover ratio for comparative purposes. Recall that most asset values listed on the balance sheet reflect historical costs rather than current values. Inflation and depreciation have caused the values of many assets that were purchased in the past to be seriously understated. Therefore, if an old hospital that had acquired much of its plant and equipment years ago is compared to a new hospital with the same physical capacity, the old hospital, because of a much lower book value of fixed assets, would report a much higher turnover ratio. This difference in fixed asset turnover is more reflective of the inability of financial statements to deal with inflation than of any inefficiency on the part of the new hospital's managers.

Total Asset Turnover Ratio   The *total asset turnover ratio* measures the turnover, or utilization, of all of a business's assets. It is calculated by dividing total revenues by total assets:

$$\text{Total asset turnover} = \frac{\text{Total revenues}}{\text{Total assets}} = \frac{\$117,476}{\$151,278} = 0.78 \text{ times.}$$

Industry average $= 0.97$.

Thus, each dollar of total assets generated 78 cents in total revenue. Riverside's total asset ratio is below the industry average but not as far below as its fixed asset turnover ratio. Thus, relative to the industry, the hospital is utilizing its current assets better than its fixed assets. Such judgments could be confirmed by examining Riverside's current asset turnover.[4]

Days in Patient Accounts Receivable   *Days in patient accounts receivable* is used to measure effectiveness in managing receivables. This measure of financial performance, which is sometimes classified as a liquidity ratio rather than an asset management ratio, has many names, including *average collection period (ACP)* and *days' sales outstanding (DSO)*. It is computed by dividing net patient accounts receivable by average daily patient revenue to find the number of days that it takes an organization, on average, to collect its receivables:[5]

$$\text{Days in patient accounts receivable} = \frac{\text{Net patient accounts receivable}}{\text{Net patient service revenue}/365}$$

$$= \frac{\$21,840}{\$108,600/365} = 73.4 \text{ days.}$$

Industry average $= 64.0$ days.

In the calculation for Riverside, premium revenue has not been included because such revenue is collected before services are provided and hence does not affect receivables.

Riverside is not doing as well as the average hospital in collecting its receivables. The lower quartile value is 78.7 days, so a relatively large number of hospitals are doing worse. Still, as was discussed in Chapter 16, it is important that businesses collect their receivables as soon as possible. Clearly, Riverside's managers should strive to increase the hospital's performance in this key area.

Other Ratios

The final group of ratios examines other facets of a business's financial condition.

Average Age of Plant   The *average age of plant* gives a rough measure of the average age in years of a business's fixed assets:

$$\text{Average age of plant} = \frac{\text{Accumulated depreciation}}{\text{Depreciation expense}} = \frac{\$25,160}{\$4,130} = 6.1 \text{ years.}$$

Industry average $= 9.1$ years.

Riverside's physical assets are newer than those of the average hospital. Thus, the hospital is offering more up-to-date facilities than average, and hence it will probably have fewer capital expenditures in the near future. On the other hand, Riverside's net fixed asset valuation will be relatively high, which as pointed out earlier, biases the hospital's fixed asset and total asset turnover ratios downward. This fact raises serious questions about the interpretation of the turnover ratios calculated previously.

For investor-owned firms with publicly traded stock, some ratios can be developed that relate the firm's stock price to its earnings and book value per share. Such *market value ratios* give managers an indication of what equity investors think of the company's past performance and future prospects.

Price/Earnings Ratio

The *price/earnings (P/E) ratio* shows how much investors are willing to pay per dollar of reported profits. Suppose that the stock of General Home Care, an investor-owned home health care company, sells for $28.50, while the firm had 2007 earnings per share (EPS) of $2.20. Then, its P/E ratio would be 13.0:

$$\text{P/E ratio} = \frac{\text{Price per share}}{\text{Earnings per share}} = \frac{\$28.50}{\$2.20} = 13.0 \text{ times.}$$

Industry average = 15.2.

P/E ratios are higher for firms with high growth prospects, other things held constant, but they are lower for riskier firms. General's P/E ratio is slightly below the average of other investor-owned home health care companies, which suggests that the company is regarded as being somewhat riskier than most, as having poorer growth prospects, or both.

Market/Book Ratio

The ratio of a stock's market price to its book value gives another indication of how investors regard the company. Companies with relatively high rates of return on equity generally sell at higher multiples of book value than those with low returns. General reported $80 million in total equity on its 2007 balance sheet, and the firm had 5 million shares outstanding, so its *book value per share* is $80 / 5 = $16.00. Dividing the price per share by the book value per share gives a *market/book (M/B) ratio* of 1.8 times:

$$\text{M/B ratio} = \frac{\text{Price per share}}{\text{Book value per share}} = \frac{\$28.50}{\$16.00} = 1.8 \text{ times.}$$

Industry average = 2.1.

Investors are willing to pay slightly less for each dollar of General's book value than for that of an average home health care company.

Comparative and Trend Analysis

When conducting ratio analysis, the value of a particular ratio, in the absence of other information, reveals almost nothing about a business's financial con-

FIGURE 17.1
Riverside
Memorial
Hospital: ROE
Analysis,
2003–2007

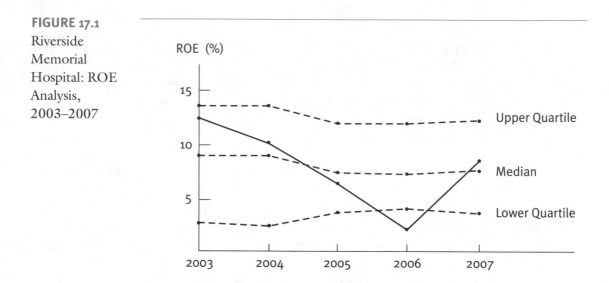

		Return on Equity (ROE)		
			Industry	
Year	Riverside	Lower Quartile	Median	Upper Quartile
2003	12.5%	2.6%	8.6%	13.3%
2004	10.0	2.5	8.6	13.3
2005	6.7	2.8	7.2	12.0
2006	2.4	4.1	7.2	12.1
2007	8.0	3.8	7.4	12.3

dition. For example, if it is known that a nursing home management company has a current ratio of 2.5, it is virtually impossible to say whether this is good or bad. Additional data are needed to help interpret the results of this ratio analysis. In the discussion of Riverside's ratios, the focus was on *comparative analysis*—that is, the hospital's ratios were compared with the average ratios for the industry. Another useful ratio analysis tool is *trend analysis,* in which the trend of a single ratio is analyzed over time. Trend analysis gives clues about whether a business's financial situation is improving, holding constant, or deteriorating.

It is easy to combine comparative and trend analyses in a single graph such as the one shown in Figure 17.1. Here, Riverside's ROE (the solid lines) and industry average ROE data (the dashed lines) are plotted for the past five years. The graph shows that the hospital's ROE was declining faster than the industry average from 2003 through 2006, but that it rose above the industry in 2007. Other ratios can be analyzed in a similar manner.

**Self-Test
Questions**

1. What is the purpose of ratio analysis?
2. What are two ratios that measure profitability?
3. What are two ratios that measure liquidity?
4. What are two ratios that measure debt management?
5. What are two ratios that measure asset management?
6. What are two ratios that measure market value?
7. How can comparative and trend analyses be used to help interpret a
   ratio?

Tying the Financial Ratios Together: Du Pont Analysis

Financial ratio analysis provides a great deal of information about a business's
financial condition, but it does not provide an overview nor does it tie any
of the ratios together. *Du Pont analysis* provides an overview of a business's
financial condition and helps managers and investors understand the relationships among several ratios.[6] Du Pont analysis, so named because managers at
the Du Pont Company developed it, combines basic financial ratios in a way
that provides valuable insights into a firm's financial performance. The analysis
decomposes return on equity (ROE), one of the most important measures of
a business's profitability, into the product of three other ratios, each of which
has an important economic interpretation. The result is the *Du Pont equation*:

$$\text{ROE} = \text{Total margin} \times \text{Total asset turnover} \times \text{Equity multiplier}$$

$$\frac{\text{Net income}}{\text{Total equity}} = \frac{\text{Net income}}{\text{Total revenue}} \times \frac{\text{Total revenue}}{\text{Total assets}} \times \frac{\text{Total assets}}{\text{Total equity}}.$$

Riverside's 2007 data are used to illustrate the Du Pont equation:

$$\frac{\$8,572}{\$107,364} = \frac{\$8,572}{\$117,476} \times \frac{\$117,476}{\$151,278} \times \frac{\$151,278}{\$107,364}$$

$$7.98\% = 7.30\% \times 0.78 \times 1.41$$

$$= 5.69\% \times 1.41.$$

In the Du Pont equation, the product of the first two terms on the right side is
return on assets (ROA), so the equation can also be written as ROE = ROA
× Equity multiplier. Riverside's 2007 total margin was 7.3 percent, so the
hospital made 7.3 cents profit on each dollar of total revenue. Furthermore,
assets were turned over (or created revenues) 0.78 times during the year, so
the hospital earned a return of 7.30% × 0.78 = 5.69% on its assets. This value
for ROA, when rounded, is the same as was calculated previously in our ratio
analysis discussion.

　　If the hospital used only equity financing, its 5.69 percent ROA would
equal its ROE. However, creditors supplied 29 percent of Riverside's capital,

while the equityholders (the community) supplied the rest. Because the 5.69 percent ROA belongs exclusively to the suppliers of equity capital, which comprises only 29 percent of total capital, Riverside's ROE is higher than its 5.69 percent ROA. Specifically, ROA must be multiplied by the *equity multiplier,* which shows the amount of assets working for each dollar of equity capital, to obtain the ROE of 7.98 percent. This 7.98 percent ROE could be calculated directly: ROE = Net income / Total equity = $8,572 / $107,364 = 7.98%. However, the Du Pont equation shows how total margin, which measures **expense control**; total asset turnover, which measures **asset utilization**; and financial leverage, which measures **debt utilization**, interact to determine ROE.

Riverside's managers use the Du Pont equation to suggest how to improve the hospital's financial condition. To influence the profit margin, Riverside must increase revenues and/or reduce costs. Thus, the hospital's marketing staff can study the effects of raising charges, or lowering them to increase volume; moving into new services or markets with higher margins; entering into new contracts with managed care plans; and so on. Furthermore, management accountants can study the expense items and, while working with department heads and clinical staff, can seek ways to reduce costs. More specific ideas regarding actions needed to improve financial condition will be gleaned from an operating indicator analysis, which is discussed later on.

Regarding total asset turnover, Riverside's analysts, while working with both clinical and marketing staffs, can investigate ways of reducing investments in various types of assets. Finally, the hospital's financial staff can analyze the effects of alternative financing strategies on the equity multiplier, seeking to hold down interest expenses and the risks of debt while still using debt to leverage up ROE.

The Du Pont equation provides a useful comparison between a business's performance as measured by ROE and the performance of an average hospital. For example, here is the comparative analysis for 2007:

$$\text{Riverside:} \qquad \text{ROE} = 7.3\% \times 0.78 \times 1.41$$

$$= \quad 5.69\% \quad \times 1.41 \approx 8.0\%.$$

$$\text{Industry average: ROE} = 5.0\% \times 0.97 \times 1.73$$

$$4.85\% \quad \times 1.73 \approx 8.4\%.$$

The Du Pont analysis tells managers and creditors that Riverside has a significantly higher profit margin, and thus better control over expenses, than does the average hospital. However, the average hospital has a better total asset turnover, and thus Riverside is getting below-average utilization from its assets. In spite of the average hospital's advantage in asset utilization, Riverside's superior expense control outweighs its utilization disadvantage because its ROA of 5.69 percent is higher than the industry average ROA of 4.85 percent. Finally, the average hospital has offset Riverside's advantage in ROA by using more financial leverage, although Riverside's lower use of debt financing decreases its risk. The end result is that Riverside gets somewhat less return on its equity capital than does the average hospital.

One potential problem with Du Pont and ratio analyses applied to not-for-profit organizations, especially hospitals, is that a large portion of their net income may come from nonoperating sources rather than from operations. If the nonoperating revenues are highly variable and unpredictable, as they often are, return on equity and the ratios as previously defined may be a poor measure of the hospital's inherent profitability. All applicable ratios, as well as the Du Pont analysis, could be recast to focus on operations by using operating revenue in lieu of total revenue.

---

1. Explain how the Du Pont equation combines several ratios to obtain an overview of a business's financial condition.
2. Why may a focus on operating revenue and operating income be preferable to a focus on total revenue and net income?

Self-Test Questions

Other Analytical Techniques

Besides ratio and Du Pont analyses, two additional financial statement analysis techniques are commonly used in financial condition analysis. In *common size analysis*, all income statement items are divided by total revenues and all balance sheet items are divided by total assets. Thus, a common size income statement shows each item as a percentage of total revenues, and a common size balance sheet shows each account as a percentage of total assets. The advantage of common size statements is that they facilitate comparisons of income statements and balance sheets over time and across companies because they remove the influence of the scale (size) of the business.

Another frequently used technique when analyzing financial statements is *percentage change analysis*. Here, the percentage changes in the balance sheet accounts and income statement items from year to year are calculated and compared. In this format, it is easy to see what accounts and items are growing faster or slower than others and thus to identify which are under control and which are out of control.

The conclusions reached in common size and percentage change analyses generally parallel those derived from ratio analysis. However, occasionally a serious deficiency is highlighted only by one of the three analytical techniques, while the other two techniques fail to bring the deficiency to light. Thus, a thorough financial statement analysis usually consists of a Du Pont analysis to provide an overview and then includes several different techniques such as ratio, common size, and percentage change analyses.[7]

Operating Indicator Analysis

Operating indicator analysis goes one step beyond financial statement analysis in that operating indicator analysis examines operating variables with the goal of **explaining** a business's financial condition. Like the financial ratios, *operating indicators* are typically grouped into major categories to make interpretation easier.

Because of the large number of indicators used in a typical operating indicator analysis, it cannot be discussed in detail here. However, to give readers an appreciation for this type of analysis, six commonly used hospital operating indicators are defined and illustrated. Note that most of the data needed to calculate operating indicators are not contained in a business's financial statements. Thus, a larger data set is required for this type of analysis, and hence it is used more by managers than by outside analysts.

Net Price Per Discharge

Net price per discharge measures the average revenue collected on each inpatient discharge. In 2007, Riverside reported $93,740,000 in inpatient service revenue and discharged 18,281 patients:

$$\text{Net price per discharge} = \frac{\text{Net inpatient revenue}}{\text{Total discharges}} = \frac{\$93,740,000}{18,281} = \$5,128.$$

$$\text{Industry average} = \$5,510.$$

Riverside collects less per discharge than the average hospital, ignoring bad debt losses. However, if Riverside's case mix, which measures the average intensity of services provided, were lower than average, perhaps its net price per discharge is appropriate, even though it is below the industry average. In fact, Riverside's case mix is slightly higher than average. Still, as we explain in a later section, the net price per discharge cannot be completely interpreted without knowing Riverside's cost per discharge.

Medicare Payment Percentage

Medicare payment percentage measures the exposure of a hospital to Medicare patients and hence to payments set by political, rather than economic, processes:

$$\text{Medicare payment percentage} = \frac{\text{Medicare discharges}}{\text{Total discharges}} = \frac{7{,}642}{18{,}281} = 41.8\%.$$

$$\text{Industry average} = 43.5\%.$$

Riverside has a somewhat lower percentage of Medicare patients than the average hospital. To the extent that Medicare payments are less than payments from other third-party payers, a higher Medicare payment percentage puts pressure on operating revenues. Conversely, if Medicare payments are higher than reimbursements by managed care plans, then, in some situations, a higher Medicare payment percentage might be good. Similar operating indicators could be constructed for Medicaid, managed care plan, and bad debt and charity care patients.

Outpatient Revenue Percentage

The *outpatient revenue percentage* measures the mix between outpatient and inpatient revenues:

$$\text{Outpatient revenue percentage} = \frac{\text{Net outpatient revenue}}{\text{Net patient service revenue}} = \frac{\$20{,}092{,}000}{\$113{,}832{,}000} = 17.6\%.$$

$$\text{Industry average} = 34.5\%.$$

Riverside has a much smaller outpatient program, relative to its size, than the average hospital. During the 1990s, most hospitals significantly expanded their outpatient programs based on the belief that such services were more profitable because Medicare paid for outpatient services on a charge basis, whereas inpatient services were paid for on a prospective basis. However, the claims of increased profitability were never proved, and Medicare has since changed to a prospective payment system for outpatient services.

Occupancy Percentage (Rate)

Occupancy rate measures the extent of utilization of a hospital's beds and hence fixed assets. As discussed in Chapter 5, because overhead costs are incurred on all assets, whether used or not, higher occupancy spreads fixed costs over more patients and hence increases per patient profitability. Based on 95,061 inpatient days in 2007, Riverside's occupancy rate was 57.9 percent:

$$\text{Occupancy percentage} = \frac{\text{Inpatient days}}{\text{Number of staffed beds} \times 365} = \frac{95{,}061}{450 \times 365} = 57.9\%.$$

$$\text{Industry average} = 44.9\%.$$

Riverside has a higher occupancy rate and hence is using its fixed assets more productively than the average hospital. It is interesting to note that this conclusion is contrary to the financial analysis interpretation of the hospital's 2007 fixed asset turnover ratio. While that ratio is affected by inflation and accounting convention, the occupancy rate is not. Hence, it is a superior measure of pure asset utilization, at least regarding inpatient assets. On this basis, it appears that Riverside's managers are doing a good job, relative to the industry, of utilizing the hospital's inpatient fixed assets.

Average Length of Stay (ALOS)

Average length of stay (ALOS), or just *length of stay (LOS)*, is the number of days that an average inpatient is hospitalized with each admission.

$$\text{ALOS} = \frac{\text{Inpatient days}}{\text{Total discharges}} = \frac{95,061}{18,281} = 5.2 \text{ days.}$$

Industry average = 4.1 days.

On average, Riverside keeps its patients in the hospital longer than the average hospital does. Riverside has a *case-mix index* of 1.28 compared with an average for the industry of 1.14. The case-mix index is a weighted average of DRG (diagnosis-related group) weights, so the higher the index, the more intense the services provided. Thus, the hospital's patients, on average, require more intensive treatment than patients in the average hospital.

Cost Per Discharge

So far, the operating analysis illustration has focused on revenue and volume measures. *Cost per discharge* measures the dollar amount of resources, on average, expended on each discharge. Because Riverside's inpatient operating expenses for 2007 were $84,865,000, its cost per discharge was $4,642:

$$\text{Cost per discharge} = \frac{\text{Inpatient operating expenses}}{\text{Total discharges}} = \frac{\$84,865,000}{18,281} = \$4,642.$$

Industry average = $5,446.

Even though Riverside's price per discharge is below average, its cost per discharge is even more so. Thus, the hospital's average margin on each discharge is more than that for the hospital industry.

As is apparent from the six operating indicators presented, operating indicator analysis goes beyond financial analysis in an attempt to identify the operating strengths and weaknesses that underlie a firm's financial performance. Although operating indicator analysis has been illustrated using the hospital industry, the concepts can be applied to any healthcare business, although the ratios selected would differ. Also, operating indicators are interpreted in the same way as financial ratios (i.e., by using comparative and trend analysis).

Self-Test Questions

1. What is the difference between financial and operating indicator analyses?
2. Why is operating indicator analysis important?
3. Describe four indicators commonly used in operating indicator analysis.

Limitations of Financial Ratio and Operating Indicator Analyses

While financial ratio and operating indicator analyses can provide a great deal of useful information regarding a business's operations and financial condition, such analyses have limitations that necessitate care and judgment. In this section, some of the problem areas are highlighted.

To begin, many large healthcare businesses operate a number of different divisions in quite different lines of business, and in such cases it is difficult to develop meaningful comparative data. This problem tends to make financial statement and operating indicator analyses somewhat more useful for providers with single service lines than for large, multiservice companies.

Next, generalizing about whether or not a particular ratio or indicator is good or bad is often difficult. For example, a high current ratio may show a strong liquidity position, which is good, or an excessive amount of current assets, which is bad. Similarly, a high asset turnover ratio may denote either a business that uses its assets efficiently or one that is undercapitalized and simply cannot afford to buy enough assets. In addition, firms often have some ratios and indicators that look good and others that look bad, which make the firm's financial position, strong or weak, difficult to determine. For this reason, significant judgment is required when analyzing financial and operating performance.

Another problem is that different accounting practices can distort financial statement ratio comparisons. For example, firms can use different accounting conventions to value cost of goods sold and ending inventories. During inflationary periods these differences can lead to ratio distortions. Other accounting practices, such as those related to leases, can also create distortions.

Finally, inflation effects can distort both firms' balance sheets and income statements. Numerous reporting methods have been proposed to adjust accounting statements for inflation, but no consensus has been reached on how to do this or even on the practical usefulness of the resulting data. Nevertheless, accounting standards encourage, but do not require, businesses to disclose supplementary data to reflect the effects of general inflation. Inflation effects tend to make ratio comparisons over time for a given company, and across companies at any point in time, less reliable than would be the case in the absence of inflation.

1. Briefly describe some of the problems encountered when performing financial statement and operating indicator analyses.
2. Explain how inflation effects created problems in the Riverside illustration.

Self-Test Questions

Economic Value Added (EVA)

Up to this point, we have focused on using different techniques to evaluate the financial condition of a business. In many situations it is useful to have a single measure that provides information on both financial condition and managerial performance. That measure is *Economic Value Added (EVA)*, which focuses on managerial effectiveness in a given year.[8] The basic formula for EVA is:

$$EVA = \text{Net operating profit after taxes (NOPAT)} - (\text{Total capital} \times \text{Corporate cost of capital}).$$

In the EVA equation, NOPAT can be thought of as revenues minus all operating costs, including taxes (if applicable), but excluding interest expense. It is actually calculated as $EBIT \times (1 - T)$. Total capital is the sum of the book values of debt and equity and hence total assets, while the corporate cost of capital is the business's cost of financing. In essence, EVA measures the dollar profit above the economic dollar cost of creating that profit. Because the calculation of EVA does not require market value data, it can be applied to both for-profit and not-for-profit businesses.[9]

To illustrate the EVA concept, consider Birmingham Health Providers, a medical group practice. The group had $1 million in NOPAT in 2007 generated from $5 million of investor-supplied debt and equity capital. The firm's corporate cost of capital was 10 percent. With these assumptions, Birmingham Health Providers's 2007 EVA was $500,000:

$$EVA = \$1 - (\$5 \times 0.10) = \$1 - \$0.5 = \$0.5 \text{ million.}$$

EVA is an estimate of a business's true economic profit for the year, and it differs substantially from accounting profitability measures such as net income. EVA represents the residual income that remains after **all costs**, including the opportunity cost of the employed equity capital, have been recognized. Conversely, accounting profit is formulated without imposing a charge for equity capital. EVA depends on both operating efficiency and balance sheet management: without operating efficiency, profits will be low; without efficient balance sheet management, there will be too many assets and hence too much capital, which results in higher-than-necessary dollar capital costs.

For investor-owned businesses, there is a direct link between EVA and the value of the business—the higher the EVA, the greater the value to owners. For not-for-profit firms, equity capital is a scarce resource that must be managed well to ensure the financial viability of the organization and hence its ability to continue to perform its stated mission. EVA lets managers know how well they are doing in managing this scarce resource because the higher the EVA in any year, the better the job managers are doing in using the organization's contributions and earnings to create value for the community.

Of course, EVA measures only economic value; any social value created by the equity capital is ignored and, therefore, must be subjectively considered. EVA can be applied to divisions as well as to entire businesses, and the charge for capital should reflect the riskiness and capital structure of the business unit, whether it is the aggregate business or an operating division.

In practice, the calculation of EVA is much more complex than presented here because many accounting issues, such as inventory valuation, depreciation, amortization of research and development costs, and the like, must be addressed properly when estimating a firm's NOPAT. In addition, non-interest-bearing debt financing should be subtracted from assets. Nevertheless, the brief discussion here illustrates that a business's true economic profitability depends on both income statement profitability and effective use of balance sheet assets. Specifically, EVA is improved by (1) increasing revenues and decreasing costs, and hence increasing NOPAT; (2) decreasing the amount of assets used to create the NOPAT; and (3) decreasing the business's capital costs. Of course, all of this is easier said than done, and there are potential negative consequences associated with these actions. Still, the EVA model provides a good (but perhaps overly simple) road map to financial excellence.

1. What is Economic Value Added (EVA), and how is it measured? 2. Why is EVA a better measure of financial performance than are accounting measures such as earnings per share and return on equity? 3. What does EVA tell managers about how to achieve good financial performance?	**Self-Test Questions**

Benchmarking

Most techniques for evaluating financial condition require comparisons to make meaningful judgments. In the previous examination of selected financial and operating indicator ratios, Riverside's ratios were compared to industry average ratios. However, like managers in most businesses, Riverside's managers go one step further—they compare their ratios not only with industry averages but also with industry leaders and primary competitors. The technique of comparing ratios against selected standards is called *benchmarking*, while the comparative ratios are called *benchmarks*. Riverside's managers benchmark against industry averages; against National/GFB Healthcare and Pennant Healthcare, which are two leading for-profit hospital businesses; and against Woodbridge Memorial Hospital and St. Anthony's, which are its primary local competitors.

To illustrate the concept, consider how Riverside's analysts present total margin data to the firm's board of trustees:

	2007		2006
National/GFB	9.8%	National/GFB	9.6%
Industry top quartile	*8.4*	*Industry top quartile*	*8.0*
St. Anthony's	8.0	St. Anthony's	7.9
Riverside	**7.3**	Pennant Healthcare	5.0
Industry median	5.0	Industry median	4.7
Pennant Healthcare	4.8	**Riverside**	**2.2**
Industry lower quartile	*1.8*	*Industry lower quartile*	*2.1*
Woodbridge Memorial	0.5	Woodbridge Memorial	(1.3)

Benchmarking permits Riverside's managers to easily see where the firm stands relative to its competition both in any given year and over time. As the data show, Riverside was roughly in the middle of the pack in 2007 with respect to its primary competitors and two large investor-owned hospital chains, although its showing was better than the average hospital. Its 2006 performance was significantly worse, so it improved substantially from 2006 to 2007. Although benchmarking is illustrated with one ratio, other ratios can be analyzed similarly. Also, for presentation purposes, charts are often used with comparative data that are color coded for ease of recognition and interpretation.

All comparative analyses require comparative data. Such data are available from a number of sources, including commercial suppliers, federal and state governmental agencies, and various industry trade groups. Each of these data suppliers uses a somewhat different set of ratios designed to meet its own needs. Thus, the comparative data source selected in a very real sense dictates the ratios that will be used in the analysis. Also, there are minor and sometimes major differences in ratio definitions between data sources—for example, one source may use a 365-day year, while another uses a 360-day year. Or one source might use operating values, as opposed to total values, when constructing ratios. It is **very important** to know the specific definitions used in the comparative data because definitional differences between the ratios being calculated and the comparative ratios can lead to erroneous interpretations and conclusions. Thus, the first task in any ratio analysis is to identify the comparative data set and the ratios to be used. Then, make sure that the ratio definitions used in the analysis match those from the comparative data set.

Self-Test Questions

1. What is benchmarking?
2. Why is it important to be familiar with the comparative data set?

Key Performance Indicators and Dashboards

Financial statement and operating indicator data are usually created on an annual (or perhaps quarterly) basis. Financial condition analyses produced from this information may include literally hundreds of *metrics* (ratios and other measures). Although annual (and quarterly) financial condition analyses are almost always performed, managers need to monitor financial condition on a more regular basis so that problem areas can be identified and corrective action taken in a timely manner. However, the type of financial condition analyses described above with, say, weekly data would overload managers, and as a result, important findings could be missed.

To help solve the data overload and timeliness problems, many health-care businesses use *Key Performance Indicators (KPIs)* and dashboards. KPIs are a **limited number** of financial and operating metrics that measure performance critical to the success of an organization. In essence, they assess the current state of the business, measure progress toward organizational goals, and prompt managerial action to correct deficiencies.

The KPIs chosen by any business depend on the line of business and its mission, objectives, and goals. In addition, KPIs usually differ by timing. For example, a hospital might have a daily KPI of number of net admissions (admissions minus discharges), while the corresponding quarterly and annual KPI might be occupancy rate. Clearly, the number of KPIs used must be kept to a minimum to allow managers to focus on the most important aspects of financial and operating performance.

Dashboards are a common way to present an organization's KPIs. The term stems from an automobile's dashboard, which presents key information (for example, speed, engine temperature, and oil pressure) about the car's performance. Often, the KPIs are shown as gauges, which allow managers to quickly interpret the indicators. The basic idea here is to allow managers to monitor the business's most important financial and operating metrics on a regular basis (daily for some metrics) in a form that is easy to read and interpret.

1. What is a Key Performance Indicator (KPI)? A dashboard? 2. How are KPIs and dashboards used in financial condition analysis?	**Self-Test Questions**

Key Concepts

The primary purpose of this chapter is to present the techniques used by managers and investors to assess a business's financial condition. The main focus is on financial condition as reflected in a business's financial statements, although operating data were also introduced to try to explain a business's current financial status. The key concepts of this chapter are as follows:

- *Financial statement analysis*, which is designed to identify a firm's financial condition, focuses on the firm's financial statements. *Operating indicator analysis*, which uses data typically found outside of the financial statements, provides insights into why a firm is in a given financial condition.

- *Financial ratio analysis*, which focuses on financial statement data, is designed to reveal the relative financial strengths and weaknesses of a company as compared to other companies in the same industry, and to show whether the business's financial condition has been improving or deteriorating over time.

- The *Du Pont equation* indicates how the total margin, the total asset turn over ratio, and the use of debt interact to determine the rate of return on equity. It provides a good overview of a business's financial condition.

- *Liquidity ratios* indicate the business's ability to meet its short-term obligations.

- *Asset management ratios* measure how effectively managers are utilizing the business's assets.

- *Debt management ratios* reveal the extent to which the firm is financed with debt and the extent to which operating cash flows cover debt service and other fixed charge requirements.

- *Profitability ratios* show the combined effects of liquidity, asset management, and debt management on operating results.

- Ratios are analyzed using *comparative analysis*, in which a firm's ratios are compared with industry averages or those of another firm, and *trend analysis*, in which a firm's ratios are examined over time.

- In a *common size analysis*, a business's income statement and balance sheet are expressed in percentages. This facilitates comparisons between firms of different sizes and for a single firm over time.

- In *percentage change analysis*, the differences in income statement items and balance sheet accounts from one year to the next are expressed in percentages. In this way, it is easy to identify those items and accounts that are growing appreciably faster or slower than average.

- *Economic Value Added (EVA)* measures the overall economic performance of a business.

- *Benchmarking* is the process of comparing the performance of a particular company with a group of benchmark companies, often industry leaders and primary competitors.

- Financial condition analysis is hampered by some serious problems, including *development of comparative data, interpretation of results*, and *inflation effects*.

- *Key Performance Indicators (KPIs)* are a limited number of *metrics* that focus on those measures that are most important to an organization's mission success. Often, KPIs are presented in a format that resembles a *dashboard*.

Financial condition analysis has its limitations, but if used with care and judgment, it can provide managers with a sound picture of a business's financial condition as well as identify those operating factors that contributed to that condition.

Questions

17.1 a. What is the primary difference between financial statement analysis and operating indicator analysis?
  b. Why are both types of analyses useful to health services managers and investors?

17.2 Should financial statement and operating indicator analyses be conducted only on historical data? Explain your answer.

17.3 One asset management ratio, the inventory turnover ratio, is defined as sales (i.e., revenues) divided by inventories. Why would this ratio be more important for a medical device manufacturer or a hospital management company?

17.4 a. Assume that Beverly Enterprises and Manor Care, two operators of nursing homes, have fiscal years that end at different times—say, one in June and one in December. Would this fact cause any problems when comparing ratios between the two companies?
  b. Assume that two companies that operate walk-in clinics both had the same December year end, but one was based in Aspen, Colorado, a winter resort, while the other operated in Cape Cod, Massachusetts, a summer resort. Would this lead to problems in a comparative analysis?

17.5 a. How does inflation distort ratio analysis comparisons, both for one company over time and when different companies are compared?
  b. Are only balance sheet accounts or both balance sheet accounts and income statement items affected by inflation?

17.6 a. What is the difference between trend analysis and comparative analysis?
  b. Which one is more important?

17.7 Assume that a large managed care company has a low return on equity (ROE). How could Du Pont analysis be used to identify possible actions to help boost ROE?

17.8 Regardless of the specific line of business, should all healthcare businesses use the same set of ratios when conducting a financial statement analysis? Explain your answer.

17.9 What is EVA, and what does it measure?

17.10 What are Key Performance Indicators (KPIs)? What is a dashboard?

Problems

17.1 a. Modern Medical Devices has a current ratio of 0.5. Which of the following actions would improve (i.e., increase) this ratio?

- Use cash to pay off current liabilities.
- Collect some of the current accounts receivable.
- Use cash to pay off some long-term debt.
- Purchase additional inventory on credit (i.e., accounts payable).
- Sell some of the existing inventory at cost.

b. Assume that the company has a current ratio of 1.2. Now which of the above actions would improve this ratio?

17.2 Southwest Physicians, a medical group practice, is just being formed. It will need $2 million of total assets to generate $3 million in revenues. Furthermore, the group expects to have a profit margin of 5 percent. The group is considering two financing alternatives. First, it can use all-equity financing by requiring each physician to contribute his or her pro rata share. Alternatively, the practice can finance up to 50 percent of its assets with a bank loan. Assuming that the debt alternative has no impact on the expected profit margin, what is the difference between the expected ROE if the group finances with 50 percent debt versus the expected ROE if it finances entirely with equity capital?

17.3 Riverside Memorial's financial statements are presented in Tables 17.1, 17.2, and 17.3.

a. Calculate Riverside's financial ratios for 2006. Assume that Riverside had $1,000,000 in lease payments and $1,400,000 in debt principal repayments in 2006. (Hint: Use the book discussion to identify the applicable ratios.)

b. Interpret the ratios. Use both trend and comparative analysis. For the comparative analysis, assume that the industry average data presented in the book is valid for both 2006 and 2007.

17.4 Consider the following financial statements for BestCare HMO, a not-for-profit managed care plan:

BestCare HMO
Statement of Operations and Change in Net Assets
Year Ended June 30, 2007
(in thousands)

Revenue:	
Premiums earned	$26,682
Co-insurance	1,689
Interest and other income	242
Total revenue	$28,613
Expenses:	
Salaries and benefits	$15,154
Medical supplies and drugs	7,507
Insurance	3,963
Provision for bad debts	19
Depreciation	367
Interest	385

Total expenses	$27,395
Net income	$ 1,218
Net assets, beginning of year	$ 900
Net assets, end of year	$ 2,118

BestCare HMO
Balance Sheet
June 30, 2007
(in thousands)

Assets

Cash and cash equivalents	$ 2,737
Net premiums receivable	821
Supplies	387
Total current assets	$ 3,945
Net property and equipment	$ 5,924
Total assets	$ 9,869

Liabilities and Net Assets

Accounts payable–medical services	$ 2,145
Accrued expenses	929
Notes payable	141
Current portion of long-term debt	241
Total current liabilities	$ 3,456
Long-term debt	$ 4,295
Total liabilities	$ 7,751
Net assets (equity)	$ 2,118
Total liabilities and net assets	$ 9,869

a. Perform a Du Pont analysis on BestCare. Assume that the industry average ratios are as follows:

Total margin	3.8%
Total asset turnover	2.1
Equity multiplier	3.2
Return on equity (ROE)	25.5%

b. Calculate and interpret the following ratios for BestCare:

	Industry Average
Return on assets (ROA)	8.0%
Current ratio	1.3
Days cash on hand	41 days
Average collection period	7 days
Debt ratio	69%
Debt-to-equity ratio	2.2

Times interest earned (TIE) ratio	2.8
Fixed asset turnover ratio	5.2

17.5 Consider the following financial statements for Green Valley Nursing Home, Inc., a for-profit, long-term care facility:

Green Valley Nursing Home, Inc.
Statement of Income and Retained Earnings
Year Ended December 31, 2007

Revenue:	
Net patient service revenue	$ 3,163,258
Other revenue	106,146
Total revenues	$ 3,269,404
Expenses:	
Salaries and benefits	$ 1,515,438
Medical supplies and drugs	966,781
Insurance and other	296,357
Provision for bad debts	110,000
Depreciation	85,000
Interest	206,780
Total expenses	$ 3,180,356
Operating income	$ 89,048
Provision for income taxes	31,167
Net income	$ 57,881
Retained earnings, beginning of year	$ 199,961
Retained earnings, end of year	$ 257,842

Green Valley Nursing Home, Inc.
Balance Sheet
December 31, 2007

Assets	
Current Assets:	
Cash	$ 105,737
Marketable securities	200,000
Net patient accounts receivable	215,600
Supplies	87,655
Total current assets	$ 608,992
Property and equipment	$ 2,250,000
Less accumulated depreciation	356,000
Net property and equipment	$ 1,894,000
Total assets	$ 2,502,992

Liabilities and Shareholders' Equity

Current Liabilities:

Accounts payable	$ 72,250
Accrued expenses	192,900
Notes payable	100,000
Current portion of long-term debt	80,000
Total current liabilities	$ 445,150
Long-term debt	$ 1,700,000

Shareholders' Equity:

Common stock, $10 par value	$ 100,000
Retained earnings	257,842
Total shareholders' equity	$ 357,842
Total liabilities and shareholders' equity	$ 2,502,992

a. Perform a Du Pont analysis on Green Valley. Assume that the industry average ratios are as follows:

Total margin	3.5%
Total asset turnover	1.5
Equity multiplier	2.5
Return on equity (ROE)	13.1%

b. Calculate and interpret the following ratios:

	Industry Average
Return on assets (ROA)	5.2%
Current ratio	2.0
Days cash on hand	22 days
Average collection period	19 days
Debt ratio	71 %
Debt-to-equity ratio	2.5
Times interest earned (TIE) ratio	2.6
Fixed asset turnover ratio	1.4

c. Assume that there are 10,000 shares of Green Valley's stock outstanding and that some recently sold for $45 per share.
   • What is the firm's price/earnings ratio?
   • What is its market/book ratio?

17.6 Examine the industry average ratios given in Problems 17.4 and 17.5 above. Explain why the ratios are different between the managed care and nursing home industries.

Notes

1. Industry average ratios are available from many sources. For example, Ingenix publishes an annual almanac that provides hospital industry data on 33 financial ratios and 43 operating indicator ratios. The ratios are reported

in several groupings, such as by hospital size and geographic location. See *www.hospitalbenchmarks.com*. The industry average ratios presented in this chapter are for illustrative use only and hence should not be used for making real-world comparisons. Also, note that in accordance with standard practice, we are calling the comparative data *averages*, but in reality they are *median* values. Median values are better for comparisons because they are not biased by extremely high or low values in the industry data set.

2. A more complete set of both financial and operating indicator ratios is available from the Health Administration Press website for this book. See ache.org/books/HCFinance4.

3. To determine the minimum proportional value that must be obtained from current assets to meet current obligations, divide the number 1 by the current ratio. For Riverside, 1 / 2.3 = 0.43, or 43%. If liquidated at 43 cents on the dollar, the hospital's current assets would provide 0.43 × $31,280,000 $13,332,000 in cash, which equals the amount of current liabilities.

4. Riverside's 2007 *current asset turnover ratio* (total revenues divided by total current assets) was 3.8, compared to an industry average of 3.6, so the hospital is slightly above average regarding current asset utilization.

5. Because information on credit sales is generally unavailable, total patient services revenue must be used. Although almost all hospital services are provided on credit because of the third-party-payer system, other healthcare businesses may not have the same high percentage of credit sales. As the proportion of cash sales increases, the days in patient accounts receivable measure loses its usefulness. Also, it would be better to use **average** receivables in the ratio, either calculated as an average of monthly figures or as (Beginning receivables + Ending receivables) / 2.

6. For pedagogic reasons, we discussed ratio analysis **before** Du Pont analysis. However, when actually conducting a financial performance analysis, most analysts would conduct the Du Pont analysis **first**. The idea here is to use Du Pont analysis to gain an overview of the business's financial condition. Then, with some understanding of the business's financial strengths and weaknesses, the ratio analysis can focus on those areas identified as critical to improving performance.

7. For more information on common size and percentage change analysis, see L. C. Gapenski, *Understanding Healthcare Financial Management* (Chicago: Health Administration Press, 2007), Chapter 13.

8. The EVA concept was developed in detail and popularized by the consulting firm of Stern Stewart and Company. For a much more complete discussion of the concept, see G. Bennett Stewart, III, *The Quest for Value* (New York: HarperBusiness, 1991). Also, note that another potential measure of managerial performance for publicly traded investor-owned businesses is *Market Value Added (MVA)*, which is the difference between the market value of equity and book value of equity. The larger the MVA, the greater the wealth created for shareholders.

9. For an excellent example of the application of EVA in setting managerial compensation within not-for-profit firms, see W. O. Cleverley and R. K. Harvey, "Economic Value Added—A Framework for Health Care Executive

Compensation," *Hospital & Health Services Administration* (Summer 1993): 215–228.

References

Beaver, W. H., and J. E. Horngren. 1991. "Ten Commandants of Financial Statement Analysis." *Financial Analysts Journal* (January–February): 9.

Boblitz, M. C. 2006. "Looking Out the Window: Market Intelligence for a View of the Real World." *Healthcare Financial Management* (July): 47–53.

Boles, K. E. 1992. "Insolvency in Managed Care Organizations: Financial Indicators." *Topics in Health Care Financing* (Winter): 40–57.

Burns, L. R., G. Gimm, and S. Nicholson. 2005. "The Financial Performance of Integrated Health Organizations." *Journal of Healthcare Management* (May/ June): 191–211.

Cleverley, W. O., and J. O. Cleverley. 2005. "Scorecards and Dashboards: Using Financial Metrics to Improve Performance." *Healthcare Financial Management* (July): 64–69.

Cleverley, W. O., and R. K. Harvey. 1990. "Profitability: Comparing Hospital Results with Other Industries." *Healthcare Financial Management* (March): 42–52.

———. 1994. "Trends in the Hospital Financial Picture." *Healthcare Financial Management* (February): 56–63.

———. 1995. "Understanding Your Hospital's True Financial Position and Changing It." *Health Care Management Review* (Spring): 62–73.

Coyne, J. S. 1985. "Measuring Hospital Performance in Multi-Institutional Organizations Using Financial Ratios." *Health Care Management Review* (Fall): 35–42.

———. 1990. "Analyzing the Financial Performance of Hospital-Based Managed Care Programs: The Case of Humana." *Journal of Health Administration Education* (Fall): 571–642.

Eastaugh, S. R. 1992. "Hospital Strategy and Financial Performance." *Health Care Management Review* (Summer): 19–32.

Finkler, S. A. 1982. "Ratio Analysis: Use with Caution." *Health Care Management Review* (Spring): 65–72.

Harkey, J., and R. Vraciu. 1992. "Quality of Health Care and Financial Performance: Is There a Link?" *Health Care Management Review* (Fall): 55–61.

Healthcare Financial Management Association (HFMA). 2004. "Back to Basics: A Self-Help Approach to Achieving Financial Success." *Healthcare Financial Management* (March): 89–97.

Lynn, M. L., and P. Wertheim. 1993. "Key Financial Ratios Can Foretell Hospital Closures." *Healthcare Financial Management* (November): 66–70.

McCue, M. J. 1991. "The Use of Cash Flow to Analyze Financial Distress in California Hospitals." *Hospital & Health Services Administration* (Summer): 223–241.

Pieper, S. K. 2005. "Reading the Right Signals: How to Strategically Manage with Scorecards." *Healthcare Executive* (May/June): 9–14.

Pink, G. H., et al. 2001. "Creating a Balanced Scorecard For a Hospital System." *Journal of Healthcare Finance* (Spring): 1–20.

Price, C. A., A. E. Cameron, and D. Price. 2005. "Distress Detectors: Measures for

Predicting Financial Distress in Hospitals." *Healthcare Financial Management* (August): 74–80.

Prince, T. R. 1991. "Assessing Financial Outcomes of Not-for-Profit Community Hospitals." *Hospital & Healthcare Administration* (Fall): 331–349.

Sherman, B. 1990. "How Investors Evaluate the Creditworthiness of Hospitals." *Healthcare Financial Management* (March): 25–31.

Sylvestre, J., and F. R. Urbancic. 1994. "Effective Methods for Cash Flow Analysis." *Healthcare Financial Management* (July): 62–72.

Watkins, A. L. 2003. "A Balanced Perspective: Using Nonfinancial Measures to Assess Financial Performance." *Healthcare Financial Management* (November): 76–80.

Wyatt, J. 2004. "Scoreboards, Dashboards, and KPIs: Keys to Integrated Performance Measurement." *Healthcare Financial Management* (February): 76–80.

Zeller, T. L., B. B. Stanko, and W. O. Cleverley. 1997. "A New Perspective on Hospital Financial Ratio Analysis." *Healthcare Financial Management* (November): 62–67.

LEASE FINANCING AND BUSINESS VALUATION

Learning Objectives

After studying this chapter, readers will be able to:

- Describe the two primary types of leases.
- Explain how lease financing affects both financial statements and taxes.
- Conduct a basic lease analysis from the perspective of the lessee.
- Discuss the factors that create value in lease transactions.
- Explain in general terms how businesses are valued.
- Conduct a business valuation using both discounted cash flow and market multiple approaches.

Introduction

This chapter contains two unrelated topics: lease financing and business valuation. *Leasing* is a substitute for debt financing and hence expands the range of financing alternatives available to businesses (and to individuals). However, leasing should be used only when it offers some advantage over conventional financing. We begin this chapter by discussing how businesses analyze lease transactions and what factors contribute to the large amount of leasing activity among healthcare businesses.

The valuation of entire businesses, as opposed to capital projects, is a critical step in the merger and acquisition process. In addition, *business valuation* plays an important role when one owner is bought out by other owners and when businesses are inherited. The second part of this chapter discusses two specific techniques used to value businesses.

Leasing Basics

Businesses generally own fixed assets, but it is the use of buildings and equipment that is important, not their ownership. One way to obtain the use of assets is to raise debt or equity capital and then use this capital to buy them. An alternative way to obtain the use of assets is by leasing. Before the 1950s, leasing was generally associated with real estate (land and buildings), but today it is possible to lease almost any kind of asset. Although leasing is used extensively in all industries, it is especially prevalent in the health services industry, primarily with medical equipment and information technology hardware and software.[1]

Note that every lease transaction has two parties: The user of the leased asset is called the *lessee*, while the owner of the property, usually the manufacturer or a leasing company, is called the *lessor*. (The term "lessee" is pronounced "less-ee," not "lease-ee," and "lessor" is pronounced "less-or.")

Leases are commonly classified into two categories: operating leases and financial leases. In this section, we discuss these informal classifications. In later sections, we will discuss the more formal classifications used by accountants in the preparation of financial statements and by the IRS.

Operating Leases

Operating leases, sometimes called *service leases,* generally provide both financing and maintenance. IBM was one of the pioneers of operating lease contracts, which are used most often for computers and office copying machines as well as for automobiles, trucks, and medical diagnostic equipment. Operating leases typically require the lessor to maintain and service the leased equipment, with the cost of maintenance built into the lease payments.

Additionally, operating leases are not fully amortized—that is, the payments required under the lease contract are not sufficient for the lessor to recover the full cost of the equipment. However, the lease contract is written for a period that is considerably shorter than the expected useful life of the leased asset, and the lessor expects to recover all costs eventually, either by lease renewal payments or by sale of the equipment.

A final feature of operating leases is that they frequently contain a *cancellation clause* that gives the lessee the right to cancel the lease and return the equipment to the lessor prior to the expiration of the lease. This is an important feature to the lessee because it means that the equipment can be returned if it is rendered obsolete by technological developments or if it is no longer needed because of a decline in the lessee's business.

Note that lease (rental) payments on operating leases can be structured in two different ways. Under *conventional* terms, fixed payments are made to the lessor periodically, usually monthly. With this type of payment, the cost to the lessee (and the return to the lessor) is known (more or less) with certainty. Under *per procedure* terms, a fixed amount is paid each time the equipment is used—for example, for each x-ray taken. Now, the cost to the lessee and return to the lessor are not known with certainty—rather, they depend on volume. In essence, a per procedure lease converts a fixed cost for the equipment, which is independent of volume, into a variable cost, which is directly related to volume. We will have more to say about per procedure leases later in the chapter.

Financial Leases

Financial leases, sometimes called *capital leases*, are differentiated from operating leases in that (1) they typically do not provide for maintenance; (2) they typically are not cancelable; (3) they are generally for a period that approximates the useful life of the asset; and hence (4) they are fully amortized.

In a typical financial lease, the lessee selects the specific item needed and then negotiates the price and delivery terms with the manufacturer. The lessee then arranges to have a leasing firm (lessor) buy the equipment from the manufacturer, and the lessee simultaneously executes a lease agreement with the lessor.

The terms of a financial lease call for full amortization of the lessor's investment, plus a rate of return on the lease that is close to the percentage rate the lessee would have paid on a secured term loan. For example, if a radiology group practice would have to pay 10 percent for a term loan to buy an x-ray machine, then the lessor would build in a return on the lease of about 10 percent. The parallel to borrowing is obvious in a financial lease. Under a secured loan arrangement, the lender would normally receive a series of equal payments just sufficient to amortize the loan and to provide a specified rate of return on the outstanding loan balance. Under a financial lease, the lease payments are set up exactly the same way—the payments are just sufficient to return the full purchase price to the lessor plus a stated return on the lessor's investment. At the end of a financial lease, the ownership of the leased asset is transferred from the lessor to the lessee.

A *sale and leaseback* is a special type of financial lease, often used with real estate, which can be arranged by a user who currently owns some asset. The user sells the asset to another party and simultaneously executes an agreement to lease the property for a stated period under specific terms. In a sale and leaseback, the lessee receives an immediate cash payment in exchange for a future series of lease payments that must be made to rent the use of the asset sold.

Although the distinction between operating and financial leases has historical significance, today many lessors offer leases under a wide variety of terms. Therefore, in practice, leases often do not fit exactly into the operating lease or financial lease categories but combine some features of each.

1. What is the difference between an operating lease and a financial lease? 2. What is a sale and leaseback? 3. How do per procedure payment terms differ from conventional terms?	**Self-Test Questions**

Tax Effects

For both investor-owned and not-for-profit businesses, tax effects can play an important role in the lease-versus-buy decision.

Investor-Owned (Taxable) Businesses

For investor-owned businesses, the full amount of each lease payment is a tax-deductible expense for the lessee **provided that the IRS agrees that a particular contract is a genuine lease**. This makes it important that lease contracts be written in a form acceptable to the IRS. A lease that complies with all of the IRS requirements for taxable businesses is called a *guideline*, or *tax-oriented*, *lease*. In a guideline lease, ownership (depreciation) tax benefits accrue to the lessor and the lessee's lease payments are fully tax deductible. A lease that does not meet the tax guidelines is called a *non-tax-oriented lease*. For this type of lease, the lessee can only deduct the implied interest portion of each lease payment. However, the lessee is effectively the owner of the leased equipment; thus, the lessee obtains the tax depreciation benefits.

The reason for the IRS's concern about lease terms is that, without restrictions, a business could set up a "lease" transaction that calls for very rapid lease payments, which would be deductible from taxable income. The effect would be to depreciate the equipment over a much shorter period than the IRS allows in its depreciation guidelines. Therefore, if just any type of contract could be called a lease and given tax treatment as a lease, then the timing of lease tax shelters could be speeded up as compared with depreciation tax shelters. This speed-up would benefit the business, but it would be costly to the government and hence to individual taxpayers. For this reason, the IRS has established specific rules that define a lease for tax purposes.

The primary point here is that if investor-owned businesses are to obtain tax benefits from leasing, the lease contract must be written in a manner that will qualify it as a true lease under IRS guidelines. Any questions about the tax status of a lease contract must be resolved by the potential lessee prior to signing the contract.

Not-for-Profit (Tax-Exempt) Businesses

Not-for-profit lessees also benefit from tax laws, but in a different way. Because not-for-profit firms do not obtain tax benefits from depreciation, the ownership of assets has no tax value. However, lessors, who are all taxable businesses, do benefit from ownership. In effect, when assets are owned by not-for-profit firms the depreciation tax benefit is lost, while when assets are leased the tax benefit is realized by the lessor rather than the lessee. This realized benefit, in turn, can be shared with the lessee in the form of lower rental payments. Note, however, that the cost of tax-exempt debt to not-for-profit firms can be lower than the after-tax cost of debt to taxable firms, so leasing is not automatically less costly to not-for-profit firms than borrowing in the tax-exempt markets or buying.

A special type of financial transaction has been created for not-for-profit businesses called a *tax-exempt lease*. The major difference between a tax-exempt lease and a conventional lease is that the implied interest portion of the lease payment is not classified as taxable income to the lessor. Thus, the return portion of the lessor's payment is exempt from federal income taxes. The rationale for this tax treatment is that the interest paid on most debt financing used by not-for-profit organizations is tax-exempt to the lender, and a lessor is, in actuality, a lender. Tax-exempt leases provide a greater after-tax return to lessors than do conventional leases, so some of this "extra" return could be passed back to the lessee in the form of lower lease payments. Thus, the lessee's payments on tax-exempt leases could be lower than when the asset is acquired by a not-for-profit business through a conventional lease.

1. What is the difference between a tax-oriented (guideline) lease and a non-tax-oriented lease?
2. Why should the IRS care about lease provisions?
3. What is a tax-exempt lease?

Self-Test Questions

Financial Statement Effects

Regardless of the type of lease, the lessee reports lease payments as an expense item on the **income statement** in the year that they are made. Furthermore, as discussed below, if the lease is a capital lease, and hence is listed on the **balance sheet**, the leased asset is depreciated each year and the annual depreciation expense is reported on the income statement.

However, under certain conditions, neither the leased asset nor the contract liabilities (present value of lease payments) appear on the lessee's balance sheet. For this reason, leasing is often called *off-balance-sheet financing*. This point is illustrated in Table 18.1 by the balance sheets of two hypothetical healthcare providers: B and L. Initially, the balance sheets of both firms are identical, and they both have debt ratios of 50 percent. Next, each firm decides to acquire a fixed asset that costs $100. Firm B borrows $100 and buys the asset, so both an asset and a liability are entered on its balance sheet, and its debt ratio rises from 50 percent to 75 percent. Firm L leases the equipment. The lease may call for fixed charges as high or even higher than the loan, and the obligations assumed under the lease may have equal or even more potential to force the business into bankruptcy, but the firm's debt ratio remains at only 50 percent.

To correct this accounting deficiency, accounting rules require businesses that enter into certain leases to restate their balance sheets to report the leased asset as a fixed asset and the present value of the future lease payments as a liability. This process is called *capitalizing* the lease, and hence such a lease is called a *capital lease*. The net effect of capitalizing the lease is to cause Firms B and L to have similar balance sheets, both of which will, in essence, resemble the one shown for Firm B.[2]

TABLE 18.1
Effects of
Leasing on
Balance Sheets

Before Asset Increase:

Firms B and L

Current assets	$ 50	Debt	$ 50
Fixed assets	50	Equity	50
Total assets	$100		$100
Debt/assets ratio			50%

After Asset Increase:

Firm B, which Borrows and Buys					Firm L, which Leases			
Current assets	$ 50	Debt	$150		Current assets	$ 50	Debt	$ 50
Fixed assets	150	Equity	50		Fixed assets	50	Equity	50
Total assets	$200		$200		Total assets	$100		$100
Debt/assets ratio			75%		Debt/assets ratio			50%

The logic here is as follows. If a firm signs a capital lease contract, its obligation to make lease payments is just as binding as if it had signed a loan agreement; the failure to make lease payments has the potential to bankrupt a firm just as the failure to make principal and interest payments on a loan can result in bankruptcy. Therefore, under most circumstances, a capital lease has the same impact on a business's financial risk as does a loan. This being the case, if a firm signs a capital lease agreement, it has the effect of raising the firm's effective debt ratio. Therefore, to maintain the firm's established target capital structure, the lease financing requires additional equity support exactly like debt financing. Another way of saying the same thing is that leasing uses up a business's *debt capacity*.

Note, however, that there are some legal differences between loans and leases, mostly involving the rights of lessors versus lenders when a business in financial distress reorganizes or liquidates under bankruptcy. In most financial distress situations, lessors fare better than lenders, so lessors may be more willing to deal with firms in poor financial condition than are lenders. At a minimum, lessors may be willing to accept lower rates of return than lenders when dealing with financially distressed businesses because the risks are lower.

If disclosure of the lease in our Table 18.1 example were not made, then Firm L's investors might be deceived into thinking that its financial position is stronger than it really is. Thus, even before businesses were required to place some leases on the balance sheet, they were required to disclose the existence of all leases longer than one year in the footnotes to their financial statements. At that time, some people argued that investors fully recognized the impact of leases and, in effect, would conclude that Firms B and L are essentially in the same financial position. Conversely, other people argued that investors would be better served if all leases were capitalized (shown directly on the balance sheet). Current accounting requirements represent a compromise between these two positions, although one that is tilted heavily toward those who favor capitalization.

A lease is classified as a capital lease and thus is shown directly on the balance sheet, if one or more of the following conditions exist:

- Under the terms of the lease, ownership of the property is effectively transferred from the lessor to the lessee.
- The lessee can purchase the property at less than its true market value when the lease expires.
- The lease runs for a period equal to or greater than 75 percent of the asset's life. Thus, if an asset has a ten-year life and the lease is written for eight years, the lease must be capitalized.
- The present value of the lease payments, when discounted at the rate of interest the lessee would have to pay if the asset were debt financed, is equal to or greater than 90 percent of the initial value of the asset. Note that any maintenance payments embedded in the lease payment must be stripped out prior to checking this condition.

These rules, together with strong footnote disclosure rules for noncapitalized (operating) leases, are sufficient to ensure that no one will be fooled by lease financing. In effect, a capital lease for a particular asset has the same economic consequences for the business as does a loan in which the asset is pledged as collateral. Thus, leases are regarded as debt for capital structure purposes, and they have roughly the same effects as debt on the financial condition of the firm.

Note that in most cases leases that meet IRS guidelines are operating leases that will not be capitalized, while leases that do not meet IRS guidelines are financial leases that will be capitalized. Remember, however, that even operating (noncapitalized) leases must be disclosed in the footnotes to the firm's financial statements.

1. Why is lease financing sometimes called off-balance-sheet financing? 2. How are leases accounted for on a business's balance sheet? On the income statement?	**Self-Test Questions**

Lease Evaluation

Leases are evaluated by both the lessee and the lessor. The lessee must determine whether leasing an asset is less costly than obtaining equivalent alternative financing and buying the asset, and the lessor must decide what the lease payments must be to produce a rate of return consistent with the riskiness of the investment. Here we will only cover the lessee's analysis.[3]

To begin, note that a degree of uncertainty exists regarding the theoretically correct way to evaluate lease-versus-purchase decisions, and some very complex decision models have been developed to aid in the analysis. However, the simple analysis given here, coupled with judgment, is sufficient to avoid situations where a lessee enters into a lease agreement that is clearly not in the business's best interests. In the typical case, the events that lead to a lease arrangement are as follows:

- The business decides to acquire a particular building or piece of equipment; this decision is based on the capital budgeting procedures discussed in Chapters 14 and 15. The decision to acquire the asset is *not* at issue in a typical lease analysis; this decision was made previously as part of the capital budgeting process. In lease analysis, we are concerned simply with whether to obtain the use of the property by lease or by purchase.
- Once the business has decided to acquire the asset, the next question is how to finance the acquisition. A well-run business does not have excess cash lying around, and even if it did, there would be opportunity costs associated with its use.
- Funds to purchase the asset could be obtained from excess cash, by borrowing, or if the business is investor-owned, by selling new equity. Alternatively, the asset could be leased.

As indicated previously, a lease is comparable to a loan in the sense that the business is required to make a specified series of payments and failure to meet these payments could result in bankruptcy. Thus, the most appropriate comparison when making lease decisions is the cost of lease financing versus the cost of debt financing, **regardless of how the asset actually would be financed if it were not leased.** The asset may be purchased with available cash if it is not leased or financed by a new equity sale, but because leasing is a substitute for debt financing, the appropriate comparison would still be to debt financing.

To illustrate the basic elements of lease analysis, consider this simplified example. Nashville Radiology Group (the Group) requires the use of an x-ray machine for two years that costs $100, and the Group must choose between leasing and buying the equipment. (The actual cost is $100,000, but let's keep the numbers simple.) If the machine is purchased, the bank would lend the Group the needed $100 at a rate of 10 percent on a two-year, simple interest loan. Thus, the Group would have to pay the bank $10 in interest at the end of each year, plus return the $100 in principal at the end of Year 2. For simplicity, assume that the Group could depreciate the entire cost of the machine over two years for tax purposes by the straight-line method if it were purchased, resulting in tax depreciation of $50 in each year. Furthermore, the Group's tax rate is 40 percent. Thus, the depreciation expense produces a tax savings, or *tax shield*, of $50 × 0.40 = $20 in each year. Also for the sake of simplicity, assume the equipment's value at the end of two years (its residual value) is estimated to be $0.

Alternatively, the Group could lease the asset under a guideline lease for two years for a payment of $55 at the end of each year. The analysis for the lease-versus-buy decision consists of (1) estimating the cash flows associated with borrowing and buying the asset, (2) estimating the cash flows associated with leasing the asset, and (3) comparing the two financing methods to determine which has the lower cost. Here are the borrow and buy flows:

Cash Flows if the Group Buys	Year 0	Year 1	Year 2
Equipment cost	($100)		
Loan amount	100		
Interest expense		($10)	($ 10)
Tax savings from interest		4	4
Principal repayment			(100)
Tax savings from depreciation		20	20
Net cash flow	$ 0	$14	($ 86)

The net cash flow is zero in Year 0, positive in Year 1, and negative in Year 2. Because the operating cash flows (the revenues and operating costs) will be the same regardless of whether the equipment is leased or purchased, they can be ignored. Cash flows that are not affected by the decision at hand are said to be *nonincremental* to the decision.

Here are the cash flows associated with the lease.

Cash Flows if the Group Leases	Year 0	Year 1	Year 2
Lease payment		($55)	($55)
Tax savings from payments		22	22
Net cash flow	$0	($33)	($33)

Note that the two sets of cash flows reflect the tax savings associated with interest expense, depreciation, and lease payments, as appropriate. If the lease had not met IRS guidelines, then ownership would effectively reside with the lessee, and the Group would depreciate the asset for tax purposes whether it was "leased" or purchased. Furthermore, only the implied interest portion of the lease payment would be tax deductible. Thus, the analysis for a nonguideline lease would consist of simply comparing the after-tax financing flows on the loan with the after-tax lease-payment stream.

To compare the cost streams of buying and leasing, we must put them on a present value basis. As we explain later, the correct discount rate is the after-tax cost of debt, which for the Group is $10\% \times (1 - T) = 10\% \times (1 - 0.4) = 6.0\%$. Applying this rate, we find the present value cost of buying to be $63.33 and the present value cost of leasing to be $60.50. Because leasing has the lower present value of costs, it is the less-costly financing alternative, so the Group should lease the asset.

This simplified example shows the general approach used in lease analysis, and it also illustrates a concept that can simplify the cash flow estimation process. Look back at the loan-related cash flows if the Group buys the machine. The after-tax loan-related flows are −$6 in Year 1 and −$106 in Year 2. When these flows are discounted to Year 0 at the 6percent after-tax cost of debt, their present value is −$100, which is the negative of the loan amount shown in Year 0. This equality results because we first used the cost of debt to estimate the future financing flows, and we then used this same rate to discount the flows back to Year 0, all on an after-tax basis. In effect, the loan amount positive cash flow and the loan cost negative cash flows cancel one another out. Here is the cash flow stream associated with buying the asset after the Year 0 loan amount and the related Year 1 and Year 2 financing flows have been removed:

Cash Flows if the Group Buys	Year 0	Year 1	Year 2
Cost of asset	($100)		
Tax savings from depreciation		$20	$20
Net cash flow	($100)	$20	$20

The present value cost of buying here is, of course, $63.33, which is the same amount we found earlier. The consistency between the two approaches will always occur regardless of the specific terms of the debt financing: As long as the discount rate is the after-tax cost of debt, the cash flows associated with the loan can be ignored.

To examine a more realistic example of lease analysis, consider the following lease-versus-buy decision that faces the Nashville Radiology Group:

- The Group plans to acquire a new computer system that will automate the Group's clinical records as well as its accounting, billing, and collection process. The system has an economic life of eight years and costs $200,000, delivered and installed. However, the Group plans to lease the equipment for only four years because it believes that computer technology is changing rapidly, and it wants the opportunity to reevaluate the situation at that time.
- The Group can borrow the required $200,000 from its bank at a before-tax cost of 10 percent.
- The system's estimated scrap value is $5,000 after eight years of use, but its estimated *residual value*, which is the value at the expiration of the lease, is $20,000. Thus, if the Group buys the equipment, it would expect to receive $20,000 before taxes when the equipment is sold in four years.
- The Group can lease the equipment for four years at a rental charge of $57,000, payable at the beginning of each year. However, the lessor will own the equipment upon the expiration of the lease. (The lease payment schedule is established by the potential lessor and the Group can accept it, reject it, or attempt to negotiate the terms.)

- The lease contract stipulates that the lessor will maintain the computer at no additional charge to the Group. However, if the Group borrows and buys the computer, it will have to bear the cost of maintenance, which would be performed by the equipment manufacturer at a fixed contract rate of $2,500 per year, payable at the beginning of each year.
- The computer falls into the MACRS five-year class life, the Group's marginal tax rate is 40 percent, and the lease qualifies as a guideline lease under a special IRS ruling.

Dollar Cost Analysis

Table 18.2 illustrates a complete dollar cost analysis. Again, our approach here is to compare the dollar cost of owning (borrowing and buying) the computer to the cost of leasing the computer. All else the same, the lower cost alternative is preferable. Part I of the table is devoted to the costs of borrowing and buying. Here, Line 1 gives the equipment's cost and Line 2 shows the maintenance expense, both of which are shown as outflows. Note that whenever an analyst is setting up cash flows on a time line, one of the first decisions to be made is what time interval will be used—that is, months, quarters, years, or some other period. As a starting point, we generally assume that all cash flows occur at the end of each year. If, at some point later in the analysis, we conclude that another interval is better, we will change it. Longer intervals, such as years, simplify the analysis but introduce some inaccuracies because all cash flows do not actually occur at year end. For example, tax benefits occur quarterly because businesses pay taxes on a quarterly basis. On the other hand, shorter intervals, such as months, often are used for lease analyses because lease payments typically occur monthly. For ease of illustration, we are using annual flows in this example.

Line 3 gives the maintenance tax savings: because maintenance expense is tax deductible, the Group saves $0.40 \times \$2,500 = \$1,000$ in taxes by virtue of paying the maintenance fee. Line 4 contains the depreciation tax savings, which equals the depreciation expense times the tax rate. For example, the MACRS allowance for the first year is 20 percent, so the depreciation expense is $0.20 \times \$200,000 = \$40,000$ and the depreciation tax savings is $0.40 \times \$20,000 = \$16,000$.

Lines 5 and 6 contain the residual value cash flows: the residual value is estimated to be $20,000, but the tax book value after four years of depreciation is $\$200,000 - \$40,000 - \$64,000 - \$38,000 - \$24,000 = \$34,000$. (See Table 18.2, Note a.) Thus, the Group is losing $14,000 for tax purposes, which results in the $0.4 \times \$14,000 = \$5,600$ tax savings shown as an inflow on Line 6. Line 7, which sums the component cash flows, contains the net cash flows associated with borrowing and buying.

Part II of Table 18.2 contains an analysis of the cost of leasing. The lease payments, shown on Line 9, are $57,000 per year; this rate, which includes maintenance, was established by the prospective lessor and offered to the

TABLE 18.2
Nashville
Radiology
Group: Dollar
Cost Analysis

	Year 0	Year 1	Year 2	Year 3	Year 4
I. Cost of Owning (Borrowing and Buying)					
1. Net purchase price	($200,000)				
2. Maintenance cost	(2,500)	($ 2,500)	($ 2,500)	($ 2,500)	
3. Maintenance tax savings	1,000	1,000	1,000	1,000	
4. Depreciation tax savings		16,000	25,600	15,200	$ 9,600
5. Residual value					20,000
6. Residual value tax					5,600
7. Net cash flow	($ 201,500)	$ 14,500	$ 24,100	$ 13,700	$ 35,200
8. PV cost of owning	($ 126,987)				
II. Cost of Leasing					
9. Lease payment	($ 57,000)	($ 57,000)	($ 57,000)	($ 57,000)	
10. Tax savings	22,800	22,800	22,800	22,800	
11. Net cash flow	($ 34,200)	($ 34,200)	($ 34,200)	($ 34,200)	$ 0
12. PV cost of leasing	($ 125,617)				

III. Cost Comparison
13. Net advantage to leasing (NAL) = PV cost of leasing − PV cost of owning
= −$125,617 − (−$126,987) = $1,370.

Notes: a. The MACRS depreciation allowances are 0.20, 0.32, 0.19, and 0.12 in Years 1 through 4, respectively.
b. In practice, a lease analysis, such as this, would be done on a monthly basis using a spreadsheet program.

Group. If the Group accepts the lease, the full amount will be a deductible expense, so the tax savings, shown on Line 10, is $0.40 \times$ Lease payment = $0.40 \times \$57,000 = \$22,800$. The net cash flows associated with leasing are shown on Line 11.

The final step is to compare the net cost of owning with the net cost of leasing, so we must put the annual cash flows associated with owning and leasing on a common basis. This requires converting them to present values, which brings up the question of the proper rate at which to discount the net cash flows. We know that the riskier the cash flows, the higher the discount rate that should be applied to find the present value. This principle was applied in both security valuation and capital budgeting analysis, and it also applies to lease analysis. Just how risky are the cash flows under consideration here? Most of them are relatively certain, at least when compared with the types of cash flows associated with stock investments or with the Group's operations. For example, the loan payment schedule is set by contract, as is the lease payment schedule. Depreciation expenses are established by law and are not subject to change, and the annual maintenance fee is fixed by contract as well. The tax savings are somewhat uncertain because they depend on the Group's future marginal tax rates. The residual value is the riskiest of the cash flows, but even here the Group's management believes that its risk is minimal.

Because the cash flows under the lease and under the borrow and purchase alternatives are both relatively certain, they should be discounted at a relatively low rate. Most analysts recommend that the firm's cost of debt financing be used, and this rate seems reasonable in our example. However, the Group's cost of debt—10 percent—must be adjusted to reflect the tax deductibility of interest payments because this benefit of borrowing and buying is not accounted for in the cash flows. Thus, the Group's effective cost of debt becomes Before-tax cost × (1 − Tax rate) = 10% × 0.6 = 6%. Accordingly, the cash flows in Lines 7 and 11 are discounted at a 6 percent rate. The resulting present values are $126,987 for the cost of owning and $125,617 for the cost of leasing, as shown on Lines 8 and 12. Leasing is the lower-cost financing alternative, so the Group should lease, rather than buy, the computer.

The cost comparison can be formalized by defining the *net advantage to leasing (NAL)* as follows:

$$NAL = PV \text{ cost of leasing} - PV \text{ cost of owning}$$

$$= -\$125,617 - (-\$126,987) = \$1,370.$$

The positive NAL shows that leasing creates more value than buying, so the Group should lease the equipment. Indeed, the value of the Group is increased by $1,370 if it leases, rather than buys, the computer system.

Percentage Cost Analysis

The Group's lease-versus-buy decision can also be analyzed by looking at the effective cost rate on the lease and comparing it to the after-tax cost rate on the loan. If the cost rate implied in the lease contract is less than the 6 percent after-tax loan cost, then there is an advantage to leasing.

Table 18.3 sets forth the cash flows needed to determine the percentage cost of the lease. Here is an explanation of the table:

- The first step is to calculate the leasing-versus-owning cash flows, which are obtained by subtracting the owning cash flows, Line 7 from Table 18.2, from the leasing cash flows shown on Line 11. The differences, shown on Line 3 of Table 18.3, are the incremental cash flows to the Group if it leases rather than buys the computer.
- Note that Table 18.3 consolidates the analysis shown in Table 18.2 into a single set of cash flows. At this point, we can discount the consolidated

	Year 0	Year 1	Year 2	Year 3	Year 4
1. Leasing cash flow	($ 34,200)	($34,200)	($34,200)	($34,200)	$ 0
2. Less: Owning cash flow	(201,500)	14,500	24,100	13,700	35,200
3. Leasing versus owning CF	$167,300	($48,700)	($58,300)	($47,900)	($35,200)

NAL = $1,370.
IRR = 5.6%.

TABLE 18.3
Nashville Radiology Group: Percentage Cost Analysis

cash flows by 6 percent to obtain the NAL of $1,370. In Table 18.2, we discounted the owning and leasing cash flows separately and then subtracted their present values to obtain the NAL. In Table 18.3, we subtracted the cash flows first to obtain a single set of incremental flows and then found their present value. The end result is the same.

- The consolidated cash flows provide a good insight into the economics of leasing. If the Group leases the computer, it avoids the Year 0 $167,300 net cash outlay required to buy the equipment, but it is then obligated to a series of cash outflows for four years. In marketing materials, leasing companies are quick to point out the fact that leasing avoids a large upfront cash outlay ($167,300, in this example). However, they are not so quick to mention that the "cost" to save this outlay is an obligation to make payments over the next four years. Leasing only makes sense financially (disregarding other factors) if the savings upfront are worth the cost over time.

- By inputting the leasing-versus-owning cash flows listed in Table 18.3 into the cash flow registers of a calculator and solving for IRR (or by using a spreadsheet's IRR function), we can find the cost rate inherent in the cash flow stream—5.6 percent. This is the equivalent *after-tax cost rate* implied in the lease contract. Because this cost rate is less than the 6 percent after-tax cost of a loan, leasing is less expensive than borrowing and buying. Thus, the percentage cost analysis confirms the dollar cost (NAL) analysis.

Some Additional Points

So far, we have discussed the main features of a lessee's analysis. Here are some additional points of relevance:

- The dollar cost and percentage cost approaches will always lead to the same decision. Thus, one method is as good as the other from a decision standpoint.
- If the net residual value cash flow (residual value and tax effect) is considered to be much riskier than the other cash flows in the analysis, it is possible to account for this risk by applying a higher discount rate to this flow, which results in a lower present value. Because the net residual value flow is an inflow in the cost of owning analysis, a lower present value leads to a higher present value cost of owning. Thus, increasing residual value risk decreases the attractiveness of owning an asset. To illustrate the concept, assume that the Group's managers believe that the computer's residual value is much riskier than the other flows in Table 18.2. Furthermore, they believe that 10 percent, rather than 6 percent, is the appropriate discount rate to apply to the residual value flows. When the Table 18.2 analysis is modified to reflect this risk, the present value cost of owning increases to $129,780, while the NAL increases to $4,163. The

riskier the residual value, all else the same, the more favorable leasing becomes because residual value risk is borne by the lessor.

- Remember that net present value (NPV) is the dollar present value of a project, assuming that it is financed using debt and equity financing. In lease analysis, the NAL is the additional dollar present value of a project attributable to leasing, as opposed to conventional (debt) financing. Thus, as an approximation of the value of a leased asset to the business, the project's NPV can be increased by the amount of NAL:

$$\text{Adjusted NPV} = \text{NPV} + \text{NAL}.$$

The value added through leasing, in some cases, can turn unprofitable (negative NPV) projects into profitable (positive adjusted NPV) projects.

Self-Test Questions

1. Explain how the cash flows are structured in conducting a dollar cost (NAL) analysis.
2. What discount rate should be used when lessees perform lease analyses?
3. What is the economic interpretation of the net advantage to leasing?
4. What is the economic interpretation of a lease's IRR?

Motivations for Leasing

Although we do not prove it here, leasing is a zero-sum game; that is, when both the lessor and the lessee have the same inputs (equal costs, tax rates, residual value estimates, and so on), a positive NAL for the lessee creates an equal but negative return (NPV) for the lessor. Thus, under symmetric conditions, it would be impossible to structure a lease that would be acceptable to both the lessee and lessor, and hence no leases would be written. The large amount of leasing activity that actually takes place is driven by differentials between the lessee and the lessor. In this section, we discuss some of the differentials that motivate lease agreements.

Tax Differentials

Many leases are driven by tax differentials. Historically, the typical tax asymmetry arose between highly taxed lessors and lessees with sufficient tax shields (primarily depreciation) to drive their tax rates very low, even to zero. In these situations, the asset's depreciation tax benefits could be taken by the lessor, and then this value would be shared with the lessee. In addition, other possible tax motivations exist, including tax differentials between not-for-profit providers with zero taxes and investor-owned lessors with positive tax rates.

The Alternative Minimum Tax (AMT)

Taxable corporations are permitted to use accelerated depreciation and other tax shelters to reduce taxable income but, at the same time, use straight-line depreciation for stockholder reporting. Thus, under the normal procedure for determining federal income taxes, many very profitable businesses report large net incomes but pay little or no federal income taxes. The *alternative minimum tax (AMT)*, which amounts to roughly 20 percent of profits as **reported to shareholders**, is designed to force profitable firms to pay at least some taxes. Those firms that are exposed to heavy tax liabilities under the AMT naturally seek ways to reduce reported income. One way is to use high-payment short-term leases, which increase the business's expenses and consequently lowers reported profits and AMT liability. Note that the lease payments do not have to qualify as a deductible expense for regular tax purposes; all that is needed is that they reduce reported income shown on the income statement.

Ability to Bear Obsolescence (Residual Value) Risk

Leasing is an attractive financing alternative for many high-tech items that are subject to rapid and unpredictable technological obsolescence. For example, assume that a small, rural hospital plans to acquire a magnetic resonance imaging (MRI) device. If it buys the MRI equipment, it is exposed to the risk of technological obsolescence. In a relatively short time, some new technology might be developed that makes the current system nearly worthless, which could create a financial burden on the hospital. Because it does not use much equipment of this nature, the hospital would bear a great deal of risk if it bought the MRI device.

Conversely, a lessor that specializes in state-of-the-art medical equipment might be exposed to significantly less risk. By purchasing and then leasing many different high-tech items, the lessor benefits from portfolio diversification; over time, some items will lose more value than the lessor expected, but these losses will be offset by other items that retain more value than expected. Also, because specialized lessors are familiar with the markets for used medical equipment, they can estimate residual values better and negotiate better prices when the asset is resold (or leased to another business) than can a hospital. Because the lessor is better able than the hospital to bear residual value risk, the lessor could charge a premium for bearing this risk that is less than the risk premium inherent in ownership.

Some lessors also offer programs that guarantee that the leased asset will be modified as necessary to keep it in line with technological advancements. For an increased rental fee, lessors will provide upgrades to keep the leased equipment current regardless of the cost. To the extent that lessors are better able to forecast such upgrades, negotiate better terms from manufacturers, and, through greater diversification, control the risks involved with such upgrades, it may be cheaper for users to ensure state-of-the art equipment by leasing than by buying.

Ability to Bear Utilization Risk

A type of lease that is gaining popularity among healthcare providers is the *per procedure lease*. In this type of lease, instead of a fixed annual or monthly payment, the lessor charges the lessee a fixed amount for each procedure performed. For example, the lessor may charge the hospital $300 for every scan performed using a leased MRI device, or it may charge $400 per scan for the first 50 scans in each month and $200 for each scan above 100. Because the hospital's reimbursement for MRI scans typically depends primarily on the amount of use, and because the per procedure lease changes the hospital's costs for the MRI from fixed to variable, the hospital's risk is reduced.

However, the conversion of the payment to the lessor from a known amount to an uncertain stream increases the lessor's risk. In essence, the lessor is now bearing the utilization (operating) risk of the MRI. Although the passing of risk often produces no net benefit, a per procedure lease can be beneficial to both parties if the lessor is better able than the lessee to bear the utilization risk. As before, if the lessor has written a large number of per procedure leases, then some of the leases will be more profitable than expected and some will be less profitable than expected; but if the lessor's expectations are unbiased, the aggregate return on all leases will be quite close to that expected.

Ability to Bear Project Life Risk

Leasing can also be attractive when a business is uncertain about how long an asset will be needed. To illustrate the concept, consider the following example. Hospitals sometimes offer services that are dependent on a single staff member—for example, a physician who performs liver transplants. To support the physician's practice, the hospital might have to invest millions of dollars in equipment that can be used only for this particular procedure. The hospital will charge for the use of the equipment, and if things go as expected, the investment will be profitable. However, if the physician dies or leaves the hospital staff, and if no other qualified physician can be recruited to fill the void, then the project must be abandoned and the equipment becomes useless to the hospital. In this situation, the annual usage may be quite predictable, but the need for the asset could suddenly cease.

A lease with a cancellation clause would permit the hospital to simply return the equipment to the lessor. The lessor would charge something for the cancellation clause because such clauses increase the riskiness of the lease to the lessor. The increased lease cost would lower the expected profitability of the project, but it would provide the hospital with an option to abandon the equipment, and such an option could have a value that exceeds the incremental cost of the cancellation clause. The leasing company would be willing to write this option because it is in a better position to remarket the equipment, either by writing another lease or by selling it outright.

Maintenance Services

Some businesses find leasing attractive because the lessor is able to provide better or less expensive (or both) maintenance services. For example, MED-TRANS, Inc., a for-profit ambulance and medical transfer service that operates in Pennsylvania, recently leased 25 ambulances and transfer vans. The lease agreement, with a lessor that specializes in purchasing, maintaining, and then reselling automobiles and trucks, permitted the replacement of an aging fleet that MEDTRANS had built up over seven years. "We are pretty good at providing emergency services and moving sick people from one facility to another, but we aren't very good at maintaining an automotive fleet," said MEDTRANS's CEO.

Lower Information Costs

Leasing may be financially attractive for smaller businesses that have limited access to debt markets. For example, a small, recently formed physician group practice may need to finance one or more diagnostic devices such as an EKG machine. The group has no credit history, so it would be relatively difficult, and hence costly, for a bank to assess the group's credit risk. Some banks might think the loan is not even worth the effort. Others might be willing to make the loan but only after building the high cost of credit assessment into the cost of the loan. On the other hand, some lessors specialize in leasing to medical practices, so their analysts have assessed the financial worthiness of hundreds, or even thousands, of such businesses. Thus, it would be relatively easy for them to make the credit judgment, and hence they might be more willing to provide the financing and charge lower rates than conventional lenders.

Lower Risk in Bankruptcy

Finally, leasing may be less expensive than buying for firms that are poor credit risks. As discussed earlier, in the event of financial distress leading to reorganization or liquidation, lessors generally have more secure claims than do lenders. Thus, lessors may be willing to write leases to firms with poor financial characteristics that are less costly than loans offered by lenders, if such loans are even available.

There are other factors that might motivate businesses to lease an asset rather than buy it. Often, the reasons are difficult to quantify, so they cannot be easily incorporated into a numerical analysis. Nevertheless, a sound lease analysis must begin with a quantitative analysis, and then qualitative factors can be considered before making the final lease-or-buy decision.

Self-Test Questions

1. What are some economic factors that motivate leasing—that is, what asymmetries might exist that would make leasing beneficial to both lessors and lessees?

2. Would it ever make sense to lease an asset that has a negative NAL when evaluated by a conventional lease analysis? Explain your answer.

Business Valuation

We now move to the second topic of this chapter, *business valuation*. Entire businesses, as opposed to individual projects, are valued for many reasons, including acquisitions, buyouts, and the assessment of taxes. Although many different approaches can be used to value businesses, we will focus on the two most commonly used in the health services industry: the discounted cash flow and market multiple approaches.

Regardless of the valuation approach, it is crucial to understand three concepts that affect valuations. First, if the valuation is for acquisition purposes, the business being valued typically will not continue to operate as a separate entity but will become part of the acquiring business's portfolio of assets. Thus, any changes in ownership form or operations that occur as a result of the proposed merger that would affect the value of the business must be considered in the analysis. Second, the goal of most valuations is to estimate the equity value of the business because most valuations are conducted to assess the value of ownership. Thus, although we use the phrase "business valuation," the ultimate goal is to value the ownership stake in the business rather than its total value. Finally, **business valuation is a very imprecise process**. The best that can be done, even by professional *appraisers* who conduct these valuations on a regular basis, is to attain a reasonable valuation rather than a precise one.

Discounted Cash Flow Approach

The *discounted cash flow (DCF) approach* to valuing a business involves the application of classical capital budgeting procedures to an entire business. To apply this approach, two key items are needed: (1) a set of statements that estimate the cash flows expected from the business and (2) a discount rate to apply to these cash flows.

The development of accurate cash flow forecasts is by far the most important step in the DCF approach. Table 18.4 contains projected profit and loss statements for Doctors' Hospital, an investor-owned hospital that is being valued by its owners for possible future sale. The hospital currently uses 50 percent debt (at book values), and it has a 40 percent marginal federal-plus-state tax rate.

Line 1 of Table 18.4 contains the forecast for Doctors' Hospital net revenues, including both patient services revenue and other revenue. Note that all contractual allowances and other adjustments to charges, including collection delays, have been considered, so Line 1 represents actual cash revenues. Lines 2 and 3 contain the cash expense forecasts, while Line 4 lists

TABLE 18.4
Doctors'
Hospital:
Projected Profit
and Loss
Statements and
Retention
Estimates
(in millions)

	2008	2009	2010	2011	2012
1. Net revenues	$105.0	$126.0	$151.0	$174.0	$191.0
2. Patient services expenses	80.0	94.0	111.0	127.0	137.0
3. Other expenses	9.0	12.0	13.0	16.0	16.0
4. Depreciation	8.0	8.0	9.0	9.0	10.0
5. Earnings before interest and taxes (EBIT)	$ 8.0	$ 12.0	$ 18.0	$ 22.0	$ 28.0
6. Interest	4.0	4.0	5.0	5.0	6.0
7. Earnings before taxes (EBT)	$ 4.0	$ 8.0	$ 13.0	$ 17.0	$ 22.0
8. Taxes (40 percent)	1.6	3.2	5.2	6.8	8.8
9. Net profit	$ 2.4	$ 4.8	$ 7.8	$ 10.2	$ 13.2
10. Estimated retentions	$ 4.0	$ 4.0	$ 7.0	$ 9.0	$ 12.0

depreciation—a noncash expense. Line 5, which is merely Line 1 minus Lines 2, 3, and 4, contains the earnings before interest and taxes (EBIT) projections for each year. Note that if the valuation were being conducted by another business that was considering making an acquisition bid for Doctors' Hospital, the revenue and expense amounts would reflect any utilization, reimbursement, and cost efficiencies that would occur as a result of the acquisition.

Note that the interest expense values shown on Line 6 include interest on current debt as well as interest on debt issued to fund growth. In addition to interest expense, any debt principal repayments that will not be funded by new debt must be reflected in Table 18.4. Because such payments are made from after-tax income, they would be placed on a line below net profit—say, on a new Line 9a. Line 7 contains the earnings before taxes (EBT), and Line 8 lists the taxes based on Doctors's 40 percent marginal rate. Note here that any tax rate changes that would result from an acquisition must be incorporated into the profit and loss statement forecasts. Line 9 lists each year's net profit.

Finally, because some of Doctors' assets are expected to wear out or become obsolete, and because the hospital must grow its assets to support projected revenue growth, some **equity funds** (shown on Line 10) must be retained and reinvested in the subsidiary to pay for asset replacement and growth. These retentions, **which would be matched by equal amounts of new debt**, are not available for distribution to shareholders.

Table 18.5 provides relevant cost of capital data for Doctors' Hospital. These data will be used to set the discount rate used in the DCF valuation. As with many healthcare valuations, there is no market beta available to help establish the cost of equity. Doctors' Hospital is investor owned but not publicly traded, while in other situations the business could be not-for-profit. However, we can obtain market betas of the stocks of the major investor-

Cost of equity	18.0%	**TABLE 18.5**
Cost of debt	10.0%	Doctors'
Proportion of debt financing	0.50	Hospital:
Proportion of equity financing	0.50	Selected Cost
Tax rate	40.0%	of Capital Data

$$CCC = [w_d \times R(R_d) \times (1 - T)] + [w_e \times R(R_e)]$$
$$= [0.50 \times 10.0\% \times (1 - 0.40)] + [0.50 \times 18.0\%]$$
$$= 3.0\% + 9.0\% = 12.0\%.$$

Note: If necessary, see Chapter 13 for a discussion of the corporate cost of capital (CCC).

owned hospital chains, and this value could be used to help estimate the cost of equity given in Table 18.5. It is important to realize that the discount rate used in the DCF valuation must reflect the **riskiness of the cash flows being discounted**. If the valuation is for acquisition purposes, and if the riskiness of the cash flows will be affected by the acquisition, then the cost of capital calculated for the business must be adjusted to reflect any expected changes in risk.

The cost of equity estimate in Table 18.5 merits additional discussion. The cost of equity estimate based on market data is applicable only to large publicly traded companies whose stock is owned by well-diversified investors. For example, in the Doctors' Hospital illustration, the cost of equity of large hospital management companies was estimated to be 14 percent. However, such companies are highly diversified both geographically and in the types of services they provide. In addition, equity (stock) ownership in such companies is very liquid—if a stockholder wants out, he or she simply calls a broker and sells the shares. Thus, a "traditional" large company cost of equity estimate does not reflect the added risks inherent in an equity position in a small, undiversified business whose stock is illiquid. Thus, it is necessary to add an additional premium to account for the added risks associated with ownership of a small company. This premium, called the *size premium*, is thought to be about 4 percentage points. Thus, Doctors' Hospital's cost of equity estimate is actually based on a 14 percent estimate for similar large companies plus a 4 percentage point size premium: 14% + 4% = 18%. If there were other factors in addition to size that would increase the risk of ownership even more, such as heavy use of new, unproven technology or extreme illiquidity or lack of portfolio diversification, an additional risk premium would be added to compensate for the unique riskiness inherent in that particular small company. We will use 18 percent as our estimate for Doctors' cost of equity, but an even higher rate probably could be justified.

At this point, there are several alternative cash flow/discount rate combinations that could be used to complete the DCF valuation. The most widely used DCF method for business valuation, the *free equity cash flow method*, focuses on cash flows that accrue solely to equityholders (owners). Free equity cash flow is defined as net profit plus noncash expenses (depreciation) less equity cash flow needed for reinvestment in the business. Table 18.6 uses the data contained in Table 18.4 to forecast the free equity cash flows for Doctors'. In valuation analyses, the term "free" means cash flows that are available to the owners after all other expenses, including asset replacement to support growth, have been taken into account.

The next step in the DCF valuation process is to choose the appropriate discount rate (opportunity cost of capital). Unlike a typical capital budgeting analysis that focuses on operating cash flows, our DCF business valuation focuses on **equity flows**. Thus, the discount rate applied must reflect the riskiness of cash flows after interest expense is deducted, which have greater risk than do operating flows. What capital cost reflects the riskiness of these higher-risk equity flows? The answer is, the cost of equity. This means that the appropriate discount rate to apply to the Table 18.6 cash flows is the **18 percent cost of equity** shown in Table 18.5, not the 12 percent corporate cost of capital.

Because we have projected only five years of cash flows, and because Doctors' Hospital will generate cash flows for many years (perhaps 20 or 30 years or more), it is necessary to estimate a *terminal value*. If the free equity cash flows given in Table 18.6 are assumed to grow at a constant rate after 2012, the constant growth model can be used to estimate the value of all free equity cash flows that would occur in 2013 and beyond. Assuming a constant 3 percent growth rate in free equity cash flow forever, the terminal value at the end of 2012 is estimated to be $76.9 million:[4]

$$\text{Terminal value} = \frac{2012 \text{ Free equity cash flow} \times (1 + \text{Growth rate})}{\text{Required rate of return} - \text{Growth rate}}$$

$$= \frac{\$11.2 \times 1.03}{0.18 - 0.03} = \frac{\$11.54}{0.15}$$

$$= \$76.9 \text{ million.}$$

Combining the free equity cash flows from Table 18.6 with the terminal value calculated above produces the following set of flows (in millions):

2007	2008	2009	2010	2011	2012
	$6.4	$8.8	$9.8	$10.2	$11.2
					76.9
					$88.1

The final step in the DCF valuation process is to discount the time line cash flows at the cost of equity—18 percent. The resulting present (2007)

	2008	2009	2010	2011	2012
1. Net profit	$ 2.4	$ 4.8	$ 7.8	$10.2	$13.2
2. Plus depreciation	8.0	8.0	9.0	9.0	10.0
3. Less retentions	4.0	4.0	7.0	9.0	12.0
4. Free equity cash flow	$ 6.4	$ 8.8	$ 9.8	$10.2	$ 11.2

TABLE 18.6
Doctors'
Hospital:
Projected Free
Equity Cash
Flows
(in millions)

value is $61.5 million. Thus, the DCF method estimates a value for Doctors' Hospital of about $60 million.

Note that the final value estimate of Doctors' Hospital probably would be higher than the DCF value. The reason is that the DCF method only values the **operations** of the business. Thus, $60 million represents the value only of the business's assets **that support operations**. Many businesses hold nonoperating assets, such as marketable securities in excess of those required for operations or real estate that will not be needed in the future to support operations. The overall value of a business is the sum of its *operational value*, as estimated by the DCF method, plus the market values of any nonoperating assets. In this example, we assume that Doctors' Hospital does not have material nonoperating assets, so a reasonable estimate of its value is $60 million.

Although we will not illustrate it here, the valuation would include a risk analysis of the cash flows that is similar to that performed on capital budgeting flows. Generally, scenario analysis (and perhaps Monte Carlo simulation) would be used to obtain some feel for the degree of uncertainty in the final estimate, which might further be used to set a valuation range rather focus on a single estimate.

Market Multiple Approach

A second method for valuing entire businesses is *market multiple analysis*, which applies a market-determined multiple to some proxy for value—typically some measure of revenues or earnings. As in the DCF valuation approach, the basic premise here is that the value of any business depends on the cash flows that the business produces. The DCF approach applies this premise in a precise manner, while market multiple analysis is more ad hoc.

To illustrate the concept, suppose that recent data of for-profit hospitals indicate that equity values average about four to five times the business's EBITDA, which means *earnings before interest, taxes, depreciation, and amortization*. Thus, we would say that the EBITDA *market multiple* is 4.5. In estimating the value of Doctors' Hospital's equity using this method, note that Doctors' 2008 EBITDA estimate is $8 million in EBIT plus $8 million in deprecation, or $16 million. Multiplying EBITDA by the 4.5 average market multiple gives an equity value of $72 million. Because of the uncertainties involved in the market multiple process, we will use $70 million as our estimate.

To illustrate another, less direct proxy, consider the nursing home industry. In recent years, prices paid for nursing home acquisitions have been in the range of $80,000 to $120,000 per bed, with an average of roughly $100,000. Thus, using number of beds as the proxy for value, a nursing home with 50 beds would be valued at $50 \times \$100,000 = \$5$ million.

Comparison of the Valuation Methods

Clearly, the valuation of any business can only be considered a rough estimate. In the Doctors' Hospital illustration, we obtained values for the business of $60 million and $70 million. Thus, we might conclude that the value of Doctors' Hospital falls somewhere in the range of $60—$70 million. In many "real-world" valuations, the range is even larger than the one in our example. Because the estimates of the two methods can differ by large amounts, it is important to understand the advantages and disadvantages of each method.

Although the DCF approach has strong theoretical support, one has to be **very concerned** about the validity of the estimated cash flows and the discount rate applied to those flows. Sensitivity analyses demonstrate that it does not take much change in the terminal value growth rate or discount rate estimates to create large differences in estimated value. Thus, the theoretical superiority of the DCF approach is offset to some degree by the difficulties inherent in estimating the model's input values.

The market multiple method is more ad hoc, but its proponents argue that a proxy estimate for a single year, such as measured by EBITDA, is more likely to be accurate than a multiple-year cash flow forecast. Furthermore, the market multiple approach avoids the problem of having to estimate a terminal value. Of course, the market multiple approach has problems of its own. One concern is the comparability between the business being valued and the firm (or firms) that set the market multiple. Another concern is how well one year, or even an average of several years, of EBITDA (or some other value proxy) captures the value of a business that will be operated for many years into the future. After all, if the valuation is for merger purposes, merger-related synergies could cause the target's EBITDA to soar in coming years.

The bottom line here is that both methods have problems. In general, business valuations should use both the DCF and market multiple methods, as well as other available methods. Then a great deal of judgment must be applied to reconcile the valuation differences that typically occur.

Self-Test Questions
1. Briefly describe two approaches commonly used to value businesses.
2. What are some problems that occur in the valuation process?
3. Which approach do you believe to be best? Explain your answer.

Key Concepts

In this chapter, we discussed both leasing decisions and business valuation. The key concepts of this chapter are:

- Lease agreements are informally categorized as either *operating leases* or *financial (capital) leases.*
- The IRS has specific guidelines that apply to lease arrangements. A lease that meets these guidelines is called a *guideline,* or *tax-oriented, lease* because the IRS permits the lessee to deduct the lease payments. A lease that does not meet IRS guidelines is called a *non-tax-oriented lease.* In such leases, ownership effectively resides with the lessee rather than the lessor.
- Accounting rules spell out the conditions under which a lease must be *capitalized* (shown directly on the balance sheet) rather than shown only in the notes to the financial statements. Generally, leases that run for a period equal to or greater than 75 percent of the asset's life must be capitalized.
- The lessee's analysis consists of a comparison of the costs and benefits associated with leasing the asset and the costs and benefits associated with owning (borrowing and buying) the asset. There are two analytical techniques that can be used: the *dollar-cost (NAL) method* and the *percentage-cost (IRR) method.*
- One of the key issues in the lessee's analysis is the appropriate discount rate. Because the cash flows in a lease analysis are known with relative certainty, the appropriate discount rate is the *lessee's after-tax cost of debt.* A higher discount rate may be used on the *residual value* if it is substantially riskier than the other flows.
- Leasing is motivated by differentials between lessees and lessors. Some of the more common reasons for leasing are (1) *tax rate differentials,* (2) *alternative minimum taxes,* (3) *residual risk bearing,* and (4) *lack of access* to conventional debt markets.
- Two approaches are most commonly used to value businesses: the *discounted cash flow approach* and the *market multiple approach.*
- The *free equity cash flow approach,* which is a commonly used DCF method, focuses on the cash flows that are available to equity investors. (The *free operating cash flow* approach focuses on cash flows that are available to service both debt and equity investors.)
- The *market multiple approach* identifies some proxy for value, such as *earnings before interest, taxes, depreciation, and amortization (EBITDA),* and then multiplies it by a multiple derived from recent market data.
- The discounted cash flow approach has the strongest theoretical basis, but its inputs—the projected cash flows and discount rate—are very difficult to estimate. The market multiple approach is somewhat ad hoc but requires a much simpler set of inputs.

This chapter concludes the book. We hope that you have found it both easy to use and useful in your quest for competency in healthcare finance.

Questions

18.1 Distinguish between operating and financial leases. Would you be more likely to use an operating lease to finance a piece of diagnostic equipment or a hospital building?

18.2 Leasing companies often promote the following two benefits of leasing. Critique the merits of each hypothesized benefit.

a. Leasing preserves a business's liquidity because it avoids the large cash outlay associated with buying the asset.

b. Leasing (with operating leases) allows businesses to use more debt financing than would otherwise be possible because leasing keeps the liability off the books.

18.3 Assume that there were no IRS restrictions on what type of transaction could qualify as a lease for tax purposes. Explain why some restrictions should be imposed.

18.4 In the Nashville Radiology Group example given in the chapter, we assumed that the lease did not have a cancellation clause. What effect would a cancellation clause have on the analysis?

18.5 Discuss some of the asymmetries that drive lease transactions.

18.6 Describe the mechanics of the discounted cash flow (DCF) approach to business valuation.

18.7 Describe the mechanics of the market multiple approach to business valuation.

18.8 Which approach do you think is best for valuing a business: the DCF approach or the market multiple approach? Explain the rationale behind your answer.

Problems

18.1 Suncoast Healthcare is planning to acquire a new x-ray machine that costs $200,000. The business can either lease the machine using an operating lease or buy it using a loan from a local bank. Suncoast's balance sheet prior to acquiring the machine is a follows:

Current assets	$ 100,000	Debt	$ 400,000
Net fixed assets	900,000	Equity	600,000
Total assets	$1,000,000	Total claims	$1,000,000

a. What is Suncoast's current debt ratio?

b. What would the new debt ratio be if the machine were leased? If it is purchased?

c. Is the financial risk of the business different under the two acquisition alternatives?

18.2 Big Sky Hospital plans to obtain a new MRI that costs $1.5 million and has an estimated four-year useful life. It can obtain a bank loan for the entire amount and buy the MRI or it can lease the equipment. Assume that the following facts apply to the decision:

- The MRI falls into the three-year class for tax depreciation, so the MACRS allowances are 0.33, 0.45, 0.15, and 0.07 in Years 1 through 4, respectively.
- Estimated maintenance expenses are $75,000 payable at the beginning of each year whether the MRI is leased or purchased.
- Big Sky's marginal tax rate is 40 percent.
- The bank loan would have an interest rate of 15 percent.
- If leased, the lease (rental) payments would be $400,000 payable at the **end of** each of the next four years.
- The estimated residual (and salvage) value is $250,000.

a. What are the NAL and IRR of the lease? Interpret each value.

b. Assume now that the salvage value estimate is $300,000, but all other facts remain the same. What is the new NAL? The new IRR?

18.3 HealthPlan Northwest must install a new $1 million computer to track patient records in its three service areas. It plans to use the computer for only three years, at which time a brand new system will be acquired that will handle both billing and patient records. The company can obtain a 10 percent bank loan to buy the computer or it can lease the computer for three years. Assume that the following facts apply to the decision:

- The computer falls into the three-year class for tax depreciation, so the MACRS allowances are 0.33, 0.45, 0.15, and 0.07 in Years 1 through 4, respectively.
- The company's marginal tax rate is 34 percent.
- Tentative lease terms call for payments of $320,000 at the **end of** each year.
- The best estimate for the value of the computer after three years of wear and tear is $200,000.

a. What are the NAL and IRR of the lease? Interpret each value.

b. Assume now that the bank loan would cost 15 percent, but all other facts remain the same. What is the new NAL? The new IRR?

18.4 Assume that you have been asked to place a value on the ownership position in Briarwood Hospital. Its projected profit and loss statements and equity reinvestment (asset) requirements are shown below (in millions):

	2008	2009	2010	2011	2012
Net revenues	$225.0	$240.0	$250.0	$260.0	$275.0
Cash expenses	200.0	205.0	210.0	215.0	225.0
Depreciation	11.0	12.0	13.0	14.0	15.0
Earnings before interest and taxes (EBIT)	$ 14.0	$ 23.0	$ 27.0	$ 31.0	$ 35.0
Interest	8.0	9.0	9.0	10.0	10.0
Earnings before taxes (EBT)	$ 6.0	$ 14.0	$ 18.0	$ 21.0	$ 25.0
Taxes (40 percent)	2.4	5.6	7.2	8.4	10.0
Net profit	$ 3.6	$ 8.4	$ 10.8	$ 12.6	$ 15.0
Asset requirements	$ 6.0	$ 6.0	$ 6.0	$ 6.0	$ 6.0

Briarwood's cost of equity is 16 percent. The best estimate for Briarwood's long-term growth rate is 4 percent.

a. What is the equity value of the hospital?

b. Suppose that the expected long-term growth rate was 6 percent. What impact would this change have on the equity value of the business? What if the growth rate were only 2 percent?

18.5 Assume that you have been asked to place a value on the fund capital (equity) of BestHealth, a not-for-profit HMO. Its projected profit and loss statements and equity reinvestment (asset) requirements are shown below (in millions):

	2008	2009	2010	2011	2012
Net revenues	$50.0	$52.0	$54.0	$57.0	$60.0
Cash expenses	45.0	46.0	47.0	48.0	49.0
Depreciation	3.0	3.0	4.0	4.0	4.0
Interest	1.5	1.5	2.0	2.0	2.5
Net profit	$ 0.5	$ 1.5	$ 1.0	$ 3.0	$ 4.5
Asset requirements	$ 0.4	$ 0.4	$ 0.4	$ 0.4	$ 0.4

The cost of equity of similar for-profit HMO's is 14 percent, while the best estimate for BestHealth's long-term growth rate is 5 percent.

a. What is the equity value of the HMO?

b. Suppose that it was not necessary to retain any of the operating income in the business. What impact would this change have on the equity value?

Notes

1. For more information about the motivating forces and extent of leasing in the hospital industry, see Louis C. Gapenski and Barbara Langland-Orban, "Leasing Capital Assets and Durable Goods: Opinions and Practices in Florida Hospitals," *Health Care Management Review* (Summer 1991): 73–81.

2. Financial Accounting Standards Board (FASB) Statement 13, "Accounting for Leases," spells out in detail both the conditions under which the lease must be capitalized and the procedures for capitalizing it.

3. For a discussion of the lessor's analysis, see Louis C. Gapenski, *Understanding Healthcare Financial Management* (Chicago: Heath Administration Press, 2007), Chapter 8.

4. The use of the constant growth model to estimate a business's terminal value could create an upward bias in the valuation estimate because it assumes that the business will be operated forever. However, the contribution of cash flows after 40–50 years to the terminal value is inconsequential, so the constant growth model does not really require constant growth into perpetuity. Still, if there is some doubt about the life of the business, it might be best to either subjectively reduce the resulting constant growth terminal value estimate or to use some other methodology to estimate the terminal value.

References

The following references are relevant to leasing:

Beggan, J. F., and L. K. McNulty. 1991. "Restrictions on Depreciation Where Tax-Exempt Entities Are Involved." *Topics in Health Care Financing* (Fall): 62–69.

Berg, I. J., and A. N. Frankel. 1988. "Equipment Leasing: How, When, and If." *Health Progress* (November 15): 22–26.

Bernstein, C. 2006. "Is Your Leasing Arrangement Paying Off?" *Healthcare Financial Management* (August): 46–50.

Conbeer, G. P. 1990. "Leasing Can Add Flexibility to High-Tech Asset Management." *Healthcare Financial Management* (July): 26–34.

Dine, D. D. 1988. "Equipment Leasing Firms Offer Deals to Hospitals." *Modern Healthcare* (November 18): 50–51.

Grant, L., and D. O'Donnell. 1990. "Watch for Pitfalls When Analyzing Lease Options." *Healthcare Financial Management* (July): 36–43.

"Leasing: Three Experts Discuss the Advantages of Equipment Leasing." 1989. *HealthWeek* (November): 51–53.

McIntire, M., and D. J. Waldron. 2006. "Funding Technology: Evaluating and Exercising the Leasing Option." *Healthcare Financial Management* (November): 92–100.

Meyers, S. C., D. A. Dill, and A. J. Bautista. 1976. "Valuation of Financial Lease Contracts." *Journal of Finance* (June): 799–819.

Rosenthal, R. A. 1992. "Creative Leasing Strategies for Medical Office Buildings." *Healthcare Financial Management* (December): 30–34.

The following references are relevant to business valuation:

Baumann, B. H., and M. R. Oxaal. 1993. "Estimating the Value of Group Medical Practices." *Healthcare Financial Management* (December): 58–65.

Becker, S., and J. Callahan. 1996. "Physician-Hospital Transactions: Developing a Process for Handling Valuation-Related Issues." *Journal of Health Care Finance* (Winter): 19–31.

Becker, S., and R. J. Pristave. 1995. "Physician-Based Transactions: The Sale of Medical Practices, Ambulatory Surgery Centers, and Dialysis Facilities." *Journal of Health Care Finance* (Winter): 13–26.

Cleverley, W. O. 1997. "Factors Affecting the Valuation of Physician Practices." *Healthcare Financial Management* (December): 71–73.

Collins, H., and G. Simpson. 1995. "Avoiding Pitfalls in Medical Practice Valuation." *Healthcare Financial Management* (March): 20–22.

Evans, C. J. 2000. "Measuring the Value of Healthcare Business Assets." *Healthcare Financial Management* (April): 58–64.

Federa, R. D., and J. S. Ketcham. 1993. "The Valuation of Medical Practices." *Topics in Health Care Financing* (Spring): 67–75.

Hahn, W. 1994. "Determining a Healthcare Organization's Value." *Healthcare Financial Management* (August): 40–44.

Harrison, J. P., M. J. McCue, and B. B. Wang. 2003. "A Profile of Hospital Acquisitions." *Journal of Healthcare Management* (May/June): 156–171.

Moore, B. E. 1999. "Nonprofit to For-Profit Hospital Transactions: All Roads Lead to the Attorney General's Office." *Journal of Health Care Financing* (Spring): 29–36.

Nanda, S., and A. Miller. 1996. "Risk Analysis in the Valuation of Medical Practices." *Health Care Management Review* (Fall): 26–32.

Reilly, R. F. 1990. "The Valuation of a Medical Practice." *Health Care Management Review* (Summer): 25–34.

Reilly, R. F., and J. R. Rabe. 1997. "The Valuation of Health Care Intangible Assets." *Health Care Management Review* (Spring): 55–64.

Rimmer, T. B. 1995. "Physician Practice Acquisitions: Valuation Issues and Concerns." *Hospital & Health Services Administration* (Fall): 415–425.

Schwartzben, D., and S. A. Finkler. 1998. "Combining Accounting Approaches to Practice Valuation." *Healthcare Financial Management* (June): 70–76.

Strode, R. D. 2004. "Hospital-Physician Joint Ventures: Threat or Opportunity." *Healthcare Financial Management* (July): 80–86.

Unland, J. J. 1989. *Valuation of Hospitals and Medical Centers.* Chicago: Health Management Research Institute.

GLOSSARY

Abandonment value. The value of a project if discontinued before the end of its physical life.

Accounting. See financial accounting or managerial accounting.

Accounting breakeven. Accounting breakeven occurs when all accounting costs are covered (zero profitability). See economic breakeven.

Accounting period. The period (amount of time) covered by a set of financial statements—often a year, but sometimes a quarter or other time period.

Accounts receivable. A balance sheet current asset created when a service is performed (or good is shipped) but payment has not been received.

Accrual accounting. The recording of economic events when a transaction takes place that leads to a cash exchange. See cash accounting.

Accrued expenses. A business liability that stems from the fact that some obligations, such as wages and taxes, are not paid immediately as the obligations are created.

Acquiring company. A business that seeks to acquire another business.

Activity-based costing (ABC). The bottom-up approach to costing that identifies the activities required to provide a particular service, estimates the costs of those activities, and finally aggregates those costs. See traditional costing.

Actual (realized) return. The return actually earned on an investment, as opposed to the return that was expected when the investment was made.

Adverse selection. Occurs when individuals or businesses that are more likely to have claims purchase insurance.

Agency costs. A direct or indirect expense that is borne by a person (or group of persons) as a result of having delegated authority to an agent. For example, the costs borne by shareholders to ensure that the company's managers are acting in their best interests.

Aging schedule. A table that expresses a business's accounts receivable by how long each account has been outstanding.

Alternative minimum tax (AMT). A provision of the federal tax code that requires profitable businesses (or individuals) to pay a minimum amount of income tax regardless of the amounts of certain deductions.

Ambulatory payment classification (APC). A set of patient procedures that forms the basis for Medicare reimbursement for hospital outpatient services.

American Institute of Certified Public Accountants (AICPA). The professional association of public (financial) accountants.

Amortization schedule. A table that breaks down the fixed payment of an installment (amortized) loan into its principal and interest components.

Amortized (installment) loan. A loan that is repaid in equal periodic amounts that include both principal and interest payments.

Annual percentage rate (APR). The stated annual interest rate when compounding occurs more frequently than annually. It is calculated by multiplying the periodic rate by the number of compounding periods per year. See effective annual rate (EAR).

Annual report. A report issued annually by a corporation to its stockholders (or stakeholders) that contains descriptive information as well as historical financial statements.

Annuity. A series of payments of a fixed amount for a specified number of equal periods.

Annuity due. An annuity with payments occurring at the beginning of each period. See ordinary annuity.

Arbitrage. The simultaneous buying and selling of the identical item in different markets at different prices, thus earning a risk-free return. See risk arbitrage.

Arrearages. Preferred dividends that have been passed (not paid).

Asset. An item that either possesses or creates economic benefit for the organization. See current asset.

Asset management ratios. Financial statement analysis ratios that measure how effectively a firm is managing its assets.

Average collection period (ACP). The average length of time it takes a business to collect its receivables. Also called days sales outstanding (DSO) and days in patient accounts receivable.

Average length of stay (ALOS). The average time a patient spends in an inpatient setting per admission. Also called length of stay (LOS).

Balance sheet. A financial statement that list a business's assets, liabilities, and equity (fund capital).

Basic earning power (BEP) ratio. Earnings before interest and taxes (EBIT) divided by total assets. The BEP ratio measures the basic return on assets (ROA), before the influence of financial leverage and taxes.

Benchmarking. The comparison of performance factors, such as financial ratios, of one company against those of other companies and industry averages. Also called comparative analysis.

Best efforts arrangement. A type of contract between an investment banker and a company issuing stock, in which the banker commits only to making its best effort to sell the issue, as opposed to guaranteeing that the entire issue will be sold. See underwritten issue.

Beta coefficient (b). A measure of the risk of one asset relative to the risk of a collection of assets. Often, beta refers to the risk of a stock relative to the risk of the overall market as measured by some stock index. See characteristic line.

Bond. Long-term debt issued by a business or government unit and generally sold to a large number of individual investors. See term loan.

Bond indenture. The loan agreement between the bond issuer and bondholders that spells out the terms of the bond.

Bond insurance. Insurance that guarantees the payment of interest and repayment of principal on a bond even if the issuing company defaults. Insured bonds are rated AAA. Also called credit enhancement.

Book depreciation. Depreciation calculated according to generally accepted accounting principles (GAAP). See depreciation.

Book value. The value of a business's assets, liabilities, and equity as reported on the balance sheet. In other words, the value in accordance with generally accepted accounting principles (GAAP). See market value.

Breakeven analysis. A type of analysis that estimates the amount of some variable (such as volume or price or variable cost rate) needed to break even. See accounting breakeven and economic breakeven.

Breakup value. The value of a business assuming its assets are sold off separately.

Budget. A detailed plan, in dollar terms, of how a business and its subunits will acquire and utilize resources during a specified period of time. See cash budget, expense budget, operating budget, and revenue budget.

Budgeting. The process of preparing and utilizing a budget. See conventional budgeting and zero-based budgeting.

Business risk. The risk inherent in the operations of a business assuming it uses zero debt (or preferred stock) financing.

Call option. A contract that gives the holder of the option the right to buy a specified asset at the specified price within the specified time period.

Call provision. A provision in a bond indenture (contract) that gives the issuing company the right to redeem (call) the bonds prior to maturity.

Callable bond. A bond having a call provision.

Capital. The funds used to finance a business.

Capital Asset Pricing Model (CAPM). An equilibrium model that specifies the relationship between a stock's value and its market risk as measured by beta. See security market line (SML).

Capital budget. A plan (budget) that outlines a company's future expected expenditures on new fixed assets (land, plant, and equipment).

Capital budgeting. The process of analyzing and choosing new fixed assets.

Capital gain (loss). The profit (loss) from the sale of certain assets at more (less) than their purchase price.

Capital gains yield. The percentage capital gain (loss), usually applied to stocks and bonds.

Capital intensity. The amount of assets required per dollar of sales (revenues), which is the reciprocal of the total assets turnover ratio.

Capital market. The financial markets for long-term capital (usually stocks and long-term debt). See money market.

Capital rationing. The situation that occurs when a business has more attractive investment opportunities than it has capital to invest.

Capital structure. The structure of the liabilities and equity section of a business's balance sheet. Often expressed as the percentage of debt financing.

Capitalizing. The process of listing a long-term asset on the balance sheet. Applies to purchased assets and some leased assets.

Capitation. A reimbursement methodology that is based on the number of covered lives as opposed to the amount of services provided. See fee-for-service.

Case-mix index. A measure of inpatient service intensity calculated by averaging the patient diagnosis related group (DRG) weights.

Cash accounting. The recording of economic events when a cash exchange takes place. See accrual accounting.

Cash budget. A schedule that lists a business's or subunit's expected cash inflows, outflows, and net cash flows for some future period. See budget, expense budget, operating budget, and revenue budget.

Cash discount. The amount by which a seller is willing to reduce the price for cash payment.

Census. The number of hospital inpatients.

Characteristic line. The simple linear regression line that results from a plot of individual investment returns on the Y-axis and portfolio returns on the X-axis. The slope of the characteristic line is the investment's beta coefficient.

Charge-based reimbursement. A reimbursement methodology based on charges (chargemaster prices).

Chargemaster. A provider's official list of charges (prices) for goods and services rendered.

Chart of accounts. A document that assigns a unique numerical identifier to every account of an organization.

Classified stock. The term used to distinguish between stock classes when a business uses more than one type of common stock.

Closely held corporation. A corporation, typically small, in which the stock is held by a small number of individuals and not publicly traded.

Coefficient of variation. A statistical measure of an investment's stand-alone risk calculated by dividing the standard deviation of returns by the expected return.

Collection policy. The procedures used by a business to collect its accounts receivable.

Combination lease. A lease that contains features of both an operating and financial lease.

Commercial paper. Unsecured short-term promissory notes (debt) issued by large financially sound businesses.

Commodity futures. Futures contracts that involve the purchase or sale of commodities such as grain, livestock, fuel, metal, and wood.

Common size analysis. A technique to help analyze a business's financial statements that uses percentages instead of dollars for income statement items and balance sheet accounts.

Community rating. Premiums that are based on the health status of the entire community as opposed to the characters of one group or individual.

Comparative analysis. The comparison of key financial and operational measures of one business with those of comparable businesses or averages. Also called benchmarking.

Compensating balance. A minimum checking account balance that a business must maintain at a bank to compensate the bank for other services or loans. When used with loans, the compensating balance often is 10 to 20 percent of the principal amount.

Compounding. The process of finding the future value of a lump sum, annuity, or series of unequal cash flows.

Conglomerate merger. A merger of businesses in unrelated lines.

Consol. Another name for perpetuity. The term stems from the government perpetual bonds called Consols issued in England in 1815.

Contra asset. A balance sheet asset account, such as accumulated depreciation, that is subtracted from another asset account.

Contribution margin. (1) The difference between per unit revenue and per unit cost (variable cost rate), and hence the amount that each unit of output contributes to cover fixed costs and ultimately flows to profit. See total contribution margin. (2) The difference between revenues and direct costs of a subunit, and hence the amount of revenue that each subunit contributes to cover indirect (overhead) costs and ultimately flows to profit.

Conventional budgeting. An approach to budgeting that uses the previous budget as the starting point. See zero-based budgeting.

Convertible bond. A bond that can be exchanged at the option of the bondholder for shares of stock of the issuing firm at a fixed price.

Copayment. The percentage of eligible medical expenses that must be paid by the insured individual. For example, 20 percent for each outpatient visit.

Corporate alliance. A cooperative venture between two businesses that is smaller in scope than a merger.

Corporate bond. Debt issued by for-profit businesses, as opposed to government or tax-exempt (municipal) bonds.

Corporate cost of capital. The discount rate (opportunity cost of capital) that reflects the overall (average) risk of the entire business. See divisional cost of capital and project cost of capital.

Corporate goals. Specified goals, including financial, that an organization strives to attain. Generally, corporate goals are qualitative in nature. See corporate objectives.

Corporate objectives. Quantitative targets that an organization sets to meet its corporate goals.

Corporate risk. A type of portfolio risk. That portion of the riskiness of a business project that cannot be diversified away by holding the project as part of the business's portfolio of projects. See market risk.

Corporation. A legal business entity that is separate and distinct from its owners (or community) and managers.

Correlation. The tendency of two variables to move together.

Correlation coefficient. A standardized measure of correlation that ranges from –1 (variables move perfectly opposite of one another) to +1 (variables move in perfect synchronization).

Cost. A resource use associated with providing, or supporting, a specific service. See fixed cost, variable cost, direct cost, and indirect cost.

Cost allocation. The process by which overhead costs are assigned (allocated) to patient services departments. See activity-based costing, cost driver, cost pool, and traditional costing.

Cost allocation method. The mathematical procedure used to allocate overhead costs to patient services departments. See direct method, reciprocal method, and step-down method.

Cost approach. A technique that uses utilization forecasts and underlying costs to set premium rates. See demographic approach and fee-for-service approach.

Cost-based reimbursement. A reimbursement methodology based on the costs incurred in providing services.

Cost behavior. The relationship between an organization's fixed costs, variable costs, and total costs. Also called cost structure or underlying cost structure. See relevant range.

Cost driver. The basis on which a cost pool is allocated; for example, square footage for facilities costs. See cost pool.

Cost of capital. A generic term for the cost of a business's financing. See corporate cost of capital.

Cost of debt. The return required (interest rate) on a business's debt financing. A component of the cost of capital.

Cost of equity. The return required on the equity investment in a business. A component of the cost of capital.

Cost pool. A group of overhead costs to be allocated; for example, facilities costs. See cost driver.

Cost shifting. The process of billing some payers a higher amount than justified by costs so that other payers can be billed a lower amount than justified by costs.

Cost structure. The relationship between an organization's fixed costs, variable costs, and total costs. Also called underlying cost structure or cost behavior. See relevant range.

Costly trade credit. That credit taken by a company from a vendor in excess of the free trade credit.

Coupon (interest) rate. The stated annual rate of interest on a bond, which is equal to the coupon payment divided by the par value.

Coupon payment. The dollar amount of annual interest on a bond.

Coverage. A debt management ratio that divides the amount of funds available to meet a set of fixed payment obligations by the amount of obligation. It measures how many dollars are available to pay each dollar of fixed obligation.

There are many different coverage ratios depending on the fixed obligations included.

Credit enhancement. Insurance that guarantees the payment of interest and repayment of principal on a bond even if the issuing company defaults. Insured bonds are rated AAA. Also called bond insurance.

Credit period. The length of time that trade credit is offered by a supplier.

Credit policy. A business's rules and regulations regarding granting credit and collecting from buyers that take the credit.

Credit rating. Ratings that are assigned by rating agencies, such as Standard & Poor's or Moody's, which measure the probability of default on a debt issue.

Credit standards. The minimum financial condition set by a seller to extend credit to a customer (buyer).

Credit terms. The statement of terms that extends credit to a buyer. For example, 2/10, net 30 means that a 2 percent discount is offered if the buyer pays in 10 days. If the discount is not taken, the full amount of the invoice is due in 30 days.

Current asset. An asset that is expected to be converted into cash within one accounting period (often a year).

Current (bond) yield. The annual coupon payment divided by the current bond price.

Current ratio. A liquidity ratio calculated by dividing current assets by current liabilities. It measures the number of dollars of current assets available to pay each dollar of current liabilities.

CVP (cost-volume-profit) analysis. A technique applied to an organization's cost and revenue structure that analyzes the effect of volume changes on costs and profits. Also called profit analysis.

Dashboard. A format for presenting a business's key performance indicators that resembles the dashboard of an automobile.

Days in patient accounts receivable. The average length of time it takes a provider to collect its receivables. Also called days sales outstanding (DSO) and average collection period (ACP).

Days sales outstanding (DSO). The average length of time it takes a business to collect its receivables. Also called average collection period (ACP) and days in patient accounts receivable.

Debenture. An unsecured bond.

Debt capacity. The amount of debt in a business's optimal (target) capital structure.

Debt ratio. A debt utilization ratio that measures the proportion of debt (versus equity) financing. Typically defined as total debt (liabilities) divided by total assets.

Decision tree. A form of scenario analysis that incorporates multiple decision points over time. The end result resembles a tree on its side with branches extending to the right.

Declaration date. The date on which a for-profit corporation's directors issue a dividend declaration statement.

Deductible. The dollar amount that must be spent on healthcare services before benefits are paid by the third-party payer. For example, $250 per year.

Default. Failure by a borrower to make a promised interest or principal repayment.

Default risk. The risk that a borrower will not pay the interest (or repay principal) as agreed upon in the loan agreement.

Default risk premium. The premium that creditors demand (add to the basic interest rate) for bearing default risk. The greater the default risk, the higher the default risk premium.

Degree of operating leverage. A measure of a business's operating leverage (the proportion of fixed costs in the cost structure). Defined as total contribution margin divided by earnings before interest and taxes (EBIT).

Demographic approach. A technique that uses population demographics and costs to set premium rates. See cost approach and fee-for-service approach.

Depreciation. A noncash charge against earnings on the income statement that reflects the "wear and tear" on a business's fixed assets. See book depreciation and Modified Accelerated Cost Recovery System (MACRS).

Derivative. A security whose value stems from the value of another asset; for example, futures and options.

Diagnosis related group (DRG). A numerical code for a single patient diagnosis. DRGs form the basis for Medicare reimbursement of hospital inpatient services.

Direct cost. A cost that is tied exclusively to a subunit, such as the salaries of laboratory employees. When a subunit is eliminated, its direct costs disappear. See indirect cost.

Direct method. A cost allocation method in which all overhead costs are allocated directly to the patient services departments with no recognition that overhead services are provided to other overhead departments. See reciprocal method and step-down method.

Discount bond. A bond that sells for less than its par value.

Discounted cash flow (DCF) analysis. The use of time value of money techniques to value investments.

Discounted payback (period). The number of years it takes for a business to recover its investment in a project when time value of money is considered. See payback (period).

Diversifiable risk. That portion of the risk of an investment that can be eliminated by holding the investment as part of a diversified portfolio. See portfolio risk.

Divestiture. The selling off of a portion of a company's assets. The opposite of acquisition.

Dividend. The periodic payment paid to owners of common and preferred stock.

Dividend irrelevance theory. The theory that the dividend amount paid has no effect on the company's stock price or cost of capital.

Dividend reinvestment plan (DRIP). A plan under which the dividends paid to a stockholder are automatically reinvested in the company's common stock.

Dividend yield. The annual dividend divided by current stock price.

Divisional cost of capital. The discount rate (opportunity cost of capital) that reflects the unique riskiness of a division within a corporation. See corporate cost of capital and project cost of capital.

Due diligence. The process of research and analysis that takes place in advance of an investment, merger, or business alliance.

Du Pont analysis. A financial statement analysis tool that decomposes return on equity into three components: profit margin, total asset turnover, and equity multiplier.

Duration. A measure of the maturity of a debt security that considers both the interest payments and the return of principal. In essence, the weighted average maturity of the security.

EBIT. Earnings before interest and taxes.

EBITDA. A common measure of earnings used in business valuation. Defined as earnings before interest, taxes, depreciation, and amortization.

Economic breakeven. Economic breakeven occurs when all accounting costs plus necessary profits are covered. See accounting breakeven.

Economic life. The number of years that maximizes the value (NPV) of a project.

Economic value added (EVA). A measure of the economic profitability of a business that considers all costs, including the cost of equity.

Economies of scale. A situation that arises when the ratio of assets (or costs) to sales decreases as sales increase (the business gets larger).

Effective annual rate (EAR). The interest rate that, under annual compounding, produces the same future value as was produced by more frequent compounding. See annual percentage rate (APR).

Efficient markets hypothesis. The theory that states that (1) stocks are always in equilibrium and (2) it is impossible for investors to consistently earn excess returns (beat the market).

Electronic claims processing. The electronic transmission and processing of reimbursement claims and payments.

Equity. The book value of the ownership position in a business.

Equivalent annual annuity. A technique for comparing the profitability of competing projects that have different lives. See replacement chain.

ESOP (employee stock ownership plan). A retirement plan in which employees own the stock of the employing company.

Ex-dividend date. The date on which the right to the dividend is lost. If a stock is bought on or after this date, the dividend is paid to the seller.

Exercise value. The difference between the price of the stock and the exercise (strike) price of an option on that stock.

Expected rate of return. The return expected on an investment when the purchase is made. See realized rate of return.

Expense budget. A budget that focuses on the costs of providing goods or services. See budget, cash budget, operating budget, and revenue budget.

External financing plan. The organization's plan for meeting its external financing needs.

Fee-for-service. A reimbursement methodology that provides payment each time a service is provided. See capitation.

Fee-for-service approach. A technique that uses utilization forecasts and fee-for-service prices to set premium rates. See cost approach and demographic approach.

Financial Accounting Standards Board (FASB). A private organization whose mission is to establish and improve the standards of financial accounting and reporting for private businesses.

Financial accounting. That field of accounting that focuses on the measurement and communication of the economic events and status of an entire organization. See managerial accounting.

Financial asset. A security such as a stock or bond that represents a claim on a business's cash flows. See real asset.

Financial distress costs. The direct and indirect costs associated with the probability of business bankruptcy. These costs play a key role in the trade-off theory of capital structure.

Financial future. A contract that provides for the purchase or sale of a financial asset some time in the future at a fixed price.

Financial intermediary. A business that buys securities with funds that it obtains by issuing its own securities. Examples include commercial banks and mutual funds.

Financial lease. A lease agreement that has a term (life) approximately equal to the expected useful life of the leased asset. See operating lease.

Financial leverage. The use of fixed cost financing such as debt and preferred stock.

Financial merger. A merger in which the companies will continue to be operated as separate entities. See operating merger.

Financial plan. That portion of the operating plan that focuses on the finance function. See strategic plan and operating plan.

Financial risk. Generically, the risk that the return on an investment will be less than expected. In a capital structure context, the additional risk placed on the business's owners (or community) when debt (or preferred stock) financing is used.

Financial statements. Statements prepared by financial accountants that convey the financial status of an organization. The three primary statements are the income statement, balance sheet, and statement of cash flows.

Financial statement analysis. The process of using data contained in a business's financial statements to make judgments about financial condition.

Fiscal year. The year covered by an organization's financial statements. It usually, but not necessarily, coincides with a calendar year.

Fixed assets. A business's long-term assets such as land, buildings, and equipment.

Fixed assets turnover (utilization) ratio. The ratio of revenues to net fixed assets. It measures the ability of fixed assets to generate sales.

Fixed cost. A cost that is not related to the volume of services supplied. For example, facilities costs (within some relevant range). See semi-fixed cost and variable cost.

Fixed rate debt. Debt that has an interest rate that is fixed for its entire life. See floating rate debt.

Flexible budget. A budget, prepared after the period is over, that combines realized volume with initial budget assumptions. See static budget.

Float. The difference between the balance shown on a business's (or individual's) checkbook and the balance shown on the bank's books.

Floating rate debt. Debt with interest payments that are linked to the rate on some other debt (or index). As the index goes up and down, so does the interest rate on the floating rate debt. See fixed rate debt.

Flotation cost. The administrative costs associated with issuing new securities, such as legal, accounting, and investment banker's fees.

Free cash flow. The cash flow available for distribution after all costs have been considered, including required investments in fixed assets.

Free trade credit. The amount of credit received from a supplier that has no explicit cost attached. In other words, credit received during the discount period.

Friendly merger. A merger that is supported by the management of the target company. See hostile merger.

Full cost pricing. For price setters, the process of setting prices to cover all costs plus a profit component. See marginal cost pricing.

Full-time equivalent (FTE). The number of employees, assuming that everyone is employed on a full-time basis.

Fund capital. Equity capital in a not-for-profit corporation.

Future value (FV). The ending amount of an investment of a lump sum, annuity, or uneven cash flow stream. See present value (PV).

Generally accepted accounting principles (GAAP). The set of guidelines that have evolved to guide the preparation and presentation of financial statements.

Global reimbursement (pricing). The payment of a single amount for the complete set of services required to treat a single episode.

Going public. The initial selling of stock to the general public by a closely held corporation. See initial public offering (IPO).

Goodwill. An accounting term for the amount paid in a business acquisition that exceeds the book value of the assets of the target business.

Gross fixed assets. The historical cost of a business's fixed assets. See net fixed assets.

Growth option. A managerial option whose value stems from the opportunity that a project creates to make other profitable investments.

Guideline lease. A lease contract that meets the Internal Revenue Service (IRS) requirements for a genuine lease, thus allowing the lessee to deduct the full amount of the lease payment from taxable income.

Hedging. A transaction undertaken to lower the risk caused by price fluctuations in such things as input commodities and interest rates.

Historical cost. In cost of capital, the average cost of a business's existing, or embedded, capital. See marginal cost. In accounting, the purchase price of an asset.

Holding company. A corporation formed for the sole purpose of owning other companies.

Horizontal merger. A merger between two companies in the same line of business.

Hostile merger. A merger that occurs in spite of the fact that the target firm's management resisted the offer. See friendly merger.

Hurdle rate. The minimum required rate of return on an investment. Also called opportunity cost rate.

Immunization. The process of structuring a debt porfolio to eliminate interest rate risk.

Income statement. A financial statement, prepared in accordance with generally accepted accounting principles (GAAP), that summarizes a business's revenues, expenses, and profitability. See profit and loss (P&L) statement.

Incremental cash flow. A cash flow that arises solely from a project that is being evaluated, and hence one that should be included in the project analysis. See nonincremental cash flow.

Indenture. A legal document that spells out the rights and obligations of both bondholders and the issuing corporation. In other words, the loan agreement for a bond.

Independent projects. Projects that are not related to one another and hence can be accepted or rejected independently. See mutually exclusive projects.

Indirect (overhead) cost. A cost that is tied to shared resources rather than to an individual subunit of an organization; for example, facilities costs. See direct cost.

Inflation premium. The premium that debt investors add to the base interest rate to compensate for inflation.

Information content (signaling) hypothesis. The theory that investors regard dividend announcements as signals of management's forecasts of future earnings.

Initial public offering (IPO). The initial sale of stock to the general public by a closely held corporation. See going public.

Insiders. The officers, directors, and major stockholders of a company.

Integrated delivery system (IDS). A single organization that offers a broad range of healthcare services in a unified manner.

Interest rate risk. The riskiness to current debtholders that stems from interest rate changes. See price risk and reinvestment rate risk.

Internal rate of return (IRR). A project return on investment (ROI) measure that focuses on expected rate of return. See net present value (NPV).

Inventory turnover (utilization) ratio. Revenues divided by inventory value. The average length of time it takes to convert inventory into revenues.

Inverted yield curve. A downward sloping yield curve. See normal yield curve.

Investment banker. The middleman between businesses that want to raise capital and the investors who supply the capital.

Investment grade bond. A bond with a BBB or higher rating. See junk bond.

Investment timing option. A managerial option to delay a project rather than to commence immediately.

Investor-owned business. A for-profit business whose capital is supplied by owners (stockholders in the case of corporations). See not-for-profit corporation.

Joint venture. The combining of parts of two different companies to accomplish a specific, limited objective.

Junk bond. A bond with a BB or lower rating. See investment grade bond.

Key performance indicator (KPI). A financial statement ratio and/or operating indicator that is considered by management to be critical to the business's financial performance.

Law of large numbers. A statistical concept that states that the standard deviation of a large number of identical probability distributions is much smaller than the standard deviation of only one of the distributions.

Length of stay (LOS). The average time a patient spends in an inpatient setting per admission. Also called average length of stay (ALOS).

Lessee. In a lease agreement, the party that uses the leased asset and makes the rental payments. See lessor.

Lessor. In a lease agreement, the party that owns the leased asset and receives the rental payments. See lessee.

Leveraged lease. A lease in which the lessor borrows a portion of the purchase price to buy the leased asset.

Liability. A fixed obligation of the business. Also, one category of balance sheet accounts. Current liabilities are those that become due (must be paid) within one accounting period (often one year).

Limited liability company (LLC). A corporate form of organization that combines some features of a partnership with others of a corporation.

Limited liability partnership (LLP). A partnership form of organization that limits the professional (malpractice) liability of its members.

Limited partnership. A partnership form of organization with general partners that have control and unlimited liability, and limited partners that have no control and limited liability.

Line of credit. A loan arrangement in which a bank agrees to lend some maximum amount to a business over some designated period.

Liquid asset. An asset that can be quickly converted to cash at its fair market value.

Liquidity. The ability of a business to meet its cash obligations as they become due.

Liquidity premium (LP). The premium that debt investors add to the base interest rate to compensate for lack of liquidity.

Lumpy assets. Fixed assets that cannot be acquired smoothly as demand grows but rather must be added in large increments. For example, hospital beds.

Managerial accounting. That field of accounting that focuses primarily on subunit (i.e., departmental) data used internally for managerial decision making.

Managerial options. Options inherent in projects that give managers the opportunity to create additional value. For example, a project to build a small outpatient surgery center provides the managerial option to expand the center should patient demand increase. Also called real options.

Marginal cost. In cost of capital, the cost of the next dollar of capital raised. See historical cost.

Marginal cost pricing. For price setters, the process of setting prices to cover only marginal costs. See full cost pricing.

Market/book ratio. The market value (price) of a stock divided by its book value, which measures the number of dollars that investors are willing to pay for each dollar of book value.

Market multiple method. A technique for valuing a business that applies a market-determined multiple to some proxy for value such as net income.

Market portfolio. A portfolio that contains all publicly traded stocks. Often proxied by some market index such as the S&P 500.

Market risk. A type of portfolio risk. That portion of the risk of a stock investment that cannot be eliminated by holding the stock as part of a diversified portfolio. Also, that portion of the riskiness of a business project that cannot be diversified away by holding the stock of the company as part of a diversified portfolio. See corporate risk.

Market risk premium (RP_M). The difference between the expected rate of return on the market portfolio and the risk-free rate. In other words, the premium above the risk-free rate that investors require to bear average risk.

Market value. The value of an asset as set by the marketplace. See book value.

Marketable securities. Securities that are held in lieu of cash. Typically very safe, short-term securities such as Treasury bills. Often called short-term investments when listed on the balance sheet.

Matching principle. The concept that expenses on an income statement must be matched (in time) with the revenues to which they are related.

Materials management. The management of the procurement, storage, and utilization of supplies inventories. Also called supply chain management.

Maturity. The amount of time until a loan matures (must be repaid).

Maturity date. The date on which the principal amount of a loan must be repaid.

Maturity matching. The matching of the maturities of assets being financed and the financing used to acquire the assets.

Maturity risk premium (MRP). The premium that debt investors add to the base interest rate to compensate for interest rate risk.

Medicaid. A federal and state government health insurance program that provides benefits to low-income individuals.

Medicare. A federal government health insurance program that provides benefits to individuals 65 and older.

Merger. The combination of two businesses into a single entity.

Miller model. A capital structure theory model that introduces the effects of personal taxes to the Modigliani and Miller (MM) model.

Mission statement. A statement that defines the overall purpose of the organization.

Modified Accelerated Cost Recovery System (MACRS). The Internal Revenue Service (IRS) system used to calculate depreciation for tax purposes. See depreciation.

Modified internal rate of return (MIRR). A project return on investment (ROI) measure similar to IRR but with a different reinvestment rate assumption. See internal rate of return (IRR).

Modigliani and Miller (MM) model. A capital structure theory model that defines the relationship between the use of debt financing and firm value. The model has two variants: one with zero taxes and one with corporate taxes. See Miller model.

Money market. The financial markets for debt securities with maturities of one year or less. See capital market.

Monte Carlo simulation. A computerized risk analysis technique that uses continuous distributions to represent the uncertain input variables.

Moral hazard. The risk that an insured individual or business will purposely take actions that increase the likelihood of a claim.

Mortgage bond. A bond issued by a business that pledges real property (land and buildings) as collateral.

Municipal bond (muni). A tax-exempt bond issued by a governmental entity such as a healthcare financing authority. See corporate bond.

Mutual fund. A company that sells shares and then uses the proceeds to buy financial instruments.

Mutually exclusive projects. Projects that are related to one another such that the acceptance of one precludes the acceptance of the other. See independent projects.

Net advantage to leasing (NAL). The discounted cash flow dollar value of a lease to the lessee. Similar to net present value (NPV).

Net assets. In not-for-profit businesses, the term often used in place of "equity."

Net cash flow. The sum of net income and noncash expenses (typically depreciation).

Net fixed assets. The value of a business's assets net of depreciation (Net fixed assets = Gross fixed assets – Accumulated depreciation). See gross fixed assets.

Net income. A business's profitability as reported on the income statement. A measure of long-run economic profitability according to generally accepted accounting principles (GAAP).

Net operating profit after taxes (NOPAT). The amount of profit a business would generate if it had no debt. Generally defined as earnings before interest and taxes (EBIT) multiplied by (1 – Tax rate).

Net present value (NPV). A project return on investment (ROI) measure that focuses on expected dollar return. See internal rate of return (IRR).

Net present social value. The present value of a project's social value. Added to the financial net present value (NPV) to obtain a project's total value.

Net working capital. A liquidity measure equal to current assets minus current liabilities. See working capital.

Nominal (stated) interest rate. The interest rate stated in a debt contract. It does not reflect the effect of compounding that occurs more frequently than annually. See effective annual rate (EAR).

Nonincremental cash flow. A cash flow that does not stem solely from a project that is being evaluated. Nonincremental cash flows are not included in a project analysis. See incremental cash flow.

Nonnormal cash flows. Project cash flows that contain one or more outflows after the inflows have begun. See normal cash flows.

Nonprofit corporation. A not-for-profit corporation.

Normal cash flows. Project cash flows that have all of the outflows occurring before all of the inflows. See nonnormal cash flows.

Normal yield curve. An upward sloping yield curve. See inverted yield curve.

Not-for-profit corporation. A corporation that has a charitable purpose, is tax exempt, and has no owners. Also called nonprofit corporation. See investor-owned business.

Occupancy rate. The percentage of hospital beds occupied.

Off-balance sheet financing. Financing used by a business that does not appear on the balance sheet. For example short-term (operating) leases.

Operating budget. A single budget that combines both the revenue and expense budgets. See budget, cash budget, expense budget, and revenue budget.

Operating indicator. A ratio that focuses on operating data rather than financial data.

Operating indicator analysis. The process of using operating indicators to help explain a business's financial condition.

Operating lease. A lease whose term is much shorter than the expected life of the asset being leased. See financial lease.

Operating leverage. The proportion of fixed costs in a business's cost structure. See degree of operating leverage.

Operating margin. Net operating income divided by total operating revenues. It measures the amount of operating profit per dollar of operating revenues, and hence focuses on the core activities of a business. See profit (total) margin.

Operating merger. A merger in which the operations of the two companies are combined into a single entity.

Operating plan. An organizational roadmap for the future, often for five years, based on the business's strategic plan. See financial plan and strategic plan.

Opportunity cost. The cost associated with alternative uses of the same asset. For example, if land is used for one project, it is no longer available for other uses, and hence an opportunity cost arises.

Opportunity cost rate. The rate of return expected on alternative investments similar in risk to an investment being evaluated. Also called hurdle rate.

Optimal capital structure. That mix of debt and equity financing that management believes to be appropriate for the business. Generally based on both quantitative and qualitative factors. Becomes the business's target capital structure.

Option. A contract that gives the holder the right to buy (or sell) an asset at a specified price within a specified period of time.

Ordinary (regular) annuity. An annuity with payments occurring at the end of each period. See annuity due.

Par value. The face (nominal) value of a security. The par value of a debt security is the amount to be repaid at maturity.

Partnership. A nonincorporated business entity that is created by two or more individuals.

Payback (period). The number of years it takes for a business to recover its investment in a project without considering the time value of money. See discounted payback (period).

Payment (PMT). In time value of money, the dollar amount of an annuity cash flow.

Payment date. The date on which a corporation pays its dividend to stockholders.

Percentage change analysis. A technique to help analyze a business's financial statements that expresses the year-to-year changes in income statement items and balance accounts as percentages.

Percent of sales method. A technique for forecasting financial statements that assumes that most income statement items and balance sheet accounts are tied directly (proportionately) to sales.

Per diem. A reimbursement methodology that pays a set amount for each inpatient day.

Periodic rate. In time value of money (discounted cash flow analysis), the interest rate per period. For example, 2 percent quarterly interest, which equals an 8 percent stated (annual) rate. See effective annual rate (EAR).

Permanent assets. The minimum amount of assets held by a business, including seasonal and cyclical periods. See temporary assets.

Permanent current assets (working capital). The dollar amount of current assets that is permanent in nature. See permanent assets.

Perpetuity. A debt security that has no stated maturity.

Poison pill. A provision in a company's charter that makes it an unattractive, hostile takeover target. For example, a provision that allows existing stockholders to buy more stock at a low price if a hostile takeover occurs.

Pooling of losses. Losses that are spread over a large group of individuals rather than borne solely by one individual.

Portfolio. A number of individual investments held collectively.

Portfolio risk. The riskiness of an individual investment when it is held as part of a large portfolio as opposed to held in isolation. There are two types of portfolio risk: corporate risk and market risk. See stand-alone risk, corporate risk, and market risk.

Post-audit. The feedback process in which the performance of projects previously accepted are reviewed and necessary actions are taken.

Preemptive right. The right that gives current shareholders the opportunity to purchase any newly issued shares (in proportion to their current holdings) before they are offered to the general public.

Preferred stock. A hybrid security issued by for-profit corporations that has characteristics of both debt and equity.

Premium tier. A category of employee health insurance coverage. For example, a two-tier system might offer individual and family coverage.

Present value (PV). The beginning amount of an investment of a lump sum, annuity, or uneven cash flow stream. See future value.

Price/earnings ratio. Price per share divided by earnings per share. It measures how much investors are willing to pay for each dollar of earnings.

Price risk. The risk that rising interest rates will lower the values of outstanding debt. See interest rate risk.

Price setter. A business that has the power to set the market prices for its goods or services. See price taker.

Price taker. A business that has no power to influence the prices set by the marketplace. See price setter.

Primary market. The market in which newly issued securities are sold for the first time. See secondary market.

Private placement. The sale of newly issued securities to a single investor or small group of investors. Private placements have lower costs and may be accomplished more quickly than a public offering. See public offering.

Probability distribution. All possible outcomes of a random event along with their probabilities of occurrence. For example, the probability distribution of rates of return on a proposed project.

Professional corporation (PC). A type of corporate business organization in which owners/managers still have professional (medical) liability. Called a professional association (PA) in some states.

Profit analysis. A technique applied to an organization's cost and revenue structure that analyzes the effect of volume changes on costs and profits. Also called CVP (cost-volume-profit) analysis.

Profit and loss (P&L) statement. A statement that summarizes the revenues, expenses, and profitability of either the entire organization or a subunit. Can be formatted in different ways for different purposes and does not conform to GAAP. See income statement.

Profit (total) margin. Net income divided by total revenues. It measures the amount of total profit per dollar of total revenues. See operating margin.

Profitability index (PI). A project return on investment (ROI) measure defined as the present value of cash inflows divided by the present value of outflows. It measures the number of dollars of inflow per dollar of outflow (on a present value basis), or the "bang for the buck."

Profitability ratios. A group of ratios that measure different dimensions of profitability, and hence the combined effects of operational decisions.

Pro forma. As applied to financial statements, a statement that is constructed under assumptions that differ from generally accepted accounting principles (GAAP). The term is also used to indicate forecasted financial statements.

Project cost of capital. The discount rate (opportunity cost rate) that reflects the unique riskiness of a project. See corporate cost of capital and divisional cost of capital.

Project scoring. An approach to project assessment that considers both financial and nonfinancial factors.

Promissory note. A document that specifies the terms and conditions of a loan. Also called loan agreement or, in the case of bonds, indenture.

Proprietorship. A simple form of business owned by a single individual. Also called sole proprietorship.

Prospective payment. A reimbursement methodology that is established beforehand by the third-party payer and, in theory, not related to costs or charges.

Provider. An organization that provides healthcare services (treats patients).

Proxy. A document giving one person the authority to act for another—typically the power to vote shares of common stock.

Proxy fight. An attempt to take control of a corporation by soliciting the votes (proxies) of current shareholders.

Public offering. The sale of newly issued securities to the general public through an investment banker. See private placement.

Publicly held corporation. A corporation whose shares are held by the general public as opposed to closely (privately) held, where the shares are held by a small number of individuals, usually the managers.

Qualitative risk assessment. A process for assessing project risk that focuses on qualitative issues as opposed to profit variability.

Ratio analysis. The process of creating and analyzing ratios from financial statement and other data to help assess a business's financial condition.

Real asset. Property such as land, buildings, and equipment that creates a business's cash flows. See financial asset.

Real options. Options inherent in projects that give managers the opportunity to create additional value. For example, a project to build a small outpatient surgery center provides the real option to expand the center should patient demand increase. Also called managerial options.

Real rate of return. The rate of return on an investment net of inflation effects.

Real risk-free rate. The rate of interest on a riskless investment in the absence of inflation.

Realized rate of return. The return actually achieved on an investment when it is sold. See expected rate of return.

Reciprocal method. A cost allocation method that completely recognizes the overhead services provided by one overhead department to another. See direct method and step-down method.

Refunding. The process of calling (redeeming) a debt security. Usually involves issuing new debt at a lower interest rate and using the proceeds to redeem existing higher interest rate debt.

Reinvestment rate risk. The risk that falling interest rates will reduce the returns earned on the reinvestment of debt interest payments (and perhaps principal repayments). See interest rate risk.

Relative value unit (RVU). A measure of the amount of resources required to provide a particular service. See resource based relative value system (RBRVS).

Relevant range. The range of output (volume) over which the organization's cost structure holds.

Replacement chain. A technique for comparing the profitability of competing projects that have different lives. See equivalent annual annuity.

Required rate of return. The minimum rate of return required on an investment considering its riskiness. Also called hurdle rate.

Required reserves. Insurance company reserves that are mandated by state regulators. See reserves.

Reserves. Funds that are accumulated by a business to protect against future adverse events. See required reserves.

Reserve borrowing capacity. The practice of businesses to use less than the true optimal amount of debt to ensure easy access to new debt at reasonable interest rates regardless of circumstances.

Residual value. The estimated market value of a leased asset at the end of the lease.

Resource based relative value system (RBRVS). The system, based on relative value units, used by Medicare to reimburse physicians. See relative value unit (RVU).

Restrictive covenant. A provision in a bond indenture (loan agreement) that protects the interests of bondholders by restricting the actions of management.

Retained earnings. That portion of net income that is retained within the business as opposed to paid out as dividends. Not-for-profit corporations must retain all earnings.

Return on assets (ROA). Net income divided by the book value of total assets. Measures the dollars of earnings per dollar of book asset investment.

Return on equity (ROE). Net income divided by the book value of equity. Measures the dollars of earnings per dollar of book equity investment.

Revenue budget. A budget that focuses on the revenues of an organization or its subunits. See budget, cash budget, expense budget, and operating budget.

Revenue cycle. The set of recurring activities and related information processing required to provide patient services and collect for those services.

Revenue recognition principle. The concept that revenues must be recognized in the accounting period when they are realizable and earned.

Revolving credit agreement. A formal line of credit extended by a lender (or group of lenders).

Rights offering. The mechanism by which new common stock is offered to existing shareholders. Each stockholder receives an option (right) to buy a specific number of new shares at a given price.

Risk-adjusted discount rate (RADR). A discount rate that accounts for the specific riskiness of the investment being analyzed.

Risk arbitrage. The buying and selling of stocks that are likely takeover targets. See arbitrage.

Risk aversion. The tendency of individuals and businesses to dislike risk. The implication of risk aversion is that riskier investments must offer higher expected rates of return to be acceptable.

Risk management. The management of the risks encountered by a business, including the minimization of both the occurrence of adverse events and the costs associated with an event should it occur.

Risk pool. A fund that is set up by an insurer that is dispersed to providers only if specified goals are met. Also called a withhold.

S corporation. A corporation with a limited number of stockholders that is taxed as a proprietorship or partnership.

Salvage value. The expected market value of an asset (project) at the end of its useful life.

Scenario analysis. (1) In general, a technique that examines alternative outcomes as opposed to only the expected outcome. (2) In project analysis, a risk assessment technique that assesses how best and worst case scenarios for uncertain input values affect profitability.

Secondary market. The market in which previously issued securities are sold.

Secured loan. A loan backed by collateral—often inventories or receivables.

Securities and Exchange Commission (SEC). The government agency that regulates the sale of securities and the operations of securities exchanges.

Security Market Line (SML). That portion of the Capital Asset Pricing Model (CAPM) that specifies the relationship between market risk and required rate of return.

Semi-fixed cost. A cost that is fixed at two or more values within the relevant range. See fixed cost and variable cost.

Sensitivity analysis. A project analysis technique that assesses how changes in single input variables, such as utilization, affect profitability.

Shelf registration. A procedure for selling securities that uses a master statement pre-filed with the Securities and Exchange Commission (SEC) to speed up the issuance process.

Sinking fund. A bond feature that calls for funds to be used to refund a portion of the issue each year until maturity.

Sole proprietorship. A simple form of business owned by a single individual. Also called proprietorship.

Spontaneously generated funds. Financing that occurs when a business's accruals and accounts payable increase automatically because of overall growth.

Stakeholder. An individual or business that has an interest, typically financial, in an organization. For example, owners (in for-profit businesses), managers, patients, and suppliers.

Stand-alone risk. The riskiness of an investment that is held in isolation as opposed to held as part of a portfolio. See portfolio risk.

Standard deviation (σ). A statistical measure of the variability of probability distribution equal to the square root of the variance.

Statement of cash flows. A financial statement that focuses on the cash flows that come into and go out of a business.

Static budget. A budget that is prepared at the beginning of a planning period. See flexible budget.

Step-down method. A cost allocation method that recognizes some of the overhead services provided by one overhead department to another. See direct method and reciprocal method.

Stop-loss insurance. Insurance taken by providers that pays some amount when individual patient expenses are higher than the specified threshold.

Strategic option. A managerial (real) option that deals with strategic issues.

Strategic plan. The foundation of the planning process. Often consists of a business's mission, scope, and objectives. See operating plan and financial plan.

Stretching. The practice of paying receivables late.

Subordinated debenture. A debt security that, in the event of bankruptcy, has a claim on assets that is below (subordinate to) other debt.

Sunk cost. A cost that has already occurred or is irrevocably committed. Sunk costs are nonincremental to project analyses, and hence should not be included.

Supply chain management. The management of the procurement, storage, and utilization of supplies inventories. Also called materials management.

Swap. An exchange of cash payment obligations. For example, one business might exchange its fixed-rate debt payments with another business that has floating-rate payments.

Synergy. A feature sought after in mergers in which the merged entity is worth more than the sum of the individual businesses.

Takeover. Occurs when an individual (or group) takes control of a business.

Target capital structure. That capital structure (mix of debt and equity) that a company strives to achieve and maintain over time. Generally the same as optimal capital structure.

Target company. A business that another company (or individual or group) seeks to acquire.

Target costing. For price takers, the process of reducing costs (if necessary) to the point where a profit is earned on the market-determined price.

Tax preference theory. A capital structure theory that holds that investors prefer capital gains over dividends because of tax differentials.

Temporary assets. Assets held temporarily by a business to meet peaks in sales due to seasonal and/or cyclical fluctuations.

Tender offer. A means to acquire a firm without gaining target management approval. Stockholders are asked to sell (tender) their shares directly to the acquiring company (or investor group).

Term loan. Long-term debt obtained from a financial institution. See bond.

Term structure. The relationship between yield to maturity and term to maturity for debt of a single risk class, say, Treasury securities. See yield curve.

Third-party payer. An entity other than the patient that pays for healthcare services. Examples include commercial insurance companies and government programs such as Medicare.

Time line. A graphical representation of time and cash flows. May be an actual line or cells on a spreadsheet.

Times-interest-earned (TIE) ratio. Earnings before interest and taxes (EBIT) divided by interest charges. Measures the number of times that a business's interest expense is covered by earnings available to pay that expense.

Total assets turnover (utilization) ratio. Total revenues divided by total assets. Measures the amount of revenue generated by each dollar of total assets.

Total contribution margin. Contribution margin multiplied by volume, or the amount of total revenues available to cover fixed costs.

Trade credit. The credit offered to businesses by suppliers (vendors) when credit terms are offered.

Trade discount. Discounts from invoice prices offered to businesses by suppliers to encourage prompt payment.

Trade-off model. A capital structure model that hypothesizes that a business's optimal capital structure balances the costs and benefits associated with debt financing.

Traditional costing. The top-down approach to costing that first identifies costs at the department level and then (potentially) assigns these costs to individual services. See activity-based costing.

Treasury security. Debt securities issued by the federal government. Treasury bills have maturities of less than one year, notes have maturities of one year to ten years, and bonds have maturities over ten years.

Trend analysis. A ratio analysis technique that examines the value of a ratio over time to see if it is improving or deteriorating. See comparative analysis.

Trustee. An individual or institution, typically a bank, that represents the interests of bondholders.

Underwriting. The process of selling new securities through an investment banker.

Underwritten issue. A new securities issue in which the investment banker agrees to buy the entire issue and then resell it to the public. See best efforts arrangement.

Variance. (1) In statistics, a measure of the variability of a probability distribution. See standard deviation. (2) In budgeting, the difference between what actually happened and what was expected to happen.

Variance analysis. A technique used in budgeting in which realized values are compared with budgeted values to help control operations.

Variable cost. A cost that is directly related to the volume of services supplied. For example, the reagent costs associated with a laboratory test. See fixed cost and semi-fixed cost.

Variable cost rate. The variable cost of one unit of output (volume).

Vertical merger. A merger between an upstream and downstream company. For example, a hospital that acquires a medical practice.

Warrant. A type of call option issued by a company that gives the holder the right to buy a stated number of shares of stock at a given price. Warrants are generally distributed with debt (or preferred stock) to induce investors to accept a lower interest rate.

Window dressing. An action taken by a business for the sole purpose of making its financial condition look better. For example, issuing long-term debt and then putting the funds into marketable securities will improve the current ratio.

Withhold. A fund that is set up by an insurer that is dispersed to providers only if specified goals are met. Also called a risk pool.

Working capital. A business's short-term (current) assets. See net working capital.

Yield curve. A plot of the term structure of interest rates (yield to maturity versus term to maturity). See term structure.

Yield to call. The expected rate of return on a debt security assuming it is held until it is called.

Yield to maturity. The expected rate of return on a debt security assuming it is held until maturity.

Zero-based budgeting. An approach to budgeting that starts with a "clean slate" and requires complete justification of all items. See conventional budgeting.

Zero-coupon bond. A bond that pays no interest. It is bought at a discount from par value, and hence its return comes solely from price appreciation.

Zero sum game. A situation wherein gains to one party are exactly matched by losses to another party. Leasing is a zero sum game when the economics of the lease are the same to both the lessee and lessor.

INDEX

ABOUT THE AUTHOR

Louis C. Gapenski, Ph.D., is a professor in both health services administration and finance at the University of Florida. He received a B.S. degree from the Virginia Military Institute; an M.S. degree from the U.S. Naval Postgraduate School; and M.B.A. and Ph.D. degrees from the University of Florida, the latter two in finance. In addition to teaching at the University of Florida, he was on the national faculty of the University of Wisconsin's Program in Administrative Medicine and has taught in programs at numerous other universities.

Dr. Gapenski is the author or coauthor of more than 20 textbooks on corporate and healthcare finance. His books are used worldwide, with Canadian and international editions as well as translations into Russian, Bulgarian, Chinese, Indonesian, Italian, Polish, Portuguese, and Spanish. In addition, he has published more than 10 journal articles related to corporate and health care finance and has authored a self-study program in healthcare finance for the American College of Healthcare Executives.

Dr. Gapenski is a member of the Association of University Programs in Health Administration, the American College of Healthcare Executives, the Medical Group Management Association, and the Healthcare Financial Management Association. He has acted as academic advisor, chaired sessions, and presented papers at numerous national meetings. Additionally, Dr. Gapenski has been an editorial board member and reviewer for many academic and professional journals.